Current Trends in Neonatology and Perinatology

Current Trends in Neonatology and Perinatology

Editor: Talia Atkins

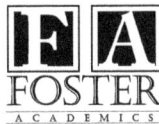

FA
FOSTER
ACADEMICS

www.fosteracademics.com

www.fosteracademics.com

FA
FOSTER
ACADEMICS

Cataloging-in-Publication Data

Current trends in neonatology and perinatology / edited by Talia Atkins.
    p. cm.
Includes bibliographical references and index.
ISBN 978-1-63242-661-1
1. Neonatology. 2. Perinatology. 3. Obstetrics. 4. Pediatrics. I. Atkins, Talia.
RJ251 .C87 2019
618.9201--dc23

Foster Academics,
118-35 Queens Blvd., Suite 400,
Forest Hills, NY 11375, USA

ISBN 978-1-63242-661-1 (Hardback)

Contents

Preface

Neonatology is a specialization within pediatrics, which encompasses the medical care of newborn infants. It focuses on the premature newborn or ones born with complications, such as low birth weight, sepsis, birth defects, birth asphyxia, pulmonary hypoplasia, etc. Infants are susceptible to a number of severe diseases as they are still adapting to extrauterine life. These may include neonatal jaundice, neonatal conjunctivitis, infant respiratory distress syndrome, neonatal sepsis, etc. Perinatology or maternal-fetal medicine is a branch of medicine that is concerned with the management of health concerns of the fetus and the mother before, after and during pregnancy. Pregnant women with chronic conditions such as diabetes, heart or kidney disease, thrombophilia, or hypertension, or those with higher risk of miscarriages, pre-eclampsia, preterm labor, and twin or triplet pregnancies are treated within the domain of perinatology. This book is compiled in such a manner, that it will provide in-depth knowledge about the current practices and procedures of neonatology and perinatology. It aims to present the new researches that have transformed these disciplines and aided their advancement. This book is a vital tool for all researching or studying neonatology and perinatology as it gives incredible insights into emerging trends and concepts.

After months of intensive research and writing, this book is the end result of all who devoted their time and efforts in the initiation and progress of this book. It will surely be a source of reference in enhancing the required knowledge of the new developments in the area. During the course of developing this book, certain measures such as accuracy, authenticity and research focused analytical studies were given preference in order to produce a comprehensive book in the area of study.

This book would not have been possible without the efforts of the authors and the publisher. I extend my sincere thanks to them. Secondly, I express my gratitude to my family and well-wishers. And most importantly, I thank my students for constantly expressing their willingness and curiosity in enhancing their knowledge in the field, which encourages me to take up further research projects for the advancement of the area.

Editor

Hearing impairment and its risk factors by newborn screening in north-western India

Zia Ul Haq Gouri[1], Deepak Sharma[2*], Pramod Kumar Berwal[3], Aakash Pandita[4] and Smita Pawar[5]

Abstract

Background: To screen the newborn by Transient evoked Otoacoustic emission and to assess the incidence of hearing damage and associated risk factors.

Method: This longitudinal prospective observational study was conducted at a tertiary care hospital in India. A total of 415 babies were included in the study. All the newborns were evaluated with Transient evoked Otoacoustic emission (TEOAE) which was done by age of 1–3 days. Auditory brain stem response audiometry (AABR) was performed at the age of three months for confirming the hearing loss in the neonates those who failed the TEOAE screening. For infants proven to have significant hearing loss in one or both ears, were denoted to an ear, nose, and throat specialist for further evaluation & rehabilitation.

Results: Out of total 415 babies included in the study, 22 neonates showed abnormal TEOAE examination. Out of these 22 neonates, hearing loss was confirmed in 18 (82 %) subjects. by AABR. The following antenatal and post-natal risk factors were associated with hearing loss: ante-partum bleeding, history of maternal blood transfusion, fetal distress, prematurity, severe birth asphyxia, NICU admission for more than 24 h and Apgar score less than five at 5 min.

Conclusion: Late identification of hearing loss presents a substantial public health burden. Early recognition and intervention prior to 6 months of age has a significant positive impact on development. A high incidence of hearing impairment seen in our study neonatal population warrants the urgent implementation of universal hearing screening of all the newborn infants in India. NICU infants admitted for more than 24 h are to have an auditory brainstem response (AABR) included as part of their screening so that neural hearing loss will not be missed.

Keywords: Transient evoked Otoacoustic emission (TEOAE), Auditory brain stem response audiometry (AABR), Newborn screening, Hearing impairment risk factor

Background

Hearing impairment has a devastating, and detrimental impact on the development of newborn infants [1]. Neonates having bilateral hearing loss or unilateral hearing loss of varying degrees above 1000 Hz develop significant long term effects on speech and language sciences [2]. Reduced auditory input also adversely affects growth of the auditory nervous system, and can negatively affect the speech perception that interferes with the increment in social, emotional, behavioral, and cognitive spheres, academic achievement, vocational alternatives, employment, and economic self-sufficiency [3]. The major difficulty with late identification of hearing loss is the effect on language development. A delay in identification can mean a delay in establishing effective communication. Professionals agree that hearing loss in infants should be detected promptlyand appropriate audiologic rehabilitation should be instituted early, to take advantage of the plasticity of developing the sensory system (critical period is 0–3 years). This exploit can lead to normal speech and speech development, social, emotional, and cognitive development, and academic achievement in the youngster [4, 5]. In addition, identifying hearing loss before it is clinically apparent, provides a baseline on which subsequent evaluation can be developed and compared. Also, medical, and surgical treatment can be initiated for conductive hearing loss to limit its progression. Timely information also provides the acceptance of hearing damage and improves the parent's readiness to

* Correspondence: dr.deepak.rohtak@gmail.com
[2]Department of Pediatrics, Pt B.D. Sharma PGIMS, Rohtak, Haryana, India
Full list of author information is available at the end of the article

begin a family centered rehabilitation program [6]. In many parts of the world routine newborn hearing screening has been implemented with varied success [7–13], but in developing world nations like ours universal screening is not available and has many obstacles to its implemenation [14, 15]. In India, there is no dedicated national program for early detection of hearing loss in newborns. Studies suggest that four out of every 1000 neonates have severe to profound hearing loss [16, 17].

The present study was designed to perform newborn hearing by Otoacoustic emission (TEOAE), determine the incidence of hearing damage in a population of at risk and not at risk neonates, and to determine various risk factor associations with learning impairment.

Methods

We conducted a prospective observational longitudinal study in a tertiary care hospital in India, Department of Pediatrics, Sardar Patel Medical College, & Associated Group of Hospitals, Bikaner (Rajasthan). The study was approved by institutional research board (IRB) of the college.

During the 8 month study period, form March, 2011 to October 2011, a total 1125 neonates were born in our hospital. We decided to enroll 415 neonates in the study. All the neonates born during the study period were divided into neonates with and without risk factors using predetermined Joint Committee statement on infant hearing screening (JCIH) criteria. Then each neonate was given a sequential number and enrolled in the study using random numbers generated by the computer for each group and enrolled till our sample size reached 415.

Inclusion criteria
All newborn babies born in our hospital from 3/11-10/11.

Exclusion criteria
Fail to get parental consent
Out of total 248 newborns having no risk factor while 167 newborn had some risk factor for hearing loss as per American Joint Committee statement on infant hearing screening (JCIH) criteria [18]. The risk factors which were assessed included

1. Low birth weight (less than 2 lb) and/or prematurity.
2. Assisted ventilation (to aid with breathing for more than 10 days after parturition).
3. Low Apgar scores with severe birth asphyxia (defined as Apgar score of three or less at 1 min of age).
4. Severe jaundice after birth requiring exchange transfusion or serum bilirubin level >20 mg/decilitre.
5. Hydrocephalus
6. Maternal illness during pregnancy (for example, German measles [Rubella]).

7. An illness or condition requiring admission of 24 h or more to a NICU.
8. Stigmata or other findings associated with a known syndrome to include a sensorineural and/or conductive hearing loss.
9. Family history of permanent childhood sensorineural hearing loss.
10. Craniofacial anomalies including those with morphological abnormalities of the pinna & ear canal.
11. In utero infection by TORCH group of organisms.
12. Respiratory distress;(presence of at least two of the following criteria-respiratory rate more than 60 per minute/subcostal or intercostal recession/expiratory grunt or groaning).
13. Meningitis and sepsis with positive CSF and blood cultures respectively.
14. Parental concern.

Informed written consent was obtained from the parents of all babies. Thorough Ear, nose, and throat examination done before doing Transient evoked Otoacoustic emission (TEOAE) that includes looking at the morphological abnormalities of the external ear. These newborns were screened for hearing impairment using the following test protocols.

- Transient evoked Otoacoustic emission (TEOAE) was employed as the first stage of screening by the age of 1–3 days.
- Auditory brain stem response audiometry (AABR) was performed at the age of three months for confirming the hearing loss if the neonates failed the TEOAE screening.

Children who had normal AABR were declared as ecologically sound & no further evaluation was suggested to these children.

All neonates were screened with TEOAE testing in a quiet room adjacent to the NICU. Otoread TEOAE screeners (Interacoustic Ltd., Assens, Denmark) was used for testing. The TEOAE was done by an audiologist who was trained in doing the TEOAE and this test was done free of cost. The Quick screen mode was used with a specially designed "stop" protocol that forced discontinuation of the protocol when "pass" criteria was met. The timing window was 12.5 milliseconds, and clicks were delivered at a rate of 80 per second. Stimuli consisted of standard transient clicks at 70 to 88 dB pSPL.

Otoacoustic emissions were judged to be present and an ear to have "pass" when signal-to-noise ratio was at least 3 dB in at least three of four frequency bands (1000, 2000, 3000, and 4000 Hz). A minimum of 60 successful sweeps was achieved in the test to be considered valid. Screening continued until passing criteria were met or 1000 successful sweeps were occurring, or for 10 min. If a baby failed an initial screen, it was repeated immediately after an effort to troubleshoot i.e. improve probe fit, clean probe contaminated by dust, decrease ambient noise, or change site of testing, calming baby by swaddling, rocking, and eating. An acceptable screen was done but once for each ear.

Follow-up testing consisted of AABR testing that was performed under conditions of natural sleep using an Evomatic 4000 evoked potential unit (Medtronic, Minneapolis, MN), a standard Ag/AgCl electrode applied on the forehead and each mastoid, and pediatric insert earphones coupled to Etymotic ER3A stimulators (Etymotic Research, Elk Grove, IL). The AABR was done by a trained audiologist and was done free of cost. Stimuli consisted of 100-millisecond rarefaction clicks and tone pips presented at a rate of 25 per second for at least 1000 presentations with alternating triggering to permit both ears to be examined simultaneously. Our cutoff values of normal were 23 to 26 dB for observable wave V for clicks and 30 dB NHL for tone pips.

For babies who failed the initial TEOAE screening, the mother, & relatives were contacted in person and counselled as to the significance of a broken screen (i.e. suggested need for further evaluation, not diagnosis of hearing loss). These neonates' parents were also contacted in between for giving them a reminder for AABR and on the day of examination, they were contacted in personnel to get the test done.

Auditory brain stem response audiometry was used to confirm the hearing loss if the neonates failed the TEOAE screening at the age of 3 months.

For infants proven to suffer substantial hearing loss in one or both ears, were referred to an Ear, nose, and throat specialist for further evaluation & rehabilitation.

Statistical analysis

All the patient data were entered into Microsoft excel sheets. The Statistical Package for the Social Sciences (SPSS) software version 16 for Windows was used for data analysis. Student's t test and Chi-square test were used for data analysis. A p value less than 0.05 was considered significant.

Results

In the present study, we have performed the initial screening of 415 newborn by TEOAE, only 22 babies had abnormal results. These 22 babies were further evaluated by AABR at age of 3 months. AABR showed 18 babies with confirmed significant hearing loss. Out of the 22 babies with abnormal results, 16 babies were in with any risk factor group and remaining babies were in without any risk factor group.

The demographic data of the study population, including gestational age, birth weight, gender stratification in with, and without risk factor groups are summarized in Table 1. During the study period neonates with suspected sepsis or clinical sepsis received cefotaxime and amikacin as a first line empirical antibiotic therapy. The newborn with asphyxial encephalopathy with sepsis, nephrotoxic drugs were avoided. The antibiotics were discontinued within 48 h if cultures were sterile. The second line of antibiotics was piperacillin tazobactum or Cefepime and antibiotics were changed as per the sensitivity pattern of the microorganism. In neonates with renal failure drug dose adjustment was performed.

Out of the 415 newborns screened with TEOAE test 22 (5.68 %) babies had abnormal screen either in single or both ears. Out of total 22 abnormal TEOAE cases, 18 (81.82 %) cases were taking in significant hearing loss with AABR while four (18.2 %) cases had normal AABR (Fig. 1).

The comparison of various risk factors between normal AABR and abnormal AABR shows that Apgar score at 5 min less than five, NICU admission, the presence of fetal distress, presence of meconium stained amniotic fluid are significantly important predictors for hearing loss (Table 2). The risk stratification of the various factors in the study population has been depicted in the pie diagram (Fig. 2).

Maternal fever was present in only 1 % patients antenatally and they all had normal hearing, while rash was present in only 0.3 % of subjects and they also had no significant hearing loss. Blood transfusion history was present in total four patients and out of them three had normal hearing screening and remaining one had significant hearing loss. APH was present in 12 patients out of

Table 1 Table showing demographics of the population -gestational age, birth weight, gender stratification in the with and without risk factor groups

Distribution of total study population according to association of risk factor		
	Without risk factor	With risk factor
Gestational age		
<30 weeks	8	10
30–33 6/7 weeks	8	20
34–36 6/7 weeks	32	29
≥37 weeks	200	108
Gender		
Male	137	93
Female	111	74
Birth weight		
<1.5 kg	7	8
1.5–2.49 kg	53	54
>2.5 kg	188	105

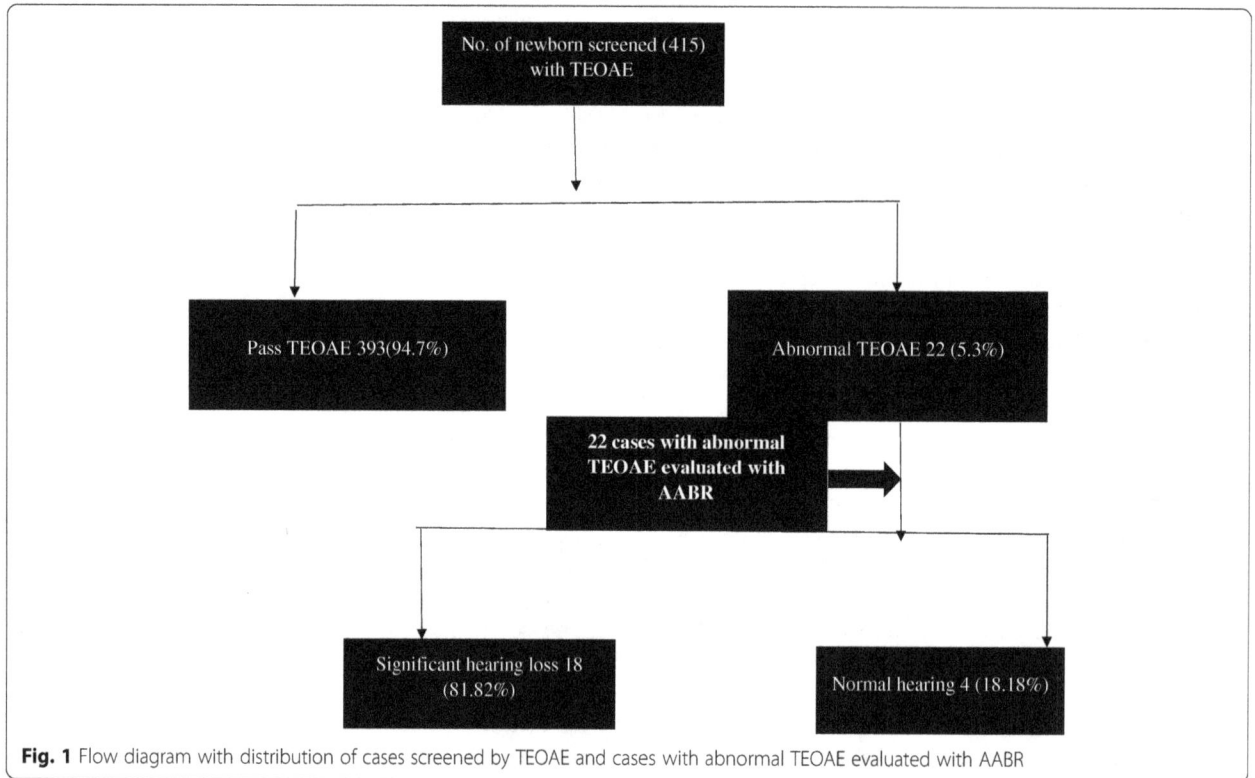

Fig. 1 Flow diagram with distribution of cases screened by TEOAE and cases with abnormal TEOAE evaluated with AABR

them ten had normal hearing and two had found significant hearing loss (Table 3).

The working cost for the institute for TEOAE was 250 Indian rupees (4 US dollars) and for AABR was 1300 Indian rupees (21 US dollars). The parents were not billed for either of the probes.

Discussion
In our survey, among 415 of the total newborns screened 94.7 % (393) cases passed on TEOAE while 5.3 % [19] cases were referred for initial screening at birth.

Nagapoornima et al. conducted a similar study in India and screened a total of 1769 infants (1490: Not at risk; 279: At risk) & reported that 10 babies were having a hearing impairment [20]. The high incidence of hearing impairment seen in our study population could be explained because of neonatal population with different geographical area and also because of different maternal antenatal risk factors. There can be also some unseen environmental and genetic and epigenetic factors responsible for the high incidence of hearing impairment in our studies.

John et al. conducted study in Christian Medical College (C.M.C.) Vellore and evaluated 500 newborns and found

Table 2 Table comparing various risk factors associated with hearing loss in BERA positive cases

	Normal hearing	Hearing loss	P value
Mean gestational age (weeks)	36.93 ± 2.41	36.71 ± 2.17	0.051
Birth weight (kg)	2.667 ± 0.50	2.747 ± 0.59	0.197
Male gender	221	9	0.550
Vaginal delivery	283	10	0.09
Apgar score at 5 min less than five	10	3	0.001
NICU admission	137	11	0.032
Fetal distress	73	9	0.009
Meconium stained amniotic fluid	28	2	0.012
Family history	15	1	0.022
Maternal age (years)	24.99 ± 3.3	25.35 ± 4.3	0.313

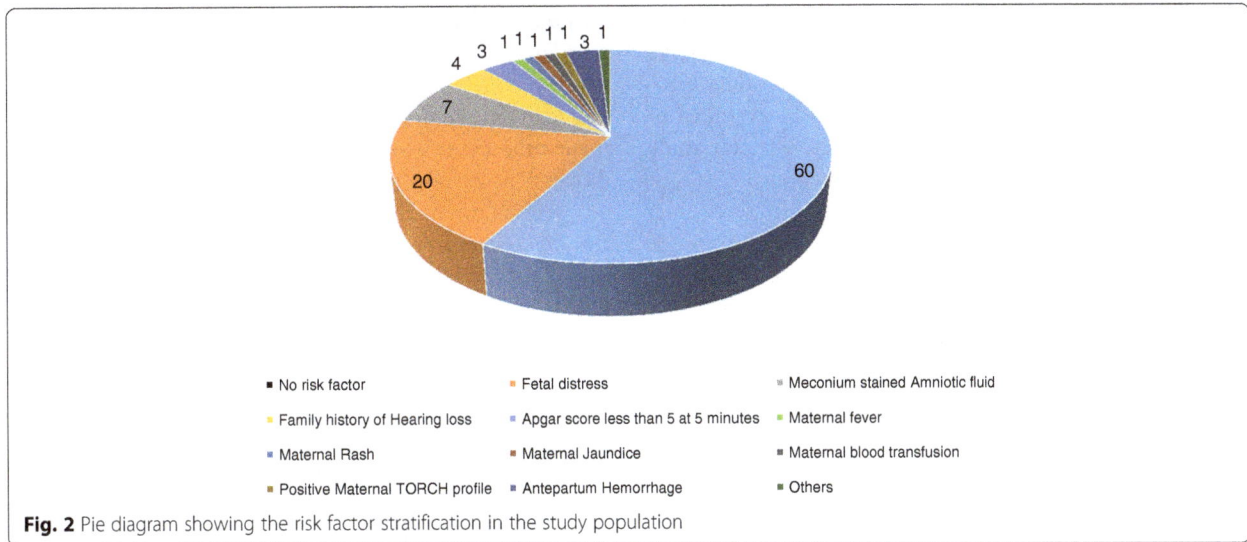

Fig. 2 Pie diagram showing the risk factor stratification in the study population

Table 3 Distribution of cases according to antenatal history in relation to significant hearing loss

Antenatal history		Significant hearing loss			χ^2	P
		Absent	Present	Total		
Fever	No	383 (99.0 %)	18 (100.0 %)	401 (99.0 %)	0.188	0.883
	Yes	4 (1.0 %)	0	4 (1.0 %)		
Rash	No	386 (99.7 %)	18 (100.0 %)	404 (99.8 %)	0.047	0.956
	Yes	1 (0.3 %)	0	1 (0.2 %)		
Jaundice	No	383 (99.0 %)	17 (94.4 %)	400 (98.8 %)	2.844	0.089
	Yes	4 (1.0 %)	1 (5.6 %)	5 (1.2 %)		
Blood Transfusion	No	384 (99.2 %)	17 (94.4 %)	401 (99.0 %)	4.019	0.045
	Yes	3 (0.8 %)	1 (5.6 %)	4 (1.0 %)		
Leaking per-vaginum	No	375 (96.9 %)	17 (94.4 %)	392 (96.8 %)	0.334	0.564
	Yes	12 (3.1 %)	1 (5.6 %)	13 (3.2 %)		
Offending drug intake	No	385 (99.5 %)	18 (100.0 %)	403 (99.5 %)	0.093	0.954
	Yes	2 (0.5 %)	0	2 (0.5 %)		
Radiation exposure	No	387 (100 %)	18 (100.0 %)	405 (100.0 %)	-	-
	Yes	0	0	0		
Other	No	384 (99.2 %)	18 (100.0 %)	402 (99.3 %)	0.141	0.987
	Yes	3 (0.8 %)	0	3 (0.7 %)		
Drug addiction	No	382 (98.7 %)	17 (94.4 %)	399 (98.5 %)	2.142	0.143
	Yes	5 (1.3 %)	1 (5.6 %)	6 (1.5 %)		
Antenatal clinics attended	No	98 (25.3 %)	5 (27.8 %)	103 (25.4 %)	0.055	0.815
	Yes	289 (74.7 %)	13 (72.2 %)	302 (74.6 %)		
Maternal TORCH profile	No	386 (99.7 %)	18 (100.0 %)	404 (99.8 %)	0.047	0.829
	Yes	1 (0.3 %)	0	1 (0.2 %)		
Pre-eclampsia	No	374 (96.6 %)	18 (100.0 %)	392 (96.8 %)	0.625	0.429
	Yes	13 (3.4 %)	0	13 (3.2 %)		
Antepartum hemorrhage	No	377 (97.4 %)	16 (88.9 %)	393 (97.0 %)	4.350	0.037
	Yes	10 (2.6 %)	2 (11.1 %)	12 (3.0 %)		

32 (6.4 %) neonates with negative response. These effects are quite comparable to our study. At the second stage screening on 32 (6.4 %) cases by Distortion Product Otoacoustic Emission DPOAE, eight (25 %) were extended to sustain a negative response [21] and similarly in our study four neonates had normal AABR in follow up.

Thomson et al. in their study of newborn screening, included 67,261 newborn from different states and 8.2 % mothers of babies were from 11–19 years age group while 23.1 % were from 20–25 years & 67.5 % mothers were a 25 + age group [22]. In our study case for maximum cases coming from 21–25 years age group was likely due to lower age for matrimony in our region as compared to the western world. We found no link between maternal age and hearing loss.

In subject done by John et al. [21], they reported that 5.2 % of cases of failed hearing screening by DOAE were from the birth weight less than 1500 g. Low birth weight is also included as a risk factor for hearing impairment in JCIH 2000 criteria [18]. A lower rate of hearing abnormalities in low birth weight in our subject population can be explained by either small sample size or high mortality in babies of low birth weight in our population. The screening should be a part of all neonates irrespective of weight, although the smallest, and tiniest neonates require AABR as a primary modality, but using only weight as a criteria is not advisable as full term neonates without any risk factors can also have hearing abnormalities.

Nagapoornima et al. [20] recorded that out of total eight cases screened with a family story of childhood sensorineural hearing loss two (25 %) cases were set up to cause hearing impairment. In our study, out of 18 cases of hearing loss, 94 % [17] cases had no family history of significant childhood hearing loss in any sibling of the child. Family history of hearing loss was present in 16 (3.8 %) children and out of these only one case had hearing handicap. This shows that although the family history is recognized as an independent risk factor for hearing loss but the neonates who don't have any family history are also prone to have hearing abnormalities hence showing the importance of universal newborn screening of all neonates irrespective of family history of hearing loss.

John et al. [21] showed that a family history of hearing loss was present in seven cases out of 500 (1.4 %) [5]. This high level of hearing loss may be due to deficiency of awareness in our region & less access to health care services.

In our study, most of the antenatal risk factor for hearing loss were found non-significant except the history of antepartum hemorrhage and history of antenatal blood transfusion in the mother. The apparent cause of these antenatal risk factors associated with hearing loss may be due to intrauterine distress to fetus followed by birth asphyxia.

In our study, we concluded that the method of delivery does not play a significant role on newborn hearing impairment.

Out of the 18 neonates with significant hearing impairment nine cases where having the antenatal sign of fetal distress in the form of either meconium stained liquor, bradycardia, or tachycardia. When comparing these data, the difference was statistically significant ($p < 0.01$). This could be explained because signs of fetal distress like meconium stained liquor, bradycardia, or tachycardia indicates fetal hypoxia, which may lead to damage to cochlear cells and neuronal pathway leading to more significant hearing abnormality. These findings also strengthen the view that these neonates with perinatal asphyxia need to be screened for hearing assessment.

In the present study, 16.7 % [3] cases out of 18 cases of significant hearing loss were found to have Apgar score ≤5. This was strongly associated risk factor for neonatal hearing loss as fetal hypoxia can damage neonates hearing system and lead to AABR abnormality.

Similar outcomes were likewise received in the survey performed by Thomson et al. [21] on newborn screening. In his study 39 (1.2 %) babies of apgar ≤5 were found to cause failure of hearing screening. Low Apgar score is also included as a risk factor for hearing impairment in JCIH 2000 criteria [18]. So our study confirms it as associated risk factor.

According to JCIH 2000 criteria [18] an illness or condition requiring admission of 24 h or more to NICU has termed as a risk factor for hearing impairment. Our study confirms the same finding. This could be because the sick neonates are exposed to various ototoxic drugs or hypoxia, which increases the chances of hearing loss. The results also tell that although the sick neonates are more likely to have a higher incidence of hearing abnormalities, but the normal neonates with no postnatal sickness or risk factors can have hearing abnormalities, hence again highlighting the need for universal screening.

In our experience from a developing country, we encountered few difficulties for newborn screening. The availability of a trained audiologist and the cost are important issues. However, both OAE and AABR are paid by the institution in the majority of places, hence all parents from the low income and low middle income countries will not be able to get their newborn infant screened. As both OAE and AABR were free to our patients could be one of the reason for hundred percent follow up of all infants. All these problems can be overcome if the government makes hearing screening compulsory, and free of cost, and many more audiologists are trained for performing newborn screens. Though the initial phase of screening implementation may be costly because getting new screening machines, training new audiologist, and setting up new rehabilitation centers, but in the long term these interventions will be more cost effective and will help in reducing the burden on society because of hearing impairments.

In the nursery, the high risk neonates are more prone to suffer hearing problems. In the various studies done it has been shown that in these neonates AABR when compared with OAE has better sensitivity and specificity which highlights that in these neonates AABR should be a primary screening modality and in normal neonates OAE can be taken as a primary modality of screening [19, 23].

Hence the results of our study show that all neonates having a turbulent course in nursery and various risk factors, needs to be screened for hearing assessment and neonates with the abnormal OAE need to be followed up. Universal screening of hearing should be done as neonates with no risk factors can also have abnormal hearing as seen in our study and it can delay the diagnosis of hearing impairment and also intervention for rehabilitation.

The limitation of our study includes small sample size, and our inability to evaluate all the risk factors of JCIH criteria. The strong point of our study includes hundred percent follow up of all the newborns who had abnormal OAE and all these neonates had AABR done. This was possible as we educated all parents regarding the consequences of impaired hearingand maintained regular contact with them.

Conclusion

Late identification of hearing loss presents a significant public health concern. However, without screening, children with hearing loss are usually not identified until 2 years of age, which results in significant delays in voice communication, language communication, social, cognitive, and emotional development. In contrast, early recognition, and intervention prior to 6 months of historic period has a significant positive impact on development.

Hence, there is an urgent need to incorporate universal neonatal hearing screening in all the neonatal health care facilities in India. While studying the facts like infrastructure limitations of our rural area where basic needs are deficient, there is a demand to employ cost-effective behavioural observation methods using calibrated noise making toys to screen all newborn infants.

Further prospective studies on a larger sample size are required to study the association of hearing impairment with various congenital syndromes and antenatal, perinatal, postnatal & demographic factors.

Competing interest
The authors declare that they have no competing interests.

Authors' contributions
Conceived and designed the experiments: ZUHG, DS, SP; Analyzed the data: DSAP. Wrote the fit draft of the manuscript: ZUHG; DS. Contributed to the writing of the manuscript: ZUHG, PKB, AP, SP. Agree with manuscript results and conclusions: ZUHG; PKB; DS; AP. Jointly developed the structure and arguments for the paper: ZUHG, PKB, DS, AP, SP. Made critical revisions and approved final version: ZUHG, PKB, DS, AP, SP. All authors reviewed and approved of the final manuscript.

Financial disclosure
This was post-graduation dissertation and no external funding was involved.

Author details
[1]Kothari Hospital and Research Center, Bikaner, Rajasthan, India. [2]Department of Pediatrics, Pt B.D. Sharma PGIMS, Rohtak, Haryana, India. [3]Department of Paediatrics, S.P. Medical College, Bikaner, Rajasthan, India. [4]Department of Pediatrics, Government Medical College, Jammu, India. [5]Department of Obstetrics and Gynaecology, Fernandez Hospital, Hyderabad, India.

References
1. US Preventive Services Task Force. Universal screening for hearing loss in newborns: US preventive services task force recommendation statement. Pediatrics. 2008;122:143–8.
2. Hall JW. Newborn Auditory Screening; Handbook of Clinical Audiology. University of Florida; U.S.A.: Allyn and Bacon Publication; 1992. p. 445–7.
3. Yoshinaga-Itano C, Coulter D, Thomson V. Developmental outcomes of children with hearing loss born in Colorado hospitals with and without universal newborn hearing screening programs. Semin Neonatol. 2001;6:521–9.
4. Moeller M. Early intervention and language development in children who are deaf and hard of hearing. Pediatrics. 2000;106, e43.
5. Kennedy CR, McCann DC, Campbell MJ, Law CM, Mullee M, Petrou S, et al. Language ability after early detection of permanent childhood hearing impairment. New Eng J Med. 2006;354:2131–41.
6. White KR. Early intervention for children with permanent hearing loss: Finishing the EHDI revolution. Volta Review. 2007;106(3):237–58.
7. Olusanya BO, Wirz SL, Luxon LM Hospital-based universal newborn hearing screening for early detection of permanent congenital hearing loss in Lagos, Nigeria. Int J Pediatr Otorhinolaryngol. 2008: 21.
8. Low WK, Pang KY, Ho LY. Universal newborn hearing screening in Singapore: the need, implementation, and challenges. Ann Acad Med Singapore. 2005;34:301–6.
9. Weichbold V, Nekahm-Heis D, Welzl-Muller K. Evaluation of the Austrian newborn hearing screening program. Int J Pediatr Otorhinolaryngol. 2006;70:235–40.
10. White KR, Vohr BR, Maxon AB, Behrens TR, McPherson MG, Mauk GW. Screening all newborns for hearing loss using transient evoked otoacoustic emissions. Int J Pediatr Otorhinolaryngol. 1994;29(3):203–17.
11. Chapchap MJ, Segre CM. Universal newborn hearing screening and transient evoked otoacoustic emission: new concepts in Brazil. Scand Audiol Suppl. 2001;53:33–6.
12. Davis A, Hind S. The newborn hearing screening programme in England. Int J Pediatr Otorhinolaryngol. 2003;67 Suppl 1:S193–6.
13. Bubbico L, Tognola G, Greco A, Grandori F. Universal newborn hearing screening programs in Italy: survey of year 2006. Acta Otolaryngol. 2008;128:1329–36.
14. Olusanya BO, Luxon LM, Wirz SL. Benefits and challenges of newborn hearing screening for developing countries. Int J Pediatr Otorhinolaryngol. 2004;68:287–305.
15. Tobe RG, Mori R, Huang L, Xu L, Han D, Shibuya K. Cost-effectiveness analysis of a national neonatal hearing screening program in China: conditions for the scale-up. PLoS One. 2013;8(1), e51990. doi:10.1371/journal.pone.0051990. Epub 2013 Jan 16. PubMed PMID: 23341887; PubMed Central PMCID: PMC3547019.
16. Rehabilitation Council of India. Status of Disability in India–2000. New Delhi: Rehabilitation Council of India; 2000. p. 172–85.
17. Government of India. Persons with Disabilities (Equal opportunities, Protection of Right and Full Participation) Act-1995. New Delhi: Ministry of Law, Justice and Company Affairs; 1996.
18. Joint Committee on Infant Hearing. Year 2000 position statement: principles and guidelines for early hearing detection and intervention programs. Pediatrics. 2000;106(4):798–217.
19. Xu FL, Xing QJ, Cheng XY. A comparison of auditory brainstem responses and otoacoustic emissions in hearing screening of high-risk neonates. Zhongguo Dang Dai Er Ke Za Zhi. 2008;10(4):460–3. PubMed.

2

Surgical site infections after cesarean delivery: epidemiology, prevention and treatment

Tetsuya Kawakita[1]* 🆔 and Helain J. Landy[2]

Abstract

Cesarean delivery (CD) is one of the most common procedures performed in the United States, accounting for 32% of all deliveries. Postpartum surgical site infection (SSI), wound infection and endometritis is a major cause of prolonged hospital stay and poses a burden to the health care system. SSIs complicate a significant number of patients who undergo CD – 2-7% will experience sound infections and 2-16% will develop endometritis. Many risk factors for SSI have been described. These include maternal factors (such as tobacco use; limited prenatal care; obesity; corticosteroid use; nulliparity; twin gestations; and previous CD), intrapartum and operative factors (such as chorioamnionitis; premature rupture of membranes; prolonged rupture of membranes; prolonged labor, particularly prolonged second stage; large incision length; subcutaneous tissue thickness > 3 cm; subcutaneous hematoma; lack of antibiotic prophylaxis; emergency delivery; and excessive blood loss), and obstetrical care on the teaching service of an academic institution. Effective interventions to decrease surgical site infection include prophylactic antibiotic use (preoperative first generation cephalosporin and intravenous azithromycin), chlorhexidine skin preparation instead of iodine, hair removal using clippers instead of razors, vaginal cleansing by povidone-iodine, placental removal by traction of the umbilical cord instead of by manual removal, suture closure of subcutaneous tissue if the wound thickness is >2 cm, and skin closure with sutures instead of with staples. Implementation of surgical bundles in non-obstetric patients has been promising., Creating a similar patient care bundle comprised evidence-based elements in patients who undergo CD may decrease the incidence of this major complication. Each hospital has the opportunity to create its own CD surgical bundle to decrease surgical site infection.

Keywords: Cesarean delivery, Chlorhexidine skin preparation, Surgical bundle, Surgical site infection, Vaginal cleansing

Background

Cesarean delivery (CD) is one of the most common procedures performed in the United States, accounting for 32% of all deliveries [1]. In 2014, nearly 1.3 million CDs were performed [1]. As with all surgical procedures, CD can be associated with SSIs, including wound infections and endometritis, as well as being associated with higher maternal morbidity and mortality with future pregnancies [2–5].

* Correspondence: tetsuya.x.kawakita@gmail.com
[1]Obstetrics and Gynecology, MedStar Washington Hospital Center, 101 Irving Street, 5B45, NW, Washington, DC 20010, USA
Full list of author information is available at the end of the article

Epidemiology
Wound complications
Wound hematoma, seroma, dehiscence

Wound hematoma and seroma are collections of blood and serum, respectively. Hematomas are usually due to failure of primary hemostasis or bleeding diathesis such as anticoagulation therapy. Vigorous coughing or severe hypertension immediately after surgery may contribute to the formation of hematoma. Wound hematoma or seroma, described in 2-5% of women after CD can cause wound dehiscence and act as a nidus for development of wound infection [6, 7]. Wound dehiscence is separation of incision and complicates 2-7% after CD [6, 7].

Wound infection

Wound infection presents with erythema, discharge, and induration of the incision, complicates 2-7% of patients and generally develops 4 to 7 days after CD [8–12]. When wound infection develops within 48 h, the offending organisms usually are groups A or B-hemolytic Streptococcus. Other common pathogens involved in wound infections are Ureaplasma urealyticum, *Staphylococcus epidermidis*, Enterococcus facialis, *Staphylococcus aureus*, *Escherichia coli*, and Proteus mirabilis [13, 14].

Necrotizing fasciitis

Necrotizing fasciitis is a rare but serious infection causing significant morbidity after CD that is characterized by rapid and progressive necrosis of subcutaneous tissue and fascia [15]. Necrotizing fasciitis is suspected with severe pain, crepitus, wooden-hard induration of the subcutaneous tissues, bullous lesions, skin necrosis or ecchymosis, and elevated serum creatine kinase level; a hallmark of necrotizing fasciitis is rapid progression of clinical manifestations [16–18]. Imaging studies such as computed tomography or magnetic resonance imaging may show edema extending along the fascial plane. The diagnosis is confirmed at the time of repeat surgery. Features suggestive include fascia that swollen and dull gray in appearance with areas of necrosis, skin necrosis with easy dissection along the fascia, or presence of gas in the soft tissues.

Type I necrotizing fasciitis results from a polymicrobial infection involving both aerobic and anaerobic bacteria; type II necrotizing fasciitis is generally caused by a single organism, group A streptococcus. In a 1997 study, necrotizing fasciitis occurred in only 0.18% of women who underwent CD; the onset occurred between 5 and 17 days following CD. The authors reported a very high mortality rate (22%) [15], which implied the importance of prompt recognition and treatment of necrotizing fasciitis.

Endometritis

Postpartum endometritis results from a polymicrobial infection of the decidua, characterized by fever ≥38.0 °C, fundal tenderness, and purulent discharge from the uterus [19]. Higher risks for endometritis are associated with CD compared to vaginal delivery [5]. Postpartum endometritis complicates 2-16% of women who underwent CD [8–12]. Risks are higher following CD performed in labor (3-11%) compared with prelabor CDs (0.5-5%), as well as in patients who had ruptured membranes compared to intact membranes (3-15% vs. 1-5%, respectively) [10, 20, 21]

Risk factors for surgical site infections following CD

Many different fisk factors for SSIs following CD have been reported (Table 1). In decreasing order of significant risk as measured by relative risks or odds ratios, risk factors include subcutaneous hematoma [8], chorioamnionitis [22–24],

Table 1 Risk factors for surgical site infection

Variables	Relative risk or odds ratios	References
Subcutaneous hematoma	11.6	8
Chorioamnionitis	5.6-10.6	21-23
American Society of Anesthesiologists class of 3 or greater	5.3	21
Tabacco	5.3	22
Incision length > 16.6 cm	4.9	24
Prenatal visit <7	4	25
Body Mass Index >35 kg/m2	3.7	26
Corticosteroid	3.1	24
Body Mass Index >30 kg/m2	2.0-2.8	21, 23, 24, 26-28
Subcutaneous tissue thickness > 3 cm	2.8	29
Second stage (vs. first stage)	2.8	30
Teaching service	2.7	8
No antibiotic prophylaxis	2.6	25
Pregestational Diabetes	1.4-2.5	26, 28, 31
Operating time ≥ 38 min	2.4	27
Hypertensive disease/Preeclampsia	1.7-2.3	21, 28
Duration of labor >12 h	2.0	23
Nulliparity	1.8	21
Twin	1.6	28
Premature rupture of membrane	1.5	28
Gestational diabetes	1.5	32
Blood loss (every 100 ml)	1.3	21
Previous cesarean delivery	1.3	32
Emergency delivery	1.3	28
Rupture of mambranes (each hour)	1.02	25

maternal comorbidities (American Society of Anesthesiologists class of 3 or greater) [22], tobacco use in pregnancy [23], incision length > 16.6 cm [25], limited prenatal care (fewer than 7 visits) [26], body mass index >30 or 35 kg/m^2 [22, 24, 25, 27–29] corticosteroid use [25], subcutaneous tissue thickness > 3 cm [30], prolonged second stage (compared with first stage) [31], teaching service [8], no antibiotic prophylaxis [26], pregestational diabetes [27, 29, 32], operating time ≥ 38 min [28], hypertensive disease/preeclampsia [22, 29], duration of labor >12 h [24], nulliparity [22], twin gestations [29], premature rupture of membranes [29], gestational diabetes [33], blood loss (increased for every increase in blood loss of 100 mL) [22], previous cesarean delivery [33], emergency delivery [29], and rupture of membranes (increased risk for every additional hour) [26].

Burden to healthcare system

Postpartum infections are a major cause of prolonged hospital stay and comprise a large burden to our health care system [12]. One study attributed costs of an additional $3700 for wound infection and an additional $4000 for endometritis (in 2008 US dollars, corresponding to $4200 and $4500 today, respectively) [34].

Prevention

Previous studies have shown that certain interventions lower SSIs. Since CD is one of the most common procedures performed worldwide, it is important for implementation of evidence-based approaches to decrease such postoperative complications. A summary of studies describing such approaches is presented in Table 2.

Preoperative management

Preoperative antibiotics

Cefazolin

Administration of a first generation cephalosporin is the mainstay of the prevention of SSIs after CD. A meta-analysis of randomized controlled trials showed that the use of first generation cephalosporin compared with no antibiotics decreased the risks for development of wound infections (Relative Risk [RR] 0.38; 95% confidence interval [CI] 0.28, 0.53) and endometritis (RR 0.42; 95% CI 0.33, 0.54) [35]. Further, lower rates of SSIs have been found with antibiotic administration of first generation cephalosporin prior to skin incision compared with administration after cord clamp [11, 36–39]. The meta-analysis by Constantine et al. reported the risk of endometritis was lowered significantly (RR 0.47; 95% CI 0.26, 0.85) [11]. Another publication of a randomized controlled trial showed lower rates of both wound infection (OR] 0.7; 95% CI 0.55, 0.90) and endometritis (OR 0.61; 95% CI 0.47, 0.79) when antibiotic prophylaxis was given prior to skin incision compared with after cord clamp [39].

Table 2 Interventions and techniques surrounding cesarean delivery

Variables	Wound infection		Endometritis	
	RR or OR	References	RR or OR	References
Preoperative elements				
First generation cephalosporin vs. none	0.38	34	0.42	34
First generation cephalosporin prior to skin incision vs. after cord clamp	0.7	11, 35-38	0.21-0.61	11, 35-38
First generation cephalosporin 2 g vs. 3 g in morbidly obese women	NS	40	-	-
Azithromycin				
In labor	0.35	9	0.62	9
Non labor	-	-	0.11	41
Chlorhexidine alcohol skin preparation vs. iodine	0.55	42, 43	NS	42
Razor hair removal vs. clippers	2.1	44	-	-
Vaginal cleansing				
Chlorhexidine vs none	NS	45	0.2	45
Iodine vs none	NS	10, 18, 46, 47	0.39	10, 18, 46, 47
In labor	NS	47	NS	47
Not in labor	NS	47	NS	47
Ruptured membranes	NS	46, 47	0.13	46, 47
Intact membranes	NS	47	NS	47
Intraoperative elements				
Uterine exteriorization	NS	49	NS	49
Manual removal of placneta vs. traction of umbilical cord	-	-	1.4-1.6	50, 51
Intraabdominal irrigation	NS	53	NS	52, 53
Closure of subcutaneous tissue if >2 cm[a]	NS	54	-	-
Subcutaneous drain	NS	55, 56	-	-
Suture skin closure vs. staple[b]	NS	6, 57, 58	-	-
Postoperative elements				
Dressing removal between 24 and 48 h vs. 6 h	NS	7	-	-

RR relative risk; OR odds ratio; NS not statistically significant; CI confidence interval
[a]Wound complications (hematoma, seroma, and infection) - RR 0.66; 95%CI 0.48, 0.91; Wound separation - RR 0.42; 95%CI 0.24, 0.75
[b]Wound complications (wound infection, hematoma, seroma, or separation of 1 cm or longer) -adjusted OR 0.43; 95%CI 0.23, 0.78; wound separation - adjusted OR 0.20; 95%CI 0.07, 0.51

The American College of Obstetricians and Gynecologists (ACOG) recommend infusion of intravenous 1 g cefazolin within 60 min prior to skin incision [40]. For women with (BMI >30 kg/m² or weight > 100 kg, a dose of 2 g cefazolin intravenous infusion is recommended [40]. Though use of higher doses have been considered in women with BMI > 40 kg/m², one retrospective study of morbidly obese women did not demonstrate a difference in SSIs comparing cefazolin doses of 2 g and 3 g [41].

Azithromycin

Recent reports have shown benefits to adding azithromycin at the time of CD. A 2008 study by Tita et al. described a lower risk of endometritis with the routine use of intravenous azithromycin compared to standard antibiotic prophylaxis (0.9% vs. 12.5%; RR 0.11; 95% CI 0.06, 0.19; P < .001) [42]. In 2016, this same author reported that adding intravenous azithromycin 500 mg to standard preoperative antibiotic prophylaxis was associated with lower risks of endometritis (3.8% vs. 6.1%; RR 0.62; 95% CI 0.42, 0.92; P = .02) and wound infection (2.4% vs. 6.6%; RR 0.35; 95% CI 0.22, 0.56; P < .001) in women undergoing non-elective CD compared with placebo. [9] The addition of preoperative azithromycin does not have any short term effects on the neonates though long term data are lacking. The randomized controlled study of azithromycin in addition to standard antibiotics did not demonstrate any differences in composite neonatal outcome, death, and NICU admission [9].

Chlorhexidine alcohol skin preparation

Skin preparation (chlorhexidine alcohol vs. iodine) has been examined by 2 randomized controlled trials with disparate results. [43, 44] Tuuli et al. compared 572 women with chlorhexidine skin preparation with 575 women with iodine skin preparation in a randomized controlled study and demonstrated a decreased rate of wound infection (RR 0.55; 95%CI 0.34, 0.90; P = .02) in patients with chlorhexidine skin preparation [43]. Results from another randomized controlled trial comparing povidone iodine alone (n = 463), chlorhexidine alone (n = 474), and both (n = 467) showed similar wound infection rates, however [44]. The reason for of the different results of these two randomized controlled trials is unclear. Nonetheless, a shift has begun towards chlorhexidine alcohol and away from povidone iodine skin preparation [18].

Use of clippers instead of razor

A 2011 Cochrane Data Base meta-analysis by Tanner et al. comparing hair removal by shaving with clipping showed a higher risk of wound infection associated with shaving (RR 2.09; 95%CI 1.15, 3.80) [45]. Use of clippers instead of razor for preoperative hair removal has been adopted by many hospitals.

Preoperative vaginal cleansing

There has been a growing interest in assessing potential benefits from preoperative vaginal cleansing. In the randomized controlled trial of 218 women comparing chlorhexidine vaginal cleansing with no vaginal cleansing by Ahmed et al., chlorhexidine vaginal cleansing compared with no vaginal cleansing was associated with a lower rate of endometritis (RR 0.2; 95% CI 0.06, 0.7) although the rate of wound infection was similar (RR 0.6; 95% CI 0.2, 1.8) [46]. Vaginal cleansing by povidone iodine also has been studied [10, 20, 47, 48]. Similar results were reported using povidone-iodine in the Cochrane Data Base meta-analysis by Haas in which vaginal preparation by povidone-iodine compared with no preparation demonstrated a lower risk of endometritis (RR 0.39; 95% CI 0.16, 0.97) with similar risks of wound infection (RR 0.99; 95% CI 0.57, 1.70) [48]. The risk reduction was particularly strong in women with ruptured membranes who had vaginal preparation by povidone-iodine compared with no preparation (RR 0.13; 95% CI 0.02, 0.66) [48].

Currently, only povidone-iodine is approved for use in the vagina, though off-label use of chlorhexidine solutions can be considered, especially in women with allergies to iodine [49]. The use of preoperative vaginal cleansing should be considered, especially in women with ruptured membranes.

Intraoperative management

Many surgical maneuvers have been taught over time without the benefit of evidence-based medicine. Below are a number of such intraoperative steps that have been evaluated recently for their merit.

Uterine exteriorization

Exteriorization of the uterus at the time of CD is often performed for better visualization to repair the uterine incision. A meta-analysis comparing repair in situ and by uterine exteriorization did not demonstrate any statistically significant differences in surgical time, intraoperative nausea or vomiting, endometritis, or wound infection [50]. The decision on whether or not to exteriorize the uterus should depend on provider preference.

Removal of placenta by traction of umbilical cord

Manual removal of the placenta compared with removal via umbilical cord traction has been associated with endometritis [51, 52]. In one meta-analysis, manual removal of the placenta was associated with a higher risk of endometritis compared with traction of umbilical cord (RR 1.64, 95% CI 1.42, 1.90) [51].

Intraabdominal irrigation

Two studies have not demonstrated a reduction of SSIs with intraabdominal irrigation of normal saline [53, 54]. In a randomized controlled trial of 236 women undergoing CD, intraabdominal irrigation did not demonstrate decreased risks of wound infection and endometritis, but was associated with intraoperative nausea (RR 1.62; 95% CI 1.15, 2.28) [53]. Similarly in a randomized controlled trial of 196 women undergoing CD, intraabdominal irrigation by normal saline did not reduce intrapartum or postpartum maternal morbidity [54]. Evidence does not support use of routine intraabdominal irrigation.

Suture closure of subcutaneous tissue if wound thickness greater than 2 cm

In a meta-analysis of randomized controlled trials, Chelmow et al. evaluated the potential benefit of suture closure of subcutaneous tissue relative to tissue thickness [55]. Their study showed a statistically significant decrease in the rate of wound complications when the subcutaneous thickness was greater than 2 cm (RR 0.66; 95% CI 0.48, 0.91). [55]. This group also found that suture closure of subcutaneous tissue was associated with a lower risk of seroma (RR 0.42; 95% CI 0.24,1.49) but not lower risks of wound hematomas (RR 1.03; 95% CI 0.38, 2.76) or wound infections (RR 0.98; 95% CI 0.65, 1.49) [55]. Current practice has adopted use of subcutaneous closure when the subcutaneous thickness measures greater than 2 cm.

Subcutaneous drain

Ramsey et al. reported a randomized controlled trial of 280 women with subcutaneous thickness 4 cm or more showing that routine subcutaneous drain was not associated with wound complications compared with standard suture reapproximation [56]. This finding was confirmed by a meta-analysis [57]. Routine subcutaneous drain is not recommended.

Suture skin closure instead of staple closure

Studies comparing suture and staple closure of the skin after CD are consistent in advising use of sutures over staples. In 2011, Tuuli et al. reported a meta-analysis of 6 studies and showed that an increased risk of wound infection or wound separation with staples (n = 803) compared with suture skin closure (n = 684) (OR 2.06; 95% CI 1.43, 2.98) [58]. A 2012 Cochrane Review of 18 trials by Mackeen et al. showed no increased risk of wound infection with staple skin closure [59]. Subsequently in 2014, a randomized controlled study of 746 women by the same group showed a lower risk of wound complications (wound infection, hematoma, seroma, or separation of 1 cm or longer) with suture skin closure compared with

staple skin closure (adjusted OR 0.43; 95% CI 0.23, 0.78) [6]. In this last study, the lower rate of wound complications was largely due to a decreased incidence of wound separation (adjusted OR 0.20; 95% CI 0.07, 0.51). Based on this evidence, routine staple skin closure is not recommended. Further studies are needed to answer if decreased risk of wound complications in suture skin closure compared with staple closure is reproducible in vertical skin incision.

Prophylactic negative pressure wound therapy

Negative pressure wound therapy (vacuum-assisted wound closure) after CD is gaining popularity, especially in obese women. Negative pressure reduces excess fluid accumulation and protects the wound from irritation caused by reducing the frequency of dressing changes to only every 3–5 days.

Data on prophylactic negative pressure wound therapy after CD are limited. A systematic review of 7 randomized trials using negative pressure wound therapy in patients with chronic open wound compared with hydrocolloid gel plus gauze or gauze soaked in normal saline or Ringer's solution did not shown improvement in wound healing [60]. Retrospective studies of prophylactic negative pressure wound therapy after CD in morbidly obese women, however, demonstrated fewer wound complications [61, 62]. A cost-benefit analysis showed that negative pressure wound therapy is only beneficial if the risk of surgical site infection is greater than 14% [63]. A large randomized controlled trials comparing prophylactic negative pressure wound therapy with standard dressing in women with obesity would be useful.

Postoperative management

Dressing removal between 24 and 48 h

Centers for Disease Control and Prevention recommend dressing removal between 24 and 48 h [64]. In a group of women who underwent scheduled CD, Peleg et al. in 2016 conducted a randomized controlled trial comparing postoperative dressing removal at 6 h (n = 160) with dressing removal at 24 h (n = 160) and showed no difference in wound complications [7]. However, the women with earlier dressing removal were more pleased or satisfied than those with later dressing removal (OR 2.35; 95% CI 1.46, 3.79). It is unknown if timing of dressing removal would make a difference in women having emergent CD or those with comorbidities such as obesity, diabetes, or hypertension.

Daily use of chlorhexidine gluconate soap after removal of dressing

Information on daily use of chlorhexidine gluconate soap after dressing removal in women after CD is limited. In a randomized nonblinded crossover trial of 7727 patients admitted in intensive care and bone marrow transplantation units, daily bathing with chlorhexidine-impregnated washcloths had a lower risk of acquisition of multidrug-resistant organisms (5.10 cases per 1000 patient days vs. 6.60 cases per 1000 patient-days; $P = .03$) and hospital acquired bloodstream infections (4.78 cases per 1000 patient days vs. 6.60 cases per 1000 patient-days; $P = .007$) [65]. Similar studies involving post-CD patients warrants further study.

Surgical bundle

Perioperative bundles of evidence-based practices to reduce SSIs have been introduced into non-obstetric surgical patients with promising results [66–68]. Similar results can be anticipated in the obstetric population. We recommend the development of SSI bundles for each hospital. Our own institution, MedStar Washington Hospital Center, began implementing a SSI bundle in December 2016 (Table 3). The study comparing the rate of SSIs prior to and after bundle implementation is underway.

Treatment

Management of wound hematoma and seroma

Small hematomas may resorb without surgical interventions, although they increase the incidence of SSI. Management of wound hematoma includes evacuation of the clot under sterile conditions, ligation or cauterization of bleeding vessels, and reclosure of the wound [69].

Seromas delay wound healing and increase the risk of SSI. Seromas under skin can be evacuated by needle aspiration. To prevent reaccumulation, compression dressings should be applied. If seromas persist, wound exploration in the operating room may be required [69].

Table 3 Surgical site infection bundle at MedStar Washington Hospital Center

Perioperative elements
Preoperative standard antibiotics
Preoperative intravenous azithromycin 500 mg
Chlorhexidine alcohol skin preparation
Use of clippers instead of razor
Vaginal cleansing by povidone-iodine
Intraoperative elements
Removal of placenta by traction of umbilical cord
Suture closure of subcutaneous tissue if wound thickness greater than 2 cm
Suture skin closure instead of staple closure
Postoperative elements
Dressing removal between 24 and 48 h
Daily use of chlorhexidine gluconate soap after removal of dressing

Management of wound infection

Management of wound infection includes antibiotics, incision and drainage, wound dressing, and delayed closure.

Antibiotics

Superficial infection such as cellulitis can be treated with antibiotics alone and do not require incision and drainage. If purulent drainage or exudates accompany cellulitis, empiric therapy should include adequate coverage for methicillin-resistant *Staphylococcus aureus* (MRSA) [70]. Options for oral antibiotics include clindamycin, trimethoprim-sulfamethoxazole, and tetracycline (doxycycline or monocycline). If cellulitis is nonpurulent (no purulent drainage or exudate and no abscess), empiric therapy to cover beta-hemolytic streptococci and methicillin-sensitive *Staphylococcus aureus* (MSSA) is recommended [71]. Options for oral antibiotics for nonpurulent cellulitis include dicloxacillin, cefadroxil, cephalexin, and clindamycin.

Incision and drainage

If the wound has purulent drainage, exudate or separation, incision and drainage to remove abscess, exudate, and hematoma is needed. If necrotic tissue is identified, sharp debridement using forceps and scalpel or scissors is needed until healthy tissue can be identified [72]. Further wound exploration to confirm the integrity of fascia is also important. Fascial dehiscence is a surgical emergency and requires further wound exploration in the Operative Room.

Wound dressings

Packing may be required if the wound has a deep defect. Commonly, wet to dry dressing changes several times daily are performed, placing moistened gauze into the wound with covering by dry gauze [73]. When the gauze is removed during the dressing change, necrotic tissue is also removed. Once necrotic tissue is completely removed and healthy granulation tissue starts to grow, dressing changes can be done less frequently. Other available dressing materials include foam, beads, alginate, hydrocolloids, and gauze with chlorhexidine, povidone iodine and mercury chloride antiseptic solution. A systematic review showed no difference in speed of wound recovery using these various types of dressing materials [74].

Delayed closure

Infected wounds should be left open to heal by secondary intention. In review of 8 prospective studies, reclosure of wound was associated with 81-100% successful healing [75]. Failures occurred in 21 of 324 reclosed wound, 16 of which were complicated by recurrent abscesses. Wound healing was faster in reclosure group compared with secondary intention (16–18 days vs. 61–72 days).

Management of necrotizing fasciitis

Treatment of necrotizing fasciitis includes early and aggressive surgical exploration and debridement of necrotic tissue in addition to broad-spectrum antibiotic therapy [76]. The goal of surgical management is debridement of necrotic tissue until healthy, viable tissue is reached. In most cases, re-exploration of wound 24–36 h after the first debridement and daily thereafter is necessary until no necrotic tissue is found.

Empiric treatment of necrotizing fasciitis should include agents effective against aerobes, including methicillin-resistant *Staphylococcus aureus*, and anaerobes. Acceptable choices for antibiotics are vancomycin, linezolid, or daptomycin combined with one of the following options 1) piperacillin-tazobactam, 2) carbapenem, 3) ceftriaxone plus metronidazole, or 4) fluoroquinolon plus metronidazole [76]. In the setting of group A streptococcal or beta-hemolytic streptococcal infection, the antibiotic regimen should be narrowed down to the combination of penicillin (4 million units every 4 h) and clindamycin (600-900 mg every 8 h). Clindamycin suppresses streptococcal toxin and cytokine production. The efficacy of intravenous immunoglobulin (IVIG) to neutralize extracellular streptococcal toxins is unclear. In a randomized controlled trial in Europe, addition of IVIG to surgical treatment and antibiotics therapy did not improve survival in women with streptococcal toxic shock syndrome [77]. In the setting of Clostridium infection, penicillin plus clindamycin is recommended [78]. The efficacy of hyperbaric oxygen therapy for clostridium infection is unclear due to the lack of data from randomized controlled trials in humans.

Management of endometritis

Endometritis is generally treated by clindamycin (900 mg intravenously every 8 h) plus gentamicin [79]. Gentamicin (5 mg/kg [ideal body weight]) compared with gentamicin (1.5 mg/kg [ideal body weight] every 8 h) is similarly efficacious, more cost effective and less task time for nurses [80–82]. Ampicillin may be added to the regimen for better coverage of enterococcus. If fever persists despite antibiotics administration, imaging of abdomen and pelvis should be considered to rule out infected hematoma and pelvic abscess.

Conclusions

SSIs following CDs represent complex clinical situations and are caused by many factors such as patient characteristics and perioperative management. In addition, SSIs comprise a burden to our health care system. Creating bundles of evidence-based elements may decrease the

rates of post-CD SSIs, as has been demonstrated in non-obstetric patients. We strongly recommend each hospital to consider the evidence-based information presented in creating its own surgical bundle to decrease the rates of SSIs after CDs.

Abbreviations

ACOG: American College of Obstetricians and Gynecologists; BMI: Body Mass Index; CI: Confidence interval; OR: Odds ratio; RR: Relative Risk

Acknowledgements

Not applicable.

Funding

None.

Authors' contributions

TK wrote the article and is corresponding author of the study. HJL critically reviewed the manuscript. Both authors read and approved the final manuscript.

Authors' information

None.

Competing interests

The authors declare that they have no competing interests.

Author details

[1]Obstetrics and Gynecology, MedStar Washington Hospital Center, 101 Irving Street, 5B45, NW, Washington, DC 20010, USA. [2]Obstetrics and Gynecology, MedStar Georgetown University Hospital, Washington, DC, USA.

References

1. Hamilton BE, Martin JA, Osterman MJK, et al. Births: final data for 2014. National vital statistics reports; vol 64 no 12. Hyattsville: National Center for Health Statistics; 2015.
2. Silver RM, Landon MB, Rouse DJ, et al. Maternal morbidity associated with multiple repeat cesarean deliveries. Obstet Gynecol. 2006;107(6):1226–32.
3. Liu S, Liston RM, Joseph KS, et al. Maternal mortality and severe morbidity associated with low-risk planned cesarean delivery versus planned vaginal delivery at term. CMAJ. 2007;176(4):455–60.
4. Deneux-Tharaux C, Carmona E, Bouvier-Colle MH, et al. Postpartum maternal mortality and cesarean delivery. Obstet Gynecol. 2006;108(3 Pt 1):541–8.
5. Burrows LJ, Meyn LA, Weber AM. Maternal morbidity associated with vaginal versus cesarean delivery. Obstet Gynecol. 2004;103:907–12.
6. Mackeen AD, Khalifeh A, Fleisher J, et al. Suture compared with staple skin closure after cesarean delivery: a randomized controlled trial. Obstet Gynecol. 2014;123(6):1169–75.
7. Peleg D, Eberstark E, Warsof SL, et al. Early wound dressing removal after scheduled cesarean delivery: a randomized controlled trial. Am J Obstet Gynecol. 2016;215(3):388.e1–5.

8. Olsen MA, Butler AM, Willers DM, et al. Risk factors for surgical site infection after low transverse cesarean section. Infect Control Hosp Epidemiol. 2008;29(6):477–84.
9. Tita AT, Szychowski JM, Boggess K, et al. Adjunctive Azithromycin prophylaxis for cesarean delivery. N Engl J Med. 2016;375(13):1231–41.
10. Haas DM, Pazouki F, Smith RR, et al. Vaginal cleansing before cesarean delivery to reduce postoperative infectious morbidity: a randomized, controlled trial. Am J Obstet Gynecol. 2010;202(3):310.e1–6.
11. Costantine MM, Rahman M, Ghulmiyah L, et al. Timing of perioperative antibiotics for cesarean delivery: a metaanalysis. Am J Obstet Gynecol. 2008; 199(3):301.e1–6.
12. Blumenfeld YJ, El-Sayed YY, Lyell DJ, et al. Risk factors for prolonged postpartum length of stay following cesarean delivery. Am J Perinatol. 2015; 32(9):825–32.
13. Martens MG, Kolrud BL, Faro S, et al. Development of wound infection or separation after cesarean delivery. Prospective evaluation of 2,431 cases. J Reprod Med. 1995;40:171–5.
14. Roberts S, Maccato M, Faro S, Pinell P. The microbiology of post-cesarean wound morbidity. Obstet Gynecol. 1993;81:383–6.
15. Goepfert AR, Guinn DA, Andrews WW, et al. Necrotizing fasciitis after cesarean delivery. Obstet Gynecol. 1997;89(3):409–12.
16. Stevens DL, Bisno AL, Chambers HF, et al. Practice guidelines for the diagnosis and management of skin and soft tissue infections: 2014 update by the infectious diseases society of America. Clin Infect Dis. 2014;59(2):147–59.
17. Sudarsky LA, Laschinger JC, Coppa GF, et al. Improved results from a standardized approach in treating patients with necrotizing fasciitis. Ann Surg. 1987;206(5):661.
18. Fitzwater JL, Tita AT. Prevention and management of cesarean wound infection. Obstet Gynecol Clin N Am. 2014;41(4):671–89.
19. Rosene K, Eschenbach DA, Tompkins LS, et al. Polymicrobial early postpartum endometritis with facultative and anaerobic bacteria, genital mycoplasmas, and Chlamydia trachomatis: treatment with piperacillin or cefoxitin. J Infect Dis. 1986;153(6):1028.
20. Reid VC, Hartmann KE, McMahon M, et al. Vaginal preparation with povidone iodine and postcesarean infectious morbidity: a randomized controlled trial. Obstet Gynecol. 2001;97:147–52.
21. Guzman MA, Prien SD, Blann DW. Post-cesarean related infection and vaginal preparation with povidone-iodine revisited. Primary Care Update OB/GYNS. 2002;9(6):206–9.
22. Tran TS, Jamulitrat S, Chongsuvivatwong V, et al. Risk factors for postcesarean surgical site infection. Obstet Gynecol. 2000;95(3):367–71.
23. Avila C, Bhangoo R, Figueroa R, et al. Association of smoking with wound complications after cesarean delivery. J Matern Fetal Neonatal Med. 2012;25:1250–3.
24. Jama FE. Risk factors for wound infection after lower segment cesarean section. Qatar Med J. 2012;2:26–31.
25. De Vivo A, Mancuso A, Giacobbe A, et al. Wound length and corticosteroid administration as risk factors for surgical-site complications following cesarean section. Acta Obstet Gynecol Scand. 2010;89(3):355–9.
26. Killian CA, Graffunder EM, Vinciguerra TJ, et al. Risk factors for surgical-site infections following cesarean section. Infect Control Hosp Epidemiol. 2001;22:613–7.
27. Wloch C, Wilson J, Lamagni T, et al. Risk factors for surgical site infection following caesarean section in England: results from a multicentre cohort study. BJOG. 2012;119(11):1324–33.
28. Opøien HK, Valbø A, Grinde-Andersen A, et al. Post-cesarean surgical site infections according to CDC standards: rates and risk factors. A prospective cohort study. Acta Obstet Gynecol Scand. 2007;86(9):1097–102.
29. Schneid-Kofman N, Sheiner E, Levy A, et al. Risk factors for wound infection following cesarean deliveries. Int J Gynaecol Obstet. 2005;90:10–5.
30. Vermillion ST, Lamoutte C, Soper DE, et al. Wound infection after cesarean: effect of subcutaneous tissue thickness. Obstet Gynecol. 2000;95(6 Pt 1):923–6.
31. Tuuli MG, Liu L, Longman RE, et al. Infectious morbidity is higher after second-stage compared with first-stage cesareans. Am J Obstet Gynecol. 2014;211(4):410.e1–6.
32. Takoudes TC, Weitzen S, Slocum J, et al. Risk of cesarean wound complications in diabetic gestations. Am J Obstet Gynecol. 2004;191(3):958–63.
33. Chaim W, Bashiri A, Bar-David J, et al. Prevalence and clinical significance of postpartum endometritis and wound infection. Infect Dis Obstet Gynecol. 2000;8:77–82.
34. Olsen MA, Butler AM, Willers DM, et al. Comparison of costs of surgical site infection and endometritis after cesarean delivery using claims and medical record data. Infect Control Hosp Epidemiol. 2010;31:872–5.
35. Smaill FM, Grivell RM. Antibiotic prophylaxis versus no prophylaxis for preventing infection after cesarean section. Cochrane Database of Systematic Reviews 2014, Issue 10. Art. No.: CD007482.
36. Sullivan SA, Smith T, Chang E, et al. Administration of cefazolin prior to skin incision is superior to cefazolin at cord clamping in preventing postcesarean infectious morbidity: a randomized, controlled trial. Am J Obstet Gynecol. 2007;196:455.e1–5.
37. Thigpen BD, Hood WA, Chauhan S, et al. Timing of prophylactic antibiotic administration in the uninfected laboring gravida: a randomized clinical trial. Am J Obstet Gynecol. 2005;192:1864–71.
38. Wax JR, Hersey K, Philput C, et al. Single dose cefazolin prophylaxis for postcesarean infections: before vs after cord clamping. J Matern Fetal Med. 1997;6:61–5.
39. Owens SM, Brozanski BS, Meyn LA, et al. Antimicrobial prophylaxis for cesarean delivery before skin incision. Obstet Gynecol. 2009;114(3):573–9.
40. American College of Obstetricians and Gynecologists. ACOG practice bulletin no. 120: use of prophylactic antibiotics in labor and delivery. Obstet Gynecol. 2011;117(6):1472–83.
41. Ahmadzia HK, Patel EM, Joshi D, et al. Obstetric surgical site infections: 2 grams compared with 3 grams of Cefazolin in morbidly obese women. Obstet Gynecol. 2015;126(4):708–15.
42. Tita AT, Hauth JC, Grimes A, et al. Decreasing incidence of postcesarean endometritis with extended-spectrum antibiotic prophylaxis. Obstet Gynecol. 2008;111(1):51–6.
43. Tuuli MG, Liu J, Stout MJ, et al. A randomized trial comparing skin antiseptic agents at cesarean delivery. N Engl J Med. 2016;374(7):647–55.
44. Ngai IM, Van Arsdale A, Govindappagari S, et al. Skin preparation for prevention of surgical site infection after cesarean delivery: a randomized controlled trial. Obstet Gynecol. 2015;126(6):1251–7.
45. Tanner J, Norrie P, Melen K. Preoperative hair removal to reduce surgical site infection. Cochrane Database Syst Rev. 2011;(11):CD004122.
46. Ahmed MR, Aref NK, Sayed Ahmed WA, et al. Chlorhexidine vaginal wipes prior to elective cesarean section: does it reduce infectious morbidity? A randomized trial. J Matern Fetal Neonatal Med. 2016;1:1–4.
47. Yildirim G, Güngördük K, Asicioğlu O, et al. Does vaginal preparation with povidone-iodine prior to caesarean delivery reduce the risk of endometritis? A randomized controlled trial. J Matern Fetal Neonatal Med. 2012;25(11):2316–21.
48. Haas DM, Morgan S, Contreras K. Vaginal preparation with antiseptic solution before cesarean section for preventing postoperative infections. Cochrane Database Syst Rev. 2014;(9):CD007892.
49. American College of Obstetricians and Gynecologists Women's Health Care Physicians, Committee on Gynecologic Practice. Committee opinion no. 571: solutions for surgical preparation of the vagina. Obstet Gynecol. 2013; 122(3):718–20.
50. Walsh CA, Walsh SR. Extraabdominal vs intraabdominal uterine repair at cesarean delivery: a metaanalysis. Am J Obstet Gynecol. 2009;200(6):625.e1–8.
51. Anorlu RI, Maholwana B, Hofmeyr GJ. Methods of delivering the placenta at caesarean section. Cochrane Database Syst Rev. 2008;(3):CD004737.
52. Atkinson MW, Owen J, Wren A, et al. The effect of manual removal of the placenta on post-cesarean endometritis. Obstet Gynecol. 1996;87(1):99–102.
53. Viney R, Isaacs C, Chelmow D. Intraabdominal irrigation at cesarean delivery: a randomized controlled trial. Obstet Gynecol. 2012;120:708.
54. Harrigill KM, Miller HS, Haynes DE. The effect of intraabdominal irrigation at cesarean delivery on maternal morbidity: a randomized trial. Obstet Gynecol. 2003;101(1):80–5.
55. Chelmow D, Rodriguez EJ, Sabatini MM. Suture closure of subcutaneous fat and wound disruption after cesarean delivery: a meta-analysis. Obstet Gynecol. 2004;103(5 Pt 1):974–80.
56. Ramsey PS, White AM, Guinn DA, et al. Subcutaneous tissue reapproximation, alone or in combination with drain, in obese women undergoing cesarean delivery. Obstet Gynecol. 2005;105(5 Pt 1):967–73.
57. Hellums EK, Lin MG, Ramsey PS. Prophylactic subcutaneous drainage for prevention of wound complications after cesarean delivery–a metaanalysis. Am J Obstet Gynecol. 2007;197(3):229–35.
58. Tuuli MG, Rampersad RM, Carbone JF, et al. Staples compared with subcuticular suture for skin closure after cesarean delivery: a systematic review and meta-analysis. Obstet Gynecol. 2011;117(3):682–90.

59. Mackeen AD, Berghella V, Larsen ML. Techniques and materials for skin closure in caesarean section. Cochrane Database Syst Rev. 2012;11: CD003577.

60. Ubbink DT, Westerbos SJ, Evans D, et al. Topical negative pressure for treating chronic wounds. Cochrane Database Syst Rev. 2008 Jul 16;(3): CD001898.

61. Swift SH, Zimmerman MB, Hardy-Fairbanks AJ. Effect of single-use negative pressure wound therapy on Postcesarean infections and wound complications for high-risk patients. J Reprod Med. 2015;60(5-6):211–8.

62. Mark KS, Alger L, Terplan M. Incisional negative pressure therapy to prevent wound complications following cesarean section in morbidly obese women: a pilot study. Surg Innov. 2014;21(4):345–9.

63. Echebiri NC, McDoom MM, Aalto MM, et al. Prophylactic use of negative pressure wound therapy after cesarean delivery. Obstet Gynecol. 2015; 125(2):299–307.

64. Mangram AJ, Horan TC, Pearson ML, et al. Guideline for prevention of surgical site infection, 1999. Hospital infection Control practices advisory Committee. Infect Control Hosp Epidemiol. 1999;20(4):250–78.

65. Climo MW, Yokoe DS, Warren DK, et al. Effect of daily chlorhexidine bathing on hospital-acquired infection. N Engl J Med. 2013;368(6):533–42.

66. Johnson MP, Kim SJ, Langstraat CL, et al. Using bundled interventions to reduce surgical site infection after major gynecologic cancer surgery. Obstet Gynecol. 2016;127(6):1135–44.

67. Keenan JE, Speicher PJ, Thacker JK, et al. The preventive surgical site infection bundle in colorectal surgery: an effective approach to surgical site infection reduction and health care cost savings. JAMA Surg. 2014;149(10):1045–52.

68. Cima R, Dankbar E, Lovely J, et al. Colorectal surgery surgical site infection reduction program: a national surgical quality improvement program–driven multidisciplinary single-institution experience. J Am Coll Surg. 2013;216(1):23–33.

69. Doherty GM. Chapter 5. Postoperative complications. In: Doherty GM, editor. CURRENT Diagnosis & Treatment: surgery, 13e. New York: McGraw-Hill; 2010.

70. Moran GJ, Krishnadasan A, Gorwitz RJ, et al. Methicillin-Resistant S. aureus infections among patients in the emergency department. N Engl J Med. 2006;355:666.

71. Liu C, Bayer A, Cosgrove SE, et al. Clinical practice guidelines by the infectious diseases society of america for the treatment of methicillin-resistant Staphylococcus aureus infections in adults and children. Clin Infect Dis. 2011;52:e18.

72. Stadelmann WK, Digenis AG, Tobin GR. Impediments to wound healing. Am J Surg. 1998;176:39S–47.

73. Ovington LGS. Hanging wet-to-dry dressings out to dry. Home Healthc Nurse. 2001;19(8):477.

74. Vermeulen H, Ubbink D, Goossens A, et al. Dressings and topical agents for surgical wounds healing by secondary intention. Cochrane Database Syst Rev 2004;(2):CD003554.

75. Wechter ME, Pearlman MD, Hartmann KE. Reclosure of the disrupted laparotomy wound: a systematic review. Obstet Gynecol. 2005;106:376–83.

76. Stevens DL, Bisno AL, Chambers HF, et al. Practice guidelines for the diagnosis and management of skin and soft tissue infections: 2014 update by the infectious diseases society of America. Clin Infect Dis. 2014;59(2):147–59.

77. Darenberg J, Ihendyane N, Sjölin J, et al. Intravenous immunoglobulin G therapy in streptococcal toxic shock syndrome: a European randomized, double-blind, placebo-controlled trial. Clin Infect Dis. 2003;37(3):333–40.

78. Stevens DL, Laine BM, Mitten JE. Comparison of single and combination antimicrobial agents for prevention of experimental gas gangrene caused by Clostridium perfringens. Antimicrob Agents Chemother. 1987;31:312–6.

79. Mackeen AD, Packard RE, Ota E, et al. Antibiotic regimens for postpartum endometritis. Cochrane Database Syst Rev 2015:CD001067.

80. Mitra AG, Whitten MK, Laurent SL, et al. A randomized, prospective study comparing once-daily gentamicin versus thrice-daily gentamicin in the treatment of puerperal infection. Am J Obstet Gynecol. 1997;177(4):786.

81. Del Priore G, Jackson-Stone M, Shim EK, et al. A comparison of once-daily and 8-hour gentamicin dosing in the treatment of postpartum endometritis. Obstet Gynecol. 1996;87(6):994.

82. Livingston JC, Llata E, Rinehart E, et al. Gentamicin and clindamycin therapy in postpartum endometritis: the efficacy of daily dosing versus dosing every 8 hours. Am J Obstet Gynecol. 2003;188(1):149.

3

New approaches to management of neonatal hypoglycemia

Paul J. Rozance* and William W. Hay Jr.

Abstract

Despite being a very common problem after birth, consensus on how to manage low glucose concentrations in the first 48 h of life has been difficult to establish and remains a debated issue. One of the reasons for this is that few studies have provided the type of data needed to establish a definitive approach agreed upon by all. However, some recent publications have provided much needed primary data to inform this debate. These publications have focused on aspects of managing low blood glucose concentrations in the patients most at-risk for asymptomatic hypoglycemia—those born late-preterm, large for gestational age, small for gestational age, or growth restricted, and those born following a pregnancy complicated by diabetes mellitus. The goal of this review is to discuss specific aspects of this new research. First, we focus on promising new data testing the role of buccal dextrose gel in the management of asymptomatic neonatal hypoglycemia. Second, we highlight some of the clinical implications of a large, prospective study documenting the association of specific glycemic patterns with neurodevelopmental outcomes at two years of age.

Keywords: Neonatal hypoglycemia, Dextrose gel, Continuous glucose monitoring, Infant of a diabetic mother, Late preterm, Small for gestational age, Large for gestational age, Intrauterine growth restriction

Background

Hypoglycemia is one of the most frequently encountered problems in the first 48 h of life, and low glucose concentrations are perhaps the most common biochemical abnormality seen by providers caring for newborns. Unfortunately, the optimal strategy for managing this problem remains elusive and is a matter of differing interpretations of the available literature [1–8]. New data to inform the optimal management of these newborns is urgently needed [9]. Especially controversial is the management of asymptomatic but at-risk newborns, most commonly those with a history or physical exam consistent with being born late-preterm, large for gestational age (LGA), small for gestational age (SGA), or growth restricted, or an infant of a diabetic mother (IDM). The reason for this controversy is that numerous studies have shown that, with the exception of the LGA group, these newborns have worse neurodevelopmental outcomes than healthy term babies [10–13] and that in some of these groups, worse neurodevelopmental outcomes are associated

with the presence of neonatal hypoglycemia [12]. To date, no study has shown that preventing or treating the hypoglycemia in these groups leads to better outcomes, making it uncertain whether hypoglycemia has a causal role in producing the worse outcomes. In fact, the statement made by the AAP in 1993 remains accurate today, "... there is no evidence that asymptomatic hypoglycemic infants will benefit from treatment [14]." The goal of this review is to discuss recent primary research that has added important new data to consider when devising strategies to manage this group of newborns. These recent data hold promise for optimizing our approach to managing neonatal hypoglycemia, especially in the at-risk groups noted above.

Asymptomatic neonatal hypoglycemia

The newborns most at risk for, and most frequently screened for, asymptomatic hypoglycemia include late preterm, LGA, SGA, and/or intrauterine growth restricted (IUGR) infants, and IDMs [4]. Frequent milk feedings with repeated glucose measurements is the current standard treatment for asymptomatic hypoglycemia in these groups of patients [4]. This approach allows mothers and babies to remain together, provides nutrient substrates

* Correspondence: Paul.Rozance@ucdenver.edu
Perinatal Research Center, Department of Pediatrics, University of Colorado School of Medicine, 13243 E 23rd Ave, MS F441, Aurora, CO 80045, USA

to support gluconeogenesis as it develops, and ensures that the hypoglycemia resolves. If hypoglycemia persists despite frequent milk feedings, a continuous intravenous dextrose infusion may be indicated. The following approach to the rate of dextrose infusion for asymptomatic hypoglycemia can be considered. A dextrose infusion rate of 3–5 mg/kg/min can be used for IDMs, as this avoids overstimulation of insulin secretion and accounts for the larger fat mass that these infants have. A dextrose infusion rate of 4–7 mg/kg/min can be used for most term and near term infants. A dextrose infusion rate of 6–8 mg/kg/min often is necessary in IUGR infants. This accounts for their greater brain/body weight ratio and physiological observations made in animal models of IUGR of both increased peripheral insulin sensitivity and increased insulin secretion as their postnatal physiology is normalized and insulin-suppressive catecholamine secretion is reduced [15–20]. Glucose concentrations must be followed closely as some of these IUGR infants, especially those very preterm, also can have hyperglycemia, due to reduced insulin secretion capacity, diminished muscle mass for glucose disposal, and persistent glucose production [17, 18, 20–30]. A continuous intravenous dextrose infusion, usually preceded by an intravenous dextrose bolus (200 mg/kg given over 5 min), also is indicated if these newborns develop symptomatic hypoglycemia. In fact, partial or complete resolution of the symptoms with correction of glucose concentrations is considered proof that the symptoms were caused by the low glucose concentrations [31]. Intravenous dextrose infusions, however, are not benign; they cause discomfort and stress due to the placement of an intravenous catheter, admission to a NICU, and physical separation of the mother and newborn which risks impairing the timely and successful establishment of breastfeeding and bonding. Preventing these complications of intravenous dextrose infusions, while safely managing asymptomatic low glucose concentrations, has many potential benefits.

Dextrose gel

To this end, Harris, et al. undertook a large, randomized, placebo-controlled, double-blinded study of buccal dextrose gel for the treatment of asymptomatic hypoglycemia, defined as a plasma glucose less than 47 mg/dL (2.6 mmol/L) irrespective of postnatal age [32]. The dextrose gel (200 mg/kg) or placebo gel was massaged into the infant's dried buccal mucosa and the infant was encouraged to feed. If the baby still had a low glucose concentration 30 min after gel administration, or if the baby developed recurrent hypoglycemia, the treatment with study gel continued for a total of six doses over 48 h. The specific characteristics of the populations studied included late preterm (35–36 weeks gestational age), LGA (>90th percentile or >4500 g), SGA/IUGR (<10th percentile or <2500 g), and IDM newborns. In these

groups dextrose gel decreased the number of episodes of hypoglycemia, decreased the recurrence rate of hypoglycemia, increased exclusive breastfeeding rates at discharge, and decreased the need for admission to the neonatal intensive care (NICU) unit to treat hypoglycemia. The number of newborns needed to treat to prevent one admission to the NICU for hypoglycemia was only eight. It is important to note that in this study the newborns, regardless of randomization, were still managed with aggressive oral feeding (mostly breastmilk) to treat hypoglycemia. There were no adverse events reported and continuous interstitial glucose monitoring (to which the care providers were blinded) did not identify more frequent, clinically unrecognized episodes of rebound or recurrent hypoglycemia in the dextrose gel group, thereby establishing short term safety. Of note, overall admission rates to the NICU for all causes were not statistically significantly different between groups (38 % in the dextrose gel group vs. 46 % with placebo gel). The most likely cause of the lack of effect on overall NICU admission rates, despite the reduction in NICU admissions to treat hypoglycemia, is simply that the sample size was too small to show a difference in this secondary outcome.

Despite these encouraging short term results, there was some concern that the dextrose gel treatment might have adversely impacted long term neurodevelopmental outcomes. Reasons for concern included a potential delay in definitive treatment with intravenous dextrose, rapid overcorrection and iatrogenic hyperglycemia, and increased variability in glucose concentrations [33, 34]. Information from continuous glucose monitoring sensors (CGMS), which was blinded to the caregivers, was reassuring regarding these concerns. When the researchers looked at the CGMS data, however, they found that the time to achieve an interstitial glucose concentration greater than 47 mg/dL (2.6 mmol/L) with dextrose gel was as rapid as has been reported for correction with intravenous dextrose given at 8 mg/kg/min–about twenty minutes [35]. CGMS data also showed that rebound hypoglycemia was rare in both groups and the incidence of recurrent hypoglycemia was less in the dextrose gel group. While these data support the safety and efficacy of he dextrose gel established by intermittent glucose sampling, CGMS was only used in a subset of the patients in this study. Therefore, it is important that two year outcomes have recently been published [36]. 78 % of the original hypoglycemic cohort was available for assessment of outcomes at two years of age. Fortunately, there were no differences between the dextrose gel group and placebo group for neurosensory impairment, processing difficulties, or secondary growth and developmental outcomes. The high rates of abnormal outcomes in both groups is concerning and should prompt further research into optimal management of these patients [36].

When considering the adoption of dextrose gel into clinical practice, it must be remembered that although the study was quite large and included a broad representation of the main at-risk groups, it was a single center study. A multi-centered trial confirming these results would broaden the applicability of this therapy. This issue is highlighted by the results for improved rates of exclusive breast feeding at two weeks of age [32]. The rates of exclusive breastfeeding at this age are quite high in this New Zealand population. Whether this benefit would be replicated in populations with higher or lower rates of breast feeding is unknown. However, if a new trial included hospitals without a NICU, the benefits of dextrose gel might also include lower transfer rates of these patients to hospitals that have intensive care capabilities. It also is important to note that the definition of hypoglycemia and treatment cut-off were both 47 mg/dL (2.6 mmole/L), irrespective of gestational and postnatal age. This definition does not take into account the age related changes in mean and lower limits of normal glucose concentrations that occur in the first days of life [37]. The definition of hypoglycemia, screening frequency, and screening duration also may vary from what is used in some clinical practices [4, 8]. Clinicians should ensure that they have accounted for these differences when considering adoption of dextrose gel into clinical practice. Not only was screening for hypoglycemia quite frequent, in this study the clinicians used a very reliable point of care device. This device uses the gold standard glucose oxidase method for measurement of plasma glucose concentrations, which is much more accurate than bedside glucometers [38]. Glucose concentrations were measured at one hour of age, then before feeds every 3–4 h for the first 24 h of age, and then before feeds every 6–8 h for the next 24 h. This protocol identified 46 % of the enrolled patients as hypoglycemic, who were included in the study. This relatively high incidence of neonatal hypoglycemia in this population likely is due to the rigorous and frequent screening protocol, the method used to measure glucose concentrations, the higher glucose concentration threshold that was used to define hypoglycemia compared to other published guidelines [4], and a definition of hypoglycemia that does not exclude infants who have low glucose concentrations during the normal physiological nadir that occurs in normal infants in the first hours of life [7, 37].

Other important considerations are that the dextrose gel treatment was tested in infants who were at-risk for hypoglycemia but were otherwise well-appearing and asymptomatic [32]. The results cannot be applied to infants with severe, symptomatic, and recurrent hypoglycemia, and/or if the infant is not in one of the at-risk groups studied. Furthermore, the dextrose gel did not eliminate the need for intravenous dextrose therapy. Over 10 % of infants treated with dextrose gel in this study had an episode of rebound hypoglycemia and over 20 % had an episode of recurrent hypoglycemia after a documented normal glucose concentration. While these rates were similar to or better than those in the placebo group, practitioners should not be using this therapy without close follow up of subsequent glucose concentrations, clinical signs of hypoglycemia, and documentation of resolution of the hypoglycemia [4, 8]. Despite these limitations, the therapy appears safe and effective at preventing NICU admissions for hypoglycemia and it may be appropriate for some hospitals to adopt into clinical practice. Indeed, such efforts are already being described with promising results [39, 40]. Making guidelines for managing low glucose concentrations in the first days of life safe and easy to follow, while at the same time promoting increased maternal-infant interactions and increased breastfeeding rates, is critical for all practitioners caring for newborns. Buccal dextrose gel appears to have a promising role in achieving these goals and caregivers can be more confident that the early benefits of dextrose gel are not associated with worse two year neurodevelopmental outcomes [36].

Continuous glucose monitoring

Another interesting feature of the dextrose gel study is the use of CGMS to continuously monitor interstitial glucose concentrations. One important observation is that many episodes of hypoglycemia, documented by both blood obtained per their low glucose concentration screening protocol and CGMS measurements, resolved spontaneously, and were not associated with bedside nursing observations of clinical signs that might be interpreted as symptoms of hypoglycemia. Thus, while CGMS remains a research tool, this observation demonstrates the potential for CGMS to reduce unnecessary treatment for hypoglycemia. For example, CGMS may identify patients in whom their low glucose concentrations have resolved prior to commencement of interventions. However, there also is the potential for CGMS to increase unnecessary treatment for hypoglycemia. For the clinician, CGMS or any other method that continuously provides glucose concentration data will present a challenge to the way we think about hypoglycemia. Instead of an intermittent variable, caregivers will be provided with a continuous variable, analogous to the transition from intermittent blood gas measurements to continuous pulse oximetry for monitoring blood oxygenation. Furthermore, CGMS in this population, as well as in more preterm newborns, will identify numerous episodes of low glucose concentrations that are not identified by intermittent routine blood sampling [41, 42]. In fact, in the populations studied by Harris, et. al., 81 % of all episodes of hypoglycemia were recognized with CGMS only and not by routine clinical blood sampling [42]. There is very little information about the clinical significance of these episodes for long term outcomes, including which should be treated and whether such treatment would improve outcomes. It is possible, therefore, that identifying these episodes of hypoglycemia with CGMS could increase overtreatment of clinically insignificant low glucose concentrations. This risk might outweigh the benefits of documenting more episodes of low glucose concentrations and avoiding treatment of those that resolve spontaneously, as well as the early detection of serious, recurrent hypoglycemia in patients with hyperinsulinemic hypoglycemia and other metabolic disorders [43]. The uncertainty regarding the balance of the risks and benefits of using CGMS or similar devices for the continuous monitoring of neonatal glucose concentrations in this population highlights the need for further studies in this area. Such studies will have to be designed to clarify relationships between continuous glucose concentrations, symptomatic hypoglycemia, responses to treatment, associated medical conditions, and neurodevelopmental outcomes.

Identifying and treating asymptomatic hypoglycemic newborns

There is very little evidence to inform how often glucose concentrations should be screened in the asymptomatic at-risk newborn or the glucose concentration threshold one should use for treatment. Also unknown are the degree and duration of hypoglycemia necessary to cause permanent neurological injury [9]. Especially important is the question of how to identify the rare infant in which asymptomatic hypoglycemia is the first presentation of a rare and persistent disorder of hypoglycemia such as congenital hyperinsulinemic hypoglycemia, fatty acid oxidation disorders, hypopituitarism, and glycogen storage diseases [8]. In 2011 the AAP published clinical guidelines to address some of these concerns, with special attention to management of hypoglycemia in the first 24 h of life [4]. They suggested that late preterm, LGA, SGA/IUGR, and IDM newborns should be fed by one hour of age and have their glucose checked 30 min after the feeding. Glucose monitoring should then continue before feeds through 12 h of age for LGA and IDM patients as long as pre-feed plasma glucose concentrations remain greater than 40 mg/dL (2.2 mmol/L). It was suggested that late preterm and SGA infants should be screened before feeds for 24 h. In 2012 Harris, et al. published the incidence of hypoglycemia during this same 24 h period, again defining as plasma glucose concentrations <47 mg/dL (2.6 mmol/L) irrespective of age in this same group of newborns [44]. They used a

more frequent screening protocol, measuring glucose concentrations one hour after birth and then before feeds every 3–4 h for the first 24 h of life, but also added screening every 3–8 h for the second 24 h of life. While the incidence of hypoglycemia in this population was quite high (51 %), more important were the observations that, of the patients with hypoglycemia, 37 % had their first episode after having had three plasma glucose concentrations greater than 47 mg/dL (2.6 mmol/L) and 6 % had their first episode after 24 h of age [44]. Another important observation in this study was that there were no differences among the at-risk groups studied in the incidence or timing of the hypoglycemia. While the long term clinical significance of these episodes of hypoglycemia, whether first identified in the first 24 h or later, remains unclear, it may be a reasonable approach to simplify screening protocols so that screening frequency and duration are the same for all at-risk groups [44, 45].

The definition of hypoglycemia and the threshold for treatment and continued management are controversial as well. A plasma glucose concentration of 47 mg/dL (2.6 mmol/L) was used in multiple studies by Harris, et al. as their threshold for diagnosis and treatment [32, 34, 36, 42, 44]. The 2011 guideline by the AAP states that once hypoglycemia is identified, treatment should commence with feeding or intravenous dextrose infusion and a target plasma glucose concentration of greater than 45 mg/dL (2.5 mmol/L) should be used [4]. In 2015 the Pediatric Endocrine Society published new recommendations regarding the management of hypoglycemia in newborns [8]. While the main goals of these recommendations were to help clinicians distinguish between physiologically low glucose concentrations in normal newborns and those that persist beyond the first 48 h of life and might place the infant at risk for neurological injury, this group made the recommendation that in the first 48 h of life the target threshold plasma glucose concentration for treatment should be 50 mg/dL (2.8 mmol/L). This group also made the case that neurogenic symptoms occur in newborns below the same glucose concentrations as in adults (55–65 mg/dL [3.1–3.6 mmol/L]) [7, 8]. Thus, they also make the recommendation that in specific patients higher glucose target thresholds of 60 mg/dL (3.3 mmol/L) and 70 mg/dL (3.9 mmol/L) should be used [8]. To date, there is no data to rationally define selection of any one of these lower limit threshold glucose concentration values, in terms of which treatment to use, acute risks vs. benefits, or impact on longer term neurodevelopmental outcomes.

The variability among the recommendations of these different publications reflects the need for further research. A recent publication from the same group that performed the dextrose gel study has provided some data [34], but this was not a study that randomized newborns to different glucose treatment thresholds. However, what they found was that, regardless of treatment with or without the dextrose gel, asymptomatic patients in the main at-risk groups (late preterm, LGA, SGA/IUGR, IDM) had similar neurodevelopmental outcomes at two years of age whether they had hypoglycemia (<47 mg/dL [2.6 mmol/L]) identified in the first seven days of life or not [34]. This assumes that the infants were screened in the first 48 h by the rigorous protocol described above and that when identified, the newborns were treated to achieve or exceed a target plasma glucose concentration of 47 mg/dL (2.6 mmol/L). The main conclusion that one can make from these data is that in this specific patient population with frequent screening and identification of hypoglycemia, using a target plasma glucose concentration of 47 mg/dL (2.6 mmol/L) results in neurodevelopmental outcomes similar to those at-risk patients who did not have an episode of hypoglycemia [34]. However, it cannot be emphasized enough that the plasma glucose concentration defining hypoglycemia was arbitrarily set at 47 mg/dL (2.6 mmol/L) and does not take into account evolution of glucose concentrations and their variability in the first week of life [7]. A plasma glucose concentration of 47 mg/dL (2.6 mmol/L) will likely be less clinically relevant at 6 h of age compared to four days of age, when low glucose concentrations should have increased spontaneously [7].

In the study by McKinlay, et al. the rate of neurodevelopmental delay was not different in the group that experienced a hypoglycemic event (33 %) compared to the group that did not (36 %) [34]. But these rates are high, and some might argue that the threshold for treatment should be even higher than 47 mg/dL (2.6 mmol/L). However, the lack of two year neurodevelopmental outcome data in a concurrently tested group of healthy term control children makes this conclusion premature. It could be that the novel and highly sophisticated techniques that were used to detect abnormal outcomes are so sensitive as to give a high false positive rate and that if a group of healthy term control infants were tested at the same time, they too would have unexpectedly high rates of abnormal outcomes. More importantly, there are significant risks to a more aggressive screening and treatment strategy. These include increased frequency of blood sampling, use of formula supplementation, admission to the NICU and separation from the mother, complications of intravenous catheters, and side effects of any therapies used to raise glucose concentrations. These risks must be balanced against the potential harm due to asymptomatic hypoglycemia, progression to symptomatic hypoglycemia, and delay in diagnosis and treatment of serious metabolic disorders.

The authors also noted three important associations in their data that should provide some caution with respect to increasing glucose treatment thresholds and goals. One is that newborns who did not have a plasma glucose lower than 54 mg/dL (3.0 mmol/L) had worse outcomes than those newborns who did. By CGMS data, the average difference in glucose concentrations between those with worse outcomes and those with better outcomes was only 2.9 mg/dL (0.16 mmol/L). A second important association noted was that those newborns who had more time with plasma glucose concentrations outside the range of 54–72 mg/dL (3.0–4.0 mmol/L) did worse in terms of the highly sensitive neurodevelopmental outcomes than those who had more time within this concentration range. Clearly, these first two associations are in conflict if one were to attempt to change clinical practice based on these observations. Most likely these conflicting associations show that sicker neonates are more metabolically unstable and have worse two year neurodevelopmental outcomes, not that the increased glucose concentration variability necessarily caused the worse outcomes – though this possibility cannot be excluded.

The final important association identified is that, of the hypoglycemic newborns, those with worse outcomes had a steeper rise in their glucose concentrations after treatment with dextrose. This brings up the possibility that in these at-risk asymptomatic newborns with low glucose concentrations, when one decides to commence therapy with intravenous dextrose, it is reasonable to simply start the patient on a continuous glucose infusion rate and not precede this with the traditional 200 mg/kg intravenous dextrose bolus. Previous studies have shown that within 20–30 min hypoglycemic newborns treated without the 200 mg/kg bolus dextrose and only a continuous infusion of dextrose achieve glucose concentrations similar to those treated with the dextrose bolus followed by the same continuous dextrose infusion rate [35]. Given that no study has shown that treatment of asymptomatic hypoglycemia in these patients, no matter how rapid, improves outcomes, it seems that avoiding the steeper rise in glucose concentrations which were associated with worse outcomes in the McKinlay, et al. study is warranted. Other important points to consider when evaluating this study are that severe and symptomatic hypoglycemia was rare. Similarly, hyperglycemia also was rare, as only three patients had a plasma glucose concentration greater than 144 mg/dL (8 mmol/L). It also should be emphasized again that the only patients studied were those who were asymptomatic and late preterm, LGA, SGA/IUGR, and IDM infants [34]. The conclusions, including the abandonment of the 200 mg/kg dextrose bolus, cannot necessarily be extrapolated to other groups, especially those with symptomatic

Table 1 Recommendations for the management of neonatal hypoglycemia

1. Buccal dextrose gel should be considered as part of a strategy for managing asymptomatic neonates with low glucose concentrations.

2. For asymptomatic neonates with low glucose concentrations requiring intravenous dextrose, bolus glucose infusions may be replaced by simply starting the patient on a continuous dextrose infusion.

3. Continuous glucose monitoring should be considered in research protocols to assess the benefits and risks of different glycemic patterns for outcomes.

hypoglycemia or a defined or suspected serious metabolic hypoglyyemia disorder, such as congenital hyperinsulinemic hypoglycemia or genetic conditions that lead to excessive glucose utilization (fatty acid oxidation disorders) or insufficient glucose production (hypopituitarism). Nevertheless, abandoning the dextrose bolus might be beneficial in infants of diabetic mothers and those with hyperinsulin-like conditions who respond to rapid increases in glucose concentration with excessive insulin secretion, potentially establishing a rebound hypoglycemia if the continuous dextrose infusion is not high enough.

Conclusions

Unfortunately, no recently published studies define one ideal strategy to diagnose and appropriately treat potentially damaging low glucose concentrations in neonates. In order to determine the best management strategy, a randomized trial comparing two different strategies with appropriate long term follow up is required, as proposed by Boluyt, et al. in 2006 [46]. Continued use of CGMS as a research tool to demonstrate the impact of different glycemic patterns on long term outcomes in hypoglycemia newborns will be very helpful in this type of study [34, 43]. However, short of this type of study we can look at recently published information and consider two potential changes in how neonatal hypoglycemia is managed (Table 1). One is consideration of dextrose gel as part of a treatment protocol for neonatal hypoglycemia. The second is abandonment of the 200 mg/kg intravenous dextrose bolus for the treatment of asymptomatic, hypoglycemic late preterm, LGA, SGA/IUGR, and IDM newborns.

Abbreviations
CGMS: Continuous glucose monitoring sensor; IDM: Infant of a diabetic mother; IUGR: Intrauterine growth restriction; LGA: Large for gestational age; SGA: Small for gestational age.

Competing interests
The authors declare that they have no competing interests.

Authors' contributions
PJR wrote the first draft of the manuscript. PJR and WWH conceived of the review, edited the manuscript and approved the final version.

Acknowledgements
The authors would like to thank Dr. Laura Brown for insightful discussions regarding the content of this manuscript.
The article is a review of very recent publications regarding the management of neonatal hypoglycemia. The new data focus on asymptomatic hypoglycemia in late preterm babies, IDM's, IUGR/SGA babies and LGA babies. More specifically, the use of dextrose gel in the management of these infants and the potential for worse outcomes with over aggressive correction of hypoglycemia are discussed. We have considered these new data in the context of previous publications and recommendations. We make some recommendations to clinicians regarding implementation of new strategies for the management of neonatal hypoglycemia taking into account these new data.

Declarations
Dr. Rozance has a consulting relationship with Xoma Corporation.

Funding
PJR is supported by NIH Grants R01 DK088139 (PJR PI; WWH Co-I) and WWH is supported by NIH Grants T32 HD007186 (WWH PI and PD) and NIH K12 HD068372 (WWH, PD). The content is solely the responsibility of the authors and does not necessarily represent the official views of the NIDDK or NICHD.

References
1. Boardman JP, Wusthoff CJ, Cowan FM. Hypoglycaemia and neonatal brain injury. Arch Dis Child Educ Pract Ed. 2013;98:2–6.
2. Hawdon JM. Definition of neonatal hypoglycaemia: time for a rethink? Arch Dis Child Fetal Neonatal Ed. 2013;98:F382–3.
3. Rozance PJ, Hay WW. Hypoglycemia in newborn infants: features associated with adverse outcomes. Biol Neonate. 2006;90:74–86.
4. Adamkin DH. Postnatal glucose homeostasis in late-preterm and term infants. Pediatrics. 2011;127:575–9.
5. Adamkin DH. Neonatal hypoglycemia. Curr Opin Pediatr. 2016;28:150–5.
6. Adamkin DH, Polin R. Neonatal hypoglycemia: is 60 the new 40? The questions remain the same. J Perinatol. 2016;36:10–2.
7. Stanley CA, Rozance PJ, Thornton PS, De Leon DD, Harris D, Haymond MW, Hussain K, Levitsky LL, Murad MH, Simmons RA, Sperling MA, Weinstein DA, White NH, Wolfsdorf JI. Re-evaluating "transitional neonatal hypoglycemia": mechanism and implications for management. J Pediatr. 2015;166:1520–5.
8. Thornton PS, Stanley CA, De Leon DD, Harris D, Haymond MW, Hussain K, Levitsky LL, Murad MH, Rozance PJ, Simmons RA, Sperling MA, Weinstein DA, White NH, Wolfsdorf JI. Recommendations from the Pediatric Endocrine Society for Evaluation and Management of persistent hypoglycemia in neonates, infants, and children. J Pediatr. 2015;167:238–45.
9. Hay Jr WW, Raju TN, Higgins RD, Kalhan SC, Devaskar SU. Knowledge gaps and research needs for understanding and treating neonatal hypoglycemia: workshop report from Eunice Kennedy Shriver National Institute of Child Health and Human Development. J Pediatr. 2009;155:612–7.
10. Arcangeli T, Thilaganathan B, Hooper R, Khan KS, Bhide A. Neurodevelopmental delay in small babies at term: a systematic review. Ultrasound Obstet Gynecol. 2012;40:267–75.
11. Brand PL, Molenaar NL, Kaaijk C, Wierenga WS. Neurodevelopmental outcome of hypoglycaemia in healthy, large for gestational age, term newborns. Arch Dis Child. 2005;90:78–81.
12. Stenninger E, Flink R, Eriksson B, Sahlen C. Long-term neurological dysfunction and neonatal hypoglycaemia after diabetic pregnancy. Arch Dis Child Fetal Neonatal Ed. 1998;79:F174–9.
13. von Beckerath AK, Kollmann M, Rotky-Fast C, Karpf E, Lang U, Klaritsch P. Perinatal complications and long-term neurodevelopmental outcome of infants with intrauterine growth restriction. Am J Obstet Gynecol. 2013;208:130–6.
14. American Academy of Pediatrics Committee on Fetus and Newborn. Routine evaluation of blood pressure, hematocrit, and glucose in newborns. Pediatrics. 1993;92:474–6.
15. Barry JS, Rozance PJ, Brown LD, Anthony RV, Thornburg KL, Hay WW Jr. Increased fetal myocardial sensitivity to insulin-stimulated glucose metabolism during ovine fetal growth restriction. Exp Biol Med (Maywood). 2016. [Epub ahead of print].

16. Leos RA, Anderson MJ, Chen X, Pugmire J, Anderson KA, Limesand SW. Chronic exposure to elevated norepinephrine suppresses insulin secretion in fetal sheep with placental insufficiency and intrauterine growth restriction. Am J Physiol Endocrinol Metab. 2010;298:E770–8.

17. Limesand SW, Rozance PJ, Zerbe GO, Hutton JC, Hay Jr WW. Attenuated insulin release and storage in fetal sheep pancreatic islets with intrauterine growth restriction. Endocrinology. 2006;147:1488–97.

18. Limesand SW, Rozance PJ, Smith D, Hay Jr WW. Increased insulin sensitivity and maintenance of glucose utilization rates in fetal sheep with placental insufficiency and intrauterine growth restriction. Am J Physiol Endocrinol Metab. 2007;293:E1716–25.

19. Macko AR, Yates DT, Chen X, Green AS, Kelly AC, Brown LD, Limesand SW. Elevated plasma norepinephrine inhibits insulin secretion, but adrenergic blockade reveals enhanced beta-cell responsiveness in an ovine model of placental insufficiency at 0.7 of gestation. J Dev Orig Health Dis. 2013;4:402–10.

20. Thorn SR, Brown LD, Rozance PJ, Hay Jr WW, Friedman JE. Increased hepatic glucose production in fetal sheep with intrauterine growth restriction is not suppressed by insulin. Diabetes. 2013;62:65–73.

21. Brown LD, Rozance PJ, Thorn SR, Friedman JE, Hay Jr WW. Acute supplementation of amino acids increases net protein accretion in IUGR fetal sheep. Am J Physiol Endocrinol Metab. 2012;303:E352–64.

22. Brown LD. Endocrine regulation of fetal skeletal muscle growth: impact on future metabolic health. J Endocrinol. 2014;221:R13–29.

23. Brown LD, Rozance PJ, Bruce JL, Friedman JE, Hay Jr WW, Wesolowski SR. Limited capacity for glucose oxidation in fetal sheep with intrauterine growth restriction. Am J Physiol Regul Integr Comp Physiol. 2015;309:R920–8.

24. Limesand SW, Jensen J, Hutton JC, Hay Jr WW. Diminished beta-cell replication contributes to reduced beta-cell mass in fetal sheep with intrauterine growth restriction. Am J Physiol Regul Integr Comp Physiol. 2005;288:R1297–305.

25. Limesand SW, Rozance PJ, Macko AR, Anderson MJ, Kelly AC, Hay Jr WW. Reductions in insulin concentrations and beta-cell mass precede growth restriction in sheep fetuses with placental insufficiency. Am J Physiol Endocrinol Metab. 2013;304:E516–23.

26. Rozance PJ, Hay WW Jr. Pancreatic islet hepatocyte growth factor and vascular endothelial growth factor A signaling in growth restricted fetuses. Mol Cell Endocrinol. 2016. [Epub ahead of print].

27. Thorn SR, Regnault TRH, Brown LD, Rozance PJ, Keng J, Roper M, Wilkening RB, Hay WW, Jr., Friedman JE. Intrauterine growth restriction increases fetal hepatic gluconeogenic capacity and reduces messenger ribonucleic acid translation initiation and nutrient sensing in fetal liver and skeletal muscle. Endocrinology. 2009;150:3021–30.

28. Wesolowski SR, Hay WW Jr. Role of placental insufficiency and intrauterine growth restriction on the activation of fetal hepatic glucose production. Mol Cell Endocrinol. 2015. [Epub ahead of print].

29. Yates DT, Green AS, Limesand SW. Catecholamines mediate multiple fetal adaptations during placental insufficiency that contribute to intrauterine growth restriction: lessons from hyperthermic sheep. J Pregnancy. 2011;2011:740408.

30. Yates DT, Clarke DS, Macko AR, Anderson MJ, Shelton LA, Nearing M, Allen RE, Rhoads RP, Limesand SW. Myoblasts from intrauterine growth-restricted sheep fetuses exhibit intrinsic deficiencies in proliferation that contribute to smaller semitendinosus myofibres. J Physiol. 2014;592:3113–25.

31. Whipple AO, Frantz VK. Adenoma of islet cells with hyperinsulinism: a review. Ann Surg. 1935;101:1299–335.

32. Harris DL, Weston PJ, Signal M, Chase JG, Harding JE. Dextrose gel for neonatal hypoglycaemia (the Sugar Babies Study): a randomised, double-blind, placebo-controlled trial. Lancet. 2013;382:2077–83.

33. Alexandrou G, Skiold B, Karlen J, Tessma MK, Norman M, Aden U, Vanpee M. Early hyperglycemia is a risk factor for death and white matter reduction in preterm infants. Pediatrics. 2010;125:e584–91.

34. McKinlay CJ, Alsweiler JM, Ansell JM, Anstice NS, Chase JG, Gamble GD, Harris DL, Jacobs RJ, Jiang Y, Paudel N, Signal M, Thompson B, Wouldes TA, Yu TY, Harding JE. Neonatal glycemia and neurodevelopmental outcomes at 2 years. N Engl J Med. 2015;373:1507–18.

35. Lilien LD, Pildes RS, Srinivasan G, Voora S, Yeh TF. Treatment of neonatal hypoglycemia with minibolus and intraveous glucose infusion. J Pediatr. 1980;97:295–8.

36. Harris DL, Alsweiler JM, Ansell JM, Gamble GD, Thompson B, Wouldes TA, Yu TY, Harding JE. Outcome at 2 years after dextrose gel treatment for neonatal hypoglycemia: follow-up of a randomized trial. J Pediatr. 2016;170:54–9.

37. Srinivasan G, Pildes RS, Cattamanchi G, Voora S, Lilien LD. Plasma glucose values in normal neonates: a new look. J Pediatr. 1986;109:114–7.

38. Woo HC, Tolosa L, El-Metwally D, Viscardi RM. Glucose monitoring in neonates: need for accurate and non-invasive methods. Arch Dis Child Fetal Neonatal Ed. 2014;99:F153–7.

39. Bennett C, Fagan E, Chaharbakhshi E, Zamfirova I, Flicker J. Implementing a protocol using glucose Gel to treat neonatal hypoglycemia. Nurs Womens Health. 2016;20:64–74.

40. Stewart CE, Sage EL, Reynolds P. Supporting 'Baby Friendly': a quality improvement initiative for the management of transitional neonatal hypoglycaemia. Arch Dis Child Fetal Neonatal Ed. 2015. [Epub ahead of print].

41. Beardsall K, Vanhaesebrouck S, Ogilvy-Stuart AL, Vanhole C, Palmer CR, van Weissenbruch M, Midgley P, Thompson M, Thio M, Cornette L, Ossuetta I, Iglesias I, Theyskens C, de Jong M, Ahluwalia JS, de Zegher F, Dunger DB. Early insulin therapy in very-low-birth-weight infants. N Engl J Med. 2008; 359:1873–84.

42. Harris DL, Battin MR, Weston PJ, Harding JE. Continuous glucose monitoring in newborn babies at risk of hypoglycemia. J Pediatr. 2010;157:198–202.

43. Hay Jr WW, Rozance PJ. Continuous glucose monitoring for diagnosis and treatment of neonatal hypoglycemia. J Pediatr. 2010;157:180–2.

44. Harris DL, Weston PJ, Harding JE. Incidence of neonatal hypoglycemia in babies identified as at risk. J Pediatr. 2012;161:787–91.

45. Rozance PJ, Hay Jr WW. Neonatal hypoglycemia–answers, but more questions. J Pediatr. 2012;161:775–6.

46. Boluyt N, van Kempen A, Offringa M. Neurodevelopment after neonatal hypoglycemia: a systematic review and design of an optimal future study. Pediatrics. 2006;117:2231–43.

Optimizing maternal and neonatal outcomes with postpartum contraception: impact on breastfeeding and birth spacing

Aparna Sridhar[1*] and Jennifer Salcedo[2]

Abstract

Postpartum contraception is important to prevent unintended pregnancies. Assisting women in achieving recommended inter-pregnancy intervals is a significant maternal-child health concern. Short inter-pregnancy intervals are associated with negative perinatal, neonatal, infant, and maternal health outcomes. More than 30% of women experience inter-pregnancy intervals of less than 18 months in the United States. Provision of any contraceptive method after giving birth is associated with improved inter-pregnancy intervals. However, concerns about the impact of hormonal contraceptives on breastfeeding and infant health have limited recommendations for such methods and have led to discrepant recommendations by organizations such as the World Health Organization and the U.S. Centers for Disease Control and Prevention. In this review, we discuss current recommendations for the use of hormonal contraception in the postpartum period. We also discuss details of the lactational amenorrhea method and effects of hormonal contraception on breastfeeding. Given the paucity of high quality evidence on the impact on hormonal contraception on breastfeeding outcomes, and the strong evidence for improved health outcomes with achievement of recommended birth spacing intervals, the real risk of unintended pregnancy and its consequences must not be neglected for fear of theoretical neonatal risks. Women should establish desired hormonal contraception before the risk of pregnancy resumes. With optimization of postpartum contraception provision, we will step closer toward a healthcare system with fewer unintended pregnancies and improved birth outcomes.

Keywords: Breastfeeding, Contraception, Inter-pregnancy interval, Lactation, Postpartum

Background

Postpartum contraception is important to prevent unintended pregnancies and short intervals between pregnancies. The appropriate method and timing of contraception initiation following a birth, miscarriage or pregnancy termination depends on multiple factors such as a patient's personal preferences, medical history, risk for pregnancy, breastfeeding preferences, and access to contraceptive services. The most important role of postpartum contraception is to help a woman achieve the desired interval before the next pregnancy in order to optimize her health and that of her young children. Theoretical concerns regarding the impact of contraception on breastfeeding must be appropriately weighed against well-supported impacts on inter-pregnancy intervals and the woman's informed decisions regarding her reproductive health.

Inter-pregnancy interval and perinatal outcomes

Assisting women in achieving recommended inter-pregnancy intervals (IPIs), defined as the time interval between a live birth and the beginning of the next pregnancy, is a significant maternal-child health concern. Short IPIs are associated with negative perinatal, neonatal, infant, and maternal health outcomes. The concept of an ideal inter-pregnancy interval emerged from a report published by World Health Organization (WHO) in 2005. Based on the best available evidence at that time, the experts reached a consensus of 24 months as the IPI. This interval was consistent with the joint WHO

* Correspondence: asridhar@mednet.ucla.edu
[1]Department of Obstetrics and Gynecology, David Geffen School of Medicine at University of California Los Angeles, California, USA
Full list of author information is available at the end of the article

and United Nations Children's Emergency Fund (UNICEF) recommendation that women breastfeed for at least 2 years [1].

Recommendations from the WHO report, "Effect of Interpregnancy Interval on Adverse Perinatal Outcomes," were evaluated using the Perinatal Information System Database of the Latin American Center for Perinatology and Human Development from 1985 to 2004. Compared to infants with IPIs of 18–23 months, those born to women with intervals shorter than 6 months had an increased risk of many adverse neonatal and perinatal outcomes [2]. A systematic review by Conde-Agudelo et al. that included 77 studies conducted in countries across six continents analyzed the association of IPIs with outcomes such as preterm birth, low birth weight, small size for gestational age (SGA) at birth, fetal death, and early neonatal death. For IPIs shorter than 6 months, there were significantly increased risks for preterm birth (Odds Ratio = 1.40), SGA (Odds Ratio =1.26), and low birth weight (Odds Ratio = 1.61). Intervals of 6 to 17 months were also associated with a significantly greater risk for these three adverse perinatal outcomes. Additionally, among women with previous low-transverse caesarean sections who underwent trials of labor, there was noted to be increased risk of uterine rupture with IPIs less than 16 months [3]. Another recent study analyzing all live births between 1991 and 2010 in California concluded that women with IPIs of less than 1 year following live birth were at increased risk for preterm birth [4]. No conclusions on the impact of IPI on maternal mortality and morbidity were able to be drawn in the WHO's report due to limited available data [1].

Unfortunately, data from the 2015 National Vital Statistics Report and the National Survey of Family Growth demonstrate that in the United States 30% of women experience IPIs of less than 18 months. Short IPIs in the U.S. are inversely associated with maternal age, with more than two thirds (67%) of teenagers between ages 15–19 experiencing IPIs of less than 18 months [5].

Postpartum endocrine changes
To understand the timing and mechanisms by which women resume risk of pregnancy following delivery, it is important to review the cascade of endocrine changes that take place after parturition. Immediately following delivery, the inhibitory effect of the estrogen and progesterone levels of pregnancy decreases and the pulsatile activity of the pituitary follicular stimulating hormone (FSH) and luteinizing hormone (LH) resumes [6]. In non-lactating women, studies evaluating urinary pregnanediol levels have reported a mean first ovulation ranging from 45 to 94 days postpartum, with the earliest ovulation reported 25 days after delivery [7, 8]. Consequently, women are assumed to be protected from pregnancy for 4 weeks following delivery. Similarly, studies

looking at ovulation after abortion suggest that most women ovulate before resuming menses, with mean time to ovulation of 22 days [9]. Lactation extends the period of postpartum infertility. Nerve impulses arising from the nipple and areola due to infant suckling release prolactin from the hypothalamus. This, in turn, suppresses the pulsatile release of gonadotropin-releasing hormone (GnRH) by the hypothalamus, likely by increasing beta-endorphin production. The pulsatile secretion of GnRH is necessary to stimulate the cells in anterior pituitary to produce FSH and LH needed for ovulation. Thus continued suckling and lactation provide protection from pregnancy [10].

Lactational amenorrhea method
The lactational amenorrhea method (LAM) is the specific name given to use of breastfeeding as a dedicated method of contraception. For breastfeeding to serve as an effective method of contraception, the woman must be exclusively or nearly exclusively breastfeeding (at least 85% of infant feeding coming from breastfeeding), be within the first 6 months following delivery, and remain amenorrheic. Some experts additionally believe that milk expression by hand or pump does not retain the same fertility-inhibiting effect as infant nursing [11]. Clinical studies of the contraceptive effect of LAM have demonstrated cumulative 6-month life-table perfect-use pregnancy rates of 0.5 – 1.5% among women who relied solely on LAM. A Cochrane review published in 2015 estimated the typical use failure rate of LAM to be 0.45 – 7.5% [12–15].

Although LAM is a highly effective temporary method of contraception, rates of the exclusive breastfeeding required for its effectiveness are low in the United States. Data from the National Immunization Survey describes an 80% incidence of breastfeeding initiation, declining to a 4 weeks postpartum exclusive breastfeeding rate of 54%, which declines to 20% at 6 months [16]. According to this data, exclusive breastfeeding rates at 3 months were lower in non-white, unmarried women with lower socio-economic status compared to non-Hispanic white, well educated, married women [16]. Among the individual states, Montana had the highest (60%) and Mississippi the lowest (21%) exclusive breastfeeding rates at 3 months in 2013 [17].

Historically, women have also been assumed to experience protection from pregnancy during the traditionally recommended 6-week period of pelvic rest following delivery. While 6-weeks may have been historically recommended to accommodate the expected time period of uterine involution, and due to its concurrent timing with the historically recommended 6-week postpartum visit, no evidence supports any specific interval of post-delivery abstinence. McDonald et al. [18] analyzed a prospective cohort of approximately 1500 nulliparous women to investigate the timing of resumption of vaginal sex after childbirth and noted that 41% of women admitted to resuming intercourse by 6 weeks, while 65 and 78% endorsed vaginal sex by 8 and 12 weeks postpartum, respectively. Spontaneous vaginal birth with an episiotomy or laceration, forceps- or vacuum-assisted vaginal birth, cesarean section, and breastfeeding are negatively associated with resumption of intercourse following delivery, while young age (<25 years) and living with a partner are associated with earlier resumption of intercourse [18].

Contraception provision postpartum

Given that women resume risk for pregnancy from 4 weeks to 6 months postpartum, effective contraceptive methods must be available to assist women in reaching recommended IPIs. Figure 1 demonstrates currently available contraceptive methods in the U.S. and their associated effectiveness in typical use. Provision of any contraceptive method within 90 days of giving birth is associated with improved IPIs [19]. However, use of long-acting reversible contraception methods (LARC) such as intrauterine devices (IUDs) and the subcutaneous contraceptive implant, both with effectiveness that is generally not reduced by user error, have been shown to substantially improve IPIs compared to other methods. More specifically, women using LARC methods after delivery have 3.89 times the likelihood of reaching recommended birth spacing intervals compared to women using condoms only, while women using user-dependent hormonal methods (pill, patch, vaginal ring and injection) have 1.89 times the likelihood of achieving recommended spacing compared to barrier method users [19, 20].

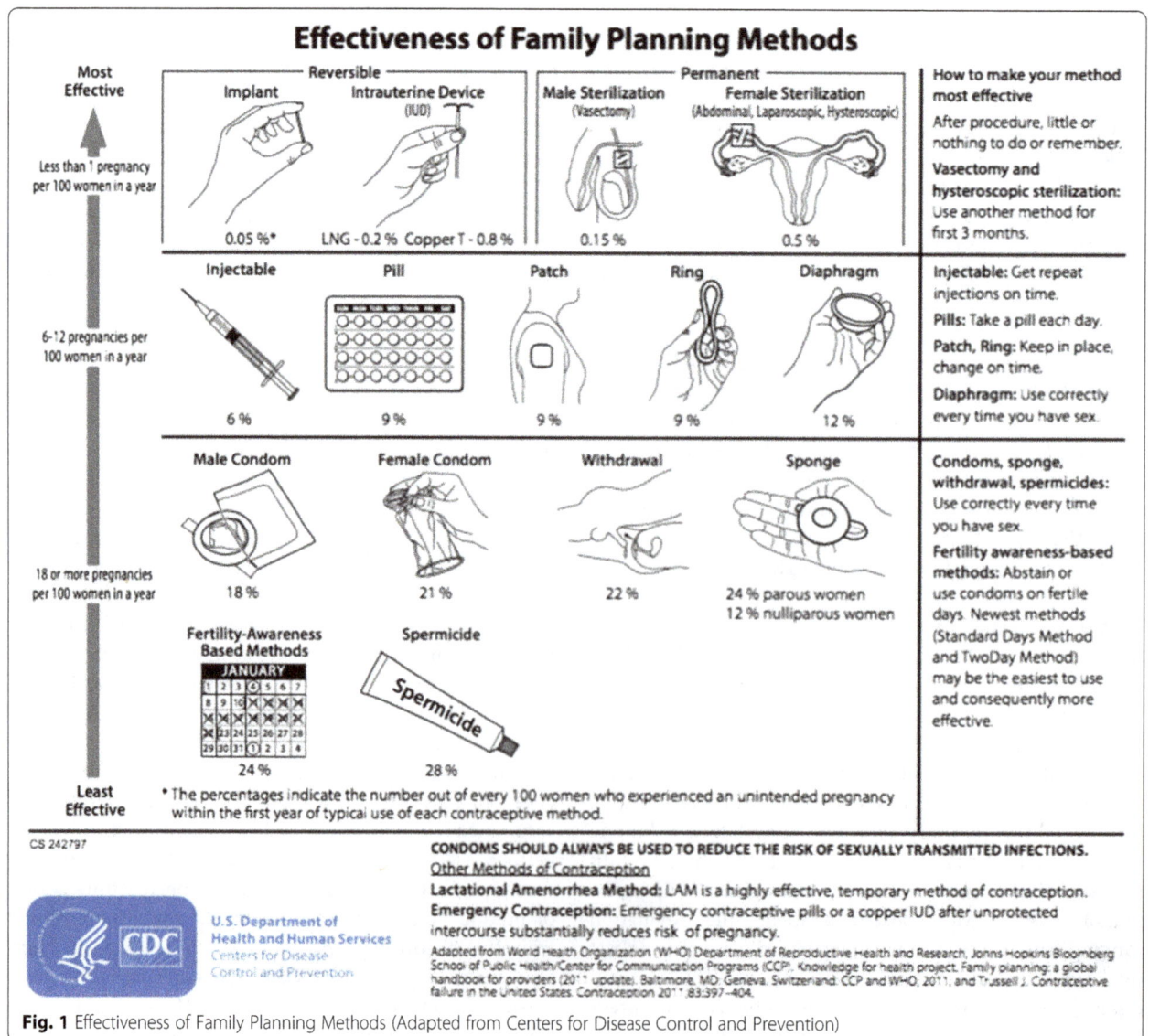

Fig. 1 Effectiveness of Family Planning Methods (Adapted from Centers for Disease Control and Prevention)

Recommendations by the World Health Organization and Centers for Disease Control and Prevention

Despite evidence that early initiation of postpartum contraception increases IPIs, concerns about the impact of hormonal contraceptives on breastfeeding and infant health have limited recommendations for such methods and have lead to discrepant recommendations by organizations such as the World Health Organization (WHO) and the U.S. Centers for Disease Control and Prevention (CDC). While both the WHO and CDC generally agree that the initiation of estrogen-containing methods should be delayed for 3–6 weeks postpartum (depending on a woman's medical risk factors) until the risk of venous thromboembolism (VTE) decreases to approximately the non-pregnant baseline, the WHO has issued more conservative recommendations than the CDC regarding use of both estrogen-containing and progestin-only methods by breastfeeding women [21, 22].

In the WHO Medical Eligibility Criteria for Contraceptive Use (MEC), Fifth Edition [23] estrogen-containing contraceptives (including combined oral contraceptives, the patch, and the vaginal ring) are considered to pose unacceptable health risks (Category 4) when used by breastfeeding women within the first 6 postpartum weeks. These methods are considered by the WHO to have theoretical or proven risks that usually outweigh their advantages (Category 3) until breastfeeding women are at least 6 months postpartum. In contrast, in the U.S. Centers for Disease Control and Prevention Medical Eligibility Criteria for Contraceptive Use (CDC MEC), the advantages of using such estrogen-containing methods

are stated to generally outweigh the theoretical or proven risks (Category 2) for women without complicating medical conditions starting 6 weeks after delivery [21] (Table 1).

In the following sections we provide a detailed review of the impact of each hormonal contraceptive method on breastfeeding outcomes.

a) Combined oral contraceptives

A CDC review of combined oral contraceptives from 2015 included 15 articles from 13 studies evaluating the impact of estrogen-containing oral contraceptive pills on breastfeeding and associated infant outcomes. Unfortunately, applicable studies were noted to be of only poor to fair methodological quality and many were from earlier decades when the estrogen-content of combined oral contraceptives was substantially higher than in modern pills [24]. In this review, no studies found significant impact on infant weight gain when combined oral contraceptives (COCs) were initiated at 6 weeks or later postpartum, and none found negative impact on other infant health outcomes regardless of the timing of COC initiation [24]. However, the results of studies examining the impact of COCs on breastfeeding performance were inconsistent [24]. A study by the WHO in 1984 assigned women to a COC containing 30 micrograms of ethinyl estradiol and 150 micrograms of levonorgestrel or a progestin-only pill containing 75 micrograms of norgestrel, started after 6 weeks postpartum. Breast milk volume was quantified following pump expression. Mean breast milk volume was lower in the COC group at 9, 16

Table 1 Medical Eligibility Criteria [CDC/WHO]

Method	<10 min	<48 h	<21 days	21 to <30 days	30-42 days	42 days-6 months	>6 months
Breastfeeding Women	Category [CDC/WHO]						
Combined hormonal contraceptives	4/4	4/4	4/4	3/4	2[a]/4	2/3[c]	2/2
Progestin-only pills	2/2	2/2	2/2	2/2	1/2	1/1	1/1
DMPA	2/3	2/3	2/3	2/3	1/3	1/1	1/1
Etonogestrel implant	2/2	2/2	2/2	2/2	1/2	1/1	1/1
Levonorgestrel intrauterine device	2/2	2/2	2/3	2[b]/3[b]	1[b]/1[b]	1/1	1/1
Copper intrauterine device	1/1	2/1	2/3	2[b]/3[b]	1[b]/1[b]	1/1	1/1
Nonbreastfeeding Women	Category [CDC/WHO]						
Combined hormonal contraceptives	4/3[d]	4/3[d]	4/3[d]	2[a]/2[a]	2[a]/2[a]	1/1	1/1
Progestin-only pills	1/1	1/1	1/1	1/1	1/1	1/1	1/1
DMPA	1/1	1/1	1/1	1/1	1/1	1/1	1/1
Etonogestrel implant	1/1	1/1	1/1	1/1	1/1	1/1	1/1
Levonorgestrel intrauterine device	1/1	2/1	2/3	2[b]/3[b]	1[b]/1[b]	1/1	1/1
Copper intrauterine device	1/1	2/1	2/3	2[b]/3[b]	1[b]/1[b]	1/1	1/1

[a] CDC & WHO Category 3 for women with other risk factors for VTE: 35 years old or older, previous VTE, thrombophilia, immobility, peripartum transfusion, peripartum cardiomyopathy, obesity, peripartum hemorrhage, cesarean delivery, preeclampsia, or smoking
[b] Refers to 28 days for intrauterine device insertion timing
[c] Refers to women who are primarily breastfeeding
[d] WHO Category 4 for women with other risk factors for VTE

and 24 weeks by 18–25 mL. However, no differences were noted between groups on use of supplemental infant nutrition [25]. In 2012, Espey et al. performed a randomized controlled trial of breastfeeding women following term delivery who desired to initiate oral contraception. At two weeks postpartum women initiated either a combined pill of 35 mcg ethinyl estradiol and 1 mg norethindrone ($n = 64$) or a progestin-only pill (POP) containing 35 micrograms of norethindrone ($n = 63$) [26]. There was no significant difference between the COC and POP groups in the primary outcome of breastfeeding continuation over the 6 months of follow-up, nor were there differences found in infant growth parameters, satisfaction with breastfeeding or oral contraceptive use, perception of milk supply adequacy, formula supplementation, or reasons cited for discontinuing breastfeeding or oral contraceptive pills [26]. Given that in non-breastfeeding women without contraindications to estrogen, combined oral contraceptives have been found to have better efficacy, higher continuation rates, and fewer side effects than POPs, and that 35 micrograms is the highest estrogen content in commonly used COCs, the authors conclude that it is reassuring that combined pills do not have a major impact on breastfeeding continuation or infant growth and a larger equivalency study should be performed to clarify the clinical impact of COCs on lactation [26]. No randomized controlled trials are available that evaluate the other estrogen-containing contraceptives available in the U.S., the contraceptive patch and vaginal ring, which have different hormonal content and absorption profiles than combined oral contraceptive pills [25].

b) Progestin only contraceptives

In contrast to estrogen-containing contraceptives, the WHO considers the benefits of progestin-only oral contraceptives and the progestin-containing contraceptive implant to generally outweigh risks of these methods during the first 6 postpartum weeks for breastfeeding women (Category 2), but recommends that the contraceptive injection (depot medroxyprogesterone acetate [DMPA] in the U.S.) be initiated no sooner than 6 weeks postpartum [23]. In contrast, the CDC considers the benefits of all progestin-only systemic methods to outweigh potential risks during the first 30 days postpartum for breastfeeding women (Category 2), and states that all such methods may be used without restriction (Category 1) 30 days following delivery [21].

While the WHO acknowledges that available evidence does not support a negative effect of progestin-only contraceptives on breastfeeding performance, and has generally demonstrated no negative impacts on infant growth or development, concern over lack of evidence on potential longer-term pediatric impacts have led to conservative recommendations for hormonal contraceptive use, particularly for contraceptive injections during the early postpartum period [23]. Animal data has suggested some effect of progesterone on the developing brain, but whether such effects are present in humans, and of what potential consequences, are unclear [23, 27]. Although limited comparative studies have not noted a difference in breastfeeding or infant outcomes with exposure to progestin-injections compared to other progestin-only methods, the higher maternal systemic hormone levels attained with progestin-injections (compared to other systemic progestin-only methods) have led the WHO Guideline Development Group to be concerned about infant hormone exposure during use of these methods, particularly in the first 6 weeks [23]. Additionally, given the paucity of high quality evidence in this area, WHO and CDC expert opinion may understandably differ based on issues such as the difference in exclusive breastfeeding rates between U.S. women and those in less developed parts of the world and the availability of safe alternatives to breast milk for infant and early childhood nutrition.

While the steroids progesterone and nestorone are orally inactive, progestin-containing contraceptives currently used in the United States contain orally active progestins [28]. The amount of progestin transferred to an infant through breast milk by hormonal contraceptive users is variable. For contraceptive implant users, the mean concentration of etonogestrel in breast milk ranges from 405 to 548 pmol/L, approximately one-half the maternal plasma concentration, which results in transferring of approximately 75–120 nanograms of hormone per day to the fully breastfed infant [28, 29]. This daily progestin dose is similar to the range estimated for progestin-only pills, which is approximately twice that of levonorgestrel-releasing IUDs. It is significantly lower than that received by infants whose mothers use progestin injectables, which is in the range of 1–13 micrograms, approximately 88% of the serum concentration [28, 30–32].

The issue of infant exposure to exogenous hormones is further complicated by the fact that newborns are initially unable to either absorb or metabolize exogenous hormones, followed by an ability to metabolize more effectively than absorb, then an ability to do both successfully by about 24 weeks of gestation [33]. For women using levonorgestrel-releasing IUDs, compared to non-hormonal IUDs, no differences were noted in infants' serum electrolytes, protein, creatinine, iron, cholesterol, or liver enzyme levels [31]. Similarly, no differences in the biochemical markers of FSH, LH, testosterone, or immunoglobin differences were noted between male infants of progestin-only pill users or users of a progestin-implant compared to non-hormonal contraceptive users [34, 35].

An updated review on progestin-only contraceptives and breastfeeding by Phillips et al. in 2015 noted that 11 non-randomized trials and observational studies found either no effect or a positive effect on breastfeeding outcomes with use of progestin-injectables initiated within the first 6 weeks postpartum [36] Similarly, eight observational studies on progestin-only pills and breastfeeding found either no differences or improved breastfeeding outcomes when pills were initiated within 6 weeks postpartum [36]. A randomized controlled trial noted no difference in infant weight gain at 14 days compared to infants not exposed to hormonal contraception [37, 38]. Similarly, in studies examining infant growth effects when progestin-only methods are initiated after 6 weeks postpartum, most have noted no differences, although small differences in both directions have been found [39].

In a study by Reinprayoon et al., women who initiated an etonogestrel implant while fully breastfeeding were found to have similar breast milk volume, composition, rates of initiation and timing of supplemental feedings, and infant growth characteristics as women who initiated a non-hormonal IUD [29]. Similarly, for women using a levonorgestrel-releasing IUD, compared to women using non-hormonal IUDs, mean duration of breastfeeding was found to be similar, although slightly fewer women were still breastfeeding at 75 days in the levonorgestrel group. No differences were noted in the growth, health, or developmental milestones measured [32].

In addition to infant hormone exposure during the first 6 weeks postpartum, some experts have expressed concern that immediate postpartum initiation of hormonal contraceptives prior to the natural postpartum decline of progesterone may have greater impact on breastfeeding performance than methods initiated even in the early weeks postpartum. Most recently, a randomized trial by Chen et al. comparing postplacental to delayed levonorgestrel IUD insertion at 6–8 weeks noted that women in the delayed group were more likely to still be breastfeeding at 6 months postpartum, although no differences in breastfeeding initiation or continuation at 6–8 weeks or at 3 months was seen [40]. This difference persisted when women who never breastfed were excluded and when only primiparous women without previous breastfeeding experience were considered [40]. A biologic etiology for this difference only seen at 6 months is difficult to ascertain given the low systemic levels of levonorgestrel found in levonorgestrel-IUD users and the fact that any impact of exogenous hormones on breastfeeding would seem most plausible at or surrounding breastfeeding initiation.

Such a negative impact of immediate hormonal LARC placement on breastfeeding outcomes has not been found in studies evaluating the etonogestrel contraceptive implant [41, 42]. For instance, a study comparing initiation of the contraceptive implant within 3 days postpartum, compared to 4–8 weeks postpartum, found no significant difference between full or any breastfeeding at any time point, breast milk creamatocrit, or a clinically significant difference in time to lactogenesis [42]. Another study that used deuterium (an isotope of hydrogen that is used as a tracer) to compare milk intake between infants whose mothers had a Nexplanon placed within 48 h of delivery to those using no contraceptive method found no difference in milk intake at any time within 6 weeks and no difference in newborn weight between groups during the follow-up period [43].

Data on the impact of DMPA administration before postpartum discharge is mixed but generally reassuring. While a study of Peruvian women noted that women who initiated DMPA more than 72 h postpartum were more likely than both women who initiated DMPA within 72 h postpartum and those who didn't initiate DMPA postpartum to be exclusively breastfeeding at 3 months, DMPA use overall was associated with higher exclusive breastfeeding rates at 3 months compared with non-use [44]. The authors of this study postulated that increased contact with healthcare providers by women who initiated DMPA more than 72 h following delivery may have provided additional opportunities for breastfeeding support [44]. In contrast, a prospective non-randomized trial comparing progestin-only contraceptive administration before postpartum discharge with non-hormonal methods found that women who initiated DMPA before postpartum discharge saw no difference in breastfeeding continuation rates at 2 weeks or 6 weeks, and no difference in discontinuation due to perceived inadequate milk supply, despite the fact that women in the DMPA group were less likely to breastfeed based on their younger age and lower gravidity and parity [45]. Study authors concluded that women who choose hormonal methods are likely to be different in breastfeeding likelihood than women who initiate non-hormonal methods or no method [45]. Similarly, a retrospective cohort study by Brownell et al. found no significant difference in breastfeeding cessation within 2 or 6 weeks postpartum between women who initiated DMPA before postpartum discharge (a mean of 37 h following delivery) and women who did not initiate DMPA, but did note that the DMPA group was significantly less likely to have a timed breastfeeding goal (such as planning to breastfeed until a particular infant age or developmental milestone) and to report social support for breastfeeding. These findings support the idea that women who choose to initiate hormonal contraception before postpartum discharge may be different in important ways from women who make other postpartum contraceptive choices [46]. The American College of Obstetricians & Gynecologists (ACOG) recognizes that clinical judgment must weigh the need for contraception against the theoretical neonatal risks and endorses early initiation of DMPA postpartum in indicated clinical situations, such as a high risk of being lost to postpartum follow-up [47].

c) Emergency contraceptive pills

In addition to routine contraception, emergency contraception is a promising component of a comprehensive contraceptive strategy to reach recommended birth spacing intervals. Emergency contraceptive pills (ECPs) are pills taken as soon as possible, and within 120 h, after unprotected or inadequately protected intercourse in order to reduce the risk of pregnancy when a routine contraceptive method was not used or was not used correctly. Two types of dedicated ECP products are available in the U.S. They are progestin-only ECPs comprised of 1.5 mg levonorgestrel, and 30 mg of uliprital acetate, which is a progestin-receptor modulator. Both medications work by delaying or preventing ovulation and neither has evidence for post-fertilization effects [48]. Uliprital acetate has been found to be more efficacious overall, and specifically for overweight and obese women and women who require ECPs for intercourse occurring close to ovulation [49, 50]. In both the WHO and CDC MEC, levonorgestrel ECPs are classified as Category 1 for all users [21, 23]. However, the WHO MEC classifies use of uliprital acetate by breastfeeding women as Category 2 and recommends that women avoid breastfeeding for 1 week following use, discarding breast milk during that time, based on the package labeling for UPA which states that, "Use of ella® by breastfeeding women is not recommended," since it is "unknown if uliprital acetate is excreted in human milk [23, 51]." In contrast, the CDC MEC classifies uliprital acetate use by breastfeeding women as Category 1, but recommends that breast milk be expressed and discarded for 24 h following use. Since there are no studies evaluating the impact of uliprital acetate exposure on infants [52], the recommendation to discard breast milk for 24 h is based on rapidly declining levels of uliprital acetate and its metabolite measured in breast milk during this time period.

Professional organizations such as the ACOG and the American Academy of Pediatrics (AAP) recommend advance prescription of emergency contraceptive pills to all reproductive aged women [53, 54]. In a randomized trial of breastfeeding Egyptian women who planned to use LAM and delay a next conception by at least 1 year, women in the standard LAM counseling group were significantly more likely than women in the levonorgestrel ECP advanced provision group to experience pregnancy within 6 months postpartum (of which 80% were unplanned and/or undesired), despite similar rates of unprotected intercourse after expiration of LAM criteria in both groups [55]. Unfortunately, knowledge of emergency contraception by postpartum women is low. In a study of inner city postpartum women, only 36% had heard of emergency contraception, only 19% could name or describe a method of emergency contraception, and only 7% could identify correct timing of ECP use [56]. Of those who were aware of emergency contraception, only 44% thought it was safe, despite CDC MEC Category 1–2 classification, and 32% incorrectly believed that it served as an abortifacient [56]. However, two-thirds of women in the study stated that they would be willing to use emergency contraception in the future [56].

System based barriers for postpartum contraception use

Despite the effectiveness of currently available contraception, U.S. women seeking to establish postpartum contraception currently face a myriad of systems barriers. Of women who indicate a plan for postpartum IUD placement, only 23–60% undergo insertion as planned [57, 58]. Women are often denied inpatient LARC placement due to the fact that reimbursement for all delivery-related care is generally based on a global fee that does not carve out the cost of LARC devices or insertions [59, 60]. This reimbursement scheme severely disincentivizes hospitals to supply and dispense LARC devices, which typically have wholesale costs upwards of $600 [59]. While Medicaid and most private insurance plans have been able to separate out reimbursement for sterilization during a delivery-related hospitalization, currently only a small minority of states have been able to address the issue for LARC devices, and primarily only for Medicaid-covered patients [59, 60]. Interestingly, this slow systems-based change takes place in a setting in which substantial cost-savings to public programs facilitating inpatient LARC placement has been demonstrated [60]. Further barriers are encountered by women who receive delivery-related care in Catholic hospitals, which currently represent one-sixth of all hospital beds in the U.S., as these facilities do not permit placement of LARC devices for the purpose of contraception [59].

Additionally, postpartum women often receive inconsistent, and sometimes incorrect, information from various members of the healthcare team regarding the safety and impact of contraception on breastfeeding. For instance, in a recent survey by Dunn et al., while 77% of lactation consultants reported offering advice about postpartum contraception and its impact on breastfeeding, the vast majority stated that progestin-only methods used in the first 21 days following delivery had theoretical or proven risks that outweighed benefits or presented unacceptable health risks (equivalent to MEC Category 3 or Category 4), which is inconsistent with medical professional guidelines and the best available evidence [61]. Specifically, 76.3% stated that progestin-only pills ought to be avoided during this time period, while 90.1% stated the same for DMPA and 92.1% for the etonogestrel implant [61]. The inconsistencies found in this study are particularly concerning, given that lactation consultants are generally considered the premier experts on breastfeeding on postpartum inpatient units where many women are finalizing contraceptive choices for initiation before discharge.

Conclusion

Regardless of age and intended family size, unintended pregnancy can occur at any point in a woman's reproductive life. As women spend the majority of their reproductive years attempting to avoid unintended pregnancy, contraception counseling is an important aspect women's healthcare, especially for those who have recently experienced pregnancy. There are very few non-hormonal contraceptive options available in the United States, and most are associated with high failure rates in typical use. Healthcare providers must communicate with women about the typical use failure rates of contraceptives and assist patients in initiating the most effective method that best fits their medical situation and preferences. Providers must also be familiar with USMEC and US Selected Practice Recommendations for Contraceptive Use in order to initiate and manage post-pregnancy contraception safely and appropriately [21]. Further, many women use contraceptive methods for their non-contraceptive benefits and may need to initiate or resume methods for such purposes postpartum. The USMEC clarifies that recommendations refer to the safety of contraceptive methods when used for contraceptive purposes and do not apply to the use of contraceptive methods for treatment of medical conditions (as the eligibility criteria may differ in such circumstances) [21].

Women may wish to discuss contraception both prenatally and after hospital discharge. A multicenter randomized controlled study evaluating antenatal discussion of planned postpartum contraception failed to demonstrate significant effect on contraceptive use or subsequent pregnancy rates [62]. An evaluation of postpartum contraception educational method by the Cochrane database also failed to identify specific strategies that work universally to improve awareness of women in this regard. Thus, to date, research has not reached a consensus on the optimal timing and method to discuss postpartum contraception with patients [63].

Despite the paucity of high quality evidence of the impact on hormonal contraception on breastfeeding outcomes, and the strong evidence for improved health outcomes with achievement of recommended birth spacing intervals, some authors have gone as far as to suggest that conducting a controlled trial to evaluate the effects of timing of hormonal contraception initiation on lactation would be unethical given the primacy of non-hormonal methods in breastfeeding and the fact that hormonal contraceptives could theoretically have negative impacts [64]. However, other authors have advocated strongly that the real risk of unintended pregnancy and its consequences must not be neglected for fear of the theoretical neonatal risks, and that women should establish desired hormonal contraception before the risk of pregnancy resumes, which is generally 4 weeks following delivery unless criteria for the lactational amenorrhea method is met [65].

Women who desire a contraceptive method should have it available as soon as possible. Advanced provision of EC is recommended by professional societies and may serve an important role postpartum. Systems barriers to women's ability to achieve recommended birth spacing must be addressed. With optimization of postpartum contraception provision, we will step closer toward a healthcare system with fewer unintended pregnancies and improved birth outcomes.

Abbreviations

CDC MEC: Centers for Disease Control and Prevention Medical Eligibility Criteria for Contraceptive Use; CDC: Centers for Disease Control and Prevention; COC: Combined oral contraceptives; DMPA: Depot medroxyprogesterone acetate; ECP: Emergency contraceptive pills; FSH: Follicular stimulating hormone; GnRH: Gonadotropin-releasing hormone; IPI: Inter-pregnancy interval; IUD: Intrauterine device; LAM: Lactational amenorrhea method ; LARC: Long-acting reversible contraception; LH: Luteinizing hormone; POP: Progestin-only pill; SGA: Small size for gestational age; UNICEF: United Nations Children's Emergency Fund ; VTE: Venous thromboembolism; WHO MEC: World Health Organization Medical Eligibility Criteria for Contraceptive Use; WHO: World Health Organization

Acknowledgement

None.

Funding

Not applicable (This is a review).

Author's contribution

Both authors Dr. Aparna Sridhar and Dr. Jennifer Salcedo have made equal contribution to the conception and design, or acquisition of data, or analysis and interpretation of data. They both have been involved in drafting the manuscript or revising it critically for important intellectual content. Both authors haven given final approval of the version to be published. Each author has participated sufficiently in the work to take public responsibility for appropriate portions of the content. Both authors have agreed to be accountable for all aspects of the work in ensuring that questions related to the accuracy or integrity of any part of the work are appropriately investigated and resolved. Both authors read and approved the final manuscript.

Competing interests

The authors have no competing interests to disclose.

Author details

[1]Department of Obstetrics and Gynecology, David Geffen School of Medicine at University of California Los Angeles, California, USA. [2]Department of Obstetrics, Gynecology & Women's Health, University of Hawaii John A. Burns School of Medicine, Hawaii, USA.

References

1. World Health Organization. Department of Reproductive Health and Research. Geneva: World Health Organization; 2005.
2. Conde-Agudelo A, Belizán JM, Norton MH, Rosas-Bermúdez A. Effect of the interpregnancy interval on perinatal outcomes in Latin America. Obstet Gynecol. 2005;106(2):359–66.
3. Conde-Agudelo A, Rosas-Bermúdez A, Kafury-Goeta AC. Birth spacing and risk of adverse perinatal outcomes: a meta-analysis. JAMA. 2006;295(15):1809–23.
4. Shachar BZ, Mayo JA, Lyell DJ, Baer RJ, Jeliffe-Pawlowski LL, Stevenson DK, Shaw GM. Interpregnancy interval after live birth or pregnancy termination and estimated risk of preterm birth: a retrospective cohort study. BJOG. 2016;123(12). doi:10.1111/1471-0528.14165. [Epub ahead of print].
5. Copen CE, Thoma ME, Kirmeyer S. Interpregnancy intervals in the United States: data from the birth certificate and the national survey of family growth. Natl Vital Stat Rep. 2015;64(3):1–10.
6. Hodgen GD. Perspectives in human reproduction. Hum Reprod. 1988;3(4): 573–6.
7. Gray RH, Campbell OM, Zacur HA, Labbok MH, MacRae SL. Postpartum return of ovarian activity in nonbreastfeeding women monitored by urinary assays. J Clin Endocrinol Metab. 1987;64(4):645–50.
8. Jackson E, Glasier A. Return of ovulation and menses in postpartum nonlactating women: a systematic review. Obstet Gynecol. 2011;117(3): 657–62.
9. Stoddard A, Eisenberg DL. Controversies in family planning: timing of ovulation after abortion and the conundrum of postabortion intrauterine device insertion. Contraception. 2011;84(2):119–21.
10. McNeilly AS. Neuroendocrine changes and fertility in breast-feeding women. Prog Brain Res. 2001;133:207–14.
11. Kazi A, Kennedy KI, Visness CM, Khan T. Effectiveness of the lactational amenorrhea method in Pakistan. Fertil Steril. 1995;64(4):717–23.
12. Labbok MH, Hight-Laukaran V, Peterson AE, Fletcher V, von Hertzen H, Van Look PF. Multicenter study of the lactational amenorrhea method (LAM): efficacy, duration, and implications for clinical application. Contraception. 1997;55(6):327–36.
13. Pérez A, Labbok MH, Queenan JT. Clinical study of the lactational amenorrhoea method for family planning. Lancet. 1992;339(8799):968–70.
14. Ramos R, Kennedy KI, Visness CM. Effectiveness of lactational amenorrhoea in prevention of pregnancy in Manila, the Philippines: non-comparative prospective trail. BMJ. 1996;313(7062):909–12.
15. Van der Wijden C, Manion C. Lactational amenorrhoea method for family planning. Cochrane Database Syst Rev. 2015;10:CD001329. doi:10.1002/14651858.CD001329.pub2.
16. https://www.cdc.gov/breastfeeding/data/NIS_data/. Accessed 1 July 2016.
17. https://www.cdc.gov/breastfeeding/nis_data/rates-any-exclusive-bf-state-2013.htm Rates of Any and Exclusive Breastfeeding by State among Children Born in 2013 Accessed 1 Jul 2016.
18. McDonald EA, Brown SJ. Does method of birth make a difference to when women resume sex after childbirth? BJOG. 2013;120(7):823–30. doi:10.1111/1471-0528.12166. Epub 2013 Feb 27.
19. Thiel de Bocanegra H, Chang R, Menz M, Howell M, Darney P. Postpartum contraception in publicly-funded programs and interpregnancy intervals. Obstet Gynecol. 2013;122(2 Pt 1):296–303.
20. Thiel de Bocanegra H, Chang R, Howell M, Darney P. Interpregnancy intervals: impact of postpartum contraceptive effectiveness and coverage. Am J Obstet Gynecol. 2014;210(4):311. e1-8.
21. Curtis KM, Tepper NK, Jatlaoui TC, et al. U.S. Medical Eligibility Criteria for Contraceptive Use, 2016. MMWR Recomm Rep. 2016;No. RR-3:1–104.
22. Jackson E, Curtis KM, Gaffield ME. Risk of venous thromboembolism during the postpartum period. Obstet Gynecol. 2011;117:691–703.
23. WHO Medical Eligibility Criteria for Contraceptive Use http://who.int/reproductivehealth/publications/family_planning/MEC-5/en/. Accessed 1 July 2016

24. Tepper NK, Phillips SJ, Kapp N, Gaffield ME, Curtis KM. Combined hormonal contraceptive use among breastfeeding women: an updated systematic review. Contraception. 2016;94(3):262–74.
25. Tankeyoon M, Dusitsin N, Chalapati S, Koetsawang S, Saibiang S, Sas M, Gellen JJ, Ayeni O, Gray R, Pinol A, et al. Effects of hormonal contraceptives on milk volume and infant growth. WHO special programme of research, development and research training in human reproduction task force on oral contraceptives. Contraception. 1984;30(6):505–22.
26. Espey E, Ogburn T, Leeman L, Singh R, Schrader R. Effect of progestin compared with combined oral contraceptive pills on lactation: a double-blind randomized controlled trial. Obstet Gynecol. 2012;119(1):5–13.
27. Lopez LM, Grey TW, Stuebe AM, Chen M, Truitt ST, Gallo MF. Combined hormonal versus non hormonal versus progestin-only contraception in lactation. Cochrane Database Syst Rev. 2015;20(3):CD003988. doi:10.1002/14651858.CD003988.pub2.
28. Diaz S. Contraceptive implants and lactation. Contraception. 2002;65(1):39–46.
29. Reinprayoon D, Taneepanichskul S, Bunyavejchevin S, et al. Effects of the etonogestrel-releasing contraceptive implant (Implanon) on parameters of breastfeeding, compared to those of an IUD. Contraception. 2000;62(5):239–46.
30. Fraser IS. A review of the use of progestogen-only minipills for contraception during lactation. Reprod Fertil Dev. 1991;3(3):245–54.
31. Koetsawang S, Nukulkarn P, Fotherby K, Shrimanker K, Mangalam M, Towobola K. Transfer of contraceptive steroids in milk of women using long-acting gestagens. Contraception. 1982;25:321–31.
32. Heikkila M, Haukkamaa M, Luukkainen T. Levonorgestrel in milk and plasma of breast-feeding women with a levonorgestrel-releasing IUD. Contraception. 1982;25(1):41–9.
33. Patel SB, Toddywalla VS, Betrabet SS, Kulkarni RD, Patel ZM, Mehta AC, Saxena BN. At what 'infant-age' can levonorgestrel contraceptives be recommended to nursing mothers? Adv Contracept. 1994;10(4):249–45.
34. Shikary ZK, Betrabet SS, Toddywala WS, Patel DM, Datey S, Saxena BN. Pharmacodynamic effects of levonorgestrel (LNG) administered either orally or subdermally to early postpartum lactating mothers on the urinary levels of follicle stimulating hormone (FSH), luteinizing hormone (LH) and testosterone (T) in their breast-fed male infants. Contraception. 1986;34:403–12.
35. Abdulla KA, Elwan SI, Salem HS, Shaaban MM. Effect of early postpartum use of the contraceptive implants, Norplant, on the serum levels of immunoglobulins of the mothers and their breastfed infants. Contraception. 1985;32:261–6.
36. Phillips SJ, Tepper NK, Kapp N, Nanda K, Temmerman M, Curtis KM. Progestogen-only contraceptive use among breastfeeding women: a systematic review. Contraception. 2016;94(3):226–52.
37. Giner Velazquez J, Cortes Gallegos V, Sotelo Lopez A, Bondani G. Effect of daily oral administration of 0.350 mg of norethindrone on lactation and on the composition of milk. Ginecol Obstet Mex. 1976;40:31–9.
38. Tankeyoon M, Dusitsin N, Chalapati S, Koetsawang S, Saibiang S, Sas M, et al. Effects of hormonal contraceptives on milk volume and infant growth. WHO special programme of research, development and research training in human reproduction task force on oral contraceptives. Contraception. 1984;30:505–22.
39. Shaamash AH, Sayed GH, Hussien MM, Shaaban MM. A comparative study of the levonorgestrel-releasing intrauterine system Mirena versus the Copper T380A intrauterine device during lactation: breast-feeding performance, infant growth and infant development. Contraception. 2005; 72:346–51.
40. Chen BA, Reeves MF, Creinin MD, Schwarz EB. Postplacental or delayed levonorgestrel intrauterine device insertion and breast-feeding duration. Contraception. 2011;84:499–504.
41. Brito MB, Ferriani RA, Quintana SM, Yazlle ME, Silva de Sá MF, Vieira CS. Safety of the etonogestrel-releasing implant during the immediate postpartum period: a pilot study. Contraception. 2009;80:519–26.
42. Gurtcheff SE, TurokDK SG, Murphy PA, GibsonM JKP. Lactogenesis after early postpartum use of the contraceptive implant: a randomized controlled trial. Obstet Gynecol. 2011;117:1114–21.
43. Braga GC, Ferriolli E, Quintana SM, Ferriani RA, Pfrimer K, Vieira CS. Immediate postpartum initiation of etonogestrel-releasing implant: A randomized controlled trial on breastfeeding impact. Contraception. 2015;92:536–42.
44. Matias SL, Nommsen-Rivers LA, Dewey KG. Determinants of exclusive breastfeeding in a cohort of primiparous periurban Peruvian mothers. J Hum Lact. 2012;28(1):45–54.

Optimizing maternal and neonatal outcomes with postpartum contraception: impact on breastfeeding...

33

45. Halderman LD, Nelson AL. Impact of early postpartum administration of progestin-only hormonal contraceptives compared with nonhormonal contraceptives on short-term breast-feeding patterns. Am J Obstet Gynecol. 2002;186(6):1250–6.

46. Brownell EA, Fernandez ID, Fisher SG, Howard CR, Ternullo SR, Lawrence RA, et al. The effect of immediate postpartum depot medroxyprogesterone on early breastfeeding cessation. Contraception. 2013;87:826–43.

47. ACOG practice bulletin. No. 73: use of hormonal contraception in women with coexisting medical conditions. Obstet Gynecol. 2006;107:1453–72.

48. Gemzell-Danielsson K, Berger C, Lalitkumar PGL. Emergency contraception – mechanisms of action. Contraception. 2013;87(3):300–8.

49. Glasier AF, Cameron ST, Fine PM, Logan SJ, Casale W, Van Horn J, et al. Ulipristal acetate versus levonorgestrel for emergency contraception: a randomized non-inferiority trial and meta-analysis. Lancet. 2010;375:555–62.

50. Glasier AF, Cameron ST, Blithe D, Scherrer B, Mathe H, Levy D, et al. Can we identify women at risk of pregnancy despite using emergency contraception? Data from randomized trials of ulipristal acetate and levonorgestrel. Contraception. 2011;84:363–7.

51. Ella prescribing information: https://www.accessdata.fda.gov/drugsatfda_docs/label/2010/022474s000lbl.pdf. Accessed 1 July 2016.

52. EllaOne prescribing information: http://www.ellanow.com/pdf/ella-full-prescribing-information.pdf. Accessed 1 Jul 2016.

53. ACOG practice bulletin. No. 112: Emergency contraception. Obstet Gynecol. 2010;115(5):1100–9.

54. American Academy of Pediatrics Policy Statement. Emergency contraception. Pediatrics. 2012;130:1174–82.

55. Shaaban OM, Hassen SG, Nour SA, Kames MA, Yones EM. Emergency contraceptive pills as a backup for lactational amenorrhea method (LAM) of contraception: a randomized controlled trial. Contraception. 2013;87:363–9.

56. Jackson R, Schwarz EB, Freedman L, Darney P. Knowledge and willingness to use emergency contraception among low-income post-partum women. Contraception. 2000;61:351–7.

57. Ogburn JA, Espey E, Stonehocker J. Barriers to intrauterine device insertion in postpartum women. Contraception. 2005;72(6):426–9.

58. Salcedo J, Moniaga N, Harken T. Limited uptake of planned intrauterine devices during the postpartum period. South Med J. 2015;108(8):463–8.

59. Aiken AR, Creinin MD, Kaunitz AM, Nelson AL, Trussell J. Global fee prohibits postpartum provision of the most effective reversible contraceptives. Contraception. 2014;90(5):466–7.

60. Rodriguez MI, Evans M, Espey E. Advocating for immediate postpartum LARC: increasing access, improving outcomes, and decreasing cost. Contraception. 2014;90:468–71.

61. Dunn K, Bayer LL, Mody SK. Postpartum contraception: an exploratory study of lactation consultants' knowledge and practices. Contraception. 2016;94:87–92.

62. Smith KB, et al. "Is postpartum contraceptive advice given antenatally of value?". Contraception. 2002;65:237–43.

63. Lopez, L.M., Hiller, J.E., Grimes, D.A., Chen, M. (2012). "Education for contraceptive use by women after childbirth." Cochrane Database of Systematic Reviews 2012, Issue 8. Art. No.: CD001863. DOI: 10.1002/14651858.CD001863.pub3.

64. Kennedy KI, Short RV, Tully MR. Premature introduction of progestin-only contraceptive methods during lactation. Contraception. 1997;55:347–50.

65. Rodriguez MI, Kaunitz AM. An evidence-based approach to postpartum use of depot medroxyprogesterone acetate in breastfeeding women. Contraception. 2009;80:4–6.

5

Prevention and treatment of neonatal nosocomial infections

Jayashree Ramasethu🄳

Abstract

Nosocomial or hospital acquired infections threaten the survival and neurodevelopmental outcomes of infants admitted to the neonatal intensive care unit, and increase cost of care. Premature infants are particularly vulnerable since they often undergo invasive procedures and are dependent on central catheters to deliver nutrition and on ventilators for respiratory support. Prevention of nosocomial infection is a critical patient safety imperative, and invariably requires a multidisciplinary approach. There are no short cuts. Hand hygiene before and after patient contact is the most important measure, and yet, compliance with this simple measure can be unsatisfactory. Alcohol based hand sanitizer is effective against many microorganisms and is efficient, compared to plain or antiseptic containing soaps. The use of maternal breast milk is another inexpensive and simple measure to reduce infection rates. Efforts to replicate the anti-infectious properties of maternal breast milk by the use of probiotics, prebiotics, and synbiotics have met with variable success, and there are ongoing trials of lactoferrin, an iron binding whey protein present in large quantities in colostrum. Attempts to boost the immunoglobulin levels of preterm infants with exogenous immunoglobulins have not been shown to reduce nosocomial infections significantly. Over the last decade, improvements in the incidence of catheter-related infections have been achieved, with meticulous attention to every detail from insertion to maintenance, with some centers reporting zero rates for such infections. Other nosocomial infections like ventilator acquired pneumonia and staphylococcus aureus infection remain problematic, and outbreaks with multidrug resistant organisms continue to have disastrous consequences. Management of infections is based on the profile of microorganisms in the neonatal unit and community and targeted therapy is required to control the disease without leading to the development of more resistant strains.

Keywords: Nosocomial, Infection, Newborn, Prevention, CLABSI, VAP

Background

Advances in neonatal care have lead to the increasing survival of smaller and sicker infants, but nosocomial infections (NI), also known as health care associated or hospital acquired infections continue to be a serious problem. Late-onset sepsis (LOS), or sepsis acquired after 72 h of life, with the exception of Group B streptococcal or Herpes simplex virus infection, is usually hospital acquired, particularly in infants who are hospitalized from birth. These infections are associated with increased mortality rates, immediate and long term morbidity, prolonged hospital stay and increased cost of care [1–3]. Efforts to eradicate neonatal NI have had limited success in some areas, but many remain intransigent, and outbreaks with multi – drug resistant organisms (MDRO) continue to occur in neonatal intensive care units (NICUs) worldwide.

Risk of NI in preterm, late preterm and term infants

Prematurity is the most important risk factor for NI. In the United States, surveillance data over almost 2 decades from the National Institute of Child Health and Human Development (NICHD) Neonatal Network show that 20–25% of very low birth weight (VLBW, birth weight ≤ 1500 g) infants who survived beyond 3 days were found to have one or more episodes of blood culture proven sepsis, with the majority being caused by gram-positive organisms, predominantly coagulase-negative staphylococci (CONS) (Table 1) [1–3].

Correspondence: jr65@gunet.georgetown.edu
Division of Neonatal Perinatal Medicine, Department of Pediatrics, MedStar Georgetown University Hospital, Washington DC 20007, USA

Table 1 Distribution of organisms responsible for late-onset sepsis

Organism	VLBW infants NICHD NRN 1991–1993[1]	VLBW infants NICHD NRN 1998–2000[2]	VLBW infants NICHD NRN 2002–2008[3]
Incidence of LOS	25	21	25
Gram-positive			
Staphylococcus coagulase-negative	55	48	53
Staphylococcus aureus	9	8	11
Enterococcus/Group D strep	5	3	4
Group B streptococcus	2	2	2
Other	2	9	7
Gram-negative			
Enterobacter	4	3	3
Escherichia coli	4	5	5
Klebsiella	4	4	4
Pseudomonas	2	3	2
Other	4	1	2
Fungi			
Candida albicans	5	6	5
Candida parapsilosis	2	4	2
Other	2	2	1

Numbers are expressed in percentages
Abbreviations NICHD NRN National Institutes of Child Health and Human Development Neonatal Research Network, VLBW Very low birth weight, birth weight ≤1500 g

The rate of infections was inversely related to birth weight and gestational age, with 50% of the infections occurring in infants born at <25 weeks or weighing less than 750 g at birth. Considerable center to center variability in the incidence of late-onset sepsis has been noted with rates of LOS ranging from 10.6 to 31.7%, despite adjusting for birth weight, GA, race and sex [2].

There has been some progress recently in tackling neonatal NI. NICHD surveillance data showed that rates of LOS decreased from 2005 to 2012 for infants of each gestational age, (eg for infants born at 24 weeks, it decreased from 54 to 40%, and for those born at 28 weeks, the decrease was from 20 to 8%) [4]. Comparable decreases in the rates of LOS in preterm VLBW infants was noted in 669 North American Hospitals in the Vermont Oxford Network, with rates of LOS decreasing from 21% in 2000 to 15% by 2009 [5]. A similar analysis of LOS in preterm infants born at <32 weeks gestation in 29 NICUs in the Canadian Neonatal Network showed that 15% of infants developed LOS, with 80% of these infection being gram-positive, chiefly CONS [6].

The incidence of LOS in late preterm infants, born at 34 to 36 weeks gestational age and in term infants is much lower. A large study of more than 100,000 late preterm infants admitted to 248 NICUS in the United States between 1996 and 2007 showed an incidence of 6.3 episodes of LOS per 1000 NICU admissions; with 59.4% caused by gram-positive organisms, predominantly CONS, 30.7% by gram-negative organisms and 7.7% by yeast [7]. In term infants (≥37 weeks gestational age) discharged from NICUs from 1997 to 2010, the rate of late-onset bloodstream infections was 2.7/1000 admissions, with similar pathogens [8].

Apart from prematurity, prolonged duration of parenteral alimentation with delayed enteral nutrition, intravascular catheterization, extended respiratory support on ventilators, gastrointestinal surgery, and use of broad spectrum antibiotics are recognized risk factors for neonatal NI [2]. The very devices that sustain life and provide sustenance to premature and/or sick newborns admitted to the NICU may become channels for bacterial invasion, with fragile skin, and immaturity of immune systems exacerbating the risk.

The most common NI in NICUs are bloodstream infections, often catheter -related (central line associated bloodstream infection, CLABSI), followed by Ventilator-Associated Pneumonias (VAP), surgical site infections and less frequently catheter associated urinary tract infections, and ventricular shunt infections. Skin and soft tissue infections may also be hospital acquired in newborn infants [9].

Outbreaks of NI have been related to overcrowding, understaffing, and contamination of equipment, environment, medications, and even breast milk [10–13].

Organisms responsible for infections

The microorganisms responsible for NI may be the patient's own microflora, present on the skin, nasopharynx and gastrointestinal tract, or the transmission of microorganisms from visitors and caretakers. Recent studies have shown that infants with a less diverse gut microbiome harbor pathogenic bacteria in the gastrointestinal tract which may translocate across the epithelial barrier, predisposing them to late-onset bloodstream infections [14, 15].

Table 1 shows the distribution of organisms responsible for LOS in NICHD Neonatal Network NICUs over the years. In resource-limited countries, gram-negative bacteria such as E. Coli, Klebsiella, Acinetobacter and Pseudomonas are the predominant bacteria responsible for NI in neonatal units, and a very high prevalence of antibiotic resistance has been described [16].

Although much attention has been paid to hospital acquired bacterial infections, with the availability of better diagnostic methods, nosocomial viral infections are increasingly being recognized. Respiratory syncytial virus, influenza and parainfluenza viruses are well known for nosocomial transmission, but rhinovirus has recently been identified as an important nosocomial pathogen in preterm infants [17]. Nosocomial viral respiratory infections result in escalation of respiratory support, prolonging length of stay, hospitalization costs and also lead to affected infants requiring home oxygen twice as often as unaffected infants [17]. Rotavirus, adenovirus and norovirus have been responsible for outbreaks of gastrointestinal illness in NICU patients, and have been implicated in clusters of NEC cases [18]. Human parechovirus infections can present with sepsis like syndromes, indistinguishable from bacterial infection, and with symptoms of meningoencephalitis. In a prospective cohort study of preterm infants with suspected LOS over an 18 month period, 13% of infants tested were found to have evidence of parechovirus by reverse transcriptase polymerase chain reaction, confirmed by DNA sequencing [19].

Prevention of neonatal NI

The "All or None" approach of process quality is an important concept to understand and implement in prevention of NI [20]. NI are usually multifactorial and preventative strategies entail multiple interventions or a series of steps which operate synergistically. Partial execution of a series of steps may be ineffective. For example, insertion of a central line using strict aseptic techniques would be vitiated by improper line care, resulting in CLABSI. Hence, the proposal of "bundles" – a set of evidence based processes, that when instituted as a group, improve outcomes. This has been found to be particularly effective in reducing CLABSIs in NICUs [21].

Among the interventions to prevent neonatal NI, some that appear quite simple (hand hygiene, feeding maternal breast milk) have been shown to be surprisingly effective, while others have not lived up to their theoretical promise (intravenous immunoglobulin), and a few are still being evaluated (lactoferrin). The cornerstone of infection prevention in any setting is hand hygiene.

Hand hygiene

Hand hygiene is the single most important intervention in interrupting the transmission of microorganisms and thus preventing NI. Bacterial counts on hands of health care workers range from 3.9×10^4 to 4.6×10^6 colony forming units/cm^2, and may include pathogens such as staphylococcus aureus, klebsiella pneumoniae, enterobacter, acinetobacter and candida [22]. Viable organisms are present on the skin squames that humans shed daily, and these contaminate patient clothing, bed linen and furniture, with transmission by health care workers' hands if they are not cleaned before and after patient contact. Although this intervention appears simple, implementation is often more challenging than expected, with low compliance rates even in intensive care areas [21]. There is now a global effort to improve hand hygiene compliance with the WHO "Clean Care is Safer

Care" campaign [23]. A multipronged effort is required to improve compliance, with education of education of health care workers, performance feedback, reminders, use of automated sinks and introduction of an alcohol based hand rub [24]. It is believed that the introduction of the alcohol based hand rub has revolutionized hand hygiene practice, since it takes less time, improves compliance and has shown to be effective in many settings. Table 2 illustrates the mode of action and efficacy of commodities commonly used for hand hygiene. Apart from health care workers, parents and siblings may also be responsible for transmission of infection [25], so hand hygiene should be emphasized for all visitors/caregivers in the NICU.

Artificial finger nails worn by health care providers have been associated with persistent carriage of Pseudomonas aeruginosa, Klebsiella pneumoniae and fungi, and linked to outbreaks with these organisms in intensive care settings [26, 27]. The Hospital Infection Control Practices Advisory Committee (HICPAC) guidelines recommend that health care providers with direct patient contact in intensive care areas should not wear artificial nails [28]. It is unclear if the use of nail polish is associated with NI [29].

Early feeding and human milk

Since the seminal paper by Narayanan et al. in 1984 that showed that feeding raw unpasteurized maternal milk was associated with lower rates of sepsis in low birth weight infants in India [30], numerous studies in industrialized countries have confirmed that feeding human milk is associated with lower rates of sepsis and necrotizing enterocolitis in preterm and very low birth weight infants [31–33]. Early enteral feeding, within 2 to 3 days of life, has been associated with lower rates of NI, without increasing rates of necrotizing enterocolitis [34]. In addition, human milk is better tolerated than bovine formula, and is associated with establishment of complete enteral nutrition at a faster rate, allowing early discontinuation of central catheters [35]. The advantages of maternal breast milk in preventing NI have not been duplicated by the use of donor milk [31]. Human milk contains secretory antibodies, phagocytes, lactoferrin and prebiotics which improve host defense and gastrointestinal function. A recent review delineates compositional and bioactive differences between mother's own milk and donor milk which may account for the differences in outcome [36]. It is important to note that human milk can also be associated with outbreaks of infection in NICUs, either due to milk sharing [13] or contamination of equipment such as milk warmers, or collection pumps [12].

Table 2 Hand hygiene: materials and efficacy

Agent	Plain soap	Antimicrobial soap with chlorhexidine	Alcohol based hand sanitizer
Mode of action	Detergent effect and mechanical friction	Cationic bisguanide, disrupts cell membranes	Disrupts membranes, denatures proteins, cell lysis
Reduction of bacterial load on hands	0.6 to 1.1 $\log_{10}$ CFU	2.1 to 3.0 $\log_{10}$ CFU; has persistent residual antiseptic activity on the skin which may last up to 30 min.	3.2 to 5.8 $\log_{10}$ CFU
Effective against	Dirt, organic material	Gram-positive cocci	Gram-positive cocci, gram-negative bacilli, mycobacterium tuberculosis, fungi, viruses
Less effective against		Gram-negative bacilli, fungi and viruses, mycobacteria, spore forming bacteria such as Clostridium difficile	Clostridium difficile, Hepatitis A, rotavirus, enteroviruses, adenovirus, spores
Comments	Trauma caused by frequent skin washing may lead to chapping of skin and shedding of resistant flora		Optimal antimicrobial activity at concentration of 60–90%

(from ref [21] and [28])

Central line care

Central venous catheters provide stable intravenous access to sick or low birth weight infants who need long term intravenous nutrition or medications, and umbilical arterial catheters are used for blood sampling and continuous blood pressure monitoring. These central lines are ubiquitous, and usually essential in the NICU, but increase the risk of NI by breaching the protective skin barrier and due to the propensity of many microorganisms to form a biofilm [37]. CLABSI are a subset of NI, defined by the Centers for Disease Control and Prevention's National Healthcare Safety Network (NHSN) as a bloodstream infection in which the initial positive culture occurs at least 2 days after placement of a central line that is in situ or was removed less than 2 days before the positive culture, and the positive blood culture was not attributable to infection at another site [38]. Evidence based care of central lines has resulted in a decrease of CLABSI over the last decade (Table 3). These care "bundles" are not complicated, but require training, commitment, and constant vigilance to maintain compliance. There is still significant heterogeneity in CLABSI prevention practices in NICUs in the United States, and in other countries, with some centers using chlorhexidine for skin antisepsis or for dressings and some centers restricting the use of chlorhexidine to larger infants based on United States Food and Drug Administration guidelines [39, 40]. Nevertheless, from 2007 to 2012, rates of CLABSIs decreased in NICUs in the United States from 4.9 to 1.5 per 1000 central line days [41], with some centers achieving sustained reductions to zero rates [42, 43]. In lower resource countries, CLABSI rates in NICUs participating in the International Nosocomial Infection Control Consortium are reported to be 10 to 20 times higher than those in NICUs reporting data to the CDC NHSN [44].

Fluconazole prophylaxis

Candida species colonize the skin and mucous membranes of 60% of critically ill neonates and can rapidly progress to invasive infection, with fungal infections being the 3rd most common cause of NI in neonates [45, 46]. Prematurity, low birth weight, use of cephalosporin antibiotics, exposure to more than 2 antibiotics, exposure to H2 blockers, gastrointestinal surgery, parenteral nutrition use >5 days, use of lipid emulsion for >7 days, lack of enteral feeding and presence of a central catheter have all been associated with increased risk of invasive candidiasis, and in extremely low birth weight infants (< 1000 g), invasive candidiasis has been associated with 73% mortality or neurodevelopmetal impairment [47]. Fungal infection accounted for 9% of cases of LOS in VLBW infants in 1996 [1], but more recent studies indicate that invasive candidiasis has decreased in NICUs in the United States since 1997, probably secondary to the widespread use of fluconazole prophylaxis and decreased use of broad spectrum antibacterial antibiotics [48]. In a study of data from 709,325 infants at 322 NICUS managed by the Pediatrix Medical Group from 1997 to 2010, the annual incidence of invasive candidiasis among infants with a birth weight of 750–999 g decreased from 24.2 to 11.6 episodes per 1000 patients, and from 82.7 to 23.8 episodes per 1000 patients among infants with a birth weight <750 g. Fluconazole prophylaxis increased among all VLBW infants over the years, with the largest increase among infants weighing <750 g at birth, increasing from 3.8 per 1000 infants in 1997 to 110.6 per 1000 infants in 2010. The use of broad spectrum antibacterial antibiotics decreased concomitantly in all infants, from 275.7 per 1000 patients in 1997 to 48.5 per 1000 patients in 2010 [48].

Prophylactic antifungal therapy reduces colonization of the skin, gastrointestinal and respiratory tracts and

Table 3 Guidelines for prevention of intravascular catheter associated infections

Education and training:

    Educate health care personnel regarding indications for intravascular catheter use, proper procedures for the insertion and maintenance of intravascular catheters and appropriate infection control measures

    Periodically reassess knowledge of and adherence to guidelines for all personnel involved in the insertion and maintenance of intravascular catheters

    Designate only trained personnel who demonstrate competence for the insertion and maintenance of central intravascular catheters.

Catheter placement and duration of use

    Weigh the risks and benefits of placing a central venous catheter.

    Evaluate daily if catheter is still necessary

    Promptly remove any intravascular catheter that is no longer essential

    Remove and do not replace umbilical artery catheters if any signs of catheter-related bloodstream infection, vascular insufficiency in the lower extremities or thrombosis are present. Optimally umbilical catheters should not be left in place > 5 days.

    Remove and do not replace umbilical venous catheters if any signs of CLABSI or thrombosis are present. Umbilical venous catheters should be removed as soon as possible but can be used up to 14 days if managed aseptically.

Placing catheters

    Hand hygiene should be performed before and after palpating catheter insertion sites as well as before and after inserting, replacing, or dressing an intravascular catheter.

    Maintain aseptic technique for insertion and care of intravascular catheters.

    Maximum sterile barrier precautions including the use of a cap, mask, sterile gown, sterile gloves and a sterile large drape are necessary for the insertion of a central venous catheter.

    A minimum of a cap, mask, sterile gloves and a small sterile fenestrated drape should be used during peripheral arterial catheter insertion.

    Prepare insertion site with povidone iodine/chlorhexidine containing antiseptic (no recommendation can be made about the safety of chlorhexidine in infants < 2 months)

    Use sterile gauze or sterile, transparent semi-permiable dressing to cover catheter site.

    Do not use topical antibiotic ointment or creams on insertion sites because of potential to promote fungal infections and antimicrobial resistance.

    Do not administer systemic antimicrobial prophylaxis routinely before insertion or during use of an intravascular catheter to prevent catheter colonization or CLABSI.

Dressing catheters

    Use sterile gloves when changing the dressing

    Replace catheter site dressing if the dressing becomes damp, loose or visibly soiled.

Catheter care

    Use the minimum number of ports or lumens essential for management of the patient

    Do not submerge the catheter or catheter site in water.

    Minimize contamination risk by scrubbing the access port with an appropriate antiseptic (chlorhexidine, povidone iodine, an iodophor, or 70% alcohol) and accessing the port only with sterile devices.

    Replace tubing used to administer blood, blood products, or fat emulsions (those combined with amino acids and glucose or infused separately) within 24 h of initiating the infusion.

from ref [38]

prevents invasive candida infection in high risk preterm infants [46, 47, 49]. Prophylaxis with intravenous fluconazole at 3 mg/kg twice a week, has been recommended for preterm infants with birth weight < 1000 g or gestational age ≤ 27 weeks gestation, starting within the first 2 days after birth, and continued until there is no necessity for central and peripheral intravenous access. In infants weighing 1000–1500 g, prophylaxis may be considered by individual NICUs with high rates of invasive candidiasis [49]. There has been no evidence of development of resistance to fluconazole with this regimen in neonates, although increasing fluconazole resistance has been documented in adult intensive care units. Oral

nystatin has also been shown to be effective for prophylaxis [50], but it cannot be used when infants have ileus, necrotizing enterocolitis or intestinal perforation, all conditions with a high risk of invasive candida infection.

The use of routine fluconazole prophylaxis has been challenged more recently, in a randomized controlled trial in infants weighing <750 g at birth, which showed that although invasive candidiasis occurred less frequently in the fluconazole group (3% [95% CI: 1 to 6%]) versus the placebo group (9% [95% CI: 5–14%]), there was no difference in the composite endpoint of death and invasive candidiasis or in the rates of neurodevelopmental impairment [51].

Use of topical emollients

Topical emollients such as vegetable oils or aquaphor have been postulated to improve skin integrity and barrier function and thereby prevent invasive infection. A recent Cochrane meta-analysis of 18 primary publications involving 3089 infants did not provide evidence that the use of emollient therapy prevents invasive infection or death in preterm infants in high, middle or low income settings [52].

Ventilator-Associated Pneumonia (VAP)

Ventilator-associated pneumonia is defined by using a combination of clinical, radiologic and laboratory criteria in a patient who has been on assisted ventilation through an endotracheal or tracheostomy tube for at least 48 h before the onset of illness. However, these criteria are subjective and frequently have common characteristics with other diseases, particularly in low birth weight infants with chronic lung disease. Rates of VAP range from 0 to more than 50 per 1000 ventilator days in various publications, reflecting differences in study patients and definitions. It is also unclear if cultures of tracheal secretions are truly representative of VAP or only indicate colonization. In 2012, the Neonatal and Pediatric Ventilator Associated Events working group recognized that the current VAP surveillance definition is of questionable utility and meaning in the neonatal population and refinements are being sought [53]. While absolute definitions may be lacking, it is well known that endotracheal intubation leads to impairment of mucociliary clearance and the potential for colonization of the endotracheal tube and trachea, from both endogenous and exogenous sources, which may then descend further and result in pneumonitis [54]. Endogenous sources of colonization are oropharyngeal secretions, and aspiration of stomach contents. Exogenous sources include transmission of infection from a health care workers' hands, contamination of suction apparatus, airway circuits, humidifiers, etc. In neonatal patients diagnosed with VAP, polymicrobial and gram-negative organisms appear to be predominant, although staphylococcus aureus and candida have also been noted [55].

VAP prevention "bundles", similar to CLABSI prevention bundles, have been used in adult ICUs with success, but many of the interventions are not applicable in neonates [54]. Interventions with potential benefit in neonates are indicated in Table 4. There are few studies showing the impact of infection control measures in reducing VAP rates in NICUs [56, 57].

Adjuvant therapy

Immunoglobulin therapy

Preterm infants are deficient in immunoglobulin G (IgG) since transplacental transport of maternal IgG is truncated by early delivery, and endogenous production

Table 4 Interventions to prevent VAP in Neonates

Definite or probable benefit	Unclear benefit
Caregiver education	Oral care with antiseptic or colostrum
Hand hygiene	Elevation of head of bed
Wear gloves when in contact with secretions	In-Line (closed) suctioning
Minimize days of ventilation	
Prevent unplanned extubation-avoid reintubation	
Suction orophaynx	
Prevent gastric distension	
Change ventilator circuit only when visibly soiled or malfunctioning	
Remove condensate from ventilator circuit frequently	

Modified from ref [54]

starts only around the third month of life. Polyclonal intravenous immunoglobulin (IVIG) has been evaluated to determine if passive immunotherapy is efficacious in preventing neonatal NI in preterm or low birth weight (<2500 g birth weight) patients. A 2013 Cochrane review summarizing 19 studies enrolling almost 5000 preterm and/or low birth weight patients concluded that when all studies were combined, there was a 3% reduction in sepsis and a 4% reduction in one or more episodes of any serious infection, but was not associated with reductions in other clinically important outcomes, including mortality [58]. The Cochrane review's final statement was "the decision to use prophylactic IVIG will depend on the costs and the values assigned to the clinical outcomes", and that no additional trials to test the efficacy of previously studied IVIG preparations are warranted.

Since Staphylococci, especially CONS, are responsible for the majority of late-onset infections in VLBW infants, IVIG preparations containing various type specific antibodies targeting different antigenic sites were developed, but studies of these products (Veronate or INH-A21: antibody against microbial surface components recognizing adhesive matrix molecules, Altastaph: antibody against capsular polysaccharide antigen type 5 and 8, and Pagibaximab: anti-lipoteichoic human chimeric monoclonal antibody) have also shown disappointing results [59, 60]. IgM-enriched immunoglobulins are being evaluated as adjuvant therapy for VLBW infants with proven sepsis, but not for prophylaxis [61].

Lactoferrin

Lactoferrin is an iron – binding glycoprotein present in mature human milk at a concentration of 1 to 3 g/L and in colostrum at 7 g/L. Lactoferrin limits the amount of iron available to pathogenic bacteria, promotes growth of commensal bacteria, and with lysozyme, another antibacterial present in human milk, is involved in the destruction of gram negative bacteria [36]. Delay in establishing enteral nutrition exacerbates the low lactoferrin levels in preterm infants. Bovine lactoferrin, which is 70% homologous with human lactoferrin, has high antimicrobial activity, and is available commercially as a food supplement, has shown promise in reducing the incidence of late-onset sepsis in VLBW infants, particularly in infants weighing <1000 g at birth [62]. There are ongoing trials which may provide additional evidence of the effectiveness of this intervention before this becomes common practice [63].

Probiotics

In babies born at term by vaginal delivery, the gut is colonized with probiotic bacteria from the mother such as lactobacilli and bifidobacteria which are crucial to the development of the intestinal mucosal immune system. Preterm neonates have abnormal intestinal colonization, often with pathogenic bacteria and have low numbers of probiotic bacteria. Efforts to repopulate the preterm infant's gut with probiotics in an effort to decrease late-onset sepsis have resulted in variable success, and metanalysis of trials have given inconsistent results. A Cochrane metanalysis in 2014 of 16 eligible trials with 5338 patients concluded that probiotic supplementation did not result in statistically significant reduction of LOS in preterm infants [64]. A more recent metanalysis of 37 randomized controlled trials with 9416 patients showed that probiotics significantly reduced the risk of LOS (13.9% versus 16.3%, number needed to treat =44), but of all the studies analyzed, the two largest trials did not show a significant reduction in the rates of LOS with probiotics [65]. In the ProPrems study [66], 1099 preterm VLBW infants in Australia and New Zealand were randomized to receive a probiotic combination of Bifidobacterium infantis, Streptococcus thermophilus and Bifidobacterium lactis or placebo. Breast milk feeding rates were high (96.9%) among these infants. No significant difference was found in definite late onset sepsis or all cause mortality, but the rate of Stage 2 necrotizing enterocolitis was reduced (2% versus 4.4%). The Probiotics in Preterm Infants Study Collaborative (PiPs trial) [67] in the United Kingdom recruited 1315 infants of whom 650 were administered the probiotic Bifidobacteium breve BBG-001. There was no significant difference in the incidence of LOS in the probiotic patients (11%) versus the controls (12%) and the rates of NEC were also similar.No adverse effects have been noted in these trials, but there have been case reports of bacteremia in preterm infants originating from probiotic therapy [68]. Despite numerous trials and metanalyses, questions remain about the effectiveness of probiotics, the strains to be used, appropriate dosage, etc.

Prebiotics

Human milk oligosaccharides (HMO) are complex carbohydrates which promote the growth of beneficial commensals like Bifidobacterium and Bacteroides in the healthy breast fed term infants' intestine. Most pathogenic Enterobacteriaceae lack specific glucosidases to utilize these oligosaccharides as a food source. In addition, HMOs have structural homology to many cell surface glycans and act as decoys by binding luminal bacteria that are then unable to bind to the luminal enterocytes. HMOs produced by mothers may vary in structure and may influence the intestinal microbiota of their infants [69]. Prebiotics are non-digestible dietary products that selectively stimulate the growth or activity of beneficial commensal bacteria similar to HMOs, but the complexity of this approach to altering gut microbiota is only just beginning to be understood [70]. Synthetic prebiotics such as short chain galacto oligosaccharides, long chain fructo-oligosaccharides, inulin, lactulose are available and have been used in combinations to mimic natural human milk oligosaccharides. A metanalysis of 7 trials including 417 patients showed that supplementation with prebiotics resulted in significantly higher growth of beneficial microbes but did not decrease the incidence of sepsis, NEC or reduce the time to full feeding [71].

Synbiotics

A synbiotic is a product that contains both a probiotic microbe and a prebiotic substrate. There is experimental evidence that the simultaneous administration of probiotics and prebiotics can improve survival of the probiotic bacteria, but there is no clinical evidence yet that synbiotics are useful in preventing neonatal NI [72].

Antibiotic stewardship

Empirical antibiotic use is widespread in neonatal intensive care units. A recent review of over 50,000 patients in 127 California NICUs showed a 40 fold variation in antibiotic prescribing practices, despite similar burdens of proven infections, NEC, surgical volume and mortality [73]. Prolonged initial empirical antibiotic treatment in preterm infants has been associated with increased rates of LOS, NEC and death, with each additional empirical treatment day associated with measureable increase in risk [74, 75]. Perinatal and early empiric antibiotic use has been associated with lower bacterial diversity in the developing microbiome of the neonate, and increased colonization with potentially pathogenic Enterobacteriaceae, which may precede bloodstream infection in preterm infants [14, 15, 76, 77]. Widespread antibiotic use, particularly with broad spectrum cephalosporins potentiates the development of resistant strains, and increased colonization and invasive disease due to candida [78].

The gravity of this scenario has been recognized and given impetus to develop local and national antibiotic stewardship programs [79]. However, a prospective longitudinal study of neonatal infections and antibiotic use over 25 years in a tertiary NICU showed that emergence of cephalosporin resistant gram-negative bacterial infection was not prevented by responsible antibiotic use, indicating that the relationship between antimicrobial use and drug resistance is complex and that other factors may be involved [80].

Management of neonatal nosocomial infections

Infants in the NICU may deteriorate rapidly when they develop NI, so vigilance and high index of suspicion for sepsis is essential. Management includes appropriate diagnostic tests including blood, and whenever possible, cerebrospinal fluid cultures, followed by antibiotic therapy and supportive care.

Initial antibiotic therapy is empirical and targeted against the most likely organisms, based on the clinical presentation, available epidemiological information on the pathogen profile in the neonatal unit where the patient is being treated and in the community [81, 82]. Antibiotic therapy should be narrowed down or modified as soon as culture and antibiotic susceptibility results are available. In infants suspected to have CLABSI, most NICUs use a regimen of vancomycin and gentamicin as initial therapy, to cover the possibility of CONS or a gram-negative infection. However, the use and overuse of vancomycin as the first line of treatment for suspected LOS in NICU patients has led to the emergence of vancomycin resistant enterococci. There is a recommendation that neonatal units consider starting empirical treatment with oxacillin or flucloxacillin instead of vancomycin, together with an aminoglycoside such as gentamicin in infants who are suspected to have CLABSI, but are not severely ill, since CONS sepsis is rarely severe and there would be time to switch to vancomycin if the strain is resistant to the initial treatment [82]. There is no evidence that a delay in vancomycin therapy increases mortality in infants with CONS sepsis [83]. On the other hand, inadequate empirical therapy for MRSA bloodstream infection has been associated with increased mortality, so the judicious selection of initial antibiotics remains critical, but still challenging, since clinical signs are usually non-specific [84]. Gram-negative septicemia and candidemia are often associated with hypotension, thrombocytopenia and acidosis. When gram-negative sepsis is strongly suspected or confirmed, or in the presence of gram-negative meningitis, the addition or substitution of a 3rd generation cephalosporin is justified. Pipercillin–tazobactam may be considered to provide coverage for resistant gram-negative organisms. In infections with extended spectrum beta-lactamase (ESBL) producing organisms, or in critically ill infants with complicated intra-abdominal infections, a carbapenem antibiotic may be considered [82, 85]. A combination of antibiotics is usually used in critically ill infants with necrotizing enterocolitis (NEC) or complicated intra-abdominal infections, where polymicrobial infection with aerobic and anaerobic microorganisms is probable [85]. Results of the ongoing Phase 2/3 study (SCAMP study, NCT 01994993) of different antibiotic regimens for complicated intra-abdominal infections in infants may help guide future therapy. Anaerobic therapy with clindamycin, metronidazole, carbapenems etc. in infants with NEC has been associated with an increase in intestinal strictures, but with lower mortality in infants with surgical NEC [86]. Invasive neonatal candidiasis is treated with amphotericin B deoxycholate, fluconazole or micafungin [87], although some authors suggest reserving fluconazole only for prophylaxis and using amphotericin for treatment to prevent the emergence of resistant strains [49].

In addition to appropriate antibiotics, consideration should be given to removal of central lines since there is an increased risk of infectious complications and persistently positive cultures if the central line is not removed promptly in bacteremic patients or in patients with candidemia [88]. One positive blood culture for Staph aureus, or Gram-negative rods or Candida warrants removal of the central line. Medical management without central line removal may be considered if there is one positive CONS culture, but if cultures are repeatedly positive, the central catheter should be removed, with placement of a new catheter if required, once cultures are negative.

Supportive care for infants with NI includes respiratory, hemodynamic, hematological and nutritional support in the NICU, and close follow up post–discharge with early intervention services since these infants are at increased risk for neurodevelopmental delays [89].

Control of outbreaks

Apart from endemic infections, outbreaks of bacterial, fungal and viral infections have been reported in NICUs, with serious consequences for patients, huge economic burdens and staffing issues [10, 11, 90]. An analysis of a world wide database of health care associated infections (https://www.outbreak-database.com) showed that NICUs account for 38% of outbreaks in ICUs and 18% of all published outbreaks, and this probably represents only the tip of the iceberg [10]. Klebsiella, Staphylococcus, including MRSA, Serratia, and Enterobacter species were responsible for the majority of reported outbreaks. ESBL producing Enterobacteriaceae have emerged as major pathogens responsible for outbreaks of infection in NICUs with associated significant mortality [11]. A recent review of 75 studies reported 1185 cases of colonization and 860 infected with 16% mortality in infected infants. Klebsiella pneumoniae was the most frequently implicated pathogen. The source of the outbreak was unknown in 57% of the reports; the most commonly identified source was admission of an ESBL colonized infant with subsequent horizontal dissemination. Understaffing was identified as a major risk factor in most studies, but the intervention most commonly implemented to terminate outbreaks was enhanced infection control measures including hand hygiene, contact precautions, patient cohorting/isolation, and environmental cleaning. In 23% of reports, the outbreak of ESBL infection led to ward closure. Most units do not routinely screen infants for ESBL infection. Some countries have adopted more rigorous routine screening measures to identify infants colonized with pathogens, in order to prevent horizontal transmission [91].

Staphylococcus aureus is the second most common cause of late-onset sepsis in VLBW infants [3], and is often implicated in outbreaks [10]. Neonates quickly become colonized after birth from their adult caregivers, and colonization may be precursor to invasive infection. In one study, 34% of mothers were colonized with Staphylococcus aureus, and, the cumulative incidence of S. aureus acquisition in infants born to carrier mothers was 42.6/100 within 72–100 h after birth, rising to 69.7/100 at 1 month follow up [92]. The emergence and rapid rise of methicillin resistant staphylococcus aureus (MRSA) infections caused considerable alarm, but large studies have shown that methicillin sensitive staphylococcus aureus (MSSA) causes more infections and more deaths than MRSA and infection prevention strategies should consider MSSA as well as MRSA [93]. Strategies to prevent MRSA transmission in NICUs have included identifying and cohorting colonized neonates, placing them on contact precautions, enhanced hand hygiene compliance, decolonization of colonized neonates and/or health care workers with topical mupirocin, and use of chlorhexidine baths for patients as well as for health care workers [94]. Following two outbreaks of Staphyloccus aureus infections, one NICU instituted a regimen of prophylactic mupirocin applied to all infants admitted to the NICU throughout hospitalization and found that both MRSA and MSSA colonization decreased from 60% to < 5% [95]. In another level 3 NICU, rigorous attempts at preventing colonization and transmission were inadequate with infants developing infection before being identified as colonized or after attempting decolonization [96].

Conclusion

The prevention and treatment of nosocomial infections continues to be a complex process with no easy solutions. There have been improvements in some areas with documented improvement in rates of CLABSI, but a number of infections remain difficult to control or eradicate. There are isolated case reports as well as outbreaks of infection with increasingly resistant strains or infections with unusual pathogens. Although there are limitations to the diagnostic and therapeutic arsenal available presently to tackle these infections, much can be achieved by attention to simple preventive measures such as hand hygiene and use of maternal breast milk.

Abbreviations

CLABSI: Central line associated bloodstream infection; CONS: Coagulase-negative staphylococcus; ESBL: Extended spectrum beta-lactamase; HMO: Human milk oligosaccharides; LOS: Late-onset sepsis; MDRO: Multi-drug resistant organisms; MRSA: Methicillin resistant staphylococcus aureus; MSSA: Methicillin sensitive staphylococcus aureus; NEC: Necrotizing enterocolitis; NI: Nosocomial infections; NICHD NRN: National Institute of Child Health and Human Development Neonatal Research Network; NICU: Neonatal intensive care unit; VAP: Ventilator-associated pneumonia; VLBW: Very low birth weight (birth weight <1500 g)

Acknowledgements

None.

Funding

None.

Authors' contributions

Sole author, not applicable.

Authors' information

On title page.

Competing interests

None.

References

1. Stoll BJ, Gordon T, Korones SB, et al. Late-onset sepsis in very low birth weight neonates: a report from the National Institute of Child Health and Human Development Neonatal Research Network. J Pediatr. 1996;129:63–71.
2. Stoll BJ, Hansen N, Fanaroff AA, et al. Late-onset sepsis in very low birth weight neonates; the experience of the NICHD Neonatal Research Network. Pediatrics. 2002;110:285–91.
3. Boghossian NS, Page GP, Bell EF, et al. Late-onset sepsis in very low birth weight infants from singleton and multiple gestation births. J Pediatr. 2013; 162:1120–4.
4. Stoll BJ, Hansen NI, Bell EF, et al. Trends in care practices, morbidity and mortality of extremely preterm neonates, 1993–2012. JAMA. 2015;314:1039–51.
5. Horbar JD, Carpenter JH, Badger GJ, et al. Mortality and neonatal morbidity among infants 501–1500 grams from 2000 to 2009. Pediatrics. 2012;129: 1019–26.
6. Shah J, Jeffries AL, Yoon EW, et al. Risk factors and outcomes of late-onsetbacterial sepsis in preterm neonates born at <32 weeks gestation. Am J Perinatol. 2015;32:675–82.

7. Cohen-Wolkowiez M, Moran C, Benjamin DK. Early and late-onset sepsis in late preterm infants. Pediatr Infect Dis J. 2009;28:1052–6.

8. Testoni D, Hayashi M, Cohen-Wolkowiecz M, et al. Late-onset bloodstream infections in hospitalized term infants. Pediatr Infect Dis J. 2014;33:920–3.

9. Nelson MU, Gallagher PG. Methicillin -resistant Staphylococus aureus in the neonatal intensive care unit. Semin Perinatol. 2012;36:424–30.

10. Gastmeier P, Loui A, Stamm-Balderjahn S, et al. Outbreaks in neonatal intensive care units-they are not like others. Am J Infect Control. 2007;35:172–6.

11. Stapleton PJM, Murphy M, McCallion N, Brennan M, Cunney R, Drew RJ. Outbreaks of extended spectrum beta-lactamase producing Enterobacteriaceae in neonatal intensive care units: a systematic review. Arch Dis Child Fetal Neonatal Ed. 2016;101:F72–8.

12. Engur D, Cakmak BC, Turkmen MK, Telli M, Eyigor M, Guzunier M. A milk pump as a source for spreading Acinetobacter baumannii in a neonatal intensive care unit. Breastfeed Med. 2014;9:551–4.

13. Nakamura K, Kaneko M, Abe Y, et al. Outbreak of extended spectrum β-lactamase producing Escherichia coli transmitted through breast milk sharing in a neonatal intensive care unit. J Hosp Infect. 2016;92:42–6.

14. Smith A, Saiman L, Zhou J, et al. Concordance of gastrointestinal tract colonization and subsequent bloodstream infections with gram-negative bacilli in very low birth weight infants in the neonatal intensive care unit. Pediatr Infect Dis J. 2010;29:831–5.

15. Madan JC, Slari RC, Saxena D, et al. Gut microbial colonization in premature neonates predicts neonatal sepsis. Arch Dis Child Fetal Neonatal Ed. 2012; 97:F456–62.

16. Srivastava S, Shetty N. Healthcare – associated infections in neonatal units: lessons from contrasting worlds. J Hosp Infect. 2007;65:292–306.

17. Zinna S, Lakshmanan A, Tan S, et al. Outcomes of nosocomial viral respiratory infections in high risk neonates. Pediatrics. 2016;138(5):e20161675.

18. Civardi E, Tzialla C, Baldani F, Strocchio L, Manzoni P, Stronati M, et al. Viral outbreaks in neonatal intensive care units: what we do not know. Am J Infect Control. 2013;41:854–6.

19. Davis J, Fairley D, Christie S, et al. Human parechovirus infection in neonatal intensive care. Pediatr Infect Dis J. 2015;34:121–4.

20. Nolan T, Berwick DM. All or none measurement raises the bar on performance. JAMA. 2006;295:1168–70.

21. Fisher D, Cochran KM, Provost LP, et al. Reducing central line – associated blood stream infections in North Carolina NICUs. Pediatrics. 2013;132:e1664–71.

22. Bolon MK. Hand hygiene: an update. Infect Dis Clin N Am. 2016;310:591–607.

23. World Health Organization. WHO guidelines for hand hygiene in health care; first global patient safety challenge: clean care is safer care. Geneva: WHO Press, World Health Organization; 2009.

24. Luangasanatip N, Hongsuwan M, Limmathurotsakul D, et al. Comparative efficacy of interventions to promote hand hygiene in hospital: systematic review and network meta-analysis. BMJ. 2015;351:h3728. doi:10.1136/bmj.h3728.

25. Morel AS, Wu F, Dell-Latta P, et al. Nosocomial transmission of methicillin – resistant Staphyoloccus aureus from a mother to her preterm quadruplet infants. Am J Infect Control. 2002;30:170–3.

26. McNeil SA, Foster CL, Hedderwick SA, Kauffman CA. Effect of hand cleansing with antimicrobial soap or alcohol based gel on microbial colonization of artificial fingernails worn by health care workers. Clin Infect Dis. 2001;32:367–72.

27. Moolenaar RL, Crutcher JM, San Joaquin VH, et al. A prolonged outbreak of pseudomonas aeruginosa in a neonatal intensive care unit: did staff fingernails play a role in disease transmission. Infect Control Hosp Epidemiol. 2000;21:80–3.

28. CDC MMWR Morbidity and Mortality Weekly Report. Guideline for hand hygiene in health care settings. Recommendations of the healthcare infection control practices advisory committee and the HICPAC/SHEA/APIC/IDSA Hand Hygiene Task Force. 2002; 51: No RR-16.

29. Arrowsmith VA, Taylor R. Removal of nail polish and finger rings to prevent surgical infection. Cochrane Database Syst Rev. 2014;8:CD003325.

30. Narayanan I, Prakash K, Murthy NS, Gujral VV. Randomized controlled trial of effect of raw and holder pasteurized human milk and of formula supplements on incidence of neonatal infection. Lancet. 1984;8412:1111–3.

31. Schanler RJ, Lau C, Hurst NM, Smith EO. Randomized trial of donor milk versus preterm formula as substitutes for mothers' own milk in the feeding of extremely premature infants. Pediatrics. 2005;116:400–6.

32. Furman L, Taylor G, Minich N, Hack M. The effect of maternal milk on neonatal morbidity of very low birth weight infants. Arch Pediatr Adolesc Med. 2003; 157:66–71.

33. Patel AL, Johnson TJ, Engstrom JL, et al. Impact of early human milk on sepsis and health care costs in very low birth weight infants. J Perinatol. 2013;33:514–9.

34. Flidel-Rimon O, Friedman S, Lev E, et al. Early enteral feeding and nosocomial sepsis in very low birth weight infants. Arch Dis Child Fetal Neonatal Ed. 2004; 89:F289–292.

35. Ronnestad A, Abrahamsen TG, Medbo S, et al. Late – onset septicemia in a Norwegian national cohort of extremely premature infants receiving very early full human milk feeding. Pediatrics. 2005;115:e269–76.

36. Meier P, Patel A, Esquerra-Zwiers A. Donor human milk update: evidence, mechanisms, and priorities for research and practice. J Pediatr. 2017;180:15–21.

37. Wilkins M, Hall-Stoodley L, Allan RN, Faust SN. New approaches to the treatment of biofilm – related infections. J Infect. 2014;69(Suppl1):S47–52.

38. Marschall J, Mermel LA, Fakih M, et al. Strategies to prevent central line associated bloodstream infections in acute care hospitals: 2014 update. Infection Cont Hosp Epidemiol. 2014;35:753–71.

39. Hocevar SN, Lessa FC, Gallgher L, Conover C, Gorwitz R, Iwamoto M. Infection prevention practices in neonatal intensive care units reporting to the national healthcare safety network. Infect Control Hosp Epidemiol. 2014;35:1126–32.

40. Taylor JE, McDonald SJ, Tan K. A survey of central venous catheter practices in Australian and New Zealand tertiary neonatal units. Aust Crit Care. 2014; 27:36–42.

41. Patrick SW, Kawai AT, Kleinman K, et al. Health-care associated infections among critically ill children in the US, 2007–2012. Pediatrics. 2014;134:705–12.

42. Shepherd EG, Kelly TJ, Vinsel JA, et al. Significant reduction of central line associated bloodstream infections in a network of diverse neonatal nurseries. J Pediatr. 2015;167:41–6.

43. Erdei C, MacAvoy LL, Gupta M, Pereira S, McGowan EC. Is zero central line associated bloodstream infection rate sustainable? A 5 year perspective. Pediatrics. 2015;135:e1485–93.

44. Rosenthal VD, Al-Abdely HM, El-Kholy AA, et al. International Nosocomial Infection control consortium report, data summary of 50 countries for 2010–2015: device associated module. Am J Infect Control. 2016;44:1495–1504.

45. Kaufman D, Boyle R, Hazen KC, Patrie JT, Robinson M, Donowitz LG. Fluconazole prophylaxis against antifungal colonization and infection in preterm infants. New Engl J Med. 2001;345:1660–6.

46. Manzoni P, Stolfi I, Pugni L, et al. A multicenter randomized trial of prophylactic fluconazole in preterm neonates. N Engl J Med. 2007;356:2483–95.

47. Benjamin Jr DK, Stoll BJ, Fanaroff AA, et al. Neonatal candidiasis among extremely low birth weight infants: risk factors, mortality rates, and neurodevelopmental outcomes at 18 to 22 months. Pediatrics. 2006;117: 84–92.

48. Aliaga S, Clark RH, Laughon M, et al. Changes in the incidence of candidiasis in neonatal intensive care units. Pediatrics. 2014;133:236–242.

49. Kaufman DA. "Getting to zero": preventing invasive Candida infections and eliminating infection-related mortality and morbidity in extremely preterm infants. Early Hum Dev. 2012;88S2:S45–9.

50. Aydemir C, Oguz SS, Dizdar EA, et al. Randomized controlled trial of prophylactic fluconazole versus nystatin for the prevention of fungal colonisation and invasive fungal infection in very low birth weight infants. Arch Dis Child Fetal Neonatal Ed. 2011;96:F164–8.

51. Benjamin Jr DK, Hudak ML, Duara S, et al. Effect of fluconazole prophylaxis on candidiasis and mortality in premature infants: a randomized clinical trial. JAMA. 2014;311:1742–9.

52. Cleminson J, McGuire W. Topical emollient for preventing infection in preterm infants. Cochrane Database Syst Rev. 2016;1:CD 001150.

53. Dudeck MA, Edwards JR, Allen-Bridson K, et al. National Healthcare Safety Network report, data summary for 2013, Device associated module. Am J Infect Control. 2015;43:206–21.

54. Garland JS. Strategies to prevent ventilatorassociated pneumonia in neonates. Clin Perinatol. 2010;37:629–43.

55. Apisarnthanarak A, Holzman-Pazgal G, Hamvas A, Olsen MA, Fraser VJ. Ventilator – associated pneumonia in extremely preterm neonates in an neonatal intensive care unit: characteristics, risk factors, and outcomes. Pediatrics. 2003;112:1283–9.

56. Azab SF, Sherbiny HS, Saleh SH, et al. reducing ventilator associated pneumonia in neonatal intensive care unit using "VAP prevention Bundle" : a cohort study. BMC Infect Dis. 2015;15:314.

57. Rosenthal VD, Rodriguez-Calderon ME, Rodriguez-Ferrer M, et al. Findings of the International Nosocomial Infection Control Consortium (INICC), Part II:

impact of a multidimensional strategy to reduce ventilator associated pneumonia in neonatal intensive care units in 10 developing countries. Infect Control Hosp Epidemiol. 2012;33:704–10.

58. Ohlsson A, Lacy JB. Intravenous immunoglobulin for preventing infection in preerm and/or low birth weight infants. Cochrane Database Syst Rev. 2013;2:CD000361.

59. Shah PS, Kaufman DA. Antistaphylococcal immunoglobulins to prevent staphylococcal infections in very low birth weight infants. Cochrane Database Syst Rev. 2009;2:CD006449.

60. Patel M, Kaufman DA. Anti-lipoteichoic acid monoclonal antibody (pagibaximab) studies for the prevention of staphylococcal bloodstream infections in preterm infants. Expert Opin Biol Ther. 2015;15:595–600.

61. Capasso L, Borrelli AC, Parrella C, et al. Are IgM enriched immunoglobulins an effective adjuvant in septic VLBW infants. Ital J Pediatr. 2013;39:63.

62. Manzoni P, Rinaldi M, Cattani S, et al. Bovine lactoferrin supplementation for prevention of late-onset sepsis in very low birth weight neonates. A randomized trial. JAMA. 2009;302:1421–8.

63. The ELFIN Trial Investigators Group. Lactoferrin immunoprophylaxis for very preterm infants. Arch Dis Child Fetal Neonatal Ed. 2013;98:F2–4.

64. Al Faleh K, Anabrees J. Probiotics for prevention of necrotizing enterocolitis in preterm infants. Cochrane Database Syst Rev. 2014;4:CD005496.

65. Rao SC, Athayle-Jape GK, Deshpande GC, Simmer KN, Patole SK. Probiotic supplementation and late-onset sepsis in preterm infants: a meta-analysis. Pediatrics. 2016;137:e20153684.

66. Jacobs SE, Tobin JM, Opie GF, et al. Probiotic effects on late onset sepsis in very preterm infants: a randomized controlled trial. Pediatrics. 2013;132: 1055–62.

67. Costoloe K, Hardy P, Juszczak E, et al. Bifidobacterium breve BBG-001 in very preterm infants: a randomized controlled phase 3 trial. Lancet. 2016;387: 649–60.

68. Bertelli C, Pillonel T, Torregrossa A, et al. Bifidobacterium longum bacteremia in preterm infants receiving probiotics. Clin Infect Dis. 2015;15:924–7.

69. Underwood MA, Gaerlan S, DeLeoz LA, et al. Human milk oligosaccharides in premature infants: absorption, excretion and influence on the intestinal microbiota. Pediatr Res. 2015;78(6):670–7.

70. Vongbhavit K, Underwood MA. Prevention of necrotizing enterocolitis though manipulation of the intestinal microbiota of the premature infant. Clin Therapeutics. 2016;38:716–32.

71. Srinivasjois R, Rao S, Patole S. Prebiotic supplementation in preterm neonates: updated systematic review and meta-analysis of randomized controlled trials. Clin Nutr. 2013;32:958–65.

72. Underwood MA, Salzman NH, Bennett SH, et al. A randomized placebo controlled comparison of two prebiotic-probiotic combinations in preterm infants: impact on weight gain, intestinal microbiota, and fecal short chain fatty acids. J Pediatr Gastroenterol Nutr. 2009;48:216–25.

73. Schulman J, Dimand RJ, Lee HC. Neonatal intensive care unit antibiotic use. Pediatrics. 2015;135:826–33.

74. Cotten CM, Taylor S, Stoll B, et al. Prolonged duration of initial empirical antibiotic treatment is associated with increased rates of necrotizing enterocolitis and death for extremely low birth weight infants. Pediatrics. 2009;123:58–66.

75. Kuppala V, Meinzen-Derr J, Morrow A, Schibler KR. Prolonged initial antibiotic treatment is associated with adverse outcomes on premature infants. J Pediatr. 2011;159:720–5.

76. Greenwood C, Morrow AL, Lagomarcino AJ, et al. Early empiric antibiotic use in preterm infants is associated with lower bacterial diversity and higher relative abundance of Enterobacter. J Pediatr. 2014;165:23–9.

77. Arboleya S, Sanchez B, Milani C, et al. Intestinal microbiota development in preterm neonates and effect of perinatal antibiotics. J Pediatr. 2015;166:538–44.

78. Clark RH, Bloom BT, Spitzer AR, Gerstman DR. Empirical use of ampicillin and cefotaxime, compared with ampicillin and gentamicin for neonates at risk for sepsis is associated with an increased risk of neonatal death. Pediatrics. 2006;117:67–74.

79. Vermont Oxford Network iNICQ 2017. Choosing Antibiotics Wisely https:// public.vtoxford.org/quality-education/inicq-2017-choosing-antibiotics-wisely/. Accessed 2 Nov 2016.

80. Carr D, Barnes EH, Gordon A, Isaacs D. Effect of antimicrobial antibiotic resistance and lat onset neonatal infections over 25 years in an Australian tertiary neonatal unit. Arch Dis Child Fetal neonatal Ed. 2016; 0: F1-F7.

81. Obiero CW, Seale AC, Berkley JA. Empiric treatment of neonatal sepsis in developing countries. Pediatr Infect Dis J. 2015;34:659–61.

82. Van den Anker JN. How to optimize the evaluation and use of antibiotics in neonates. Early Hum Dev. 2014;90S1:S10–2.

83. Ericson JE, Thaden J, Cross HR, et al. No survival benefit with empiricial vancomycin therapy for coagulase – negative staphylococcal bloodstream infections in neonates. Pediatr Infect Dis J. 2015;34:371–5.

84. Thaden JT, Ericson JE, Cross H, et al. Survival benefit of empirical therapy for staphylococcus aureus bloodstream infections in infants. Pediatr Infect Dis J. 2015;34:1175–9.

85. Cohen-Wolkowiez M, Poindexter B, Bidegain M, et al. Safety and effectiveness of meropenem in infants with suspected or complicated intra-abdominal infections. Clin Infect Dis. 2012;55:1495–502.

86. Autmizguine J, Hornik CP, Benjamin Jr DK, et al. Anaerobic antimicrobial therapy after necrotizing enterocolitis in VLBW infants. Pediatrics. 2015;135: e117–25.

87. Botero-Calderon L, Benjamin Jr DK, Cohen-Wolkowiez M. Advances in the treatment of invasive neonatal candidiasis. Expert Opiin Pharmacother. 2015;16:1035–48.

88. Benjamin Jr DK, Miller W, Garges H, et al. Bacteremia, central catheters, and neonates: when to pull the line. Pediatrics. 2001;107:1272–6.

89. Stoll BJ, Hansen NI, Adams-Chapman I, National Institute of Child Health and Human Development Neonatal Research Network, et al. Neurodevelopmental and growth impairment among extremely low-birth-weight infants with neonatal infection. JAMA. 2004;292(19):2357–65.

90. Song X, Perencevich E, Campos J, Short BL, Singh N. Clinical and economic impact of methicillin – resistant Staphylococcus aureus colonization or infection on neonates in intensive care units. Infect Control Hosp Epidemiol. 2010;31:177–82.

91. Dawczynski K, Proquitte H, Roedel J, et al. Intensified colonization screening according to the recommendations of the German Commission for Hospital Hygiene and Infectious Diseases Prevention (KRINKO): identification and containment of a Serratia marcescens outbreak in the neonatal intensive care unit, Jena, Germany, 2013–2014. Infection. DOI: 10.1007/s15010-016-0922-y.

92. Leshem E, Maayan-Metzger A, Rahav G, et al. Transmission of Staphylococcus aureus from mothers to newborns. Pediatr Infect Dis J. 2012;31:360–3.

93. Ericson JE, Popola VO, Smith B, et al. Burden of invasive Staphylococcus aureus infections in hospitalized infants. JAMA Pediatr. 2015;169:1105–11.

94. Gerber SI, Jones RC, Scott MV, et al. Management of outbreaks of methicillin resistant Staphylococcus aureus infection in the neonatal intensive care unit: a consensus statement. Infect Control Hosp Epidemiol. 2006;27:139–145.

95. Delany HM, Wang E, Melish M. Comprehensive strategy including prophylactic mupirocin to reduce Staphylococcus aureus colonization and infection in high risk neonates. J Perinatol. 2013;33:313–8.

96. Popoola VO, Budd A, Wittig SM, et al. MRSA transmission and infections in a neonatal intensive care unit despite active surveillance cultures and decolonization-challenges for infection prevention. Infect Control Hosp Epidemiol. 2014;35:412–8.

6

A physiologic approach to cord clamping: Clinical issues

Susan Niermeyer ⓘ

Abstract

Background: Recent experimental physiology data and a large, population-based observational study have changed umbilical cord clamping from a strictly time-based construct to a more complex equilibrium involving circulatory changes and the onset of respirations in the newly born infant. However, available evidence is not yet sufficient to optimize the management of umbilical cord clamping.

Findings: Current guidelines vary in their recommendations and lack advice for clinicians who face practical dilemmas in the delivery room. This review examines the evidence around physiological outcomes of delayed cord clamping and cord milking vs. immediate cord clamping. Gaps in the existing evidence are highlighted, including the optimal time to clamp the cord and the interventions that should be performed before clamping in infants who fail to establish spontaneous respirations or are severely asphyxiated, as well as those who breathe spontaneously.

Conclusion: Behavioral and technological changes informed by further research are needed to promote adoption and safe practice of physiologic cord clamping.

Keywords: Umbilical cord, Placental transfusion, Resuscitation, Respiration, Infant, Newborn, Infant, Premature

Background

"In the time of Hippocrates the cord was not cut until the placenta was delivered....Since the time of Levret it has been established as a general rule, among accoucheurs, to separate the child from the mother as soon as it has passed through the vulva, and that it is never necessary to wait for the expulsion of the foetal appendages. At first view the conduct of the ancients appears to be more rational and more physiological than that of the moderns; it seems that the placenta ought immediately to follow the foetus, or at least be separated from the uterus before the cord can be prudently cut; that before it is divided, the circulation ought to be permitted gradually to take on its new type, which soon becomes similar to that of the adult; but in reality it is not perceived that the present mode of practice produces the least inconvenience to the foetus, and is certainly better for the mother." [1]

– Prof. A.A. Velpeau, 1829 [1]

Correspondence: susan.niermeyer@ucdenver.edu
Section of Neonatology, University of Colorado School of Medicine, 13121 E. 17th Avenue, Mail Stop 8402, Aurora, CO 80045, USA

For centuries, lively debate has surrounded the question of when to clamp and cut the umbilical cord of the newly born infant, and practices have ranged from one extreme to the other. From the time of the Ancient Greeks, midwives have described the value of waiting to clamp the cord until pulsations stop or until the placenta is delivered [1]. This approach is taken to its furthest modern extent in Lotus birth, when the umbilical cord and placenta remain attached to the infant until natural separation at the umbilicus occurs after several days. As Prof. Velpeau pointed out in his Treatise on Midwifery in 1829, a different practice arose among *accoucheurs*, male midwives or obstetricians, who perceived that immediate cord clamping and cutting offered benefit to the mother and posed no "inconvenience" to the newborn [1]. Recently, the obstetrical practice of immediate cord clamping has been modified by policy statements from the American College of Obstetricians and Gynecologists (ACOG), the Royal College of Obstetricians and Gynaecologists, and the The Royal College of Midwives [2–4]. The ACOG statement received endorsement from the American Academy of Pediatrics [5]; the International Liaison

Table 1 Targets for further research on physiologic umbilical cord clamping

Population

    Extremely low birth weight/extremely preterm infants

    Infants with evidence of asphyxia – antepartum/intrapartum

    Infants born in low-resource settings

Intervention (delayed cord clamping with multiple covariates)

    Antenatal corticosteroid administration before preterm birth

    Type of maternal anesthesia

    Uterine activity (contractions or operative delivery without labor)

    Administration of uterotonic relative to cord clamping

    Onset of respirations relative to cord clamping

        Spontaneous

        Assisted ventilation

    Position of infant relative to placenta

    Duration of delay before clamping

Comparison

Delay in cord clamping with and without resuscitation

    Initial steps (drying, clearing airway, specific stimulation to breathe)

    Positive-pressure ventilation

        Sustained inflation

        CPAP

        Intermittent positive-pressure ventilation

Umbilical cord milking vs. delayed cord clamping

    Active milking (length of cord segment, rate, number of passes)

    Draining of cord segment

Outcome

Need for resuscitation

Physiologic characteristics during postnatal stabilization

    Temperature

    Blood pressure

    Blood glucose

    Need for volume expanders/pressors (per defined criteria)

    Regional blood flow – e.g. cerebral

Hemoglobin/hematocrit/iron status

Blood volume

Need for transfusion (per defined criteria)

Complications of prematurity

    Intracranial hemorrhage/periventricular leukomalacia

    Necrotizing enterocolitis

    Bronchopulmonary dysplasia/duration of supplemental oxygen

    Patent ductus arteriosus

Hyperbilirubinemia

    Premature and term infants

    Populations at high risk (genetic variations)

    Settings with limited access to phototherapy

Table 1 Targets for further research on physiologic umbilical cord clamping (Continued)

Polycythemia

    Term infants and growth-restricted infants

    Technique-specific differences (delayed clamping vs. umbilical cord milking)

Neurodevelopment

    Toddler, preschool, elementary school outcomes

    Sex-specific differences

    Correlation with iron status

    Brain microstructure/development (advanced imaging i.e. MRI)

Behavior

    Prevalence/duration of exclusive breastfeeding

Mortality

Maternal obstetrical outcomes

    Physiologic characteristics postpartum

    Postpartum hemorrhage

    Intraoperative complications

Committee on Resuscitation recommended delayed cord clamping for infants who do not require immediate resuscitation [6]; and the World Health Organization (WHO) reiterated their recommendation to delay cord clamping for 1–3 min while initiating simultaneous essential newborn care [7]. Still, all current practice guidelines vary slightly in their emphasis and details, and all suggest that delayed cord clamping may not be feasible or desirable in every situation, especially when immediate resuscitation is required. This review will relate recent experimental physiology data to clinical studies, examine the practical dilemmas faced by clinicians, and identify gaps in knowledge as well as directions for further research to more fully define a physiologic approach to cord clamping.

Findings
Physiology of umbilical cord clamping

Physiologic data from experimental animals have changed the frame of reference for umbilical cord clamping from a strictly time-based construct to a more complex equilibrium between the circulatory changes accompanying the onset of respirations and completion of the circulatory and respiratory functions of the placenta. In an accompanying article, Hooper et al. describe in detail the differences in heart rate, right ventricular output, carotid artery pressure and flow, and pulmonary and ductus arteriosus blood flow encountered with immediate cord clamping before onset of respirations vs. delay in cord clamping until after ventilation in anesthetized preterm lambs [8, 9].

At birth, the function of respiration shifts from the placenta to the infant's lungs, as they expand first with air and then with a large increase in pulmonary blood flow. During fetal life, placental blood passes through the umbilical vein and ductus venosus to the right atrium, where it primarily streams across the foramen ovale to provide preload for the left ventricle (Fig. 1). Systemic fetal venous return also enters the right atrium and passes into the right ventricle; however, only a small percentage of total right ventricular output passes through the lungs. Most right ventricular output diverts via the ductus arteriosus to the descending aorta where it perfuses fetal organs or returns to the placenta via the umbilical arteries. When breathing begins, much more of the right ventricular output flows to the lungs and placental blood maintains ventricular preload. As the pulmonary circuit fills, pulmonary blood return to the left atrium gradually increases to serve as preload for the systemic circulation. In the process, pulmonary vascular resistance falls, right heart pressure falls, and the foramen ovale functionally closes [10, 11]. When the umbilical cord remains intact as a healthy infant begins breathing, the shift in respiratory function from placenta to lungs is accompanied by a physical shift in blood volume from the placenta to the newly born infant to maintain circulatory equilibrium as the pulmonary vascular bed opens.

If the umbilical cord is clamped before breathing begins, systemic blood pressure rises with loss of the low-resistance placental circuit and still-high pulmonary vascular

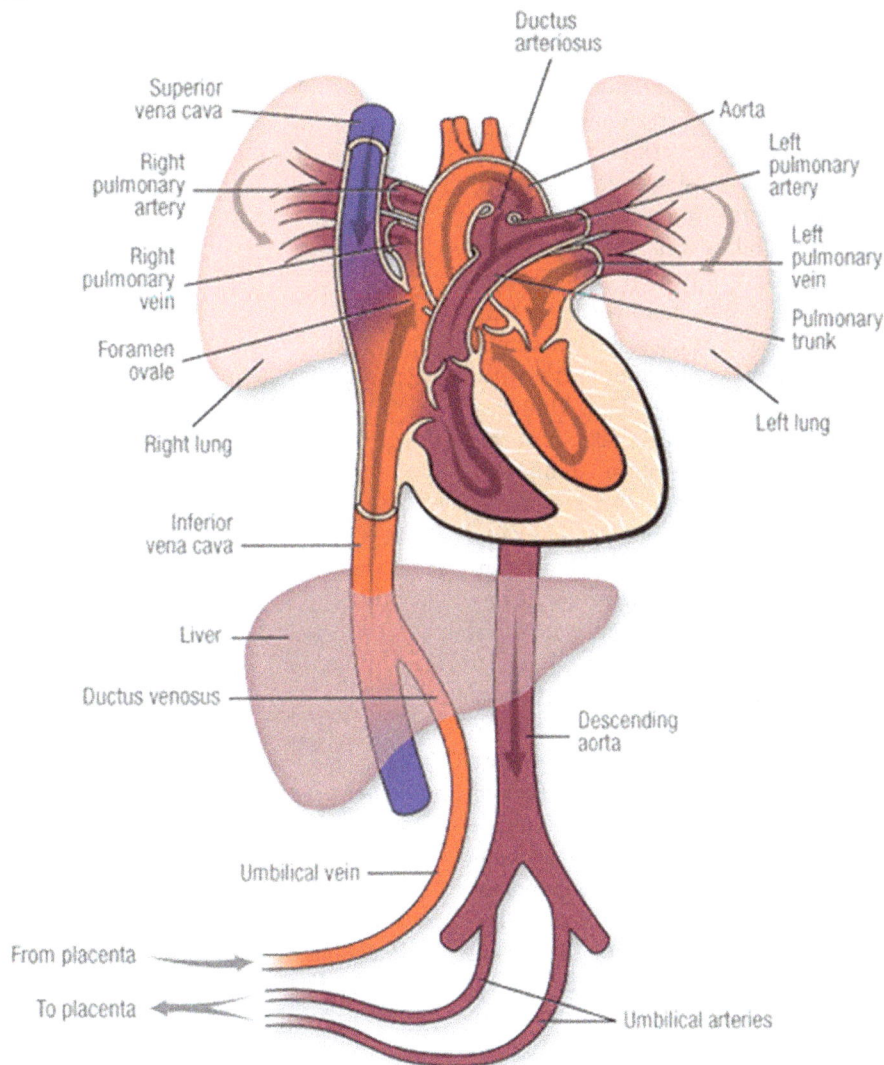

Fig. 1 Schematic of the fetal circulation (http://www.heart.org/HEARTORG/Conditions/CongenitalHeartDefects/SymptomsDiagnosisofCongenitalHeartDefects/Fetal-Circulation_UCM_315674_Article.jsp)

resistance preventing left-to-right flow through the ductus arteriosus. There follows a loss of preload to the left ventricle which results in a steep fall in cardiac output [12]. If there is delay in establishing respirations, hypoxemia also ensues, potentially resulting in postnatal hypoxic-ischemic conditions. Compensatory mechanisms move circulating volume from the peripheral to central circulation. Only when pulmonary vascular resistance falls does pulmonary blood flow increase through right ventricular outflow and left-to-right shunting through the ductus arteriosus. Pulmonary venous return to the left atrium then restores left ventricular preload, cardiac output, and systemic pressure [9, 13].

Reaching the point of circulatory equilibrium in the transition from placental to pulmonary respiration requires a variable amount of time, depending on the individual circumstances at birth. Various lines of data from early physiological studies suggest that the transition usually lasts several minutes [14]. In ventilated lambs, pulmonary blood flow reaches a maximum only after 5–10 min [15]. Measurement of residual placental blood volume in human infants describes rapid transfer of blood initially, followed by slower rate of transfer documented through 3 min or more [16] (Fig. 2). Measurements of actual umbilical vein flow by dye dilution follow a similar pattern in healthy term infants, with high flow in the first 2 min, followed by a variable decrease [17]. More recent studies show a similar pattern of increase in infant weight after birth when the umbilical circulation remains intact [18]. Umbilical Doppler blood flow patterns immediately after birth are highly variable, but flow may continue up to 10 min [19]. Electrical impedance measurements show an increase in cardiac output through 3–5 min in the majority of infants [20]. Experimental and clinical physiological data are generally consistent in suggesting that reaching circulatory equilibrium requires several minutes, even under ideal circumstances.

A single large, population-based observational study of infants in a resource-limited setting in Tanzania reported an association between the timing of umbilical cord clamping relative to the onset of spontaneous respirations and the outcomes of death or admission to a special care area [21]. The cohort of 12,730 term and preterm infants was selected on the criterion that all established spontaneous respirations and received only routine care. They were judged to be healthy and strong by the delivering midwives. Independent observers documented the timing of key interventions and infant responses at all deliveries. Variation in the time of umbilical cord clamping occurred as the facility transitioned from the previous practice of immediate cord clamping to a new routine of cord clamping delayed for 1–3 min. Special care in the neonatal area was limited to administration of antibiotics and

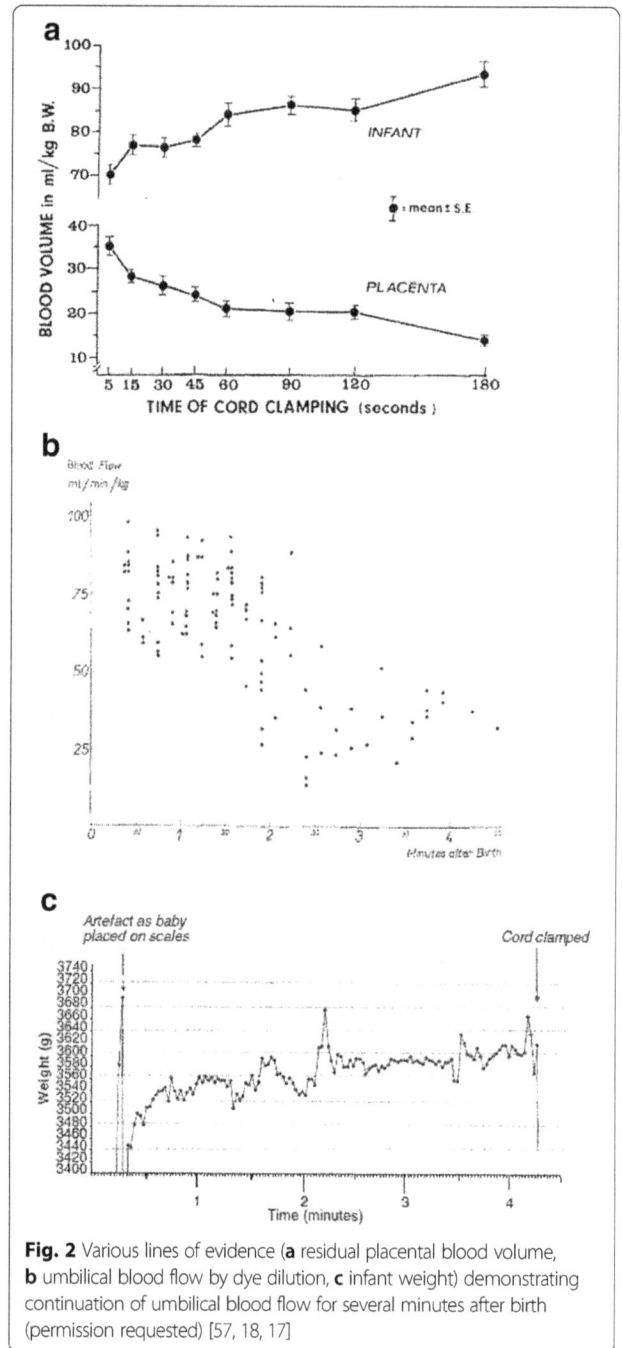

Fig. 2 Various lines of evidence (**a** residual placental blood volume, **b** umbilical blood flow by dye dilution, **c** infant weight) demonstrating continuation of umbilical blood flow for several minutes after birth (permission requested) [57, 18, 17]

intravenous fluids. Logistic modelling showed the risk of death/admission to the special care area by 24 h was consistently higher if cord clamping occurred before spontaneous respirations. Risk of death or admission decreased by 20 % for every 10-s delay in cord clamping after spontaneous respiration up to 2 min. Death/admission occurred more frequently in infants of low birth weight (<2500 g) and preterm gestational age; however the described relationship held in both normal weight and low birth weight infants. In a setting where cardiorespiratory or even general supportive care was not available to buffer physiologic derangements, the impact of cord clamping before onset of respirations manifested as increased risk of death and instability, and delay in cord clamping through 2 min had a dose-dependent effect of decreasing that risk.

Although the physiological data and clinical data from resource-limited settings indicate a clear and important relationship between onset of respirations and the timing of cord clamping, the situations faced by clinicians are complex and variable. Available literature does not yet provide sufficient high-quality evidence to address management with complications such as intrapartum asphyxia, fetal growth restriction, or extreme prematurity. While some data on physiologic outcomes exist, primary outcomes have more commonly related to hemoglobin/hematocrit and volume of placental transfusion. Thus, there are gaps in the existing evidence to guide management, and clinicians face a number of dilemmas, including:

- Timing – What is the optimal time to clamp the cord in term and preterm infants who breathe spontaneously, fail to establish spontaneous respirations, or are severely asphyxiated? Should resuscitative interventions be performed during the interval before clamping to stimulate breathing or begin assisted ventilation?
- Technique – does umbilical cord milking offer equivalent or superior outcomes to delayed cord clamping? What is the interplay of umbilical cord milking and onset of respirations?
- To be determined – what gaps in knowledge, skills, and technological support impede the adoption and safe practice of physiologic cord clamping in the clinical setting?

Timing: optimizing the relationship between cord clamping and onset of respirations

"If a careful attention be paid to what happens after an ordinary birth, it will be seen that the pulsations grow weaker and soon disappear in the cord, beginning at the placenta, and that after a few minutes it may be cut without being followed by the least hemorrhage. This remarkable phenomenon which is attributed to the change of direction of the iliac arteries, and to the difficulty experienced by the blood in passing into the aorta through the ductus arteriosus, and into the cord through the umbilical arteries, always takes place where everything occurs in a natural and regular order, but in reality depends upon the circumstance that the attractive force exerted by the placenta upon the blood, is replaced by that of the respiratory organ, and that the after-birth is no

longer anything more than an inert substance, without vitality, which is abandoned by the blood, as it abandons a gangrenous or asphyxiated limb." [2]

The clinician is faced with a number of uncertainties before the delivery of a newborn. Will the lungs be mature? Will the baby cry and breathe spontaneously? Will an acute intrapartum hypoxic-ischemic event or an obstetrical circumstance preclude delayed cord clamping? The answers to each of these may become apparent only at the moment of delivery, yet they all potentially influence management of umbilical cord clamping and immediate care of the newly born infant. The available evidence relating to physiologic outcomes for term and preterm infants who breathe spontaneously can help guide clinical practice. The limited data from babies who are born in either primary or secondary apnea help to frame gaps in knowledge and suggest practical approaches to management and further research.

Spontaneous cry in term infants

The healthy term infant who cries spontaneously and breathes well often accomplishes the crucial first moments of circulatory transition with an intact umbilical cord, even when clamping is not deliberately delayed. Early physiological studies of residual placental blood volume demonstrated that a relatively larger proportion of the fetoplacental blood volume resides in the fetus at term as compared to earlier in gestation. Spontaneous cry before umbilical cord clamping significantly increases the volume of placental transfusion and hematocrit [22]. The curve of blood volume transferred vs. time as constructed by Yao highlights that more than half of the total blood transfer occurs within the first minute [16]. Among healthy term infants delivered vaginally, position at the perineum or on the mother's abdomen/chest does not significantly affect the volume of placental transfusion when clamping is delayed until 2 min [23]. Umbilical vein flow, as measured by dye dilution, is fastest in the first 1–2 min and slows variably thereafter [17]. Doppler ultrasound of umbilical blood flow patterns immediately after birth reveals highly variable flow duration and direction in both the umbilical artery and vein. Flow continues longer than previously described, with flow documented in some cases at the time of cord clamping between 5 and 10 min. In addition, the presence of cord pulsations does not necessarily signify ongoing flow, and cessation of pulsations can occur with or without flow [19].

Most literature examining clinical outcomes of delayed cord clamping in term infants reports primary outcomes related to volume of placental transfusion and/or hematocrit and relatively few secondary physiological endpoints. Meta-analysis of trials in term infants confirms that not only are acute measures of blood volume and hematocrit generally improved among infants with delayed clamping, but indices of iron status in infancy are also improved [24]. This has important implications in the prevention of iron-deficiency anemia and the associated sequelae of impaired cognitive, motor and behavioral development. While the global burden of iron deficiency anemia is greatest in sub-Saharan Africa and Southeast Asia, improvement in hematologic indices occurs even in highly developed industrialized countries such as Sweden [25]. Although short-term neurodevelopmental outcome showed no difference, follow-up at 4 years of a cohort of term Swedish infants with clamping delayed until 3 min shows improved processing speed, fine motor and personal-social scores compared to infants with immediate clamping [26, 27]. Another behavioural outcome of potential significance is the observation of improved rates of exclusive or predominant breastfeeding after hospital discharge [28]. One postulated linking mechanism is improved physiologic stability and alertness in the hour immediately after birth, promoting successful early initiation of breastfeeding, which in turn increases the duration of breastfeeding and the likelihood of exclusive breastfeeding through 4 months of life [29]. Studies of skin temperature in the days after birth support improved physiologic stability in late-clamped term infants and give indirect evidence for peripheral cutaneous vasoconstriction among those with early clamping. Infants with cord clamping delayed until pulsations stopped (average 3 min and 38 s) show significantly higher heel and palm temperatures than the group with immediate clamping, but no difference in epigastric or rectal temperatures [30]. Physiologic studies of cardiac and haematological indices show transient alterations consistent with increased circulating red cell volume but no systematic evidence of increased need for special care (i.e. for hyperviscosity/polycythemia or respiratory distress) [31–34].

In practice there is evidence to support a delay of two minutes or more, while providing routine care, before clamping the umbilical cord of the healthy term newborn. There is presently no accepted clinical sign indicating that circulatory equilibrium has been achieved between the newly born infant and the placenta. The midwifery literature describes "flattening" of the cord (Fig. 3) as a correlate for completion of the placental transfusion [35] and cessation of pulsation also has been used as an endpoint. Position at the introitus or on the mother's abdomen appears equivalent for the vigorous term infant [23]. Routine care at vaginal delivery, including thorough drying, any necessary clearing of the airway, thermal protection (skin-to-skin contact with mother), and monitoring of breathing, can occur during the delay before clamping and cutting the cord. At caesarean section, the infant can be placed between the mother's legs on the sterile field and routine care can be provided with warmed, sterile towels for drying. Although skin-to-skin contact cannot occur during the delay at caesarean section, the infant can be positioned skin-to-skin with the mother above the anesthesia barrier drape immediately after dividing the cord. This requires that the mother be alert under regional anesthesia and supported by the continuous presence of a nurse to monitor the infant's condition and safe positioning [36].

Variable establishment of respirations in preterm infants

"I once received a human foetus, at the sixth month of pregnancy, enclosed within its membranes. The umbilical arteries continued to beat strongly as long as the membranes were unruptured; but they fell into inertia as soon as the lungs and chest, upon coming in contact with the air, attempted to perform some respiratory movements. And do we not every day see the blood flow or stop spontaneously in the same child, accordingly as the respiration is free or embarrassed?" [3]

The preterm infant who is healthy may cry and breathe spontaneously or may have delayed onset of spontaneous respirations or shallow, irregular breathing after birth [37]. When general anesthesia at preterm delivery is necessary for maternal medical or obstetrical conditions, the newly

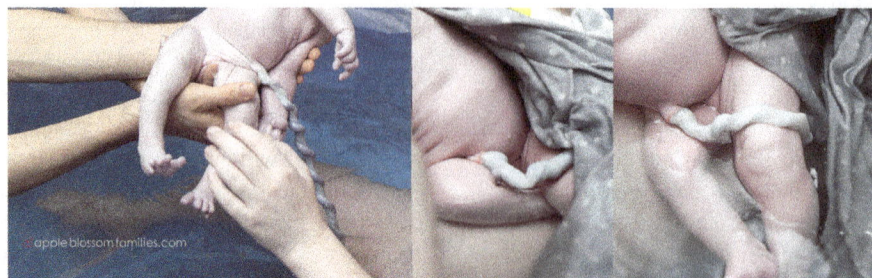

Fig. 3 Change in appearance of the umbilical cord from birth, to 12 and 23 min after birth, with umbilical cord intact and completion of third stage of labor at 30 min (appleblossomfamilies.com, Morag Hastings, photographer)

born infant may be completely apneic, although not asphyxiated, and require positive-pressure ventilation for lung expansion. Preterm infants manifest increased vulnerability to end-organ injury in the cerebral and intestinal circulations (intracranial haemorrhage and necrotizing enterocolitis), making ventilation of the lung prior to umbilical cord clamping and smooth cardiovascular transition theoretically even more desirable. Yet, very few human studies have explored the physiologic changes around respiration and cord clamping in preterm births.

Much of the literature reporting clinical outcomes of delayed cord clamping in preterm infants reports primary outcomes related to volume of placental transfusion and hemoglobin/hematocrit with some additional secondary physiological endpoints. Multiple small, randomized controlled trials and several meta-analyses confirm higher hematocrit at birth and decreased need for transfusion during hospitalization [38]. There is also evidence for improved cardiovascular stability, with higher mean blood pressure at 1 and 4 h after birth [39–42], higher measured blood volume [43, 44] and higher superior vena cava flow [45, 46]. Two major preterm morbidities, intracranial hemorrhage (all grades) and necrotizing enterocolitis, occur less frequently among infants who received delayed cord clamping. However, severe intracranial haemorrhage (grades III and IV) and mortality to discharge do not differ between groups. Temperature on admission to a newborn area does not differ; the rate of hyperbilirubinemia treated with phototherapy and the peak serum bilirubin are higher after delayed cord clamping, but criteria for treatment vary widely [38]. Two randomized trials have reported neurodevelopmental outcome (Bayley II scores), at 7 or 18–24 months age, showing no difference in Mental Developmental Index < 70, but very wide confidence intervals [47].

Two large observational studies with comparison groups report intermediate physiologic outcomes as part of quality improvement programs introducing delayed cord clamping for preterm infants [48, 49]. Very-low-birth-weight (VLBW) infants with delayed cord clamping received less delivery room resuscitation (supplemental oxygen, bag and mask ventilation, intubation, compressions, medications) compared to the immediate cord clamping group (61 vs. 79 %, $p = 0.01$), but there was no difference between groups among low-birth-weight (LBW) infants (30 vs. 27 %). The second study reported no difference in the need for ventilation in the delivery room among infant 24–34 weeks gestation [49]. Blood pressure in the first 2 days of life was higher in LBW late-clamped infants, but not different between the VLBW groups [48]. Mean temperature was in the normal range but higher for infants compliant with delayed cord clamping, and the incidence of temperature < 36.3C was decreased in this group [49]. In both studies, health care providers could clamp the cord if they felt it necessary; 6 of 249 infants [48] had delayed clamping abandoned to begin immediate resuscitation, and 12 of 236 infants [49] remained apneic and inactive after 20 s of assessment, prompting delayed clamping to be abandoned.

For the clinician, there is insufficient strong evidence to guide either the length of the delay before clamping the umbilical cord or the extent of resuscitative interventions provided to preterm infants during a delay. In many trials, no resuscitative intervention was provided; in other studies, infants were provided the initial steps of resuscitation (drying, positioning and clearing the airway as needed, specific stimulation to breathe i.e. rubbing the back) [43, 48]. Theoretical and practical challenges merit carefully controlled trials of beginning positive-pressure ventilation with intact umbilical circulation. Although positive-pressure ventilation may be necessary to aerate the lung and increase pulmonary blood flow, experimental animal studies suggest excessive end-expiratory pressure or mean airway pressure may not only cause lung injury, but may also impair cardiovascular transition and result in potential cerebral injury [50].

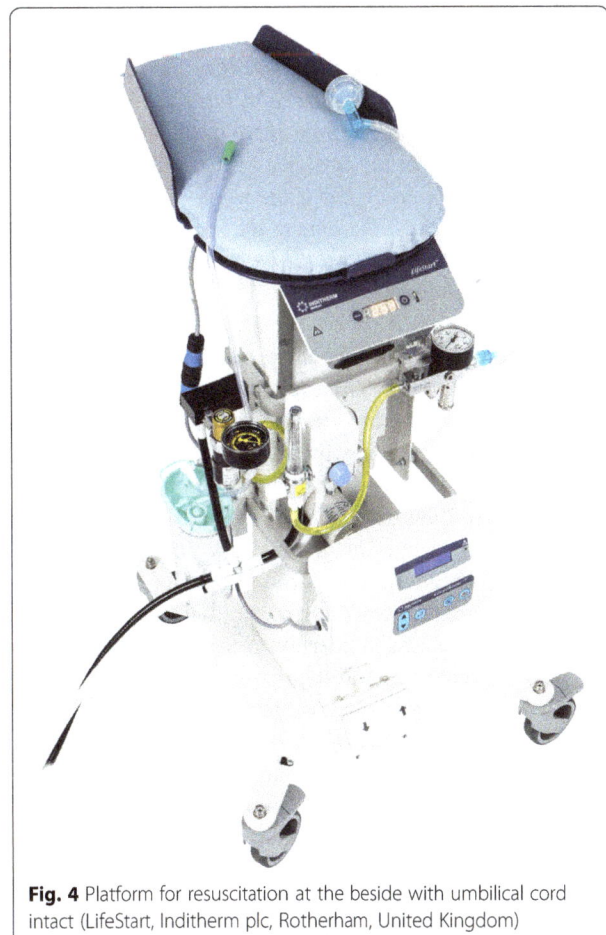

Fig. 4 Platform for resuscitation at the beside with umbilical cord intact (LifeStart, Inditherm plc, Rotherham, United Kingdom)

The physical arrangement necessary to provide positive-pressure ventilation calls for collaboration between providers caring for the mother and those caring for the newly born infant. A small trial has demonstrated the feasibility and acceptability of a compact, adjustable resuscitation platform (Fig. 4) which can be positioned close to the perineum at normal and assisted vaginal birth or the abdominal incision at caesarean section [51]. Alternatively, a flat, dry, firm surface can be positioned at the perineum on the unbroken delivery bed or on the mother's legs at caesarean section. Use of a t-piece device for ventilation or CPAP limits the equipment introduced into the field of the delivery or the sterile field at caesarean section. Delayed cord clamping may require modification of routines for thermal protection with polyethylene wrap or bags. However, contemporary observational cohorts suggest that improved placental transfusion may help maintain body temperature [48, 49]. Randomized controlled trials using a package of interventions addressing cord clamping, initial support of breathing/positive-pressure ventilation, low supplemental oxygen, and thermal protection will be challenging, but vital to ascertain the real potential of these interventions combined.

Asphyxia and secondary apnea in term or preterm infants

"Where there is reason to believe that the placenta still maintains a part of its natural relations with the womb, and especially where there is still some tremour, some pulsation in the cord, we may follow the advice... not to cut it too soon; but if the womb be well contracted, if the adhesions of the placenta be evidently destroyed, it would be better to separate the fœtus at once from its mother." [4]

The asphyxiated term or preterm infant presents unique physiological circumstances around umbilical cord clamping. Early literature suggests that antepartum asphyxia is accompanied by in utero transfer of blood volume from the placenta to the fetal circulation [52–54]. Data from dye-dilution studies of the umbilical circulation in term asphyxiated infants support lower flow rates immediately after birth compared to healthy controls [55]. In contrast, acute intrapartum asphyxial events, such as tight nuchal cord or shoulder dystocia, may be accompanied by cord occlusion and hypovolemia. In either setting, with severe hypoxia-ischemia, the myocardium and the cerebral circulation may be particularly vulnerable to further insult from immediate clamping of the cord. The resultant loss of preload and transient decrease in cardiac output are likely to produce bradycardia, swings in cerebral perfusion, and further interruption in blood flow to the renal, gastrointestinal, and pulmonary circulation. Although the volume of blood transferred after birth may be reduced or increased compared to non-asphyxiated infants, the maintenance of a patent umbilical circulation at least until ventilation has been established may limit further injury. However, chest compressions in the setting of intact umbilical circulation theoretically could fail to generate the diastolic pressure vital for coronary perfusion and return of spontaneous circulation because of the large, low-resistance vascular bed in the placenta [56]. There is also theoretical concern that hydrostatic pressure resulting from the relative position of infant and placenta may exert a substantial effect on the direction/volume of blood transfer in the setting of asphyxia [57].

Management of umbilical cord clamping in the asphyxiated term or preterm infant has received little attention in recent randomized controlled trials; usually the need for immediate resuscitation has constituted a criterion for exclusion. The logistic challenges of conducting an extensive resuscitation, including possible need for immediate intubation, chest compressions, and umbilical line placement for medication administration, argue for use of a specialized resuscitation platform for initial management proximate to the field of delivery. Once the initial steps of resuscitation and lung expansion have been accomplished, the infant can be relocated for more extensive interventions.

Technique: cord milking as an alternative to delayed cord clamping

"In the time of Aristotle the midwives were in the habit of forcing the blood contained in the cord into the belly of the fœtus before they tied it, and pretended by means of this practice, which has been revived at the commencement of the present century, to restore strength and vigour to feeble children." [5]

Cord milking offers an alternative to delayed cord clamping for facilitation of placental transfusion. Cord milking typically involves compressing the blood from a 20–30 cm segment of cord into the infant over 2–3 s; usually this procedure is repeated three times, allowing the umbilical vessels to refill from the placental side between milking [58]. To maximize transfer of blood, coils in the umbilical cord must be untwisted first. When there is great urgency, the cord can be immediately clamped close to the placental side, suspended over the infant on the resuscitation platform, and milked or passively drained as resuscitative interventions begin. Measurement of residual blood volume in the umbilical cords of extremely preterm infants estimates the volume contained in a 30-cm segment of cord at approximately 17 mL/kg [59]. The residual volume tended to be reduced in the cords of infants with low weight for gestational age.

The evidence base for umbilical cord milking is more limited than that for delayed umbilical cord clamping. Meta-analysis of five small randomized controlled trials in preterm infants < 33 weeks shows higher initial levels of hemoglobin and hematocrit, as well as lower incidence of intracranial haemorrhage of all grades in infants who received umbilical cord milking as compared to immediate clamping [60]. One recent trial reports that preterm infants in the umbilical cord milking group had higher heart rate over the first 2 min, higher oxygen saturation in the first minutes with less supplemental oxygen, and reduced need for supplemental oxygen at 36 weeks [61]. Preterm infants < 32 weeks born by caesarean delivery show higher superior vena cava flow in the first 12 h with umbilical cord milking as compared to 45–60 s of delay in cord clamping [62]. The meta-analysis finds no difference in mortality before discharge, hypotension requiring volume or inotropes, need for transfusion, severe intraventricular haemorrhage, peak serum bilirubin or need for phototherapy [60]. Only one study followed infant to 24 months for developmental outcome, finding no difference in rates of disability [47]. Two small randomized controlled trials in infants > 35 weeks report higher hemoglobin immediately after birth. Of 224 total infants, none had symptomatic polycythemia. There was no difference in the peak serum bilirubin or the need for phototherapy [63, 64].

In practice, umbilical cord milking offers the primary advantage of speed. The actions can be completed in a matter of seconds, the maneuvers are readily accomplished at caesarean section, and the baby can be immediately transferred to the pediatric team for any needed resuscitation. Entire surgical teams do not need to pause during a caesarean section, and the obstetrical provider at a vaginal delivery can immediately move to controlled cord traction. The action of milking the cord requires some standardization of practice, however, as the helical spirals of the cord create obstruction to blood flow if not untwisted prior to milking. The length of the segment milked, speed, and number of repetitions of milking have been established by pragmatic choice rather than controlled experiments. Transfer of blood occurs as a bolus rather than a process of equilibration as with delayed cord clamping; milking often is accomplished in 15 s or less [61]. If respirations have not been established prior to clamping the cord, the volume of blood retained in the infant's circulation may not be as large as if the pulmonary circulation has expanded. Hemodynamic fluctuations similar to those described with immediate cord clamping theoretically could occur; the

hemodynamic significance of retrograde flow in the umbilical arteries also is unclear. Additional concerns arise around potential volume overload in infants who have experienced hypoxic-ischemic events during labor and increased products of endothelial activation entering the infant's circulation with milking of the umbilical arteries [65].

To be determined: gaps in knowledge and practice

"Instead of coming into the world pale, anemic, or exsanguinous, the child is sometimes born in quite a contrary condition; its skin is of a bluish red or liver colour, of various degrees of intensity, especially on the face, and appears as if thickened.....The apoplectic state is met with, especially in strong children, after long and difficult labours, the application of the forceps, and pelvis labours, either spontaneous or artificial; where the child has remained for several hours under the influence of the uterine contractions after the discharge of the waters; where it has presented in a bad position; where it is too large to pass with ease through the various passages; where a loop of the cord strictures its neck, or is itself in any way compressed, and particularly where any of these accidents occur coincidently with a previous plethoric state. When a child is born in this state we should make haste to disengorge its vascular system..." [6]

When is physiological cord clamping not feasible or beneficial?

Widely varying conditions have been considered as exclusions from delayed cord clamping or umbilical cord milking in published trials. Hemorrhagic complications during labor (i.e. placental abruption and placenta previa) and cord abnormalities or accidents (true knot, prolapse, avulsion) may physically interrupt placental transfer. Tight nuchal cord which cannot be reduced conventionally may be reduced by using the somersault maneuver, permitting delayed clamping or cord milking [66]. In multiple gestations with evidence of placental connections (monochorionic placentation, twin-twin-transfusion syndrome) or discordant growth, facilitating placental transfusion poses theoretical risk to the second twin and potential to exaggerate polycythemia/hypervolemia. Hemolytic disease has been viewed as a contraindication because delayed clamping increases the volume of sensitized red blood cells; however the relative risks/benefits of hypovolemia and hemodynamic lability at birth vs. larger bilirubin load have not been carefully studied.

Questions arise around a number of maternal and fetal conditions which might represent relative contraindications to facilitated placental transfusion. Growth restriction, especially if a result of chronic intrauterine hypoxia, may be associated with higher risk for polycythemia and hyperviscosity. Maternal diabetes and pre-eclampsia also represent circumstances associated with intrauterine hypoxia. Non-vigorous infants born through meconium-stained amniotic fluid have historically undergone immediate intubation for tracheal suctioning, prompting immediate cord clamping. Programs focusing on prevention of maternal-to-child transmission of HIV previously advocated immediate clamping as part of the package of interventions; in the absence of any evidence or logical mechanism of increased viral transmission, WHO recommendations now explicitly advocate delayed cord clamping in this situation [7].

What factors determine the volume/rate of blood transfer and what clinical indicators can aid in establishing the point of hemodynamic equilibrium?

During either delayed cord clamping or umbilical cord milking in the clinical setting there is little certainty about the volume, rate, or direction of blood transfer. The onset of spontaneous respirations and opening of the pulmonary vascular bed are now recognized as major determinants of placental blood transfer. However, other factors have been demonstrated to influence the equilibrium of placental transfusion, including uterine contractions (or their absence at caesarean section), administration of uterotonics, physical position of the newly born infant relative to the placenta, gestational age, and antepartum/intrapartum hypoxic-ischemic conditions [67]. A variety of experimental techniques have been used in human infants to document blood flow and net transfer. Highly accurate scales have been used to document the time course and estimate the volume of placental transfusion with delayed cord clamping [18]. In the 1960s impedance plethysmography was used to study the relative contributions of lung aeration and pulmonary blood flow during delayed cord clamping [68]. Modern electrical impedance tomography (EIT) converts impedance signals into images and may offer the prospect of studying lung recruitment and the dynamics of delayed cord clamping simultaneously and noninvasively. Doppler flow measurement has proven feasible for the measurement of umbilical cord flow, as well as cardiac output, regional blood flow, and tissue perfusion. Near-infrared spectroscopy offers insight into cerebral hemodynamics with non-invasive, bedside methods [11, 69]. Experimental animal studies offer the possibility of multiple simultaneous and direct measures of blood flow, pressure, volume as well as advanced imaging using such techniques as scintigraphy and magnetic resonance imaging (MRI). More attention could also focus on description of clinical correlates of adequate placental transfusion, such as capillary refill in the infant or appearance of the umbilical cord. In parallel with lung recruitment, the timing of cord clamping as a patient-defined strategy deserves further research to define useful measures and clinical signs of physiological equilibrium [70].

What changes in infrastructure and human behaviour are necessary?

While uncertainties still exist around the best approach to achieve physiologic cord clamping, incremental changes in practice are now possible [71, 49, 48]. The model of gradual transition in circulation and respiratory function from the placenta to the lungs should serve as the model for collaboration between obstetrical and pediatric providers at a birth. Both disciplines need to communicate and formulate a plan before birth to accomplish a smooth transition; both need to be involved in monitoring third stage of labor in the mother and signs of circulatory transition and equilibrium in the newly born infant; both need to promptly detect and respond to deviations from the normal postnatal course. Waiting is difficult, especially waiting without action for a process that is largely invisible and incompletely understood. Active monitoring of umbilical cord appearance/pulsatility as well as uterine contractions/placental detachment and active provision of routine care or the initial steps of resuscitation turn passive waiting into action and provide shared learning and experience with clinical signs of physiologic transition and equilibrium. Although umbilical cord milking also eliminates passive waiting, controlled comparisons of delayed cord clamping vs. umbilical cord milking are necessary before it can be established that cord milking and rapid clamping/cutting pose "not....the least inconvenience" for the newly born infant.

Delay in term infants has often been limited to one minute, which may be insufficient to complete the process of placental transfer to a point of equilibrium. Observational studies in term infants to determine optimal timing should examine carrying out the steps of routine care with the newly born infant on mother's abdomen to safely prolong the delay and set the stage for early initiation of breastfeeding. However, in many settings, maintenance of skin-to-skin contact in the first hour and facilitation of breastfeeding demand considerable change in provider workflow to provide adequate support and monitoring of mother and baby.

Delay in umbilical cord clamping of premature infants in many studies has been in the range of 30–45 s only; these studies very likely have not captured the full potential benefit of delayed cord clamping to preterm infants. Assuring thermal protection and providing the initial steps of resuscitation to preterm infants during delay in cord clamping can safely prolong the delay and possibly achieve onset of respirations in the majority of infants. Performing the initial steps of routine care or resuscitation during delay deserves comparison with umbilical cord milking.

Delivery of positive-pressure ventilation to achieve lung expansion before umbilical cord clamping calls for re-design of communication and the physical interaction between obstetric and pediatric providers, as well as the equipment for resuscitation. Although equipment for suctioning and ventilation can be readily adapted to space and sterility constraints, monitoring currently proves more cumbersome. Disposable colorimetric carbon dioxide detectors may offer a useful summative indicator for both ventilation and pulmonary blood flow; delivery of carbon dioxide to the alveoli requires pulmonary blood flow and delivery of carbon dioxide to the detector requires unobstructed pulmonary ventilation. Color change has been shown to be useful in detecting airway obstruction during bag and mask ventilation and predictive of restoration of normal heart rate in the setting of bradycardia immediately after delivery [72]. There is considerable potential for further development of monitoring, such as transthoracic impedance and quantitative end-tidal carbon dioxide, that would give real-time information on progress of the physiologic transition after birth.

In resource-limited settings, the balancing outcomes of temperature stability and hyperbilirubinemia deserve close consideration. Thermal protection during delay in umbilical cord clamping may require different strategies where control of environmental temperature and use of chemical warming mattresses are limited. It is unclear if delayed cord clamping in preterm infants would increase demand for phototherapy beyond available capacity in areas where specialty care is limited.

Directions for further research
What are the broader implications of physiologic umbilical cord clamping for neonatal clinical research?
Research is now needed to investigate how the beneficial effects of physiologic transition can be maximized (Table 1). With respect to umbilical cord clamping, this means re-orientation of research to clearly document the timing of cord clamping in relation to the onset of respirations in all studies and to place new emphasis on collection of immediate and intermediate cardiovascular outcomes as well as long-term neurodevelopmental outcomes in both term and preterm infants. The results of large randomized clinical trials comparing delayed and immediate clamping are needed to improve the low quality of evidence now aggregated from multiple small trials with variable patient populations, few extremely preterm infants, and variable interventions and outcome measures. The Cord Trial in the United Kingdom is

comparing clamping within 20 s to clamping after at least 2 min among births < 32 weeks gestation [73]. The Australian Placental Transfusion Study compares clamping within 10 s to clamping after 1 min with the infant held below the level of the placenta. Comparative trials of delayed cord clamping vs. cord milking can help define the relative advantages of each method. Experimental physiology studies of umbilical cord milking could help further define the hemodynamics of that practice. Trials that specifically examine initiation of positive-pressure ventilation and/or continuous positive airway pressure with the umbilical cord intact are underway. Packages of interventions that include other aspects of physiologic transition (thermal control, minimizing oxygen exposure and intubation, facilitating lung recruitment with positive-pressure ventilation, skin-to-skin contact for moderate and late preterm infants) should be tested for their potential to achieve more-than-additive benefit.

Conclusions
The existing literature on delayed cord clamping and cord milking has consistently demonstrated benefit in facilitating placental transfusion. Improved physiologic stability in transition (blood pressure), reduced need for transfusion, and lower incidence of intracranial haemorrhage and necrotizing enterocolitis are valuable improvements in outcome. Several studies, of both delayed cord clamping and cord milking, have shown reduced need for resuscitative interventions. Although these outcomes fall short of the overarching goals of improved neurodevelopmental outcome and reduced mortality in intensive care settings, they offer promise. And, under circumstances where medical support available to newly born infants is severely limited, delayed cord clamping shows a positive relationship with decreased mortality.

Recent experimental and population-based studies highlight the interaction between onset of respirations and timing of umbilical cord clamping. These have changed the concept of delayed cord clamping from one of a defined time interval only to one of facilitation of physiologic transition after birth. Before clear guidance is available for clinicians on how best to facilitate this transition, more research is needed. For the term infant who breathes spontaneously, a delay of at least 2–3 min appears necessary to optimize circulatory transition and placental transfusion. More evidence is needed about the interventions that should be performed during delay in cord clamping among infants who fail to breathe after birth. Preterm and very low birth weight infants as well as infants who have experienced hypoxic-ischemic events are of special interest, as they have generally been excluded from past studies. Data on umbilical cord milking are limited, and comparison between delayed cord clamping and cord milking is especially important.

Endnotes

[1]Velpeau, AA. Traité elementaire de l'art des accouchements; ou, Principes de tokologie et d'embryologie [Elementary treatise on the art of midwifery; or, Principles of tokology and embryology], 3rd Edition English translation of the 1829 French text, Philadelphia: Lindsay & Blakiston, 1845, page 550, section 1209.

[2]Ibid, page 552, section 1213.

[3c]Ibid, page 553, section 1213.

[4]Ibid, page 559, section 1222.

[5]Ibid, page 551, section 1212.

[6]Ibid, page 562-3, section 1227–9.

Abbreviations
ACOG: American College of Obstetricians and Gynecologists; CPAP: Continuous positive airway pressure; EIT: Electrical impedance tomography; MRI: Magnetic resonance imaging; WHO: World Health Organization.

Competing interests
The author declares that she has no competing interests.

Author's contributions
The author contributed to the conception and design of the review, reviewed and interpreted the data, prepared the manuscript, approved the final version to be published, and assumes responsibility for the contents. The author read and approved the final manuscript.

Author's information
SN is Professor of Pediatrics in the Section of Neonatology of the University of Colorado School of Medicine and serves as a volunteer evidence reviewer for the International Liaison Committee on Resuscitation.

Acknowledgements
None.

References
1. Velpeau AA. Traité elementaire de l'art des accouchements; ou, Principes de tokologie et d'embryologie [Elementary treatise on the art of midwifery; or, Principles of tokology and embryology]. 3rd ed. Philadelphia: Lindsay & Blakiston; 1829.
2. Committee on Obstetric Practice American College of Obstetricians and Gynecologists. Committee Opinion No.543: Timing of umbilical cord clamping after birth. Obstet Gynecol. 2012;120(6):1522–6.
3. Royal College of Obstetricians and Gynaecologists, Scientific Advisory Committee. Clamping of the umbilical cord and placental transfusion, Scientific Impact Paper No. 14, 2015. [http://rcog.org.uk/globalassets/documents/guidelines/scientific-impact-papers/sip-14.pdf] Accessed: 27 August 2015.
4. The Royal College of Midwives Guideline Advisory Group. Evidence Based Guidelines for Midwifery-Led Care in Labour. Third Stage of Labour. 2012. [https://www.rcm.org.uk/sites/default/files/ThirdStageofLabour.pdf] Accessed: 27 August 2015.
5. American Academy of Pediatrics. Statement of endorsement. Timing of umbilical cord clamping after birth. Pediatrics. 2013;131(4):e1323. doi:10.1542/peds.2013-0191.
6. Perlman JM, Wyllie J, Kattwinkel J, Atkins DL, Chameides L, Goldsmith JP, et al. Part 11: Neonatal resuscitation: 2010 International Consensus on Cardiopulmonary Resuscitation and Emergency Cardiovascular Care Science With Treatment Recommendations. Circulation. 2010;122(16 Suppl 2):S516–38.
7. World Health Organization, USAID, MCHIP. Delayed clamping of the umbilical cord to reduce infant anaemia. 2013 [http://apps.who.int/iris/bitstream/10665/120074/1/WHO_RHR_14.19_eng.pdf?ua=1] Accessed: 27 August 2015.
8. Hooper SB. Maternal Health, Neonatology and Perinatology. 2015.
9. Bhatt S, Alison BJ, Wallace EM, Crossley KJ, Gill AW, Kluckow M, et al. Delaying cord clamping until ventilation onset improves cardiovascular function at birth in preterm lambs. J Physiol. 2013;591(Pt 8):2113–26.
10. Lind J. Human fetal and neonatal circulation: some structural and fuctional aspects. Eur J Cardiol. 1977;5(3):265–81.
11. van Vonderen JJ, Roest AA, Siew ML, Walther FJ, Hooper SB, te Pas AB. Measuring physiological changes during the transition to life after birth. Neonatology. 2014;105(3):230–42.
12. Peltonen T. Placental transfusion - advantage and disadvantage. Eur J Pediatr. 1981;137:141–6.
13. van Vonderen JJ, Roest AA, Siew ML, Blom NA, van Lith JM, Walther FJ, et al. Noninvasive measurements of hemodynamic transition directly after birth. Pediatr Res. 2014;75(3):448–52.
14. Rudolph AM. Fetal and neonatal pulmonary circulation. Ann Rev Physiol. 1979;41:383–95.
15. Crossley KJ, Allison BJ, Polglase GR, Morley CJ, Davis PG, Hooper SB. Dynamic changes in the direction of blood flow through the ductus arteriosus at birth. J Physiol. 2009;587(Pt 19):4695–704.
16. Yao AC, Moinian M, Lind J. Distribution of blood between infant and placenta after birth. Lancet. 1969;2(7626):871–3.
17. Stembera ZK, Hodr J, Janda J. Umbilical blood flow in healthy newborn infants during the first minutes after birth. J Obstet Gynecol. 1965;91:568–74.
18. Farrar D, Airey R, Law GR, Tuffnell D, Cattle B, Duley L. Measuring placental transfusion for term births: weighing babies with cord intact. BJOG. 2011;118(1):70–5. doi:10.1111/j.1471-0528.2010.02781.x.
19. Boere I, Roest AA, Wallace E, ten Harkel AD, Haak MC, Morley CJ, et al. Umbilical blood flow patterns directly after birth before delayed cord clamping. Arch Dis Child Fetal Neonatal Ed. 2014. doi:10.1136/archdischild-2014-307144.
20. Katheria AC, Wozniak M, Harari D, Arnell K, Petruzzelli D, Finer NN. Measuring cardiac changes using electrical impedance during delayed cord clamping: a feasibility trial. Maternal Health, Neonatology and. Perinatol. 2015;1:15. doi:10.1186/s40748-015-0016-3.
21. Ersdal HL, Linde J, Mduma E, Auestad B, Perlman J. Neonatal outcome following cord clamping after onset of spontaneous respiration. Pediatrics. 2014;134(2):265–72.
22. Philip AG, Teng SS. Role of respiration in effecting transfusion at cesarean section. Biol Neonate. 1977;31(3–4):219–24.
23. Vain NE, Satragno DS, Gorenstein AN, Gordillo JE, Berazategui JP, Alda MG, et al. Effect of gravity on volume of placental transfusion: a multicentre, randomised, non-inferiority trial. Lancet. 2014. doi:10.1016/s0140-6736(14)60197-5.
24. McDonald SJ, Middleton P, Dowswell T, Morris PS. Effect of timing of umbilical cord clamping of term infants on maternal and neonatal outcomes. Cochrane Database Syst Rev. 2013;7:Cd004074. doi:10.1002/14651858.CD004074.
25. Andersson O, Hellstrom-Westas L, Andersson D, Domellof M. Effect of delayed versus early umbilical cord clamping on neonatal outcomes and iron status at 4 months: a randomised controlled trial. BMJ. 2011;343:d7157. doi:10.1136/bmj.d7157.
26. Andersson O, Domellof M, Andersson D, Hellstrom-Westas L. Effect of delayed vs early umbilical cord clamping on iron status and neurodevelopment at age 12 months: A randomized clinical trial. JAMA pediatrics. 2014. doi:10.1001/jamapediatrics.2013.4639.
27. Andersson O, Lindquist B, Lindgren M, Stjernqvist K, Domellof M, Hellstrom-Westas L. Effect of delayed cord clamping on neurodevelopment at 4 years of age: A randomized clinical trial. JAMA pediatrics. 2015;169(7):631–8.
28. Oxford Midwives Research Group. A study of the relationship between the delivery to cord clamping interval and the time of cord separation. Midwifery. 1991;7:167–76.
29. World Health Organization. Early initiation of breastfeeding. In: e-Library of Evidence for Nutrition Actions (eLENA) Accessed March 2, 2015.
30. Oh W, Lind J. Body temperature of the newborn infant in relation to placental transfusion. Acta Paediatr Scand. 1967;172:137–45.
31. Linderkamp O, Nelle M, Kraus M, Zilow EP. The effect of early and late cord-clamping on blood viscosity and other hemorheological parameters in full-term neonates. Acta Paediatr. 1992;81(10):745–50.

32. Nelle M, Zilow EP, Kraus M, Bastert G, Linderkanp O. The effect of Leboyer delivery on blood viscosity and other hemorheologic parameters in term neonates. Am J Obstet Gynecol. 1993;169(1):189–93.

33. Nelle M, Zilow EP, Bastert G, Linderkamp O. Effect of Leboyer childbirth on cardiac output, cerebral and gastrointestinal blood flow velocities in full-term neonates. Am J Perinatol. 1995;12(3):212–6. doi:10.1055/s-2007-994455.

34. Nelle M, Kraus M, Bastert G, Linderkamp O. Effects of Leboyer childbirth on left- and right systolic time intervals in healthy term neonates. J Perinat Med. 1996;24(5):513–20.

35. Mercer JS, Erickson-Owens DA. Rethinking placental transfusion and cord clamping issues. J Perinat Neonatal Nurs. 2012;26(3):202–17. quiz 18–9.

36. Stevens J, Schmied V, Burns E, Dahlen H. Immediate or early skin-to-skin contact after a Caesarean section: a review of the literature. Matern Child Nutr. 2014;10(4):456–73.

37. te Pas AB, Wong C, Kamlin CO, Dawson JA, Morley CJ, Davis PG. Breathing patterns in preterm and term infants immediately after birth. Pediatr Res. 2009;65(3):352–6.

38. Rabe H, Diaz-Rossello JL, Duley L, Dowswell T. Effect of timing of umbilical cord clamping and other strategies to influence placental transfusion at preterm birth on maternal and infant outcomes. Cochrane database syst rev. 2012;8, CD003248.

39. Kugelman A, Borenstein-Levin L, Riskin A, Chistyakov I, Ohel G, Gonen R, et al. Immediate versus delayed umbilical cord clamping in premature neonates born < 35 weeks: a prospective, randomized, controlled study. Am J Perinatol. 2007;24(5):307–15.

40. Baenziger O, Stolkin F, Keel M, von Siebenthal K, Fauchere J-C, Kundu SD, et al. The influence of the timing of cord clamping on postnatal cerebral oxygenation in preterm neonates: a randomized, controlled trial. Pediatrics. 2007;119(3):455–9.

41. Mercer JS, McGrath MM, Hensman A, Silver H, Oh W. Immediate and delayed cord clamping in infants born between 24 and 32 weeks: a pilot randomized controlled trial. J Perinatol. 2003;23:466–72.

42. Mercer JS, Vohr BR, McGrath MM, Padbury JG, Wallach M, Oh W. Delayed cord clamping in very preterm infants reduces the incidence of intraventricular hemorrhage and late-onset sepsis: a randomized, controlled trial. Pediatrics. 2006;117(4):1235–42.

43. Aladangady N, McHugh S, Aitchison TC, Wardrop CAJ, Holland BM. Infants' blood volume in a controlled trial of placental transfusion at preterm delivery. Pediatrics. 2006;117(1):93–8.

44. Strauss RG, Mock DM, Johnson KJ, Cress GA, Burmeister LF, Zimmerman MB, et al. A randomized clinical trial comparing immediate versus delayed clamping of the umbilical cord in preterm infants: short-term clinical and laboratory endpoints. Transfusion. 2008;48(4):658–65.

45. Sommers R, Stonestreet BS, Oh W, Laptook A, Yanowitz TD, Raker C, et al. Hemodynamic effects of delayed cord clamping in preterm infants. Pediatrics. 2012;129:e667. doi:10.1542/peds.2011-2550.

46. Meyer MP, Mildenhall L. Delayed cord clamping and blood flow in the superior vena cava in preterm infants: an observational study. Arch Dis Child Fetal Neonatal Ed. 2012;97(6):F484–6. doi:10.1136/F2 of 3 adc.2010.

47. Ghavam S, Batra D, Mercer J, Kugelman A, Hosono S, Oh W, et al. Effects of placental transfusion in extremely low birthweight infants: meta-analysis of long- and short-term outcomes. Transfusion. 2014;54(4):1192–8.

48. Kaempf JW, Tomlinson MW, Kaempf AJ, Wu Y, Wang L, Tipping N, et al. Delayed umbilical cord clamping in premature neonates. Obstet Gynecol. 2012;120(2 Pt 1):325–30.

49. Aziz K, Chinnery H, Lacaze-Masmonteil T. A single-center experience of implementing delayed cord clamping in babies born at less than 33 weeks' gestational age. Adv Neonatal Care. 2012;12(6):371–6.

50. Polglase GR, Miller SL, Barton SK, Kluckow M, Gill AW, Hooper SB, et al. Respiratory support for premature neonates in the delivery room: effects on cardiovascular function and the development of brain injury. Pediatr Res. 2014;75(6):682–8.

51. Thomas MR, Yoxall CW, Weeks AD, Duley L. Providing newborn resuscitation at the mother's bedside: assessing the safety, usability and acceptability of a mobile trolley. BMC Pediatr. 2014;14:135.

52. Philip AGS, Yee AB, Rosy M, Surti N, Tsamtsouris A, Ingall D. Placental transfusion as an intrauterine phenomenon in deliveries complicated by foetal distress. Br Med J. 1969;2:11–3.

53. Yao AC, Wist A, Lind J. The blood volume of the newborn infant delivered by caesarean section. Acta Paediatr Scand. 1967;56(6):585–92.

54. Yao AC, Lind J. Blood volume in the asphyxiated term neonate. Biol Neonate. 1972;21(3):199–209.

55. Stembera ZK, Hodr J, Janda J. Umbilical blood flow in newborn infants who suffered intrauterine hypoxia. Am J Obstet Gynecol. 1968;101(4):546–53.

56. Bhatt S, Polglase GR, Wallace EM, Te Pas AB, Hooper SB. Ventilation before Umbilical Cord Clamping Improves the Physiological Transition at Birth. Frontiers in Pediatrics. 2014;2:113.

57. Yao AC, Lind J. Effect of gravity on placental transfusion. Lancet. 1969;2(7619):505–8.

58. Rabe H, Jewison A, Alvarez RF, Crook D, Stilton D, Bradley R, et al. Milking compared with delayed cord clamping to increase placental transfusion in preterm neonates: a randomized controlled trial. Obstet Gynecol. 2011;117(2 Pt 1):205–11.

59. Hosono S, Hine K, Nagano N, Taguchi Y, Yoshikawa K, Okada T et al. Residual blood volume in the umbilical cord of extremely premature infants. Pediatrics International.57(1):68–71. doi:10.1111/ped.12464.

60. Al-Wassia H, Shah PS. Efficacy and Safety of Umbilical Cord Milking at Birth: A Systematic Review and Meta-analysis. JAMA pediatrics. 2015;169(1):18–25.

61. Katheria A, Blank D, Rich W, Finer N. Umbilical cord milking improves transition in premature infants at birth. PLoS ONE. 2014;9(4):e94085.

62. Katheria AC, Truong G, Cousins L, Oshiro BT, Finer NN. Umbilical cord milking versus delayed cord clamping in preterm infants. Pediatrics. 2015;136(1):61–9.

63. Erickson-Owens DA, Mercer JS, Oh W. Umbilical cord milking in term infants delivered by cesarean section: a randomized controlled trial. J Perinatol. 2012;32(8):580–4.

64. Upadhyay A, Gothwal S, Parihar R, Garg A, Gupta A, Chawla D, et al. Effect of umbilical cord milking in term and near term infants: randomized control trial. Am J Obstet Gynecol. 2013;208(2):e1–6.

65. Quan A, Leung SW, Lao TT, Man RY. 5-hydroxytryptamine and thromboxane A2 as physiologic mediators of human umbilical artery closure. J Soc Gynecol Investig. 2003;10(8):490–5.

66. Mercer JS, Skovgaard RL, Peareara-Eaves J, Bowman TA. Nuchal cord management and nurse-midwifery practice. J Midwifery Womens Health. 2005;50(5):373–9. doi:10.1016/j.jmwh.2005.04.023.

67. Linderkamp O. Placental transfusion: determinants and effects. Clin Perinatol. 1982;9(3):559–92.

68. Olsson T, Victorin L. Transthoracic impedance, with special reference to newborn infants and the ratio air-to-fluid in the lungs. Acta Paediatrica Scandinavica - Supplement. 1970;207:1.

69. Backes CH, Rivera B, Haque U, Copeland K, Hutchon D, Smith CV. Placental transfusion strategies in extremely preterm infants: The next piece of the puzzle. J Neonatal-Perinatal Med. 2014;7(4):257–67.

70. Zonneveld E, Lavizzari A, Rajapaksa A, Black D, Perkins E, Sourial M, et al. A volumetric-response sustained inflation at birth: towards a patient-defined strategy? Pediatric Academic Societies; Vancouver, BC, Canada. [http://www.abstracts2view.com/pasall/view.php?nu=PAS14L1_1180.2] Accessed: 27 August 2015.

71. McAdams RM, Backes CH, Hutchon DJR. Steps for implementing delayed cord clamping in a hospital setting. Maternal Health, Neonatology and. Perinatol. 2015;1:10. doi:10.1186/s40748-015-0011-8.

72. Blank D, Rich W, Leone T, Garey D, Finer N. Pedi-cap color change precedes a significant increase in heart rate during neonatal resuscitation. Resuscitation. 2014;85(11):1568–72.

73. Duley L, Batey N. Optimal timing of umbilical cord clamping for term and preterm babies. Early Hum Dev. 2013;89(11):905–8.

7

Continuous glucose monitoring in neonates

Christopher J.D. McKinlay[1,2]* (iD), J. Geoffrey Chase[3], Jennifer Dickson[3], Deborah L. Harris[1,4], Jane M. Alsweiler[1,2] and Jane E. Harding[1]

Abstract

Continuous glucose monitoring (CGM) is well established in the management of diabetes mellitus, but its role in neonatal glycaemic control is less clear. CGM has provided important insights about neonatal glucose metabolism, and there is increasing interest in its clinical use, particularly in preterm neonates and in those in whom glucose control is difficult. Neonatal glucose instability, including hypoglycaemia and hyperglycaemia, has been associated with poorer neurodevelopment, and CGM offers the possibility of adjusting treatment in real time to account for individual metabolic requirements while reducing the number of blood tests required, potentially improving long-term outcomes. However, current devices are optimised for use at relatively high glucose concentrations, and several technical issues need to be resolved before real-time CGM can be recommended for routine neonatal care. These include: 1) limited point accuracy, especially at low or rapidly changing glucose concentrations; 2) calibration methods that are designed for higher glucose concentrations of children and adults, and not for neonates; 3) sensor drift, which is under-recognised; and 4) the need for dynamic and integrated metrics that can be related to long-term neurodevelopmental outcomes. CGM remains an important tool for retrospective investigation of neonatal glycaemia and the effect of different treatments on glucose metabolism. However, at present CGM should be limited to research studies, and should only be introduced into routine clinical care once benefit is demonstrated in randomised trials.

Keywords: Neonatal hypoglycaemia, Neonatal hyperglycaemia, Interstitial glucose, Continuous glucose monitoring, Hyperinsulinaemia

Background

Continuous glucose monitoring (CGM) is well established in the management of diabetes mellitus, but its role in neonatal care is less clear. CGM has provided important insights about neonatal glucose metabolism [1, 2], and there is increasing interest in its clinical use, particularly in preterm neonates and in those in whom glucose control is difficult. Neonatal glucose instability, including hypoglycaemia and hyperglycaemia, has been associated with poorer neurodevelopment [3], and serial blood glucose monitoring by heel lancing is invasive, with potential adverse effects on neurodevelopment [4]. CGM offers the possibility of adjusting treatment in real time to account for individual metabolic requirements while reducing the number of blood glucose measurements required, potentially improving long-term outcomes [5]. However, several technical issues need to be resolved before CGM can be recommended for routine neonatal care, including accuracy, calibration, sensor drift and plasma-interstitial time delay.

The clinical interpretation of CGM is also challenging. Neonatal studies using CGM have revealed that variability in glucose concentrations is common both during neonatal transition [1, 3] and in enterally fed preterm infants [5–9]. However, the clinical significance of these findings is uncertain, and in the absence of well-established guidelines there is a risk that CGM could lead to unnecessary or even harmful intervention [3]. Further, while CGM provides more information than intermittent blood testing, it is also less accurate. CGM parameters, therefore, need to be conceptualised as dynamic and integrated rather than as

* Correspondence: c.mckinlay@auckland.ac.nz
[1]Liggins Institute, University of Auckland, Private Bag 92019, Victoria St West, Auckland 1142, New Zealand
[2]Department of Paediatrics: Child and Youth Health, University of Auckland, Auckland, New Zealand
Full list of author information is available at the end of the article

static thresholds, and there is little information about how such parameters should be interpreted.

It is important that clinicians understand the limitations and implications of this rapidly evolving technology before it is adopted into clinical practice. This paper will review: 1) CGM technologies for neonatal care; 2) insights from CGM about neonatal glucose metabolism; and 3) the current evidence for the clinical application of CGM in neonatal intensive care.

CGM technology for neonatal care
Types of CGM
CGM devices measure the glucose concentration of the interstitial fluid, either in subcutaneous tissue or in transdermal fluid (Table 1). Subcutaneous biosensors are of two types: microdialysis fibres and amperometric needle electrodes. Microdialysis involves insertion into the subcutaneous tissue of a thin hollow fibre that is composed of a semipermeable membrane through which an isotonic fluid containing no glucose is infused [10]. Glucose from the interstitium diffuses into the fluid stream and is measured by an external enzymatic probe. These devices have had only limited use in neonates in research settings [11, 12], and there are currently no commercial systems available.

Subcutaneous needle CGM systems consist of a fine needle sensor connected to a non-implantable transmitter that powers the sensor and sends raw data to a monitor, either by cable or Bluetooth. Some systems display the resulting output in real-time on the monitor or another linked device; others store the data for later downloading. The challenge for sensor manufacturers is to combine all the components of an enzymatic ampometric system into a single needle [13]. Ampometric sensors measure current flowing from an oxidation (electron producing) reaction at a working electrode to a reduction (electron consuming) reaction at a counter electrode. The working electrode is coated with glucose oxidase which catalyses the oxidation of glucose when a voltage is applied, resulting in transfer of electrons to a chemical mediator, usually hydrogen peroxide. A reference electrode is used to ensure a stable voltage is applied to the working electrode, but reference and counter electrodes are often combined. In addition, subcutaneous sensors require a barrier membrane to limit glucose access to the sensor because of the deficiency of oxygen in the subcutaneous environment relative to glucose supply. Each manufacturer has their own proprietary method for combining these elements within the needle sensor.

Two main CGM brands have been used in neonates, Medtronic Minimed (Northridge, CA, United States) and DexCom (San Diego, CA, United States), both of which manufacture retrospective and real-time devices. However, it should be noted that none of these devices have been approved for clinical use in neonates. The needle electrodes and transmitters have generally been placed on the lateral thigh in neonates (Fig. 1), and have been used for up to 7 days [1, 14]. Some, but not all babies appear to experience brief pain on insertion of the needle electrode, but sensors are subsequently well tolerated in most neonates, and complications are rare [1, 15].

Raw signal data from the electrode is generated approximately every 10 s, and is averaged and processed to give a glucose reading every 5 min, thus providing near-continuous output. Notably, these devices do not display

Table 1 Methodologies for continuous glucose monitoring

Fluid location	Biosensor	Advantages	Disadvantages	Commercial devices currently used in neonates
Subcutaneous	Microdialysis fibre with external amperometric probe.	Most accurate.	Subcutaneous inflammation.	Not available
		Sensing element is outside the skin and so is not susceptible to biofouling.	Expensive.	
			Long lag time.	
			Discomfort.	
			Requires calibration.	
	Amperometric needle electrode.	Easier insertion.	Less accurate.	Medtronic MiniMed.
			Sensor degradation due to biofouling.	DexCom.
			Poor detection with oedema.	
			Discomfort. Most require calibration.	
Transdermal	Glucose binding protein.	No skin penetration.	Accuracy unknown.	Not yet available.
		Potentially suitable in neonates due to their high trans-epidermal water loss.		

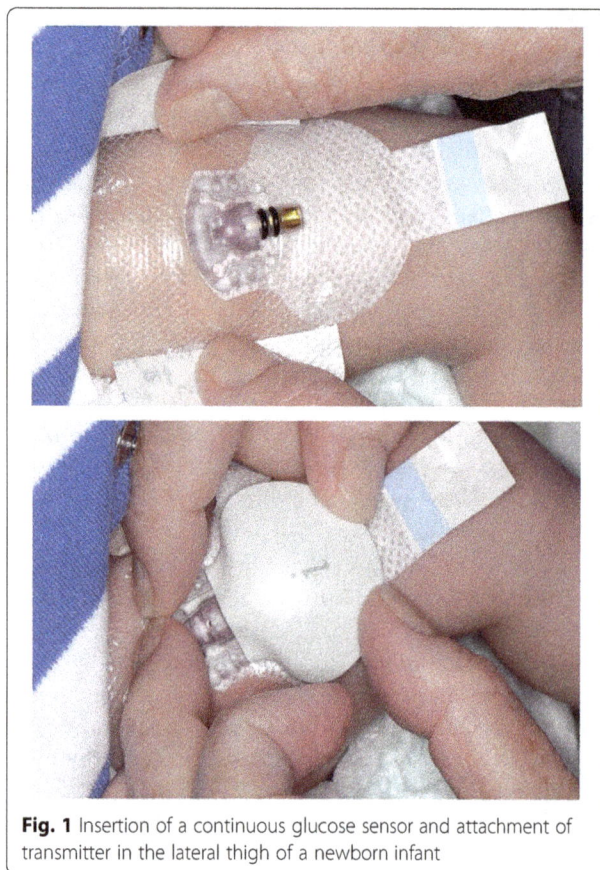

Fig. 1 Insertion of a continuous glucose sensor and attachment of transmitter in the lateral thigh of a newborn infant

data when glucose concentrations fall below 2.2 mmol/L (40 mg/dl), although retrospective analysis and calibration of the raw signal may still be possible [16]. Subcutaneous devices may also fail to give readings in the presence of significant skin oedema or dehydration, and with use of vasopressors.

Conversion of the raw signal to a glucose result requires regular input of calibration measures, i.e., current blood or plasma glucose concentrations, and thus the resulting output will reflect the calibration samples used. It is, therefore, important to understand the effect of sample type, collection method, analytical delay and assay technique on calibration values. For example, glucose concentration in whole-blood samples is usually reported to be lower than in plasma. However, immediate testing of whole arterial or capillary blood with a ward-based blood gas analysers can yield very similar glucose concentrations to laboratory analysis of plasma derived from the same samples, with a mean processing delay of 30 min [17].

Transdermal sensors are still in development, but in the future, may be useful in neonates because of their thin skin layer [18]. They can be divided into those that rely on passive diffusion of glucose into the transdermal fluid and those that use reverse iontophoresis to induce flow of molecules through the skin by applying a small

electrical surface current. Because the concentration of glucose in the transdermal fluid is very low, signal transduction relies on specialised glucose binding proteins that undergo conformational change in the presence of glucose.

Accuracy and types of error

Like all glucose sensors, CGM accuracy is affected by random error or noise, which may vary with glucose concentration [19]. Commonly used point-of-care glucometers typically have a zero-mean error (deviation from the true value) of 10% to 30% [20, 21]. However, CGM error also contains a drift component (Fig. 2) [22]. CGM measures rely on a continuous shifting internal algorithm to generate a glucose concentration from the raw sensor signal, based on regular calibration against 'true' measurements (blood sample) which are entered into the device by the clinician or patient. In addition to random error, the reported glucose concentration can 'drift' from the true measure between calibration measurements and this may significantly impact on accuracy, particularly if there is a sudden change in glycaemic status [16]. Most devices require calibration input at least every 12 h, with more frequent calibration recommended for increased accuracy.

While random, zero-mean errors can be large in CGMs due their interstitial location and sensing method, drift is unseen and thus a major issue in monitoring and control. For example, drift may result in an apparent constant CGM glucose reading when blood glucose concentration is actually falling. Perhaps worse, drift is generally not quantified as it is not required for regulatory approval, even though it has been shown to be problematic in a number of CGM devices [16, 23]. Standard assessment statistics for sensors, such as mean absolute relative difference (MARD) [24], indicate overall error but do not delineate its various components.

A typical CGM device has a MARD of 7% to 12% [23, 25], which, in adults, can vary based on the location of the sensor and acuity of the patient [26]. Assessment of drift requires intermediate independent glucose measurements, but this undermines one of the key benefits of CGM, namely, reduced blood sampling. Further, it is likely that the level of drift changes in different clinical situations, and so it is difficult to be certain about error limits. Nevertheless, expected ranges have been modelled for several sensors and devices in adult cohorts [23, 27].

Most CGM devices are designed for type 1 or type 2 diabetes and use a multiple point weighted calibration, i.e., the algorithm takes into account a weighted average of the last several 'true' calibrating glucose concentrations entered. Multiple point calibration aims to increase accuracy over the range of calibration points recorded

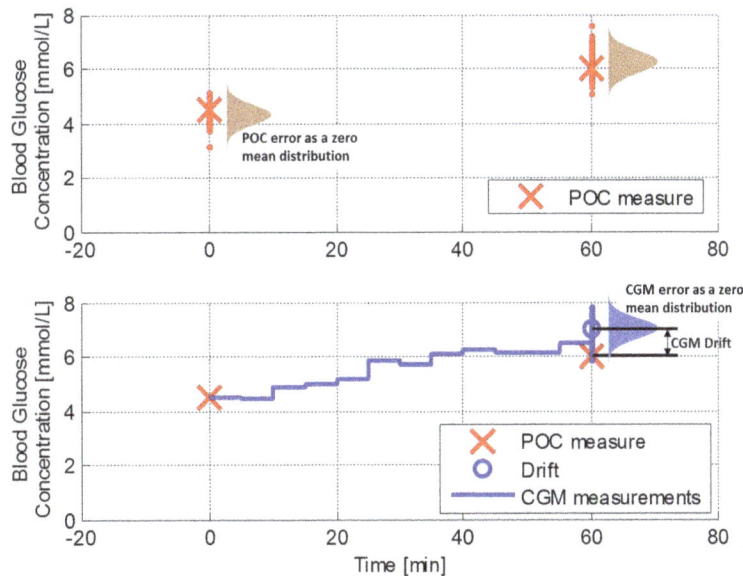

Fig. 2 Comparison of the types of measurement error for point-of-care (POC) and continuous glucose monitors (CGM), where CGMs can be prone to drift as well as a zero-centred noise

because it is assumed that less accurate point-of-care glucometers will be used for calibration [28]. However, when the blood glucose concentration deviates from the previous range of calibration values, calibration may be less accurate and errors may increase, particularly at low glucose concentrations [16].

Sensor drift results from altered access to interstitial fluid or a change in probe surface due to biofilm build up or corrosion, so that different currents are generated by the same blood glucose concentration. Multiple point calibration exacerbates this problem as each measurement can influence calibration for longer. For example, if a device is calibrated every 8 h using a three-point calibration method, each measure will influence calibration for up to 24 h.

In point-to-point calibration, the algorithm interpolates readings only between one calibration glucose measure and the next. This avoids the problem of multiple point calibration exacerbating the error due to sensor drift, and is suitable for neonatal intensive care where highly accurate glucose measurements are readily available from a blood gas machine or laboratory analyser (Fig. 3) [16], However, point-to-point calibration is not employed in currently available real-time CGM devices for clinical care. Rather, current devices use proprietary algorithms based on multiple calibration measures, and the calibration method can only be changed by the manufacturer. Fortunately, some retrospective devices, such as that produced by Medtronic MiniMed, output the actual sensor current, which is very useful in research because it allows the researcher to apply post hoc point-to-point recalibration to reduce calibration error and ameliorate drift [16].

An additional challenge in achieving accurate CGM measurements is that calibration must account for the diffusion of glucose from blood to interstitial fluid. This imposes not only a variable time delay, but also a low-pass filter effect, altering the glucose concentration dynamics between blood and interstitial fluid [29]. Further, time delay tends to increase as blood glucose concentration falls [30, 31], so that there is usually increasing positive error (CGM reading higher than true blood glucose concentration) at onset of hypoglycaemia [32]. This could lead to delayed intervention if CGM were to be used clinically to monitor for hypoglycaemia. Little is known of blood-interstitial glucose dynamics in neonates, although lag times of up to 1 h have been reported [33].

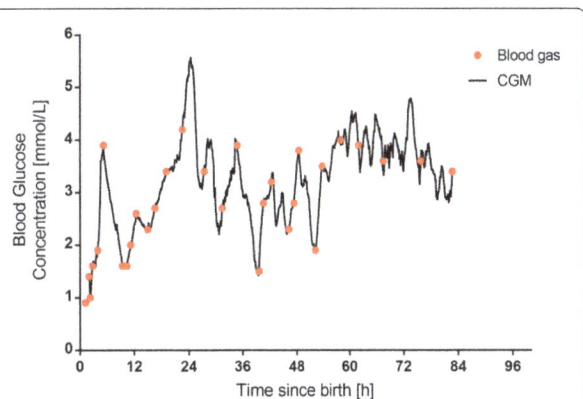

Fig. 3 Example of neonatal subcutaneous continuous glucose monitoring (CGM) with retrospective point-to-point calibration (Data from McKinlay et al. [3])

Analysis and display of CGM data

Given the measurement errors inherent in real-time CGM, it cannot be relied upon for point accuracy, particularly when looking for outlying events, such as hypoglycaemia. Further, traditional glycaemic metrics based on exceeding a specified threshold, such as hypoglycaemic episodes, have limited utility because of the potentially large zero-mean, random errors. For example, in very low birthweight infants, real-time CGM, had a positive predictive value for hypoglycaemia (blood glucose <2.6 mmol/L [<47 mg/dl]) of only 40%, and wide limits of agreement (~ ± 1.5 mmol/L [± 27 mg/dl]) [14]. In another study that measured blood glucose concentration only by point-of-care glucometer, the limits of agreement for CGM were even wider (~ ± 2.0 mmol/L [± 36 mg/dl]) [34]. Nevertheless, CGM, with its high density of data, contains a wealth of information about glycaemic status that may be of clinical importance.

An alternative approach is to focus on clusters of data points in moving windows. Although this reduces the number of independent 'measures', it minimises the impact of random errors, while still providing more frequent information than intermittent blood sampling. Direct filtering is also possible in post hoc analysis [16], but this is currently not available in real time. Guidelines for neonatal CGM analysis are yet to be established, but four main types of metrics should be considered:

i. Time within a desirable band. Studies in adult intensive care patients suggest that the cumulative quality of blood glucose control is physiologically more important than the number of extreme excursions. For example, patients who spend more time in the central blood glucose range appear to have less organ injury and better survival [35–37], although the extent to which these associations are causal is a focus of ongoing debate.

ii. Integral (area) under the glycaemic curve. This can be useful for creating alarm or guardrail systems to warn of impending clinically significant events. For example, a diminishing integral has been shown to be a better marker of impending hypoglycaemia than a rolling point average [38].

iii. Rising or falling trend. This is the rate of change over time, which can also be used to warn that a clinical threshold is about to be exceeded. It should be noted that the accuracy of trend information is different to point accuracy, and must be evaluated and monitored separately. One such tool, the Trend Compass, appears to be suitable for this purpose [39].

iv. Point-to-point change. In general, changes between each individual CGM measure should be relatively small. The distribution of these changes can be used to determine unlikely or outlying changes in sensor output [40, 41]. A large number or cluster of such extreme point-to-point changes can indicate sensor failure or a marked change in subcutaneous tissue condition, such as with oedema. Alternatively, they could be used to detect periodic events that induce larger glucose changes, such as feeding [41].

Insights from CGM about neonatal glucose metabolism

Healthy term infants

It is commonly reported that neonatal glucose concentrations decline after birth, reaching a physiological nadir at approximately 2 h [42]. However, several serial [43] and cross-sectional [44] studies in healthy, breastfed term infants have failed to demonstrate any nadir in true (laboratory) blood glucose concentrations. On the contrary, these studies suggest, albeit based on intermittent sampling, that mean blood glucose concentration remains stable at approximately 3.0 mmol/L (54 mg/dl) throughout the first 24 to 48 h, thereafter gradually rising to a mean of approximately 4.0 mmol/L (72 mg/dl) [45].

CGM offers the possibility of studying early trends in neonatal glycaemia in greater detail, including effects of feeding. Several studies have shown that this is feasible from shortly after birth, although delays between birth and sensor insertion, and the period of sensor "wetting" before the output signal stabilises, means that it is difficult to get reliable measurements in the first 2 h [1, 46]. A study is currently under way in healthy term infants that is using CGM with retrospective point-to-point recalibration based on true blood glucose concentrations, and will provide important new insights about glucose dynamics during the neonatal transition (http://hdl.handle.net/2292/32066). This is important because it has been argued that early transitional hypoglycaemia is a normal physiological phenomenon, and so does not require treatment. However, in one population study, even a single episode of neonatal hypoglycaemia was associated with poorer performance on later learning, raising the question of whether all newborns should be screened for hypoglycaemia rather than just those with risk factors for impaired metabolic adaptation [47].

At-risk term and near-term infants

A large, prospective cohort study of term and late preterm infants born at risk of neonatal hypoglycaemia (the CHYLD Study) included retrospective CGM data for ≥48 h in 75% of the cohort [3]. Analysis was based on point-to-point recalibration using all available blood glucose measures (all by blood gas analyser), thus maximising accuracy at low glucose concentrations [16]. This study showed that despite regular blood glucose testing and a clinical management protocol aimed at maintaining blood glucose ≥2.6 mmol/L [≥47 mg/dl], many infants experienced prolonged periods of low interstitial glucose (<2.6 mmol/L [<47 mg/dl]). For example, 25% of infants who developed hypoglycaemia spent at least 5 h with interstitial glucose concentrations <2.6 mmol/L [<47 mg/dl], and nearly one-quarter of infants with normal blood glucose concentrations had episodes (≥10 min) of low interstitial glucose concentrations detected only on CGM, some of which were prolonged [3].

At 2 years of age, 404 infants born at ≥35 weeks' gestation underwent detailed neurodevelopmental assessment [3]. Although hypoglycaemia was not associated with adverse outcome, CGM showed that those with neurodevelopmental impairment had higher glucose concentrations throughout the first 48 h after birth, and a steeper rise in glucose concentrations after hypoglycaemia, particularly if episodes were treated with dextrose rather than feeds alone [3]. These observations suggest that too rapid a rise or higher, less stable blood glucose concentrations during recovery from hypoglycaemia may have adverse effects on the immature brain. This is supported by animal studies showing increased generation of reactive oxygen species and neuronal injury with higher glucose concentrations after hypoglycaemia [48, 49]. Further, when this cohort was reassessed at 4.5 years of age, children who had experienced low glucose concentrations detected by CGM but not by intermittent blood testing had a four-fold increased risk of impaired executive function, whereas the risk in those identified with, and thus treated for, hypoglycaemia was increased only two-fold [50]. This suggests that these clinically undetected changes in glucose concentration may be of physiological significance. More information is needed from CGM about the effect of different treatments and feeding strategies on glycaemic response, glycaemic stability and later outcomes.

Preterm infants

Since the demonstration that CGM is feasible in very low birth weight babies [51], it has been shown in preterm babies that blood glucose concentrations can fluctuate widely [52] and intermittent blood glucose sampling commonly fails to detect episodes of both hyperglycaemia and hypoglycaemia [14, 53, 54]. Indeed, periods of hypoglycaemia and hyperglycaemia not identified through intermittent glucose blood testing alone have been detected by CGM in up to 50% of preterm babies [2, 5, 55]. Even fully enterally fed preterm babies may have large fluctuations in their glucose concentrations, varying from hypoglycaemia to hyperglycaemia within a day, and for several hours at a time [7, 54]. In one study these fluctuations were related to feed tolerance [8], and in another study episodes of hyperglycaemia were more common in girls and those with fetal growth restriction [54].

The NIRTURE trial of early insulin treatment was the first large trial ($N = 389$) that used CGM without real-time display to detect hyperglycaemia in very low birthweight babies [56]. CGM was well tolerated, even in babies as young as 23 to 24 weeks' gestation, with minimal interference of nursing cares [51]. Neonatal hyperglycaemia was found to be common, with over half of the babies having a CGM concentration of >10 mmol/L (>180 mg/dl), and was associated with low gestational age and birthweight z-score, and inotrope use [53]. It is important to note that many of the participating centres in this trial used point-of-care glucometers to calibrate the CGM devices, and this will have increased CGM random error [28]. Consequently, there was >10% difference between CGM and point-of-care measures for approximately 25% of recordings, and accuracy relative to true blood glucose (laboratory or blood gas analyser) is unknown [14].

More recently, a randomised controlled trial in very low birthweight infants demonstrated that CGM detected nearly three times as many episodes of hypoglycaemia (<2.8 mmol/L [<50 mg/dl]) during neonatal transition than intermittent blood glucose testing, and the medium duration of each episode was 95 min [5]. However, this study was also limited by use of point-of-care glucometers rather than true glucose measurements for both CGM calibration and diagnosis of hypoglycaemia.

Clinical use of CGM in neonatal intensive care

While use of CGM in neonatal intensive care is attractive to help improve neonatal glycaemic control and reduced the numbers of blood tests, there is currently little direct evidence of the benefits and risks of this technology in neonates. One small randomised trial ($N = 43$) compared real-time CGM with intermittent blood glucose monitoring in very low birthweight infants and found that CGM reduced the median duration of hypoglycemic episodes <2.8 mmol/L (<50 mg/dl) by 50% (95 vs 44 min) and the number of capillary blood samples by 25% [5]. However, infants in the CGM group also received more intravenous dextrose boluses and total carbohydrate, which could lead to higher or less stable glucose concentrations and increased total fluid intake, factors that were not reported but have been associated with increased morbidity [3, 57]. Thus in absence of clinical outcome data, including neurodevelopmental status, the overall balance of risks and benefits associated with clinical use of CGM in preterm infants remains uncertain.

There are several clinical situations in which neonatal glucose management can be particularly difficult and where optimisation of glycaemic control with CGM may be more likely to improve outcomes. These include infants with prolonged transitional hypoglycaemia, hypoxic ischaemic encephalopathy and preterm infants with hyperglycaemia. There is a paucity of data about use of CGM in these subgroups, and further studies are warranted.

Prolonged transitional hypoglycaemia

In most term and late preterm infants, hypoglycaemia resolves spontaneously within 1 to 3 days. However, a smaller group of infants experience persistent hypoglycaemia, sometimes called "perinatal stress-induced" or "prolonged transitional" hypoglycaemia, that can last for several weeks before gradually resolving [58]. These infants have dysregulation of pancreatic beta cells with associated hyperinsulinism [59], which can be difficult to manage due to rapidly changing glycaemic status. These infants likely experience significant subclinical hypoglycaemia and are at high risk of neurosensory impairment. A real-time CGM system that warned of impending hypoglycaemia in these infants would potentially allow for a more targeted approach to blood sampling, and may facilitate earlier transition to enteral feeding and reduce exposure to neuroglycopenia.

Hypoxic ischaemic encephalopathy

Dysglycaemia is common in babies with hypoxic ischemic encephalopathy [60], and both hypo- and hyperglycaemia have been associated with reduced survival and poorer neurological outcome [61]. There is, however, ongoing debate as to whether infants with initial hyperglycaemia have a more [62] or less [63] favourable response to therapeutic hypothermia. Current evidence suggests that the aim of glycaemic management in infants with hypoxic ischaemic encephalopathy should be careful avoidance of hypoglycaemia [64, 65] and maintenance of euglycaemia by regular titration of glucose delivery [65, 66]. This can be difficult to achieve with intermittent testing, unless sampling is frequent. Real-time CGM with trend information may help achieve greater glucose stability, although the effect of whole-body cooling on CGM sensor function is currently not known.

Hyperglycaemia in preterm infants

In very preterm infants, hyperglycaemia is associated with increased mortality, retinopathy of prematurity, sepsis and long-term neurodevelopmental impairment [67, 68], and animal studies indicate that this association is at least in part causal [69]. Since CGM data has shown that up to half of very low birth weight infants develop hyperglycaemia [2, 53], better detection and treatment of high glucose concentrations may improve outcomes. However, the benefits of treatment with insulin are uncertain as insulin infusions substantially increase the risk of hypoglycaemia, both in very preterm infants [56, 70] and in children in intensive care [71].

The use of combined CGM, insulin pump and computer algorithm (artificial pancreas) has been shown to be effective in type 1 diabetics in reducing the frequency and duration of hypoglycaemia [72]. Computer determined insulin dosing using calculated insulin sensitivity has promise as a management tool in hyperglycaemic preterm infants [73, 74]. However, there are currently no data on the use of CGM to inform insulin management of neonatal hyperglycaemia, although the use of CGM in conjunction with an insulin infusion was reported to reduce the number of episodes of hypoglycaemia in a baby with neonatal diabetes [75]. In paediatric intensive care, use of CGM to guide frequency of blood glucose measurements in a trial of insulin and tight glycaemic control did not prevent severe hypoglycaemia [71]. However, this study did not use calculated insulin sensitivity to guide insulin dose and CGM calibration was based only on point-of-care glucometers without point-to-point calibration. If accuracy of real-time CGM can be improved, it may become possible for very preterm infants with hyperglycaemia to be managed with an artificial pancreas to allow optimal glycaemic control.

Conclusion

CGM offers considerable potential for optimisation of glycaemia in newborn infants but several issues need to be addressed before this technology can be recommended for real-time monitoring in neonatal intensive care. First, devices should ideally be calibrated to plasma equivalent whole-blood glucose concentrations measured on a blood gas analyser using a point-to-point algorithm. Current CGM devices employ multi-point algorithms that were designed for management of diabetes mellitus in children and adults using home glucometers and at higher glucose concentrations. Real-time calibration methods that are specific to the neonatal intensive care environment are required. Second, the potential for sensor drift, which could result in apparently stable CGM values when blood glucose concentration is falling, requires further investigation, including the extent to which it occurs in neonates and its impact on clinical care. This information will be important in determining how frequently calibration should occur. Third, because CGM has limited point accuracy, clinical metrics should be based on integration of multiple GCM values with a focus on glucose stability, trends and changing metabolic patterns, rather than exceeding specific thresholds. Further research is needed to determine which metrics should be targeted for improving long-term outcomes.

Despite these limitations, retrospective CGM is already an important tool for understanding neonatal glycaemia and the effect of different treatments on glucose metabolism. Current use of CGM should be limited to research studies, and this technology should not be introduced into routine clinical care without evidence of benefit from randomised trials.

Abbreviations

CGM: Continuous glucose monitor; MARD: Mean absolute relative difference

Acknowledgements

We are grateful to members of The CHYLD Study Team who contributed to work cited in this review; the authors also acknowledge the support of the EUFP7 and RSNZ Marie Curie IRSES program, the Health Research Council (HRC) of New Zealand, The Eunice Kennedy Shriver National Institute of Child Health and Human Development, the MedTech CoRE and TEC, and NZ National Science Challenge 7, Science for Technology and Innovation. The content is solely the responsibility of the authors and does not necessarily represent the official views of the Eunice Kennedy Shriver National Institute of Child Health and Human Development or the National Institutes of Health.

Funding

No direct funding was obtained for this review.

Authors' contributions

All authors contributed to writing this review, and read and approved the final manuscript.

Competing interests

The authors declare that they have no competing interests.

Author details

[1]Liggins Institute, University of Auckland, Private Bag 92019, Victoria St West, Auckland 1142, New Zealand. [2]Department of Paediatrics: Child and Youth Health, University of Auckland, Auckland, New Zealand. [3]Mechanical Engineering, University of Canterbury, Christchurch, New Zealand. [4]Neonatal Intensive Care Unit, Waikato District Health Board, Hamilton, New Zealand.

References

1. Harris DL, Battin MR, Weston PJ, Harding JE. Continuous glucose monitoring in newborn babies at risk of hypoglycemia. J Pediatr. 2010;157(2):198–202.
2. Szymonska I, Jagla M, Starzec K, Hrnciar K, Kwinta P. The incidence of hyperglycaemia in very low birth weight preterm newborns. Results of a continuous glucose monitoring study–preliminary report. Dev Period Med. 2015;19(3 Pt 1):305–12.
3. McKinlay CJD, Alsweiler JA, Ansell JM, Anstice NS, Chase JG, Gamble GD, et al. Neonatal glycemia and neurodevelopmental outcomes at two years. N Engl J Med. 2015;373:1507–18.
4. Ranger M, Chau CM, Garg A, Woodward TS, Beg MF, Bjornson B, et al. Neonatal pain-related stress predicts cortical thickness at age 7 years in children born very preterm. PLoS One. 2013;8(10):e76702.
5. Uettwiller F, Chemin A, Bonnemaison E, Favrais G, Saliba E, Labarthe F. Real-time continuous glucose monitoring reduces the duration of hypoglycemia episodes: a randomized trial in very low birth weight neonates. PLoS One. 2015;10(1):e0116255.
6. Hume R, McGeechan A, Burchell A. Failure to detect preterm infants at risk of hypoglycemia before discharge. J Pediatr. 1999;134(4):499–502.
7. Mizumoto H, Kawai M, Yamashita S, Hata D. Intraday glucose fluctuation is common in preterm infants receiving intermittent tube feeding. Pediatr Int. 2016;58(5):359–62.
8. Nakamura T, Hatanaka D, Nakamura M, Kusakari M, Takahashi H, Kamohara T. Serial investigation of continuous glucose monitoring in a very low birth weight infant with transient late-onset hyperglycemia. Fukushima J Med Sci. 2016;62(2):108–11.
9. Mola-Schenzle E, Staffler A, Klemme M, Pellegrini F, Molinaro G, Parhofer KG, et al. Clinically stable very low birthweight infants are at risk for recurrent tissue glucose fluctuations even after fully established enteral nutrition. Arch Dis Child Fetal Neonatal Ed. 2015;100(2):F126–31.
10. Poscia A, Mascini M, Moscone D, Luzzana M, Caramenti G, Cremonesi P, et al. A microdialysis technique for continuous subcutaneous glucose monitoring in diabetic patients (part 1). Biosens Bioelectron. 2003;18(7):891–8.
11. Baumeister FA, Rolinski B, Busch R, Emmrich P. Glucose monitoring with long-term subcutaneous microdialysis in neonates. Pediatrics. 2001;108(5):1187–92.
12. Hildingsson U, Sellden H, Ungerstedt U, Marcus C. Microdialysis for metabolic monitoring in neonates after surgery. Acta Paediatr. 1996;85(5):589–94.
13. McGarraugh G. The chemistry of commercial continuous glucose monitors. Diabetes Technol Ther. 2009;11(Suppl 1):S17–24.
14. Beardsall K, Vanhaesebrouck S, Ogilvy-Stuart AL, Vanhole C, VanWeissenbruch M, Midgley P, et al. Validation of the continuous glucose monitoring sensor in preterm infants. Arch Dis Child Fetal Neonatal Ed. 2013;98(2):F136–40.
15. Harris DL, Weston PJ, Harding JE. Mothers of babies enrolled in a randomized trial immediately after birth report a positive experience. J Perinatol. 2014;34(4):280–3.
16. Signal M, Le Compte A, Harris DL, Weston PJ, Harding JE, Chase JG, et al. Impact of retrospective calibration algorithms on hypoglycemia detection in newborn infants using continuous glucose monitoring. Diabetes Tech Ther. 2012;14(10):883–90.
17. Peet AC, Kennedy DM, Hocking MD, Ewer AK. Near-patient testing of blood glucose using the Bayer Rapidlab 860 analyser in a regional neonatal unit. Ann Clin Biochem. 2002;39(Pt 5):502–8.
18. Tiangco C, Andar A, Quarterman J, Ge X, Sevilla F, 3rd, Rao G, et al. Measuring transdermal glucose levels in neonates by passive diffusion: an in vitro porcine skin model. Anal Bioanal Chem 2017;409(13):3475-3482.
19. Mauras N, Beck RW, Ruedy KJ, Kollman C, Tamborlane WV, Chase HP, et al. Lack of accuracy of continuous glucose sensors in healthy, nondiabetic children: results of the Diabetes Research in Children Network (DirecNet) accuracy study. J Pediatr. 2004;144(6):770–5.
20. Michel A, Kuster H, Krebs A, Kadow I, Paul W, Nauck M, et al. Evaluation of the Glucometer Elite XL device for screening for neonatal hypoglycaemia. Eur J Pediatr. 2005;164(11):660–4.
21. Rosenthal M, Ugele B, Lipowsky G, Kuster H. The Accutrend sensor glucose analyzer may not be adequate in bedside testing for neonatal hypoglycemia. Eur J Pediatr. 2006;165(2):99–103.
22. Facchinetti A, Sparacino G, Cobelli C. Modeling the error of continuous glucose monitoring sensor data: critical aspects discussed through simulation studies. J Diabetes Sci Technol. 2010;4(1):4–14.
23. Biagi L, Ramkissoon CM, Facchinetti A, Leal Y, Vehi J. Modeling the error of the medtronic paradigm veo enlite glucose sensor. Sensors (Basel). 2017;17(6).
24. Fonseca VA, Grunberger G, Anhalt H, Bailey TS, Blevins T, Garg SK, et al. Continuous glucose monitoring: a consensus conference of the american association of clinical endocrinologists and american college of endocrinology. Endocr Pract. 2016;22(8):1008–21.
25. Damiano ER, McKeon K, El-Khatib FH, Zheng H, Nathan DM, Russell SJ. A comparative effectiveness analysis of three continuous glucose monitors: the Navigator, G4 Platinum, and Enlite. J Diabetes Sci Technol. 2014;8(4):699–708.
26. Signal M, Thomas F, Shaw GM, Chase JG. Complexity of continuous glucose monitoring data in critically ill patients: continuous glucose monitoring devices, sensor locations, and detrended fluctuation analysis methods. J Diabetes Sci Technol. 2013;7(6):1492–506.
27. Facchinetti A, Del Favero S, Sparacino G, Castle JR, Ward WK, Cobelli C. Modeling the glucose sensor error. IEEE Trans Biomed Eng. 2014;61(3):620–9.
28. Thomas F, Signal M, Harris DL, Weston PJ, Harding JE, Shaw GM, et al. Continuous glucose monitoring in newborn infants: how do errors in calibration measurements affect detected hypoglycemia? J Diabetes Sci Technol. 2014;8(3):543–50.

29. Breton MD, Shields DP, Kovatchev BP. Optimum subcutaneous glucose sampling and fourier analysis of continuous glucose monitors. J Diabetes Sci Technol. 2008;2(3):495–500.

30. Kovatchev BP, Shields D, Breton M. Graphical and numerical evaluation of continuous glucose sensing time lag. Diabetes Technol Ther. 2009;11(3):139–43.

31. Schmelzeisen-Redeker G, Schoemaker M, Kirchsteiger H, Freckmann G, Heinemann L, Del Re L. Time delay of CGM sensors: relevance, causes, and countermeasures. J Diabetes Sci Technol. 2015;9(5):1006–15.

32. Breton M, Kovatchev B. Analysis, modeling, and simulation of the accuracy of continuous glucose sensors. J Diabetes Sci Technol. 2008;2(5):853–62.

33. Baumeister FA, Hack A, Busch R. Glucose-monitoring with continuous subcutaneous microdialysis in neonatal diabetes mellitus. Klin Padiatr. 2006; 218(4):230–2.

34. Tiberi E, Cota F, Barone G, Perri A, Romano V, Iannotta R, et al. Continuous glucose monitoring in preterm infants: evaluation by a modified Clarke error grid. Ital J Pediatr. 2016;42:29.

35. Chase JG, Pretty CG, Pfeifer L, Shaw GM, Preiser JC, Le Compte AJ, et al. Organ failure and tight glycemic control in the SPRINT study. Crit Care. 2010;14(4):R154.

36. Signal M, Le Compte A, Shaw GM, Chase JG. Glycemic levels in critically ill patients: are normoglycemia and low variability associated with improved outcomes? J Diabetes Sci Technol. 2012;6(5):1030–7.

37. Krinsley JS, Preiser JC. Time in blood glucose range 70 to 140 mg/dl >80% is strongly associated with increased survival in non-diabetic critically ill adults. Crit Care. 2015;19:179.

38. Pretty CG, Chase JG, Le Compte A, Shaw GM, Signal M. Hypoglycemia detection in critical care using continuous glucose monitors: an in silico proof of concept analysis. J Diabetes Sci Technol. 2010;4(1):15–24.

39. Signal M, Gottlieb R, Le Compte A, Chase JG. Continuous glucose monitoring and trend accuracy: news about a trend compass. J Diabetes Sci Technol. 2014;8(5):986–97.

40. Thomas F, Signal M, Chase JG. Using continuous glucose monitoring data and detrended fluctuation analysis to determine patient condition: a review. J Diabetes Sci Technol. 2015;9(6):1327–35.

41. Signal M, Le Compte A, Harris DL, Weston PJ, Harding JE, Chase JG, et al. Using Stochastic modelling to identify unusual continuous glucose monitor measurements and behaviour, in newborn infants. Biomed Eng Online. 2012;11:45.

42. Srinivasan G, Pildes RS, Cattamanchi G, Voora S, Lilien LD. Plasma glucose values in normal neonates: a new look. J Pediatr. 1986;109(1):114–7.

43. Diwakar KK, Sasidhar MV. Plasma glucose levels in term infants who are appropriate size for gestation and exclusively breast fed. Arch Dis Child Fetal Neonatal Ed. 2002;87(1):F46–8.

44. Hoseth E, Joergensen A, Ebbesen F, Moeller M. Blood glucose levels in a population of healthy, breast fed, term infants of appropriate size for gestational age. Arch Dis Child Fetal Neonatal Ed. 2000;83(2):F117–9.

45. Güemes M, Rahman SA, Hussain K. What is a normal blood glucose? Arch Dis Child. 2016;101(6):569–74.

46. Wackernagel D, Dube M, Blennow M, Tindberg Y. Continuous subcutaneous glucose monitoring is accurate in term and near-term infants at risk of hypoglycaemia. Acta Paediatr. 2016;105(8):917–23.

47. Kaiser JR, Bai S, Gibson N, Holland G, Lin TM, Swearingen CJ, et al. Association between transient newborn hypoglycemia and fourth-grade achievement test proficiency: a population-based study. JAMA Pediatr. 2015; 169(10):913–21.

48. Ennis K, Dotterman H, Stein A, Rao R. Hyperglycemia accentuates and ketonemia attenuates hypoglycemia-induced neuronal injury in the developing rat brain. Pediatr Res. 2015;77(1–1):84–90.

49. Suh SW, Gum ET, Hamby AM, Chan PH, Swanson RA. Hypoglycemic neuronal death is triggered by glucose reperfusion and activation of neuronal NADPH oxidase. J Clin Invest. 2007;117(4):910–8.

50. McKinlay CJD, Alsweiler JM, Anstice NS, Burakevych N, Chakraborty A, Chase JG, et al. A prospective cohort study of neonatal glycemia and neurodevelopmental outcomes at 4.5 years. JAMA Pediatr. 2017;171(10):1–12.

51. Beardsall K, Ogilvy-Stuart AL, Ahluwalia J, Thompson M, Dunger DB. The continuous glucose monitoring sensor in neonatal intensive care. Arch Dis Child Fetal Neonatal Ed. 2005;90(4):F307–10.

52. Beardsall K. Measurement of glucose levels in the newborn. Early Hum Dev. 2010;86(5):263–7.

53. Beardsall K, Vanhaesebrouck S, Ogilvy-Stuart AL, Vanhole C, Palmer CR, Ong K, et al. Prevalence and determinants of hyperglycemia in very low birth

weight infants: cohort analyses of the NIRTURE study. J Pediatr. 2010;157(5): 715–9.e1-3.

54. Pertierra-Cortada A, Ramon-Krauel M, Iriondo-Sanz M, Iglesias-Platas I. Instability of glucose values in very preterm babies at term postmenstrual age. J Pediatr. 2014;165(6):1146–53.e2.

55. Iglesias Platas I, Thio Lluch M, Pociello Alminana N, Morillo Palomo A, Iriondo Sanz M, Krauel VX. Continuous glucose monitoring in infants of very low birth weight. Neonatology. 2009;95(3):217–23.

56. Beardsall K, Vanhaesebrouck S, Ogilvy-Stuart AL, Vanhole C, Palmer CR, van Weissenbruch M, et al. Early insulin therapy in very-low-birth-weight infants. N Engl J Med. 2008;359(18):1873–84.

57. Oh W, Poindexter BB, Perritt R, Lemons JA, Bauer CR, Ehrenkranz RA, et al. Association between fluid intake and weight loss during the first ten days of life and risk of bronchopulmonary dysplasia in extremely low birth weight infants. J Pediatr. 2005;147(6):786–90.

58. Collins JE, Leonard JV. Hyperinsulinism in asphyxiated and small-for-dates infants with hypoglycaemia. Lancet. 1984;2(8398):311–3.

59. Hoe FM, Thornton PS, Wanner LA, Steinkrauss L, Simmons RA, Stanley CA. Clinical features and insulin regulation in infants with a syndrome of prolonged neonatal hyperinsulinism. J Pediatr. 2006;148(2):207–12.

60. Nadeem M, Murray DM, Boylan GB, Dempsey EM, Ryan CA. Early blood glucose profile and neurodevelopmental outcome at two years in neonatal hypoxic-ischaemic encephalopathy. BMC Pediatr. 2011;11:10.

61. Basu SK, Kaiser JR, Guffey D, Minard CG, Guillet R, Gunn AJ. Hypoglycaemia and hyperglycaemia are associated with unfavourable outcome in infants with hypoxic ischaemic encephalopathy: a post hoc analysis of the CoolCap Study. Arch Dis Child Fetal Neonatal Ed. 2016;101(2):F149–55.

62. Basu SK, Salemi JL, Gunn AJ, Kaiser JR. Hyperglycaemia in infants with hypoxic-ischaemic encephalopathy is associated with improved outcomes after therapeutic hypothermia: a post hoc analysis of the CoolCap Study. Arch Dis Child Fetal Neonatal Ed. 2017;102(4):299–306.

63. Chouthai NS, Sobczak H, Khan R, Subramanian D, Raman S, Rao R. Hyperglycemia is associated with poor outcome in newborn infants undergoing therapeutic hypothermia for hypoxic ischemic encephalopathy. J Neonatal Perinatal Med. 2015;8(2):125–31.

64. Wong DS, Poskitt KJ, Chau V, Miller SP, Roland E, Hill A, et al. Brain injury patterns in hypoglycemia in neonatal encephalopathy. Am J Neuroradiol. 2013;34(7):1456–61.

65. Boardman JP, Hawdon JM. Hypoglycaemia and hypoxic-ischaemic encephalopathy. Dev Med Child Neurol. 2015;57(Suppl 3):29–33.

66. McGowan JE, Perlman JM. Glucose management during and after intensive delivery room resuscitation. Clin Perinatol. 2006;33(1):183–96.

67. van der Lugt NM, Smits-Wintjens VE, van Zwieten PH, Walther FJ. Short and long term outcome of neonatal hyperglycemia in very preterm infants: a retrospective follow-up study. BMC Pediatr. 2010;10:52.

68. Mohsen L, Abou-Alam M, El-Dib M, Labib M, Elsada M, Aly H. A prospective study on hyperglycemia and retinopathy of prematurity. J Perinatol. 2014; 34(6):453–7.

69. Alsweiler JM, Harding JE, Bloomfield FH. Neonatal hyperglycaemia increases mortality and morbidity in preterm lambs. Neonatology. 2013;103(2):83–90.

70. Alsweiler JM, Harding JE, Bloomfield FH. Tight glycemic control with insulin in hyperglycemic preterm babies: a randomized controlled trial. Pediatrics. 2012;129(4):639–47.

71. Agus MS, Wypij D, Hirshberg EL, Srinivasan V, Faustino EV, Luckett PM, et al. Tight glycemic control in critically ill children. N Engl J Med. 2017;376(8): 729–41.

72. Phillip M, Battelino T, Atlas E, Kordonouri O, Bratina N, Miller S, et al. Nocturnal glucose control with an artificial pancreas at a diabetes camp. N Engl J Med. 2013;368(9):824–33.

73. Le Compte A, Chase JG, Lynn A, Hann C, Shaw G, Wong XW, et al. Blood glucose controller for neonatal intensive care: virtual trials development and first clinical trials. J Diabetes Sci Technol. 2009;3(5):1066–81.

74. Le Compte AJ, Lynn AM, Lin J, Pretty CG, Shaw GM, Chase JG. Pilot study of a model-based approach to blood glucose control in very-low-birthweight neonates. BMC Pediatr. 2012;12:117.

75. Beardsall K, Pesterfield CL, Acerini CL. Neonatal diabetes and insulin pump therapy. Arch Dis Child Fetal Neonatal Ed. 2011;96(3):F223–4.

8

Introducing eHealth strategies to enhance maternal and perinatal health care in rural Tanzania

Angelo Nyamtema[1,2,3]*[iD], Nguke Mwakatundu[1], Sunday Dominico[1], Mkambu Kasanga[1], Fadhili Jamadini[1], Kelvin Maokola[1], Donald Mawala[1], Zabron Abel[2], Richard Rumanyika[1,4], Calist Nzabuhakwa[1,5] and Jos van Roosmalen[1,6,7]

Abstract

Background: Globally, eHealth has attracted considerable attention as a means of supporting maternal and perinatal health care. This article describes best practices, gains and challenges of implementing eHealth for maternal and perinatal health care in extremely remote and rural Tanzania.

Methods: Teleconsultation for obstetric emergency care, audio teleconferences and online eLearning systems were installed in ten upgraded rural health centres, four rural district hospitals and one regional hospital in Tanzania. Uptake of teleconsultation and teleconference platforms were evaluated retrospectively. A cross sectional descriptive study design was applied to assess performance and adoption of eLearning.

Results: In 2015 a total of 38 teleconsultations were attended by consultant obstetricians and 33 teleconferences were conducted and attended by 40 health care providers from 14 facilities. A total of 240 clinical cases mainly caesarean sections (CS), maternal and perinatal morbidities and mortalities were discussed and recommendations for improvement were provided. Four modules were hosted and 43 care providers were registered on the eLearning system. For a period of 18–21 months total views on the site, weekly conference forum, chatroom and learning resources ranged between 106 and 1,438. Completion of learning modules, acknowledgment of having acquired and utilized new knowledge and skills in clinical practice were reported in 43–89% of 20 interviewed health care providers. Competencies in using the eLearning system were demonstrated in 62% of the targeted users.

Conclusions: E-Health presents an opportunity for improving maternal health care in underserved remote areas in low-resource settings by broadening knowledge and skills, and by connecting frontline care providers with consultants for emergency teleconsultations.

Keywords: EHealth, eLearning, Teleconference, Teleconsultation, Rural settings, Maternal health, Tanzania

Background

Tanzania has one of the highest maternal mortality ratios (MMR 398/10⁵ live births) and one of lowest densities of skilled health care providers in the world, an element which is critical to enhance maternal and perinatal health [1]. Skilled health care workers (i.e. physicians, associate clinicians, nurse-midwives, and laboratory, radiology and pharmaceutical technicians) fill only 35% of the requirement, and only 55% of births in rural areas are assisted by skilled personnel compared to 87% in urban areas. This suggests not only a severe crisis of human resources for health, but also serious health inequities across the country [2, 3]. Like many other countries, Tanzania has embarked on task-sharing by using less trained mid-level care providers including clinical officers (associate clinicians) and assistant medical officers (advanced associate clinicians) [4, 5]. The World Health Organization (WHO) defines associate clinician as a professional with basic

* Correspondence: nyamtema_angelo@yahoo.co.uk
[1]Thamini Uhai Program, Dar es Salaam, Tanzania
[2]Tanzanian Training Centre for International Health, Ifakara, Tanzania
Full list of author information is available at the end of the article

competencies to diagnose and manage common medical, maternal, child health and surgical conditions [6]. Advanced level associate clinician is defined as a professional with advanced competencies to diagnose and manage the most common medical, maternal, child health and surgical conditions, including obstetric and gynaecological surgery (e.g. caesarean sections). Although evidence shows that mid-level care providers can perform related tasks, task sharing must be aligned with broader strengthening of knowledge and clinical skills, mentorship and support if sustainable provision of quality health care is to be achieved [7].

Worldwide consensus exists that eHealth, the use of information and communication technologies (ICT) for health, has the potential to significantly improve management of patients, conducting research, educating health care providers, tracking diseases and monitoring public health [8]. EHealth can be used to improve knowledge, competencies, accountability and effectiveness; mentorship provision and health system's ability to manage its commodities, equipment and health care workers [9]. Increasing uptake of mobile ICT in Tanzania constitutes new opportunities to support maternal and perinatal health care interventions. Tanzania's eHealth strategy 2013, through its well-articulated strategic objectives, emphasizes the need to improve quality of health service delivery in rural settings through eHealth solutions [3].

Recognizing the potential of ICT in addressing challenges in provision of quality maternal health care, the Thamini Uhai program designed and implemented an eHealth platform with a goal to support national efforts to address the crisis of skilled care providers and improve maternal health care delivery [3]. Our platform aimed at improving knowledge and clinical decision-making skills of mid-level care providers, support emergency care and formulate an eHealth model solution for maternal health care in underserved rural settings. This study describes the Thamini Uhai program's best practices, gains and challenges of implementing eHealth for maternal health care in extremely remote and rural Tanzania.

Methods
Project areas
The project established an eHealth platform to support fifteen health facilities (ten upgraded health centres [HC], four rural district hospitals and one regional referral hospital) located in three regions (Kigoma, Morogoro and Pwani) in Tanzania. Nine upgraded HC were located in the hardest to reach rural areas in seven districts. Upgrading of HC involved constructing and equipping maternity blocks, operating theatre, laboratories, staff houses and installing solar panels, standby generators

and water supply systems, and training associate clinicians in CEmONC and anaesthesia. The details of the support other than the eHealth platform have been reported elsewhere [10].

ICT infrastructure design
The eHealth platform had three components: 1) mobile teleconsultations for obstetric emergency care; 2) an audio teleconferencing model; and 3) an online eLearning platform. The mobile teleconsultation platform was designed to enable health care providers, working in Thamini Uhai-supported facilities, to call experienced obstetricians and discuss obstetric emergencies in which further guidance or advice was needed to help providers make the right decisions. Health care providers in the supported facilities and consultant obstetrician/gynaecologists were connected through toll-free mobile phones by way of a closed user group. Duty rosters for consultant obstetricians were developed and all calls made for consultation were documented. This service was available 24 hours a day, seven days a week.

An audio teleconferencing model was established in 2012 and health care providers in the supported facilities, consultant obstetrician/gynaecologists, and anaesthesiologists were routinely connected through toll-free mobile phones by way of a closed user group. This model applied the concept of case study-based learning, a form of problem-based learning, using challenging obstetric cases encountered over the previous week to increase knowledge and understanding and develop generic skills and encourage self-reflection in maternal health care. During the teleconference one person from each facility reported the weekly number of deliveries, caesarean sections, vacuum-assisted vaginal deliveries, number and reasons for obstetric referrals. Severe morbidities, fresh stillbirths, very early neonatal and maternal deaths were reported in length and management and justifications (indications) for interventions were discussed. Selection of these cases was based on the fact that they might be preventable based on changes in care, resources, education, or medical access. The contents of these teleconferences were documented and disseminated to the relevant stakeholders for action-oriented feedback.

An online eLearning platform was established in 2014. The learning sessions were hosted in a web-based eLearning application called Moodle. To address the challenge in internet connectivity in rural settings, Multi-Protocol Label Switching (MPLS) Virtual Private Network was installed in all supported facilities to enable users in remote facilities to connect with the application server in Dar es Salaam through laptops. Network Address Translation (NAT) enabled accessibility of the application through the web. Each facility was equipped with at least one laptop through the local contact person.

A total of four sessions were hosted in the eLearning platform. These included caesarean section, spinal anaesthesia (which included two tailor-made education films), management of postpartum haemorrhage and neonatal resuscitation. This 'virtual classroom' also enabled health care providers to access presentations and up-to-date peer-review journal articles. The system also allowed registered users to use integrated online fora to share clinical challenges and successes with fellow colleagues and senior experts across the 15 health facilities.

Study design, study population and sampling technique

A retrospective study design was applied to evaluate the mobile teleconsultation platform and audio teleconferencing model. A cross sectional descriptive study design was applied to evaluate the performance and adoption of online eLearning platform. The study population for online eLearning platform were health care providers working in supported health facilities. Only those health care providers who were available on the day of study were included in the study. Considering the diversity of the topics of learning sessions in the online eLearning platform, purposive selection of health care providers for interview was preferred and applied. Because of the time limitations placed on the study, at least one care provider was selected from each health facility to demonstrate skills on using eLearning platform.

E-learning system evaluation framework

To evaluate performance and adoption of the eLearning system the Method Evaluation Model (MEM) was used. MEM was chosen because it incorporates all aspects of evaluation including user performance, perceptions of usefulness, intentions to use and user behaviour towards the system (Fig. 1) [11].

In the MEM model, efficiency is measured by the extent to which use of the eLearning system by health care providers is effort free, whereas actual effectiveness is measured by the extent to which use of the eLearning system improves the quality of learning. Perceived ease

of use and perceived usefulness represented user's perceptions about the usefulness and ease of use of the eLearning platform. The third construct was the intention to use, which is the extent to which a health care provider intends to use the eLearning system in the future for learning purposes. The last construct measured actual usage of the system.

Data collection instruments

Four types of instruments for data collection were used in this study.

Instrument 1: Data collection instrument for the mobile teleconsultation platform

This instrument was used to extract the number of calls made, obstetric indications (types of emergencies) for calling, type of support provided and outcome.

Instrument 2: Data collection instrument for audio teleconferencing model

This instrument was used to collect data on the number of health facilities and health care providers who participated in each teleconference, frequency of connectivity interruptions, categories of cases (morbidity, mortality, and procedures) presented and discussed.

Instruments 3.1 and 3.2: Data collection tools for e-Learning

These were developed to gain as much information as possible regarding design and impact of the eLearning system on improving learning and health outcomes. Instrument 3.1: end-user questionnaire, which aimed at assessing provider's awareness, knowledge, perception and practice of using the e-Learning platform. Instrument 3.2: Review and analysis of the general and session specific activity report worksheets. These data were obtained by commanding the reports on the eLearning platform.

Data collection

Data collection tools for mobile teleconsultation and audio teleconferencing platforms were used to extract

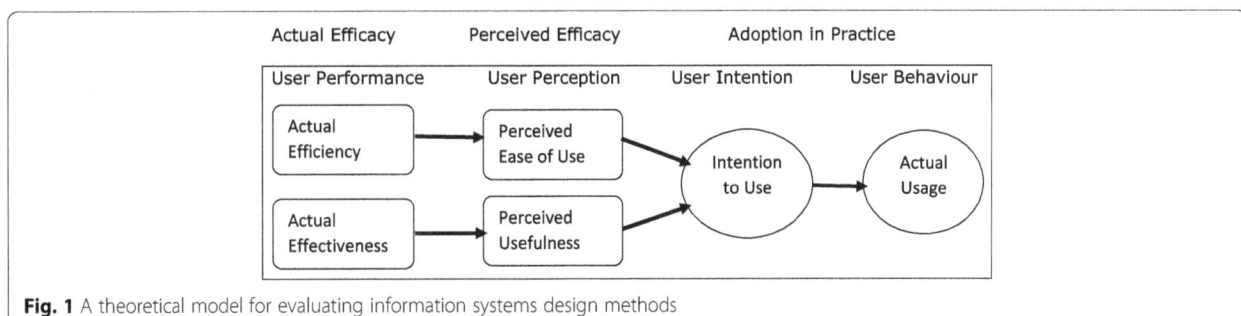

Fig. 1 A theoretical model for evaluating information systems design methods

information from the available records. Data collection for eLearning platform involved a team of experts who visited the health facilities to evaluate user performance, perceptions and intentions, and user behaviour towards the installed system.

Effectiveness of the eLearning system

To investigate users' effectiveness of using the eLearning platform, health care providers were required to demonstrate the use of the eLearning system when the investigator observed. Then the investigator, guided by instrument 3.1, observed how effectively health care providers used the module and whether they had completed, and/or had learnt new things. Furthermore, through interviews, the investigation aimed at determining whether health care providers used in practice the knowledge they had learned through the eLearning system.

Efficiency of the eLearning system

To investigate efficiency on using the eLearning platform health care providers were required to demonstrate use of the system in the presence of an observer. Seven tasks were used to assess efficiency: enter user name and password, identify features within the platform, ability to use features within the platform (site news, chatroom, learning resources), identify the four sessions in the platform, open one of the sessions, navigate through the sessions, and perform quiz questions within the platform.

Perception-based variables

Perceived ease of use is the degree to which a person believes that using the eLearning system is free of effort. In order to investigate users' perception of the eLearning platform, we asked the participants to grade the system based on how easy it was to use the system. We scaled responses on a Likert scale from 1 to 5, i.e. very difficult, difficult, neutral, easy and very easy.

Intention to use variables

Participants were asked questions designed to assess their intentions to use the eLearning system in the future for learning purposes.

Actual usage variables

To investigate actual usage of the system we retrieved data from instrument 3.2, the platform general activity and session specific reports obtained by commanding the reports on the e-Learning platform. The data included user access to the website, user participation in chats, posting and viewing various learning contents.

Data analysis

Data were cleaned and consistency checks were done using Microsoft Excel. Actual effectiveness, perceived efficacy and adoption in practice of the eLearning system were analysed using Microsoft Excel and summarized in proportions.

Results

Teleconferencing and mobile teleconsultation platforms

A total of 33 teleconferences were conducted in 2015 and 40 health care providers from 14 supported facilities took part. Participants included 14 (35%) assistant medical officers, 13 (32.5%) nurse-midwives/clinical officers trained in anaesthesia, and 13 (32.5%) additional nurse-midwives. Health facility participation ranged from 2 to 6 per teleconference with an average of 4 facilities per teleconference. The facility recording the highest level of participation was Kibiti HC in Pwani region, which participated in 82% (27) of the teleconferences (Table 1). Nyenge HC in Kigoma region did not participate in any of the teleconferences because of poor connectivity.

A total of 240 clinical cases were presented and discussed during the teleconferences. These included 7 (3%) maternal deaths, 24 (10%) perinatal deaths (fresh stillbirths and early neonatal deaths), 54 (23%) maternal and newborn morbidities and 138 (57%) caesarean sections, 12 (5%) vacuum-assisted vaginal deliveries and 5 (2%) cases of ectopic pregnancy, breech deliveries and internal podalic version for a retained second twin. Commendable performances and factors related to substandard care within the facilities were identified, discussed and recommendations for improvement were provided. During teleconferences a remarkable proportion of severe morbidities and maternal and/or perinatal deaths were attributed to inadequate, inappropriate interventions and delayed decisions. These cases were audited during physical supervision visits to the facilities and the results have been reported elsewhere [10, 12].

A total of 38 emergency teleconsultations (calls) were received and attended by consultant obstetricians/gynaecologists in 2015. These included complications of pregnancy and labour, medical conditions in pregnancy and abnormalities of menstruation. Advice on how to manage the patients was provided. A total of 33 (87%) patients were successfully managed locally and the rest (13%) were stabilized and referred to higher facilities.

Online eLearning system: views and performance

A total of 43 health care providers were registered as users and were oriented on the eLearning platform at the time of its establishment. For a period of 18 to 21 months the total views on the site ranged between 106 and 1,438 among the different options of weekly conference forum, project chatroom, caesarean section

Table 1 Frequency of participation of health facilities and connectivity interruptions during the teleconferences

Health Facility	Frequency of facility participation n (%)	Number of care providers participated at least once	Frequency of connectivity interruptions during teleconference n (%)
Health Centres			
Kibiti	27 (82%)	7	0 (0%)
Ujiji	15 (45%)	3	0 (0%)
Nguruka	12 (36%)	5	1 (8%)
Mtimbira	14 (42%)	2	2 (14%)
Mabamba	12 (36%)	4	1 (8%)
Kakonko	8 (24%)	1	0 (0%)
Mlimba	11 (33%)	6	2 (18%)
Buhingu	5 (15%)	2	1 (20%)
Mwaya	6 (18%)	1	0 (0%)
Nyenge	0 (0%)	0	0 (0%)
District Hospitals			
Kibondo	2 (6%)	2	0 (0%)
Utete	12 (36%)	4	0 (0%)
Mahenge	11 (33%)	1	1 (9%)
Kasulu	1 (3%)	1	0 (0%)
Kigoma (Maweni) RRH	2 (6%)	2	0 (0%)

Note: *RRH* regional referral hospital

resources, spinal anaesthesia resources and videos for various topics (Table 2).

Actual effectiveness of the eLearning system

Almost six months after orientation, 20 care providers (47% of the registered users) from the supported health facilities were interviewed and their competencies in using the system were assessed. Among these 10 (50%) were assistant medical officers (advanced associate clinicians), one was a clinical officer (associate clinician), seven were nurse-midwives, and two were anaesthetists.

Table 2 Summary of Thamini Uhai's eLearning system utilization from its establishment in September 2014 to May 2016.

Activity	Date of posting into system	Views as of 31 May 2016
Site views	2 Sept 2014	1,438
Weekly conference forum	4 Oct 2014	487
Project chatroom	4 Oct 2014	329
Caesarean section resources	17 Nov 2014	184
Spinal anaesthesia resources	17 Nov 2014	121
Video		
Introduction on caesarean section	17 Nov 2014	208
Caesarean section procedure	17 Nov 2014	150
Introduction on spinal anaesthesia	17 Nov 2014	106
Spinal anaesthesia procedure	17 Nov 2014	125
Modules[a]		
Postpartum haemorrhage	3 Jul 2015	38
Caesarean section	20 Oct 2014	36
Spinal anaesthesia for caesarean section	20 Oct 2014	36
Birth asphyxia and neonatal resuscitation	4 Jul 2015	36

[a]The number of views and viewers were those made by registered care providers from the supported facilities

Health care providers were grouped based on the scope of tasks they routinely performed with regards to emergency obstetric care, caesarean section and anaesthesia, and then were interviewed on the hosted modules. Between 43% and 78% of the respondents reported to have completed the modules, while 57% - 89% acknowledged to have learnt something new after reading the modules, utilized in clinical practice the lessons learned and expected to use the modules in future (Fig. 2).

Specifically, the skills that the care providers reported to have acquired through the eLearning included active management of third stage of labour, better ways of performing caesarean section, use of condom tamponade for controlling postpartum bleeding, proper preparation of pregnant women before CS and proper positioning of a pregnant woman during and after provision of anaesthesia.

Actual efficiency of the eLearning system

Sixteen health care providers were involved in the assessment of competencies in using the system. Each care provider was individually assessed whether she/ he was able to: identify features within the platform; open at least one session; navigate through the sessions; and perform a quiz within the platform. Competencies in performing these task were demonstrated by 5 – 10 (i.e. 31–62%) care providers (Fig. 3). As expected, competencies were demonstrated more in the simplest use-features of the system, like identification of features within the platform (62%), rather than in complex features like navigating through the sessions (31%).

Perceived efficacy and adoption in practice of the eLearning system

Out of twenty respondents who were interviewed for this construct, 13 (65%) perceived the eLearning system to be easy to use, whereas 3 (15%) found the system to be difficult to use and 4 (20%) were neutral. None of the respondents perceived the system to be very difficult or very easy to use. The eLearning platform was positively perceived by health care providers as one of the best platforms for sharing clinical experiences; suitable for Continuing Professional Development; inspiring the user to keep on learning; providing a good opportunity for self-assessment, learning knowledge and skills that were neither taught in medical colleges nor learnt in work settings; and that the system reminded the providers of knowledge gained in medical schools. Findings indicated that 12 (60%) of the respondents had the intention to use the system in the future whereas 6 (30%) were neutral.

Factors affecting utilization of the ICT learning platforms

Utilization of online eLearning system was affected by infrastructural and technical factors. First, there was inadequate internet and mobile phone connectivity. Second, some eLearning users had inadequate computer literacy and there was a serious lack of local IT technical support. With the exception of only one health facility there were no IT personnel to support users and the system at the local level.

Discussion

In order to ensure quality maternal and perinatal health care delivery, knowledge and skills of health care providers

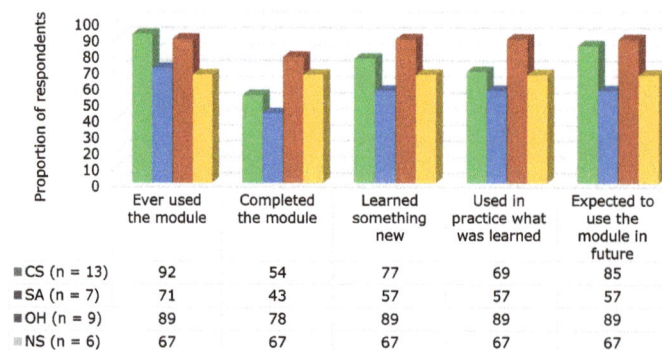

	Ever used the module	Completed the module	Learned something new	Used in practice what was learned	Expected to use the module in future
CS (n = 13)	92	54	77	69	85
SA (n = 7)	71	43	57	57	57
OH (n = 9)	89	78	89	89	89
NS (n = 6)	67	67	67	67	67

Note: CS = caesarean section module; SA = spinal anaesthesia module; OH = obstetric haemorrhage module; NS = neonatal resuscitation module

Fig. 2 The effectiveness of the eLearning system on caesarean section, spinal anaesthesia, obstetric haemorrhage and neonatal resuscitation modules

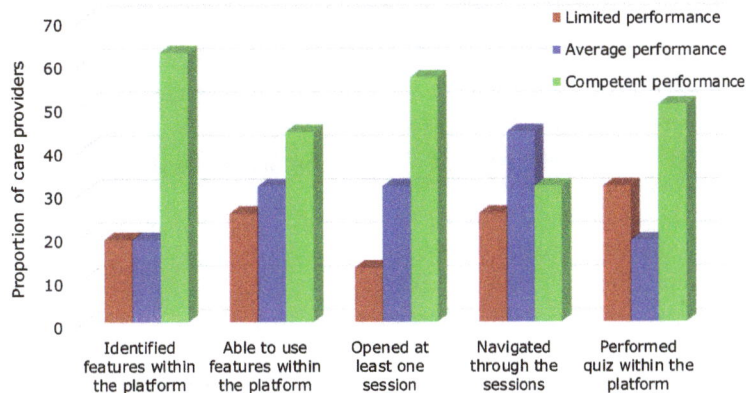

Fig. 3 Level of efficiency of health care providers in using the eLearning system

play a vital role. This underscores the importance of continuing professional development and emergency care support of frontline health care providers. Understanding the limitation of knowledge and skills of mid-level care providers working independently in underserved rural settings many advocate for the application of eHealth technologies for human resources capacity building [13, 14].

Teleconferencing and mobile teleconsultation platforms

The fact that 60% of the health centres participated in more than one third of the teleconferences, and the fact that there were few connectivity interruptions highlights the potential of the innovative audio teleconferencing platform for improving knowledge and decision-making skills, and hence the quality of maternal and perinatal health care. The teleconference platform used real event cases (real patients with problems) that were encountered over the past week for learning. Real case studies were the preferred teaching method because they enhance active engagement of learners in professional reasoning in the midst of case decision-making and allow learners to know how expert clinicians think through the case. There were no reports of any negative consequences associated with presenting real event case studies with bad outcomes suggesting acceptability of this learning method. Studies indicate that case studies are powerful and effective training tools, and are a popular mechanism to improve the adult learning experience particularly in medicine [15]. Although 38 emergency calls (teleconsultations) were made and attended by consultant obstetricians in 2015, there is still a need to strengthen and support clinical decision-making for mid-level care providers considering the short period of their training programs, limited knowledge and skills but also the gaps identified during the teleconferences. Considering that life experiences strongly affect learning, teleconsultation encouraged immediate use of newly acquired knowledge.

Integration of mobile phone technology into the health care system provided care providers with new ways of learning and opportunities to apply knowledge, thereby enhancing clinical problem-solving and enhanced accountability/personal responsibility in care. Like other studies our findings suggest that mobile phone technology can be used for continuing professional development and may enhance clinical decision making even in underserved rural areas in low-resource settings [14, 16].

E-learning platform
Efficacy of the eLearning system

In this study users reported a remarkable level of effectiveness and demonstrated an appreciable degree of competencies on the e-Learning system. Specifically, e-Learning platform users reported to have acquired a wide range of clinical skills which are critical in the management of women with obstetric complications and when providing anaesthesia. Knowledge and skills acquired by the users can partly explain improved maternal and perinatal outcomes in the project areas which have been reported elsewhere [10, 12]. Our findings suggest that an e-Learning strategy can be used to refresh health care providers with current practices and support development of clinical competencies which are essential for life saving maternal and perinatal health care [17]. However, the fact that the 13–31% of care providers demonstrated limited performance in using the eLearning system suggests further investigation to determine why the system worked with some and not others. Some studies have reported that eLearning can be as effective as or even more effective than face-to-face instruction and can be more efficient if effective techniques are used, especially for the development of knowledge and critical thinking, and decision making skills [9, 18, 19].

Perceived efficacy and adoption in practice of the eLearning system

The fact that health care providers perceived the eLearning platform positively with regards to its usefulness and ease of use, and that they were ready to use it in the future suggest that they were satisfied and that the e-Learning platform was acceptable. Acceptability of the platform was also manifested by a significant number of views made on the weekly conference forum, caesarean section and spinal anaesthesia resource folders. Like other studies, our findings suggest that a well-designed e-Learning platform can promote and motivate learners to become more engaged with the content [17].

These results come from rural areas, suggesting that e-Learning can help to broaden the skills of existing professionals, reach those who live in geographically isolated areas and reduce costs of learning-related travel. Considering the acute shortage of care providers, eLearning is beneficial to the health care system in that health care workers do not need to leave their work places for training. E-Learning platform allows learning at work and at home, so that learners can broaden their skills whilst continuing to provide crucial services to their communities [20]. The fact that mid-level care providers working in rural areas are the backbone of almost all national health goals in most low-resource countries, it is essential to equip them with adequate clinical knowledge and skills for optimum service delivery. Like other reports, these results suggest that a wider use of eLearning might help to address the need for capacity building of frontline health care workers [14, 21, 22].

Establishing an eHealth platform in extremely remote and rural health facilities for continuing professional development and supporting obstetric emergency care is an appropriate and effective intervention, has proven feasible and is currently operational. This report is an inspiring testimony on how to integrate eHealth into the existing health care system for human resource capacity building in the most isolated remote and rural areas in low-resource countries.

eHealth implementation challenges in rural settings

Although these results suggest a great potential for scaling up eHealth solutions in rural Tanzania, the use of online eLearning is facing infrastructural and technical factors that need to be overcome. These factors included inadequate computer literacy, lack of local IT technical support and inadequate internet connectivity. To optimize eLearning systems for continuing professional development, basic computer application training programs should be introduced and where available strengthened in educational curricula in secondary schools and colleges. The fact that availability of broadband in rural sub-Saharan Africa is still restricted, learning content needs to

be available both online and offline. Local health facilities in remote settings can be outfitted with desktop computers and laptops where eLearning modules for essential skills updates can be uploaded.

Limitations of the study

This study describes considerable practices on eHealth for supporting maternal and perinatal health care but does not robustly evaluate the impact of these interventions on health outcomes. The impact of these interventions on health outcomes was not evaluated because the project combined a wide range of approaches to improve knowledge, skills including face-to-face training which were also conducted during on site supportive supervision [10]. This study also does not adequately evaluate effectiveness and efficiency of the eHealth strategies, given the methodological designs (convenience and purposive sampling, and the lack of control groups).

Conclusions

This article highlights considerable practices and gains made in using eHealth strategies for maternal and perinatal health care and offers them as a model that Ministries of Health in low-resource countries and international agencies can adopt. It calls for all stakeholders to consider the increasing penetration of mobile networks into rural and remote areas as opening up new opportunities to support the provision of quality health care by broadening knowledge and skills of frontline health care providers, and by supporting obstetric and neonatal emergency care through teleconsultations.

Abbreviations

CS: Caesarean section; HC: Health centres; ICTs: Information communication technologies; MEM: Method Evaluation Model; WHO: World Health Organization

Acknowledgements

The authors would like to thank the Ministry of Heath of the United Republic of Tanzania and all district health authorities for administrative support and for allowing this program to be conducted. We would also like to thank Patricia Bailey for proofreading support, health care providers and all people whose contributions made this work possible.

Funding

The authors would like to acknowledge the Swedish International Development Cooperation Agency, Merck for Mothers, Bloomberg Philanthropies and Fondation H&B Agerup for their generous financial support to the project.

Authors' contributions

All authors participated in the implementation of this project. SD & DM were involved in data collection. AN analysed the data and wrote the manuscript. All authors read and approved the final manuscript.

Competing interests

The authors declare that they have no competing interests.

Author details

[1]Thamini Uhai Program, Dar es Salaam, Tanzania. [2]Tanzanian Training Centre for International Health, Ifakara, Tanzania. [3]Saint Francis University College for Health and Allied Sciences, Ifakara, Tanzania. [4]Catholic University of Health and Allied Sciences, Mwanza, Tanzania. [5]Maweni Regional Hospital, Kigoma, Tanzania. [6]Leiden University Medical Centre, Leiden, The Netherlands. [7]Athena Institute, VU University Amsterdam, Amsterdam, The Netherlands.

References

1. WHO, UNICEF, UNFPA, World Bank Group. UN: Trends in Maternal Mortality: 1990 to 2015 Estimates by WHO, UNICEF, UNFPA, World Bank Group and the United Nations Population Division. Geneva: WHO; 2015.
2. United Republic of Tanzania. Tanzania Demographic and Health Survey and Malaria Indicator Survey 2015–2016.
3. United Republic of Tanzania, Ministry of Health & Social Welfare. Tanzania National eHealth Strategy: July, 2013 – June 2018.
4. Nyamtema AS, Pemba SK, Mbaruku G, Rutasha FD, van Roosmalen J. Tanzanian lessons in using non-physician clinicians to scale up comprehensive emergency obstetric care in remote and rural areas. Hum Resour Health. 2011;9:28.
5. McPakeemail B, Mensah K. Task shifting in health care in resource-poor countries. Lancet. 2008;372:870–87. doi:10.1016/S0140-6736(08)61375-6.
6. WHO. WHO recommendations: optimizing health worker roles to improve access to key maternal and newborn health interventions through task shifting. 2012. www.who.int/iris/bitstream/10665/77764/1/9789241504843_eng.pdf. Accessed 12 Mar 2016.
7. WHO. Task shifting to tackle health worker shortages. WHO/HSS/200703. 2007.
8. WHO. WHO eHealth Resolution. http://www.who.int/healthacademy/news/en/. Accessed 22 June 2016
9. Jorge GR, Michael JM, Rosanne ML. The Impact of E-Learning in Medical Education. Acad Med. 2006;81:207–12.
10. Nyamtema AS, Mwakatundu N, Dominico S, Mohamed H, Pemba S, Rumanyika R, et al. Enhancing maternal and perinatal health in under-served remote areas in sub-Saharan Africa: a Tanzanian model. PLoS ONE. 2016;11(3):e0151419. doi:10.1371/journal.pone.0151419.
11. Moody DL. The Method Evaluation Model: A Theoretical Model for Validating Information Systems Design Methods. Naples, Italy: European Conference on Information Systems; 2003.
12. Nyamtema A, Mwakatundu N, Dominico S, Mohamed H, Shayo A, Rumanyika R, et al.: Increasing the availability and quality of caesarean section in Tanzania. BJOG 2016; doi: 10.1111/1471-0528.14223
13. Lee SH, Nurmatov UB, Nwaru BI, Mukherjee M, Grant L, Pagliari C. Effectiveness of mHealth interventions for maternal, newborn and child health in low–and middle–income countries: systematic review and meta analysis. J Glob Health. 2016;6(1):010401. doi:10.7189/jogh.06.010401.
14. WHO. mHealth: New horizons for health through mobile technologies. www.who.int/goe/publications/goe_mhealth_web.pdf. Accessed 11 Jan 2017.
15. Cantillon P, Hutchinson L, Wood D. ABC of learning and teaching in medicine. London: BMJ Publishing Group; 2003.
16. Obasola OI, Mabawonku I, Lagunju I. A Review of e-Health Interventions for Maternal and Child Health in Sub-Sahara Africa. Matern Child Health J. 2015;19:1813–24. doi: 1810.1007/s10995-10015-11695-10990.
17. Clark D. Psychological myths in e-learning. Med Teach. 2002;24:598–604.
18. Means B, Toyama Y, Murphy R, Bakia M, Jones K. Evaluation of evidence-based practices in online learning: a meta-analysis and review of online learning studies: U.S. Department of Education. https://www2.ed.gov/rschstat/eval/tech/evidence-based-practices/finalreport.pdf. Accessed 11 Jan 2017.
19. Chumley-Jones HS, Dobbie A, Alford CL. Web-based learning: sound educational method or hype? A review of the evaluation literature. Acad Med. 2002;77 suppl 10:S86–93.
20. Bastable S, Gramet P, Jacobs K, Sopczyk D. Health professional as educator: principles of teaching and learning. Sudbury: Jones & Bartlett Learning; 2011.
21. WHO. eLearning as good as traditional training for health professionals: where is the evidence? http://www.who.int/hrh/news/2015/e_learning_4_hrh/en/. Accessed 10 April 2016
22. Chakravarty N, Nallala S, Mahapatra S, Chaudhury P, Sultana F, Bhattacharjee S. Blended Training for Frontline Health Functionaries: Is this the Way Ahead? Int J Prev Med. 2016;7:37. doi:10.4103/2008-7802.176002.

9

Golden hour of neonatal life: Need of the hour

Deepak Sharma

Abstract

"Golden Hour" of neonatal life is defined as the first hour of post-natal life in both preterm and term neonates. This concept in neonatology has been adopted from adult trauma where the initial first hour of trauma management is considered as golden hour. The "Golden hour" concept includes practicing all the evidence based intervention for term and preterm neonates, in the initial sixty minutes of postnatal life for better long-term outcome. Although the current evidence supports the concept of golden hour in preterm and still there is no evidence seeking the benefit of golden hour approach in term neonates, but neonatologist around the globe feel the importance of golden hour concept equally in both preterm and term neonates. Initial first hour of neonatal life includes neonatal resuscitation, post-resuscitation care, transportation of sick newborn to neonatal intensive care unit, respiratory and cardiovascular support and initial course in nursery. The studies that evaluated the concept of golden hour in preterm neonates showed marked reduction in hypothermia, hypoglycemia, intraventricular hemorrhage (IVH), bronchopulmonary dysplasia (BPD), and retinopathy of prematurity (ROP). In this review article, we will discuss various components of neonatal care that are included in "Golden hour" of preterm and term neonatal care.

Keywords: Golden hour, Neonate, Preterm, Term

Introduction

The concept of "Golden Hour" has been introduced recently in field of neonatology, highlighting the importance of neonatal care in the first 60 minutes of postnatal life [1]. The golden hour term has been adopted from adult trauma where it is used for the initial first hour of trauma management [2, 3]. Dr. R. Adams Cowley gave the concept of "Golden Hour" in emergency medicine and showed that with the use of golden hour approach there was decrease in patient mortality with better transport and patient outcome [2, 4]. Reynolds et al. was the first person to implement this concept in the neonatal care [1]. The neonatal management in the first hour of life have an important effect on both immediate and long-term outcomes of all neonates. There are many interventions that needs to be practiced in golden hour for neonatal care so that neonatal complications are minimized [5]. The prime objective of golden hour is to use evidence based interventions and treatment for better neonatal outcome, importantly for extremely low gestational age neonates (ELGAN) [6]. In the golden

Correspondence: dr.deepak.rohtak@gmail.com
National Institute of Medical Science, Jaipur, Rajasthan, India

hour, standard approach is followed derived from the best available evidence with aim of practicing gentle but timely and effective interventions with non-invasive procedures if required [7]. In this review article, we have covered the various components of golden hour approach in preterm and term neonatal care (Fig. 1 and Table 1). The details of all the interventions with current evidence can be read from other published reviews of the author [8, 9].

Antenatal counseling and team briefing

Infants born at an extremely low gestational age have a high mortality rate and are at risk of having neurodevelopmental disabilities ranging from subtle to severe in grade [10–12]. Estimated gestational age of delivery has shown strong association with neurodevelopmental outcome and it serves as the basis for antenatal counselling [11], although it has some fallacies that limits its role for using as single parameter like the rate of fetal development during the early third trimester and the inaccuracy of gestational age dating. The goal of antenatal counseling is to inform parents and assist them in decision-making over either providing resuscitation or giving only

Send required laboratory investigations
- Complete blood count
- Blood culture
- Blood glucose
- Arterial blood gas analysis/capillary blood gas
- Chest X-ray

Prevent Hypothermia
- Use Plastic wrap or bag/Plastic caps/ Cling wrap/ Radiant warmer /Thermal mattress/ Pre-warmed incubators/Warm humidified gases
- Provide skin to skin contact or Kangaroo mother care
- Keep delivery room temperature 26-28° C

Antenatal counselling and team briefing
- Reply all questions, discuss plan of management and allay anxiety of parents
- Define role and responsibility of members of resuscitation team

Therapeutic Hypothermia in term newborn with birth asphyxia

Communicate with parents regarding condition of newborn

Give support to respiratory system
- Start resuscitation with 21% oxygen in term and 21-30% in preterm neonate
- Targeted saturation
- Sustained inflation (SI)
- Heated humidified blended oxygen
- Delivery room CPAP
- T piece resuscitation
- Early rescue surfactant
- Gentle ventilation strategy

Give nutritional care
- Total parenteral nutrition (TPN) Enteral nutrition/ Breast feeding
- Prevent Hypoglycemia
- Start IV fluids if feeding can't be given
- Insert Umbilical lines or cannula

Delayed cord clamping

Give support to cardiovascular system
- Maintain normal perfusion and blood pressure
- Detect shock in compensatory phase

Prevent nosocomial infection if admitted in nursery
- Use strict asepsis methods
- Use bundle approach for insertion of central line, surfactant instillation and TPN preparation
- Antibiotic first dose if indicated

Keep necessary records
- Record resuscitation details
- Birth weight and gender
- Axillary temperature on admission to nursery
- Time of surfactant instillation/ starting therapeutic hypothermia/ umbilical catheterization
- Position of endotracheal tube, umbilical catheters and feeding tube

Fig. 1 Figure showing golden hour interventions to be done at the time of preterm and term newborn birth (Figure copyright Dr Deepak Sharma)

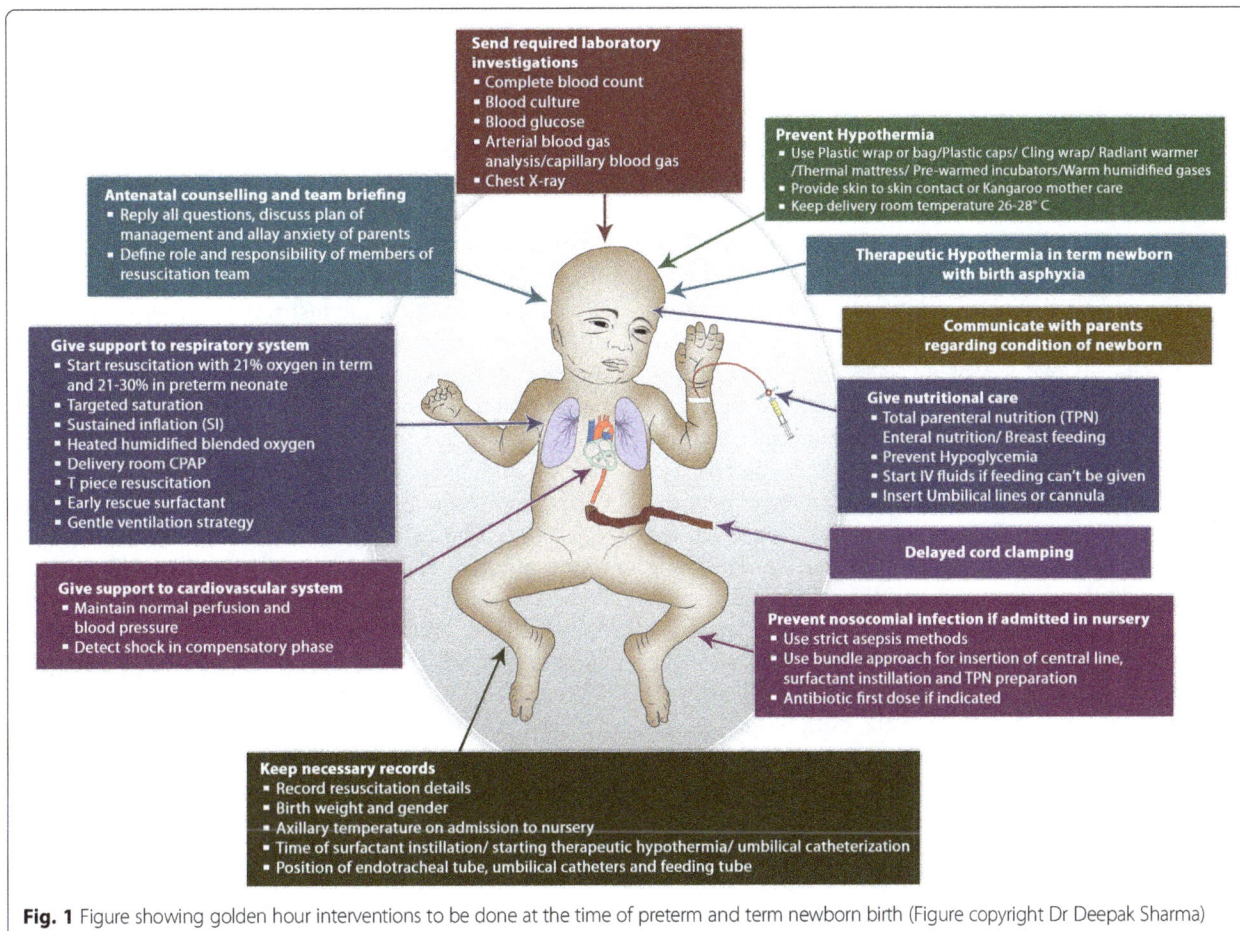

Table 1 Various components of "Golden 60 minutes" project for term and preterm newborn

S. no	Components
1	Antenatal counseling and team briefing
2	Delayed cord clamping
3	Prevention of hypothermia/temperature maintenance
4	Support to respiratory system
5	Support to cardiovascular system
6	Early nutritional care
7	Prevention of hypoglycemia
8	Initiation of breast feeding
9	Infection prevention
10	Starting of therapeutic hypothermia for birth asphyxia
11	Laboratory investigation
12	Monitoring/record
13	Communication with family

comfort care to the neonate. The parents can be offered comfort care for the newborn born at gestational below 25 weeks, but this decision needs to be made after consideration of region specific guidelines. The decision to provide comfort care will also depend upon the variables such as perceived accuracy of gestational age assignment, the presence or absence of chorioamnionitis, and the level of care available for location of delivery [13–15]. The three components of effective counseling are assessment of risks, communication of those risks, and ongoing support. Antenatal counselling especially before a preterm delivery has many benefits for parents like reducing parental anxiety, increasing knowledge, facilitating informed decision-making and making rapport with the neonatal clinicians [16, 17]. In the counselling the parents should be told about most accurate prognostic morbidity and mortality data available for their infant based on hospital-specific database or regional or national data [18, 19]. Parents also need to be informed that inspite to the best efforts, both things namely the exact prognosis or outcome for a specific infant either antenatally or immediately after delivery and prediction of long-term neurologic outcome remains limited

[20, 21]. The parents should be given appropriate time for making decision over the neonatal management [17, 22]. Evidence shows that rational, consensus periviability guidelines are well accepted and can be used for antenatal counselling by neonatologists, obstetricians, and nurses who provide care to pregnant women and infants at extremely low gestational ages [23].

The importance of antenatal counselling has been emphasized in neonatal resuscitation programme (NRP) 2015. The parents should be counselled antenatally, answering all the question asked by them about the newborn thus allaying there anxiety. This hold true for both pre-term and term neonate. If the newborn is going to be shifted to mother side than parents need to be counselled regarding breast feeding and general newborn care [13, 14] The parents should also be told about expected duration of neonatal intensive care unit (NICU) stay and morbidities which the newborn is likely to face in the postnatal life depending upon the gestational age and birth weight. The prediction of hospital stay duration will depend upon the gestational age at birth, expected morbidities and previous database of the hospital for the same gestational age neonate. The pregnancy outcome will depend upon the birth weight, gestational age, gender, use of prenatal steroids, singleton pregnancy, maternal age, maternal health, maternal nutrition, substance use, genetics, and complications during pregnancy [17, 19, 22]. The challenges of antenatal counselling includes counselling for near viability birth and fetus having antenatally diagnosed malformations. If the fetus is diagnosed with congenital malformations (e.g. congenital diaphragmatic hernia, abdominal wall defects, lung malformations, tetralogy of Fallot, hydronephrosis, or sacrococcygeal teratoma) pediatric surgeon should be brought in picture and the goal of counselling should be to inform parents regarding the implications of the fetal anomaly, reduce parental anxiety and stress and inform about the post-natal intervention like need for ventilation, hemodynamic stabilization and surgical intervention in such cases. When the fetus is diagnosed with immune hydrops fetalis than parents need to be counselled for exchange transfusion after birth and need for storage of blood antenatally so that management of the neonate is not delayed. The outcome of these neonates in such cases will depend upon the other associated malformations, lung: head ratio in case of diaphragmatic hernia, and severity of pulmonary stenosis in case of tetralogy of Fallot [24]. The parents should be counselled about the possible outcome (mortality and morbidity) keeping the past record of such newborn in the hospital [25]. Ideally both obstetrics team and neonatal team should do counselling together and present a consistent approach for the newborn as this leads to better rapport between neonatologist, obstetrician and parents.

When called for attending birth of high risk neonate than the resuscitation team should decide for the team leader and every member of the team should be given role before the delivery of the neonate so that during resuscitation there are no confusions over interventions and and thus avoiding any miss-happening. The NICU personal need to be informed for the expected neonatal admission, especially if the team is going to attend birth of any preterm neonate or high-risk term neonate. Working condition of the instruments needed during resuscitation should be checked and should be in adequate number if twins or triplets are being expected. Pre-resuscitation check list use make this equipment checking process very easy and rapid. Maternal history should be read in detail from the maternal records and required details should be noted down. The team who is going to attain the delivery of extreme premature, or term neonate with malformations (hydrops fetalis, congenital diaphragmatic hernia, upper airway malformation), should be expertise in attending such neonates and should have necessary skills for all interventions that may be required in the delivery room. During the time neonate reaches NICU, neonatal bed should be made ready and all required medications should be procured, thus avoiding delay in treatment once the shifting process is over [26, 27].

Delayed cord clamping (DCC)

Physiologically early cord clamping (ECC) have been defined as clamping of cord when still there is circulation of blood from placenta to newborn and delayed cord clamping (DCC) has been defined as clamping of cord after stoppage of placental circulation [28, 29]. When timing of cord clamping is taken in consideration for the definition of ECC and DCC, then before the mid-1950s cord clamping within one minute after birth was termed as ECC, and clamping after five minutes was defined as DCC [30]. The present studies that compared ECC and DCC, have defined ECC as cord clamping immediately or within 15 seconds of birth and DCC as cord clamping after 30 seconds to 3 min after neonatal birth [31–33]. The fetal-placental circulation contains blood that approximates to 110 -115 mL/kg of fetal body weight, with approximately 35 - 40% of total is present in the placenta at one point of time [34, 35]. In term newborn, DCC for one-minute lead to transfer of 80 ml extra blood and delay of three minutes leads to total transfer of 100 ml blood to the neonate [36]. The factor that determine the placental transfusion includes cord clamping time, uterine contractions, umbilical blood flow, newborn respiration and gravity [37]. The placental flow to fetus decrease rapidly after the neonatal birth and after three minutes of birth, placental blood flow to neonate becomes insignificant, and by 5 minutes it absolutely ceases [38]. NRP 2015 guideline recognizes the importance of DCC in newborn and thus included new recommendations over this issue. It recommends DCC clamping (delay in cord clamping for more than 30 seconds) for all preterm and term newborn not requiring resuscitation at birth. The guidelines also further states that in newborn that requires resuscitation at time of birth, DCC should not be done till further trials are done seeking the feasibility over this [13, 14]. The author inference from the available evidence is to delay the cord clamping for more than 30 seconds after the birth and should not be practiced in newborn requiring resuscitation. Newer beds equipped with neonatal resuscitation equipments are being made to implement the concept of DCC in newborn requiring resuscitation, although trials are still needed to see feasibility of such beds during neonatal resuscitation [39]. Cochrane meta-analysis studied the effect of timing of umbilical cord clamping and other strategies to influence placental transfusion in preterm birth on maternal and infant outcomes. This meta-analysis included fifteen studies and showed that DCC was associated with fewer infants requiring transfusions for anaemia (RR 0.61, 95% CI 0.46 - 0.81), less intraventricular haemorrhages (IVH) (ultrasound diagnosis all grades) (RR 0.59, 95% CI 0.41- 0.85) and lower risk for necrotizing enterocolitis (NEC) (RR 0.62, 95% CI 0.43 - 0.90) compared with ECC. The peak bilirubin concentration was significantly higher in neonates allocated to DCC compared with ECC (mean difference 15.01 mmol/L, 95% CI 5.62 - 24.40) [40]. The Cochrane meta-analysis that sought the effect of DCC in term neonates reported no significant differences in neonatal mortality, Apgar score < 7 at five minutes and neonatal admission. There was significant increase in mean birth weight in DCC (101 grams; 95% CI 45 – 157), although neonates in DCC required more phototherapy for neonatal jaundice (RR 0.62; 95% CI 0.41- 0.96). The haemoglobin concentration in infants at 24 to 48 hours was significantly higher in DCC group [41]. Thus the current evidence shows various beneficial effect of DCC except significant increase in requirement of phototherapy. There is still controversy over the correct time for DCC with many unresolved question and clinical issues for its successful implementation [30, 42].

There are concerns about practicing DCC in extreme premature and neonates requiring resuscitation, for which umbilical cord milking (UCM) has emerged as an alternative. In the umbilical vein alone there is approximately 15 to 20 mL of cord blood which can be transferred to newborn with cord milking [43]. UCM is practiced by milking 20 cm of umbilical cord 2 to 3 times before clamping at a rate of 20 cm per 2 seconds while the infant is held at or below the level of the placenta [44, 45]. The NRP 2015 guidelines are against the routine use of cord milking for newborn who are born at < 29 weeks of gestation except in a research setting [13, 14].

Prevention of Hypothermia

Hypothermia defined as temperature < 36.5 °C is a dangerous problem in newborn especially in very low birth weight (VLBW), extremely low birth weight (ELBW) and ELGAN. The reported incidence of hypothermia at time of admission to the NICU in VLBW newborn ranges from 31% to 78% [46–49]. There is 28% increase in neonatal mortality with each 1 °C fall in axillary temperature while admitted in NICU [46], and admission temperature in NICU is a strong predictor for neonatal mortality [50, 51]. The highest risk of neonatal hypothermia is within the first minutes to hours after birth as there is wide difference between in-utero and environmental temperature [52]. After the birth of newborn, there is rapid loss of heat by four mechanisms namely conduction, convection, evaporation and radiation. The neonate develop hypothermia because of larger surface area per unit body weight, high surface area to volume ratio, increased evaporative fluid losses from the skin, very large surface area of head compared to body, and presence of thin layer of subcutaneous fat thus making them susceptible to easily develop hypothermia [53, 54]. Hypothermia leads to significant increase in Apgar score less than 7, IVH, late onset sepsis, hypoglycemia and respiratory distress [50]. NRP 2015 guideline recommend maintaining temperature between 36.5 to 37.5 °C and avoiding hyperthermia (>37.5 °C) [13]. Hypothermia can be prevented by keeping delivery room temperature from 26 to 28 °C, using pre-warmed linen sheets to receive the newborn just after birth, re-warming surfaces and eliminating drafts. In the delivery room and during transportation various interventions that can be practiced to prevent hypothermia are using plastic wrap or bag [55, 56], plastic caps, cling wrap, radiant warmer, thermal mattress [57, 58], pre-warmed single/double walled incubators [59], warm humidified gases [60, 61], and skin to skin contact [59, 62, 63]. The preterm newborn just after the birth is covered with polyethylene wrap/cling wrap or transferred into vinyl bag without drying with all necessary resuscitation steps being carried out with newborn covered in wrap. The wrap/bags is to be removed only after the newborn is shifted to nursery and is stabilized [64–70]. Plastic wraps/cling wraps/plastic caps/vinyl bags prevents heat loss by evaporation, radiant warmer prevent heat loss secondary to radiation and conduction, incubator prevent heat loss by conduction, convection, radiation and evaporation, whereas skin to skin contact and warm humidified gases acts by preventing conductive heat loss. The insensible fluid losses can be decreased by placing the infant in a double walled incubators like giraffe/ humidified isolette on arrival to NICU with humidification of 70-80% [71]. NRP 2015 recommend the use of polyethylene wrap for prevention of hypothermia and early skin to skin contact in term newborn [13, 72]. The term neonate who are stable can be dried in delivery room and hat can be placed to prevent evaporative heat loss [73]. In lower and middle income countries, NRP 2015 recommend use of clean food-grade plastic bag up to the level of the neck and skin to skin contact to prevent hypothermia [13, 14]. Cochrane meta-analysis reported plastic wraps or bags, plastic caps, skin-to-skin care (SSC) and trans-warmer mattress being effective in reducing heat losses and reducing hypothermia [73].

Support to respiration

The goal of providing support to respiratory system is to help in the smooth transition of gas exchanging organ from placenta to lung. Support to respiratory system forms an important part of golden hour management. Both preterm and term newborn are prone to develop respiratory distress immediately after birth. Although the etiology of this respiratory distress could be varied, but the immediate goal of the neonatologist in delivery room should be in providing support to the respiratory system of these newborns [5]. NRP 2015 recommended that resuscitation of preterm newborns (< 35 weeks of gestation) should be started with 21 to 30% oxygen, and in newborn > 35 weeks of gestation, resuscitation should be started with room air. Use of pulse oximetry is recommended when resuscitation is anticipated, when positive pressure ventilation (PPV) is administered, when central cyanosis persists beyond the first 5 to 10 minutes of life, or when supplementary oxygen is administered. The goal of oxygen therapy is to achieve pre-ductal oxygen saturation as per the time specific interquartile range recommended in NRP (1 min 60-65%, 2 min 65-70%, 3 min 70-75%, 4 min 75-80%, 5 min 80-85% and 10 min 85-95%) [13, 14] When neonates are transported to NICU and started on invasive mode than targeted saturation should be 90-95% in the preterm infants [74–77].

As per the latest NRP 2015, newborn who are born with meconium stained amniotic fluid and are vigorous (defined as having a normal respiratory effort and normal muscle tone) should be provided routine care and the infant may stay with the mother. If the newborn is not vigorous (defined as having depressed respiratory effort and poor muscle tone), the initial steps of resuscitation should be completed under the radiant warmer. Routine tracheal intubation for tracheal suctioning in non-vigorous neonate is not recommended and PPV should be initiated if the infant is not breathing or the

heart rate is less than 100/min after the completion of initial steps. During neonatal resuscitation, endotracheal intubation is performed when bag-mask ventilation is ineffective or prolonged, when chest compressions are "anticipated" or preferably prior to onset of chest compressions, or when bag and mask ventilation is contraindicated such as congenital diaphragmatic hernia [13, 14]. Exhaled/End tidal CO_2 detection is the most reliable method of confirmation of endotracheal tube placement [78, 79]. CO_2 detector are of two type namely colorimetric devices that change color in the presence of CO_2 (colour changes from blue/purple to yellow) and capnographs that are electronic monitors displaying the CO_2 concentration with each breath and these detectors are attached to the ET tube. It gives false result when the infant is in cardiac arrest leading to unnecessary extubation and reintubation in critically ill newborns [80]. If there is no improvement in heart rate after effective resuscitation, chest compression and drugs or there is sudden deterioration of any infant on ventilation than suspicion of pneumothorax is kept. Transillumination test can be done in delivery room for detection of air leak syndrome [81]. If a pneumothorax causes significant respiratory distress, bradycardia, or hypotension, it should be relieved urgently by placing a catheter into the pleural space and evacuating the air. If the baby has ongoing respiratory distress, in the NICU thoracostomy tube can be inserted and may be attached to continuous suction. Pneumothorax can be prevented by avoiding giving too much inflating pressure and high PEEP during resuscitation [13, 14]. If there is suspicion of pulmonary hypoplasia than such infants should be started on invasive ventilation with goal of gentle ventilation and hemodynamic monitoring [24].

The aim of providing early respiratory support is to achieve functional residual capacity (FRC), provide appropriate tidal volume (4 -6 ml/kg) and minute ventilation, decrease work of breathing, avoid apnea, and to avoid invasive ventilation by providing assistive ventilation. The respiratory system can be supported by sustained lung inflation (SLI) [82–86], delivery room continuous positive airway pressure (CPAP) [87, 88], blended heated humidified oxygen, use of T piece resuscitation for providing PEEP (Peak end expiratory pressure) and PIP (Peak inspiratory pressure), early rescue surfactant (avoiding prophylactic surfactant) [75, 89–91], and use of gentle ventilation strategies [volume guarantee [92], patient triggered ventilation, permissive hypercapnia (tolerating PCo_2 upto 55- 60 mmHg provided the pH >7.2) [93, 94], targeted saturation (90-95%) in preterm [75–77], avoiding hypoxia and hyperoxia, proper humidification, early extubation and using non-invasive modes of ventilation like CPAP and non-invasive mechanical ventilation (NIMV)] [95–99].

The goal of providing PPV is to use just enough pressure to inflate and aerate the lungs so that the heart rate and oxygen saturation increase. In the delivery room we can start PPV with PIP of 20 to 25 cm H2O [Full-term babies may require a higher PIP for the first few breaths to inflate their lungs (30-40 cm H2O)], PEEP of 5 cm H2O, respiratory rate of 40- 60 breaths/minute and FiO2 of 21% in ≥ 35 weeks and 21-30% in < 35 weeks gestational age newborn. The most important indicator of successful PPV is a rising heart rate. The adequacy of PIP is see as gentle rise and fall of the chest with each breath. If there is no chest rise than ventilation corrective steps should be done (MRSOPA=Mask adjustment, Reposition head, Suction airway, Open mouth, Pressure increase, and Alternative airway). After starting of effective PPV, monitor the baby's chest movement, heart rate, and respiratory effort. FiO2 need to be adjusted based on pulse oximetry. When the heart rate is consistently more than 100 bpm, gradually reduce the rate and pressure of PPV, observe for effective spontaneous respirations, and stimulate the baby to breathe. PPV may be discontinued when the baby has a heart rate continuously over 100 bpm and sustained spontaneous breathing. After PPV is stopped, there is need for continues monitoring of the newborn oxygen saturation and breathing. Free-flow oxygen or CPAP may be required and can be weaned, as tolerated, based on pulse oximetry. PPV can be provided by self-inflating bag, flow-inflating bag and T piece resuscitator. T piece resuscitator requires a compressed gas source and pressure adjustment to deliver PIP and PEEP, hence need to be used in delivery room that have source of compressed gas. Its primary advantage is that it provides more consistent pressure with each breath than the self-inflating bag. It need to be use when there is need to deliver CPAP to a spontaneously breathing newborn, providing SLI and when there is need to deliver PIP also. Self-inflating bag doesn't need any source of compressed gas, hence can be used in resuscitation where there is no availability of compressed gas [86].

Sustained inflation (SLI) strategy leads to lung recruitment immediately after birth through delivery of brief peak pressure to the infant airways via a nasopharyngeal tube or mask, thus allowing preterm infants to achieve FRC. SLI leads to better alveolar recruitment, increase in pulmonary blood flow and decrease in pulmonary vascular resistance, movement of lung liquid out of the alveoli, and uniform lung expansion and better compliance [86]. After oropharyngeal and nasal suctioning, pressure-controlled (20-30 cmH2O) inflation is sustained for 5-15 seconds, using a neonatal mask and a T-piece ventilator, followed by the delivery of 5 cmH2O NCPAP. Patients is observed for the following 6 to 10 seconds to evaluate their cardio-respiratory function. If respiratory failure persists (that is, apnea and gasping) and/or the heart rate is >60 and <100 bpm despite NCPAP, the SLI maneuver

(again 20-30 cmH2O for 5-15 seconds) is repeated. If the heart rate remains >60 and <100 bpm after the second SLI maneuver, the infant is resuscitated following the current guidelines of the NRP [82, 83, 85, 100, 101]. The European Resuscitation Council Guidelines recommend SI for the initial ventilation of apneic term and preterm infants [102].

In a ventilated infant Oxygen saturation index (OSI = Mean airway pressure × FiO2 × 100 : SpO2) is an non-invasive method to assess severity of hypoxic respiratory failure, acute respiratory distress syndrome or acute lung injury [103]. OSI of 6.5 equals to the acute lung injury criteria, and an OSI of 7.8 equals to acute respiratory distress syndrome criteria [104]. The goal of invasive ventilation should be minimizing lung injury secondary to ventilation namely barotrauma, volutrauma, atelectotrauma, biotrauma and rheotrauma [92, 94, 105]. Volume targeted mode of ventilation has shown to cause reduction in the combined outcome of death or BPD, pneumothorax, hypocarbia and the combined outcome of periventricular leukomalacia or grade 3-4 IVH, thus making it a preferred mode over pressure control mode in neonatal ventilation [92, 106]. When nasal CPAP is compared with nasal intermittent positive pressure ventilation (NIPPV) as primary mode of respiratory support, NIPPV has found to superior to NCPAP for decreasing respiratory failure and the need for intubation and endotracheal tube ventilation among preterm infants with respiratory distress syndrome (RDS) [107]. Similarly for post-extubation respiratory support, NIPPV has shown to be superior over NCPAP in reducing the incidence of extubation failure and the need for re-intubation within 48 hours to one week [108]. Any wrong intervention done in golden hour leads to damage of the lung parenchyma, and plays an important role in development of bronchopulmonary dysplasia (BPD) in ELBW, VLBW or EGLAN [109].

Preterm neonates are born with less surfactant pool and the use of surfactant in the management of respiratory distress syndrome has revolutionized care of the preterm infants. Animal derived surfactant is preferred over protein free synthetic surfactant as it leads to greater early improvement in the requirement for ventilator support, fewer pneumothoraxes, and fewer deaths [110]. When protein containing synthetic surfactants was compared with animal derived surfactant, results of the study showed equal efficacy [111]. Surfactant should be given as "early rescue" i.e. within two hours of neonatal birth and is preferred over "late rescue" with simultaneous respiratory system support in form of either invasive ventilation or non-invasive ventilation depending upon the clinical condition of the infant [112]. The indication for giving surfactant are preterm infants born at <30 weeks' gestation who need mechanical ventilation because of severe RDS and infant showing signs of RDS and need more than 30% inspired oxygen to maintain saturations in the normal range [75]. Surfactant should be administered in the standard method of aliquots instilled into an endotracheal tube. There are multiple method of surfactant administration namely administration through catheter, side port, or suction valve; administration through dual-lumen endotracheal tube; administration through a laryngeal mask airway; nasopharyngeal administration of surfactant and INSURE. INSURE (INtubation SURfactant administration and Extubation to CPAP) is the preferred method of surfactant installation if the infant has good respiratory efforts [113, 114]. The complications of surfactant administration includes transient airway obstruction, oxygen desaturation, bradycardia, and alterations in cerebral blood flow and brain electrical activity [115]. Early surfactant replacement therapy with extubation to NCPAP compared with later selective surfactant replacement and continued mechanical ventilation with extubation from low ventilator support has shown to be associated with less need mechanical ventilation, lower incidence of BPD and fewer air leak syndromes [116]. With the use of delivery room CPAP, using "prophylactic surfactant" i.e. surfactant installation within 15 minutes of birth is not recommended in clinical practice [91]. Recently there has been research in less invasive surfactant administration (LISA) and studies have shown that it leads to lower rates of mechanical ventilation, postnatal steroids, BPD and BPD or death than the controls [117–119].

Airway obstruction is a life-threatening emergency and needs immediate management. The newborn's airway may be obstructed by thick secretions or a congenital anomaly that leads to an anatomic obstruction. If newborn with Pierre robin sequence develops labored breathing, he is turned prone on his stomach. In this position, the tongue move forward and open the airway. If prone positioning is not successful, small endotracheal tube (2.5 mm) is inserted through the nose with the tip placed deep in the posterior pharynx, past the base of the tongue, and above the vocal cords. It is not inserted into the trachea and there is no requirement of laryngoscope. This helps in relieving the airway obstruction. In these newborn who develop severe difficulty in breathing and requires resuscitation, face-mask ventilation and endotracheal intubation may be very difficult and laryngeal mask may provide a lifesaving rescue airway. In newborn choanal atresia is usually unilateral and does not cause significant symptoms in the newborn period. Newborn with bilateral choanal atresia may develop respiratory distress immediately after birth. The mouth and airway can be kept open by inserting one of the following into the baby's mouth—a feeding nipple or pacifier modified by cutting off the end (McGovern

nipple) and secured with ties around the occiput, an oral endotracheal tube positioned with the tip just beyond the tongue in the posterior pharynx, or a plastic oral (Guedel) airway. In newborn with congenital high airway obstruction (CHAOS), then there is need for special expertise and equipment for successful intubation. If the obstruction is above the level of the vocal cords than placement of a laryngeal mask may provide a lifesaving rescue airway. If the obstruction is below vocal cords than there will need for emergency tracheostomy, therefore if CHAOS is diagnosed antenatally than such babies should be born in a facility where emergency management of the airway by a trained multidisciplinary team is immediately available in the delivery room [13, 14].

The clinical course of respiratory distress also helps in differentiating the various cause of distress. In RDS there is onset of respiratory distress immediately after birth followed by gradual worsening of distress over next six hours. In air leak syndrome there will be sudden onset of hypoxia and hypercarbia, chest hyperinflation and reduced air entry. In neonate with PPHN there will be severe cyanosis, extreme liability especially on handling, tricuspid systolic murmur and differential saturation of pre-ductal and post-ductal. In MAS there will cord stained of meconium in term or post-term neonate, tachypnea, hypoxia, barrel shaped chest and PPHN. Chest X-ray done in NICU will also further help in diagnosing the etiology of respiratory distress [120, 121].

Support to cardiovascular system

The goal of giving support to cardiovascular system is to have normal capillary refill time (For 5 seconds, finger is pressed over sternum to have blanching of skin and then count seconds to see disappearance of blanching, consider abnormal when it is ≥ 3 second), heart rate and blood pressure in both preterm and term newborn [122]. The first parameter that shows effectiveness of resuscitation is improvement in heart rate. To assess the response to initial steps of resuscitation, auscultation along the left side of the chest is the most accurate physical examination method of determining a neonate's heart rate. Estimation of the heart rate is done by counting the number of beats in 6 seconds and multiplying by 10. If the newborn requires PPV during resuscitation than assessment of heart rate is done using 3 lead ECG, which is more reliable than pulse oximetry for detection of heart rate. Thus as per NRP 2015 during resuscitation of term and preterm newborns, the use of 3-lead ECG is recommended for the rapid and accurate measurement of the newborn's heart rate [13, 14]. The interventions that may be needed in delivery room for supporting cardiovascular system includes bag and mask ventilation, intubation and PPV, chest compression and rarely drugs (normal saline and adrenaline). Venous access should be established at the earliest with umbilical vein being the easiest vein to be cannulated through which medicines are given. Umbilical venous catheter (UVC) is inserted for 2 to 4 cm (less in preterm babies) until there is free flow of blood [13]. The medicine are required during resuscitation when inspite of effective ventilation and chest compression, the newborn still have a heart rate below 60 bpm. The medicine required during resuscitation are epinephrine and normal saline (0.9% NaCl). Epinephrine is given if the newborn heart rate remains below 60 bpm after 1) At least 30 seconds of PPV that inflates the lungs (moves the chest), and 2) Another 60 seconds of chest compressions coordinated with PPV using 100% oxygen. The recommended intravenous or intraosseous dose is 0.1 to 0.3 mL/kg (equal to 0.01 to 0.03 mg/kg) for 1:10,000 dilution. If epinephrine is to be given by endotracheal pathway, than the recommended dose is 0.5 to 1 mL/kg (equal to 0.05 to 0.1 mg/kg) for 1: 10,000 dilution. Newborns with hypovolemic shock from acute blood loss (eg, acute feto-maternal hemorrhage, bleeding vasa previa, extensive vaginal bleeding, fetal trauma, cord disruption, umbilical cord prolapse, and severe cord compression) may require emergency volume expansion. These newborn have features of shock like pale in color, delayed capillary refill, and/ or weak pulses. Packed red blood cells should be considered for volume replacement when severe fetal anemia is suspected. If cross-matched blood is not immediately available, then non–cross-matched, type-O, Rh-negative packed red blood cells are used. The initial dose of the selected volume expander is 10 mL/kg that needs to be given as a steady infusion over 5 to 10 minutes, followed by repeat dose if the newborn does not improve after the first dose [13, 14].

The causes of shock in preterm and term newborn includes prematurity (secondary to poor vasomotor tone, immature myocardium that is more sensitive to changes in afterload and dysregulated nitric oxide production), asphyxia, early onset sepsis (EOS), air leak syndromes, myocardial dysfunction, hypovolemia, maternal anaesthesia, fetal arrhythmias and fetal blood loss (ante-partum hemorrhage, feto-maternal hemorrhage or twin to twin transfusion syndrome) [123]. Arterial blood pressure (BP) is the most frequently monitored indicator of neonatal circulatory status but studies has shown that systemic perfusion shows poor correlation with BP [124, 125]. Groves et al. showed that in infants with reduced systemic perfusion, BP tends to have normal or high values in the first hours of life and low BP didn't correlated with poor perfusion in the first 48 h of postnatal life in sick preterm infants [126]. Lactate measurement can be done in blood gas and it is used as biomarker in diagnosing and assessing the severity of systemic hypoperfusion and can help in earlier diagnosis of shock in normotensive neonates during golden hour [127].The neonatologist should identify

shock in compensated phase and should manage it aggressively. The management includes establishing early intravenous access, judicious use of fluid resuscitation, vasopressors (dopamine or dobutamine) and other supportive care like blood transfusion for hemorrhage, and antibiotics for septic shock [122, 128].

ELBW/EGLAN and VLBW are prone to have IVH during postnatal life, and of the total IVH 50% take place on day 1 of post-natal life. Indomethacin prophylaxis has been used to reduce incidence of IVH in premature neonates [129]. Trial of Indomethacin prophylaxis in preterms (TIPP) trial which is the largest study conducted to see the effect of Indomethacin prophylaxis in ELBW reported that prophylactic indomethacin lead to the reduction in the incidence of PDA, PDA ligation, IVH (grades 3 and 4), and pulmonary hemorrhage [16, 18], but there was no reduction in the incidence of death or neurodevelopmental abnormalities [130]. Cochrane meta-analysis that included 19 trials concluded that prophylactic indomethacin reduced the incidence of symptomatic PDA, PDA surgical ligation and incidence of severe IVH but there was no effect on mortality or on a composite of death or severe neurodevelopmental disability assessed at 18 to 36 months old [131]. Hence, indomethacin is not recommended for routine prophylaxis against IVH. However, indomethacin is still being used in some neonatal units depending on clinical circumstances and personal preferences [132].

As traditional clinical and biochemical markers of perfusion have little importance in the neonatal population, therefore bed side functional echocardiography (FE) has come in picture and is used as point of care in the golden hour to find out the cause of shock and help in the management of neonatal shock. FE helps in the assessment of function of the circulatory system rather than detailed anatomy and help in rapid decision making based on real time images of central blood flow [133, 134]. Assessment of superior vena cava (SVC) flow using FE has shown to the best available method of monitoring central perfusion in the neonatal population and flow within the SVC has been considered as a good surrogate marker of cerebral perfusion [135, 136]. Thus SVC flow can be assessed in neonates who are in shock or having perinatal asphyxia [137, 138].

Persistent Pulmonary Hypertension (PPHN) is also seen sometimes in sick neonates during the golden hour. PPHN is due to increased pulmonary vascular resistance or supra-systemic pulmonary pressure leading to right-to-left shunting of blood across patent foramen ovale (PFO) and patent ductus arteriosus (PDA) leading to hypoxemia [139]. PPHN is result of either maladaptation of lung parenchyma, maldevelopment of pulmonary vasculature, underdevelopment of pulmonary vasculature or intrinsic obstruction in the pulmonary vasculature. The clinical presentation of PPHN includes labile saturations, hypoxemia, high Fio2 requirement, predominant tachypnea, saturation difference (>5-10%), or PaO2 differences (10–20 mmHg) between right upper limb and lower limbs. Echocardiography is gold standard to confirm the diagnosis, and should be performed when suspicion of PPHN is there. Right to left shunting across PDA and PFO, flattening or left deviation of the interventricular septum and tricuspid regurgitation are suggestive of PPHN [140]. The management of PPHN includes optimal oxygenation, avoiding respiratory and metabolic acidosis, normoglycemia, normal metabolic milieu, blood pressure stabilization, sedation, inhaled or intravenous prostacyclin, intravenous prostaglandin E1, pulmonary vasodilator therapy (selective like Nitric Oxide and non –selective like Sildenafil and Milrinone) and extracorporeal membrane oxygenation (ECMO). Left to right shunting at both PDA and PFO level in the golden hour should be managed with optimal lung recruitment (providing adequate PEEP) and surfactant if there is parenchymal disease. Left to right shunting at PDA and right to left shunting at PFO level indicates ductal dependent right sided heart lesion and needs Prostaglandin E1 infusion, whereas vice-versa shunting across PFO and PDA shows ductal dependent left sided heart lesion and needs Prostaglandin E1 infusion and Milrinone [141–143].

Support for nutrition

In-utero placenta provides necessary nutritional support to the fetus and as the umbilical cord is cut, the supply of nutrition is also interrupted. This makes providing support to nutrition for both term and preterm newborn a priority. In case of term newborn with no contraindications of feeding, breast feeding should be started within half hour of birth. NRP 2015 and Baby Friendly Hospital Initiative (BFHI) guidelines recommend stable newborn babies to be kept in SSC contact with mother immediately after birth and breast feeding should be done within the first half-hour following birth [13, 14, 144]. In ELBW, VLBW, EGLAN or term neonates, whom immediately feeding cannot be started, nutritional requirements needs to be taken care of. The fluid requirement of the newborn will depend upon the gestational age, and sensible/insensible water loss. The goal of fluid replacement is to provide adequate calories, protein and lipids; and compensate for the ongoing fluid losses [145]. In newborn infants the starting fluid on day 1 for birth weight < 1000 gram is 100-150 ml/kg/day, 1000-1500 gram is 80-100 ml/kg/day and for > 1500 gram is 60-80 ml/kg/day. Fluid restriction is done when there is decreased weight loss (<1%/day or a cumulative loss <5%),

decreased serum sodium in the presence of weight gain (Na < 130 meq/dl), decreased urine specific gravity <1.005 or urine osmolality <100 mosm/L and increased urine output (>3 ml/kg/hr) [146]. The results from various studies have shown that restricted water intake has a beneficial effect on the incidence of PDA, BPD, NEC and death [147]. Hyponatremia with weight loss suggests sodium depletion and needs sodium replacement. Hyponatremia with weight gain suggests dilutional hyponatremia and requires fluid restriction. Hypernatremia with weight loss suggests dehydration and management includes fluid correction over 48 hours. Hypernatremia with weight gain suggests salt and water load and needs fluid and sodium restriction [148]. The daily protein and lipid requirement in ELBW/VLBW neonates is around 4-4.5 gm/kg/day and 3 gm/kg/day respectively [149–151]. The venous access should be secured in these newborn and intravenous fluids should be started at earliest to prevent hypoglycemia. The VLBW/ELBW/ELGAN newborn should be started on total parenteral nutrition (TPN) (dextrose, lipids and protein) with in the first hour of post-natal life [152–154]. The stable preterm who don't have any contraindication of enteral feedings should be started on enteral feeds within golden hour with preference to mother milk or donor human milk [155]. The newborn who are born with surgical conditions like gastrochisis and omphalocele needs stabilization in delivery room. Sterile silastic bowel bags and/or saline-soaked gauze dressings are used to prevent damage to the exposed intestines. Handling of the bowel is minimized to prevent vascular compromise. A nasogastric tube is placed to decompress the stomach and bowel. Such newborns are sometimes born with clinical features of shock, thereafter fluid resuscitation with isotonic solutions such as normal saline or Ringer's lactate is recommended. Maintenance fluids are started (2-3 times of normal maintenance) to compensate for increased fluid loss and third space deficit. Broad-spectrum antibiotics are begun prophylactically. Any metabolic acidosis is corrected, and urgent surgical consultation is obtained [156].

The newborn who are at high risk for developing hypoglycemia after birth are premature, intrauterine growth restricted [157], sick, low birth weight, infant of diabetic mother, late preterm, large for gestational age and birth asphyxia. The neonates who are sick and have risk factor to develop hypoglycemia should get glucose level measured in golden hour [158]. The goal is to keep glucose level 50 -110 mg/dl and hypoglycemia should be managed with feeding, or dextrose infusion (glucose infusion rate (GIR) is calculated and infusion is started at GIR of 4-6 mg/kg/min in preterm and 6-8 mg/kg/min in term neonates and increased gradually to 12 mg/kg/min) as per the clinic condition of the newborn and symptoms of hypoglycemia [159, 160]. Symptomatic hypoglycemia (irritability, stupor, jitteriness, tremors, apathy, episodes of cyanosis, convulsions, intermittent apneic spells or tachypnea, weak and high pitched cry, limpness and lethargy, difficulty in feeding, and eye rolling) or glucose level < 25 mg/dl needs to be managed with bolus of 10% dextrose at 2ml/kg followed by continuous glucose infusion at GIR of 6-8 mg/kg/min. Blood sugar should be checked again after 20-30 minutes after bolus and then and then hourly until stable, to determine if additional bolus is required [161–163]. The infants who generally need GIR > 8mg/kg/min are usually severe IUGR or else having congenital hypopituitarism, adrenal insufficiency, hyperinsulinemic states, galactosemia, glycogen storage disorders, Maple syrup urine disease, Mitochondrial disorders and Fatty acid oxidation defect [164]. Recently oral 40% dextrose gel used in the management of hypoglycemia has shown to reduces the incidence of mother-infant separation for treatment and increased the likelihood of full breast feeding after discharge compared with placebo gel [165]. Hyperglycemia (defined as blood glucose level >125 mg/dl or plasma glucose level > 145 mg/dl) is also possible in golden hour. Hyperglycemia is managed by reducing the GIR and exogenous insulin is used when glucose values exceed 250 mg/dL despite decreasing GIR or when prolonged restriction of parenterally administered glucose would substantially decrease the required total caloric intake [166].

Prevention of sepsis

Neonatal sepsis and prematurity are the two most common cause of neonatal mortality and morbidity [167–169]. The clinical manifestations of neonatal sepsis are varied and needs high degree of suspicion for early diagnosis of neonatal sepsis [170–175]. Many intervention are done to prevent neonatal sepsis, but the most important are hand washing and using asepsis precautions while handling the newborn [176–180]. The newborn should be handled with strict asepsis techniques starting from the time the neonatal birth. All invasive procedures like umbilical line or peripheral cannula insertion, administration of surfactant, preparation of IV fluids, TPN, and antibiotics should be done using aseptic precautions and bundle approach should be used [181–184]. CPAP/ventilator tubing should be sterilized and sterile distill water should be used for humidification. The newborn whom antibiotics needs to be started secondary to risk factor for early onset sepsis (EOS), first dose of antibiotic need to be given as per the unit policy in the golden hour and blood culture should be sought using aseptic precautions [1]. The risk factor for EOS includes leaking per vaginum > 18 hours; maternal features of chorioamnionitis like maternal fever, maternal tachycardia, maternal leukocytosis, foul smelling liquor,

uterine tenderness, and fetal tachycardia; ≥ 3 clean vaginal examination or single unclean examination; and maternal urinary tract infection in last two weeks [185]. Placental pathological examination has also been used to confirm histologic chorioamnionitis which is defined as presence of inflammatory cells in the fetal membranes [186, 187]. Organism can be isolated by culture or PCR of the placenta, but placental cultures may be negative, even in the presence of overt histologic inflammation, thus making role of culture in diagnosis of chorioamnionitis doubtful [188]. In developing countries the most common organism responsible for early onset sepsis are Klebsiella spp., Enterobacter spp., Escherichia coli and Coagulase Negative Staphylococci [170, 189], whereas in developed countries Group B Streptococci (GBS) is most common in term, and Escherichia coli is most prevalent among premature infants [190–192]. The antibiotic therapy should be directed toward the most common causes of neonatal sepsis, including intravenous ampicillin for GBS and coverage for gram negative organisms (Aminoglycoside) and antibiotic decision should also take into consideration local antibiotic resistance patterns [193]. The total duration of antibiotics will depend upon the clinical status, results of sepsis screen and blood culture. If the blood culture shows growth of organism, antibiotics should continue for next 10-14 days; if the blood culture is sterile, sepsis screen is normal and the neonate is clinically well, antibiotics should be stopped after 48 hours and if the blood culture is negative and the neonate is well, but the sepsis screen is abnormal, then empirical antibiotics are continued for 5-7 days [194–197]. Lumbar puncture done for cerebrospinal fluid culture, biochemical and microbiological analysis is usually not recommended as routine investigation for early onset sepsis screening and it should to be done in neonates whose blood culture is positive, infants with a strong clinical suspicion of sepsis or neonate present with seizure activity, apnea, and depressed sensorium [198]. There is no role of CRP measurement in golden hour as half-life of CRP is 24 to 48 h and it takes around 10 to 12 h for level to increase, thus making CRP measurement in golden hour unreliable [199].

Fungal prophylaxis has shown to cause significant reduction in incidence of invasive fungal infection in very preterm or VLBW infants [200]. All ELBW/VLBW neonates can be started on fluconazole prophylaxis within golden hour provided the incidence of fungal sepsis is significant in the neonatal care unit (>5% at baseline) [201]. On the other hand European guidelines suggest that 2% incidence of fungal sepsis should be the threshold for implementing a fluconazole prophylaxis [202].

Mother are also sometimes infected with various viral infection at the time of neonatal birth. Such neonates needs to be managed in golden hour as per the viral infection of the mother. The neonate who are born to mother with active herpes simplex virus (HSV) genital lesions should be evaluated at 24 hours of postnatal life with HSV surface cultures (and PCRs if desired), HSV blood PCR, CSF cell count, chemistries, and HSV PCR and serum alanine transferase and should be either started on acyclovir or observed till the results of the initial tests [203, 204]. The clinical manifestation of neonatal HSV depends upon the time of acquiring infection with HSV. In-utero or congenital HSV infected neonate presents with triad of clinical manifestations at birth a). cutaneous (active lesions, scarring, aplasia cutis, hyperpigmentation or hypopigmentation) b). neurological (microcephaly, intracranial calcifications, hydranencephaly) c). ocular (chorioretinitis, microphthalmia, optic atrophy). Neonatal HSV infection acquired during the peripartum or postpartum period manifest in three forms namely Skin, eyes and mucocutaneous disease (SEM) disease [involve skin, eye, or mucocutaneous membranes]; Central nervous system (CNS) disease [involve CNS and may also have mucocutaneous involvement, but no evidence of any other organ system involvement] and disseminated disease [involve multiple organ systems including the liver, lungs, adrenals, gastrointestinal tract, CNS and the skin, eyes, or mouth] [204, 205]. The infants born to mother infected with Hepatitis-B should receive Hepatitis B immunoglobulin and single-antigen hepatitis B vaccine within 12 hours of birth. The infants who are born to HIV positive mother should be either started on exclusive breast feeding or formula feeds after discussing with parents and explaining them to avoid mixed feeding. The infants also need to be started on antiretroviral (ARV) prophylaxis with either Zidovudine or Nevirapine [206, 207].

Congenital syphilis infection occur in the newborn secondary to transmission of spirochetes across the placenta during pregnancy. The risk for congenital syphilis depends on the stage of maternal infection and the stage of infection at the time of exposure during pregnancy. The infant is examined for any physical features of congenital syphilis, dark field microscopic examination is done of any suspicious lesion or body fluids, pathological examination is done of placenta or umbilical cord and infant is evaluated with standard non-treponemal serologic tests, including venereal disease research laboratory test (VDRL) or rapid plasma (RPR) test and reactive non-treponemal tests is confirmed with a treponemal-specific test. These infants need to be started on treatment with penicillin with duration and regimen of treatment depends upon the maternal treatment received, neonatal physical examination and results of neonatal serological test [207].

There is high risk of development of antibiotic resistance with the widespread use of antibiotics thus making careful and selective use of antibiotics to the highest risk patients a universal goal. Antibiotic stewardship limits the development of antimicrobial-resistant organisms and it can be done by improving use of antibiotics. Narrow spectrum antibiotics should be used, fixed protocols should be there for starting and stopping antibiotics, start antibiotic only when clinically indicated and downgrade antibiotics after seeing blood culture sensitivity pattern are few components of antibiotic stewardship [208–210].

Therapeutic hypothermia for asphyxia

Hypoxic–ischemic encephalopathy (HIE) is encephalopathy from peripartum asphyxia with incidence of moderate-to-severe HIE being 1–3 infants per 1000 at-term livebirths in developed countries and up to 20 infants per 1000 at-term livebirths in developing countries, with worse outcome seen in severe HIE when compared to moderate HIE [211]. This difference in asphyxia incidence is because of difference in level of antenatal care received by mother. Still in developing countries, deliveries take place in nonhospital settings in absence of health care personal, thus leading to high incidence of perinatal asphyxia in these countries [212]. Term and near-term newborn, having moderate or severe asphyxia should be started on therapeutic hypothermia if they fulfill the predefined criteria's of eligibilty [213, 214]. The eligibilty criteria for starting therapeutic hypothermia are a) birth weight $\geq$ 2000 gram, post-menstrual age $\geq$ 36 weeks, b) evidence of fetal distress or neonatal distress as evidenced by one of the following: i. history of acute perinatal event (e.g., placental abruption, cord prolapse, severe fetal heart rate abnormality); ii. pH $\leq$7.0 or base deficit $\geq$16 mmol/L in cord gas or postnatal blood gas obtained within first hour of life; iii. 10-minute Apgar score of $\leq$5; iv. assisted ventilation initiated at birth and continued for at least 10 minutes, c) evidence of moderate to severe neonatal encephalopathy by examination and/or aEEG (amplitude integrated EEG) as follows: i. primary method for determining neonatal encephalopathy is physical exam (indicated by lethargy, stupor, or coma). ii. If exam shows moderate or severe encephalopathy, aEEG should be performed to provide further assessment and monitoring. iii. In circumstances in which physical exam is unreliable (e.g., muscle relaxants), an aEEG should be performed to determine if there is encephalopathy. iv. Patterns on aEEG that indicate moderate or severe encephalopathy includes the following, with minimum of 20 minutes recording time: a) severely abnormal: upper margin <10 μV b) moderately abnormal: upper margin >10 μV and lower margin <5 μV c) seizures identified by aEEG [215–217]. Neurological examination and Sarnath Staging of the newborn will help in assessment of severity of neonatal encephalopathy

[218]. Electroencephalography (EEG) or aEEG have been used in classification of severity of encephalopathy, identification of seizure, see effect of anti-convulsant on seizure frequency, identification of abnormal background activity and for inclusion of starting therapeutic hypothermia [219].

Lactate is produced during anaerobic metabolism during hypoxia and poor tissue perfusion. Serum lactate has been used to as early predictor of short-term outcome after intrapartum asphyxia [220]. Shah et al. reported that initial lactate levels are significantly higher in neonates with moderate-to-severe HIE as compared to those with mild or no HIE and the lactate levels took longer to normalize in neonates with moderate to severe HIE. Thus the author concluded that highest recorded lactate level in the first hour of life and serial measurements of lactate are important predictors of moderate-to-severe HIE [221]. In other study it was shown that high lactate level after 72 hours of therapeutic hypothermia is associated with poor neurodevelopmental outcome [222]. Moderate hypothermia (33.5 °C) for 72 h after birth is the only effective neural rescue therapy for infants born at term and near-term with moderate-to-severe HIE [223]. American academy of Paediatrics (AAP) recommends therapeutic hypothermia to be started within 6 hours of birth and continued for next 72 hours followed by gradual rewarming in next 6-8 hours [224]. Cochrane meta-analysis showed significant reduction in neonatal mortality and neurological impairment with the implementation of therapeutic hypothermia [225, 226]. Therapeutic hypothermia started within one hour of post-natal life leads to reduction in incidence of clinico-electrical seizures [227]. The neonates requiring therapeutic hypothermia should be first stabilized by providing support to respiratory and cardiovascular system if required. NRP 2015 guideline recommend that in resource abundant areas newborn born at more than 36 weeks of gestation with evolving moderate-to-severe HIE should be offered therapeutic hypothermia under clearly defined protocols [213, 214]. For resource limited countries, NRP 2015 guideline states that therapeutic hypothermia may be done if the newborn fulfills predefined criteria as defined in clinical trials and in facilities with the capabilities for multidisciplinary care and longitudinal follow-up [228]. The complications of therapeutic hypothermia that are frequently seen in neonates are increase incidence of sinus bradycardia, thrombocytopenia, subcutaneous fat necrosis, hypotension, increased fibrinolytic activity, and prolongation of prothrombin time and partial thromboplastin time tests [229, 230]. Hence goal of neonatologist in case of perinatal asphyxia is to identify the neonates fulfilling the criteria for starting therapeutic hypothermia and then starting it as early as possible, preferably in golden hour [13, 14].

Laboratory investigation

All the necessary investigations required for the management of newborn should be done in the golden hour so that there is minimal handling afterwards and decision is taken over the management plan. The investigations needs individualization as per the newborn clinical status and ante-natal risk factors. The list of various investigations includes complete blood count, blood culture, glucose, arterial blood gas (ABG) analysis/capillary blood gas, and chest X-ray (CXR). CXR helps in differentiating the various neonatal respiratory causes of distress. The CXR finding of RDS includes low lung volume, ground glass appearance, air bronchograms, reticulogranular pattern and white out lung [120]. The CXR features suggestive of TTN are prominent central perihilar vascular markings, edema of the interlobar septae, fluid in the interlobar fissures, mild cardiomegaly, minimal pleural effusion, and hyperinflation [121]. In pulmonary hypoplasia CXR will be suggestive of low lung volume on the affected side with mediastinal shift to the same side [231]. The X-ray feature suggestive of air leak syndrome will be leakage of air from the alveoli into the extra-alveolar space like pneumothorax (air collection in pleural space), pneumomediastinum (collection of air in mediastinum), pneumopericardium (collection of air around heart in pericardium), and pulmonary interstitial emphysema (PIE) (presence of air in the lung interstitium) [232–234]. CXR in meconium aspiration syndrome typically shows diffuse, asymmetric patchy infiltrates, areas of consolidation, often worse on the right, hyperinflation and sometimes presence of air leak syndrome [235]. In case of perinatal asphyxia cord blood ABG or ABG within first hour will help us decide about starting of therapeutic hypothermia. In case of immune hydrops fetalis, necessary investigations required are total serum bilirubin, direct coombs test, reticulocyte count, and hematocrit for guiding about need for partial exchange or double volume exchange transfusion (DVET) and phototherapy. Partial exchange transfusion is indicated prior to DVET when the newborn is hydropic or anemic (hematocrit <30%) [236]. Similarly CXR in case of congenital diaphragmatic hernia will tell us about the severity of lung compromise and will help us in prognostication of neonate [237].

Monitoring/Record

Monitoring and record keeping is an important part of golden hour. All the vital parameters of the newborn like heart rate, respiratory rate, capillary refill time, invasive or non-invasive blood pressure, saturation, and blood sugar should be monitored and recorded in the newborn case record. Near infrared spectroscopy (NIRS) is newly emerging technology in which bed side assessment is done of tissue blood flow/perfusion including cerebral, renal, and gastro-intestinal tract in neonates having peri-natal asphyxia, shock, cyanotic heart disease or intestinal surgeries [238–240]. NIRS has been used in management of neonates undergoing surgical correction for complex congenital heart disease. The studies shows that low cerebral regional oxygen saturation (cRSO2) correlate with poorer neurologic outcomes and increased perioperative mortality. Interventions need to be done to increase cRSO2 if there is decrease in it by ≥ 20% from a stable baseline [241]. NIRS has been used for monitoring cRSO2 in neonates during transition after birth, a period when the brain is vulnerable to injury and dysfunction [242]. It has also been used in premature newborn to see the impact of prematurity and intensive care on early brain development [243]. The other clinical usage of NIRS includes cerebral oxygenation assessment in HIE, preterm neonates with hypotension, preterm neonates with patent ductus arteriosus (PDA), preterm neonates with respiratory distress syndrome (RDS), neonates with peri/intraventricular hemorrhage (P/IVH) and preterm neonate with apneas and bradycardias [241]. Record needs to be kept of the various intervention done with their timing as this will guide us about the scope of any improvement in the aspect of timing of various interventions in the golden hour. The records keeping includes Apgar score, interventions done during resuscitation, birth weight, axillary temperature at time of admission to nursery, time of surfactant instillation, time of umbilical catheterization, time of starting ventilation and CPAP, time of starting therapeutic hypothermia, time of giving first feeds, time of starting intravenous fluids and TPN, time of giving first dose of antibiotics, complications secondary to any neonatal procedure, size and depth of endotracheal tube, umbilical catheters and depth of feeding tube fixation [1, 237].

Communication and counselling of family

This is an important aspect of golden hour and includes talking with parents and relatives of newborn for updating about the postnatal condition of newborn. The parents of term stable newborn, shifted to mother should be counselled regarding maintenance of temperature, frequency of breast feeding with emphasis on starting of early feeding and maintenance of asepsis in the newborn care. The parents of preterm and term newborns admitted in nursery or requiring referral to higher center, should be counselled regarding the present status, interventions that have been done till that time and further plan of management. All the questions of the parents should be answered patiently and counselling should be documented and all necessary consent should be taken from the parents like admission, procedure, transportation, and starting of hypothermia consents. The obstetrician who was involved in the antenatal care of the

newborn should also be informed about the condition and plan of management [237]. Post-counselling documentation should be done and is important in providing a record to which future health-care professionals can refer like starting point for later discussions or usage as a form of legal document if advance treatment preferences are being decided [244].

Transportation in Golden Hour

The infant may sometimes need transportation to health care center just after birth either because of lack of facilities for the neonatal care to the place neonate is born or because of home delivery to provide specific neonatal care. The aim of neonatal transport is to transfer a newborn infant requiring intensive care to a center where specialized resources and experience can be provided for the appropriate assessment and continuing treatment of a sick newborn infant [245]. These VLBW, ELBW, EGLAN and sometimes term neonates require transfer to tertiary centers for management and often hypothermic on reaching referral center due to lack of adequate precautions for hypothermia prevention during transport [246, 247]. In Golden hour, the neonate should be first stabilized and during transportation care should be taken for maintenance of temperature, sugar and necessary interventions need to be done for supporting heart, lungs and brain like giving ventilatory/CPAP support if required and starting of inotropes if the newborn is in shock. The infant should be started on intravenous fluids if shifting to tertiary health care center and referred hospital should be informed regarding this transport so that the neonate receives required care on reaching the center [248].

Current evidence for golden hour

The current evidence that sought the effect of golden hour in care of VLBW/ ELBW reported increase in admission temperature after implementation of golden hour project [1, 249], increase in number of infants with an admission temperature of 36.5 °C – 37.4 °C [250], decrease in the incidence of ROP and BPD [1, 249], significant improvement in time of surfactant administration, time to start dextrose and amino acids infusion [7, 249, 250], significant decrease in time to give antibiotics [7], decrease in the incidence of IVH, faster placement of umbilical catheters, significant reduction in time to reach in the NICU after delivery [251], incidence of admission glucose greater than 50 mg/dL [133]. Presently, there are no studies that have sought the role of golden hour in term neonates. We purpose flow diagram for the care of preterm and term newborn during the critical golden hour that will be helpful for management of these newborns (Fig. 2).

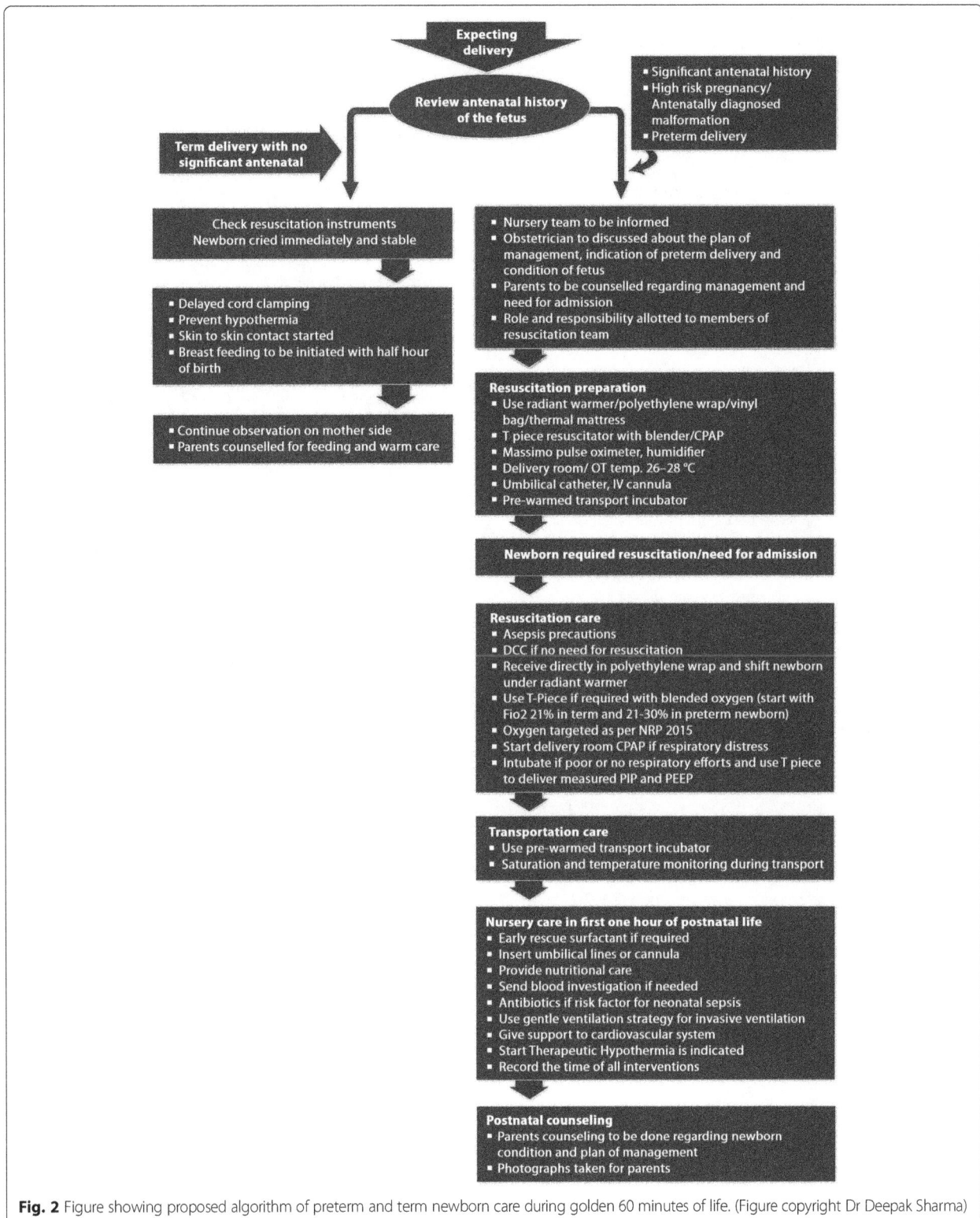

Fig. 2 Figure showing proposed algorithm of preterm and term newborn care during golden 60 minutes of life. (Figure copyright Dr Deepak Sharma)

Conclusion

The concept of "Golden hour" is new evolving strategy for better outcome of preterm and term neonates. All the health care personal should be explained about the components and importance of golden hour approach. Neonatologist attending the birth of VLBW/ELBW/ ELGAN or high-risk term neonate should be well trained in attending such deliveries and should implement all the components of golden hour during the initial first hour of post-natal life. Predelivery checklist should be followed and implemented, with teaching of the health care personal should be continuous for implementation of golden hour. The various components of golden hour include ante-natal counseling and team briefing, delayed cord clamping, prevention of hypothermia, support to respiratory and cardiovascular system, nutritional support, prevention of sepsis, therapeutic hypothermia, laboratory investigation, record keeping and counselling of parents. The current evidence supports the use of Golden hour concept by showing reduction in various neonatal morbidities like hypothermia, ROP and BPD thus showing positive impact over the survival and morbidity of the preterm and high risk term infants.

Abbreviations

AAP: American academy of Paediatrics; ABG: Arterial blood gas; ARV: Antiretroviral; BHFI: Baby Friendly Hospital Initiative; BP: Blood Pressure; BPD: Bronchopulmonary dysplasia; CHAOS: Congenital high airway obstruction; CI: Confidence interval; CNS: Central nervous system; CPAP: Continuous positive airway pressure; CSF: Cerebrospinal fluid; CXR: Chest X-ray; DCC: Delayed cord clamping; DVET: Double volume exchange transfusion; ECC: Early cord clamping; ECMO: Extracorporeal membrane oxygenation; ELBW: Extremely low birth weight; ELGAN: Extremely low gestational age neonates; EOS: Early onset sepsis; FE: Functional echocardiography; FRC: Functional residual capacity; GBS: Group B Streptococci; GIR: Glucose infusion rate; HIE: Hypoxic–ischemic encephalopathy; HSV: Herpes simplex virus; IV: Intravenous; IVH: Intraventricular hemorrhage; NEC: Necrotizing enterocolitis; NICU: Neonatal intensive care unit; NIMV: Non-invasive mechanical ventilation; NIRS: Near infrared spectroscopy; NRP: Neonatal resuscitation programme; PDA: Patent ductus arteriosus; PEEP: Peak end expiratory pressure; PFO: Patent Foramen Ovale; PIE: Pulmonary interstitial emphysema; PIP: Peak inspiratory pressure; PPHN: Persistent Pulmonary Hypertension; PPV: Positive pressure ventilation; RDS: Respiratory distress syndrome; ROP: Retinopathy of prematurity; RPR: Rapid plasma test; RR: Relative risk; SEM: Skin, eye and mucocutaneous; SLI: Sustained lung inflation; SSC: Skin-to-skin care; SVC: Superior vena cava flow; TIPP: Trial of Indomethacin prophylaxis in preterms; TPN: Total parenteral nutrition; UCM: Umbilical cord milking; VDRL: Venereal disease research laboratory test; VLBW: Very low birth weight

Acknowledgements
None

Funding
No external funding for this manuscript

Financial disclosure
None

Authors' contributions
DS made substantial contribution to conception and design of the case report. DS involved in drafting the manuscript or revising it critically for important intellectual content. DS gave final approval of the version to be published. DS agreed to be accountable for all aspects of the work in ensuring that questions related to the accuracy or integrity of any part of the work are appropriately investigated and resolved.

Competing interests
The authors declared that they have no competing interests.

References

1. Reynolds RD, Pilcher J, Ring A, Johnson R, McKinley P. The Golden Hour: care of the LBW infant during the first hour of life one unit's experience. Neonatal Netw NN. 2009 Aug;28(4):211-219; quiz 255-258.
2. Lerner EB, Moscati RM. The golden hour: scientific fact or medical "urban legend"? Acad Emerg Med Off J Soc Acad Emerg Med. 2001 Jul;8(7):758–60.
3. Sasada M, Williamson K, Gabbott D. The golden hour and pre-hospital trauma care. Injury. 1995 Apr;26(3):215–6.
4. Cowley RA, Hudson F, Scanlan E, Gill W, Lally RJ, Long W, et al. An economical and proved helicopter program for transporting the emergency critically ill and injured patient in Maryland. J Trauma. 1973 Dec;13(12):1029–38.
5. Wyckoff MH. Initial resuscitation and stabilization of the periviable neonate: the Golden-Hour approach. Semin Perinatol. 2014 Feb;38(1):12–6.
6. Vento M, Cheung P-Y, Aguar M. The first golden minutes of the extremely-low-gestational-age neonate: a gentle approach. Neonatology. 2009;95(4):286–98.
7. Lambeth TM, Rojas MA, Holmes AP. Dail RB. A Quality Improvement Initiative. Adv Neonatal Care Off J Natl Assoc Neonatal Nurses: First Golden Hour of Life; 2016 Jul 7.
8. Sharma D. Golden 60 minutes of newborn's life: Part 1: Preterm neonate. J Matern-Fetal Neonatal Med Off J Eur Assoc Perinat Med Fed Asia Ocean Perinat Soc Int Soc Perinat Obstet. 2016 Dec;1:1–12.
9. Sharma D, Sharma P, Shastri S. Golden 60 minutes of newborn's life: Part 2: Term neonate. J Matern-Fetal Neonatal Med Off J Eur Assoc Perinat Med Fed Asia Ocean Perinat Soc Int Soc Perinat Obstet. 2016 Nov;29:1–6.
10. Hoekstra RE, Ferrara TB, Couser RJ, Payne NR, Connett JE. Survival and long-term neurodevelopmental outcome of extremely premature infants born at 23-26 weeks' gestational age at a tertiary center. Pediatrics. 2004 Jan;113(1 Pt 1):e1–6.
11. Hintz SR, Kendrick DE, Vohr BR, Poole WK, Higgins RD. National Institute of Child Health and Human Development Neonatal Research Network. Changes in neurodevelopmental outcomes at 18 to 22 months' corrected age among infants of less than 25 weeks' gestational age born in 1993-1999. Pediatrics. 2005 Jun;115(6):1645–51.
12. Hack M, Taylor HG, Drotar D, Schluchter M, Cartar L, Andreias L, et al. Chronic conditions, functional limitations, and special health care needs of school-aged children born with extremely low-birth-weight in the 1990s. JAMA. 2005 Jul 20;294(3):318–25.
13. Wyckoff MH, Aziz K, Escobedo MB, Kapadia VS, Kattwinkel J, Perlman JM, et al. Part 13: Neonatal Resuscitation: 2015 American Heart Association Guidelines Update for Cardiopulmonary Resuscitation and Emergency Cardiovascular Care. Circulation. 2015 Nov 3;132(18 Suppl 2):S543–60.
14. Wyckoff MH, Aziz K, Escobedo MB, Kapadia VS, Kattwinkel J, Perlman JM, et al. Part 13: Neonatal Resuscitation: 2015 American Heart Association Guidelines Update for Cardiopulmonary Resuscitation and Emergency Cardiovascular Care (Reprint). Pediatrics. 2015 Nov;136(Suppl 2):S196–218.
15. Smith PB, Ambalavanan N, Li L, Cotten CM, Laughon M, Walsh MC, et al. Approach to Infants Born at 22 to 24 Weeks' Gestation: Relationship to Outcomes of More-Mature Infants. Pediatrics. 2012 Jun;129(6):e1508–16.
16. Brett J, Staniszewska S, Newburn M, Jones N, Taylor L. A systematic mapping review of effective interventions for communicating with, supporting and providing information to parents of preterm infants. BMJ Open. 2011 Jun 2;1(1):e000023.
17. Cummings J, COMMITTEE ON FETUS AND NEWBORN. Antenatal Counseling Regarding Resuscitation and Intensive Care Before 25 Weeks of Gestation. Pediatrics. 2015 Sep;136(3):588–595.

18. Watts JL, Saigal S. Outcome of extreme prematurity: as information increases so do the dilemmas. Arch Dis Child Fetal Neonatal Ed. 2006 May;91(3):F221–5.

19. Tyson JE, Parikh NA, Langer J, Green C, Higgins RD. National Institute of Child Health and Human Development Neonatal Research Network. Intensive care for extreme prematurity–moving beyond gestational age. N Engl J Med. 2008 Apr 17;358(16):1672–81.

20. Ambalavanan N, Baibergenova A, Carlo WA, Saigal S, Schmidt B, Thorpe KE, et al. Early prediction of poor outcome in extremely low birth weight infants by classification tree analysis. J Pediatr. 2006 Apr;148(4):438–44.

21. Singh J, Fanaroff J, Andrews B, Caldarelli L, Lagatta J, Plesha-Troyke S, et al. Resuscitation in the "gray zone" of viability: determining physician preferences and predicting infant outcomes. Pediatrics. 2007 Sep;120(3):519–26.

22. Batton DG. Committee on Fetus and Newborn. Clinical report–Antenatal counseling regarding resuscitation at an extremely low gestational age. Pediatrics. 2009 Jul;124(1):422–7.

23. Kaempf JW, Tomlinson MW, Campbell B, Ferguson L, Stewart VT. Counseling pregnant women who may deliver extremely premature infants: medical care guidelines, family choices, and neonatal outcomes. Pediatrics. 2009 Jun;123(6):1509–15.

24. Chandrasekharan PK, Rawat M, Madappa R, Rothstein DH, Lakshminrusimha S. Congenital Diaphragmatic hernia - a review. Matern Health Neonatal Perinatol. 2017;3:6.

25. Lakhoo K. Fetal counselling for surgical conditions. Early Hum Dev. 2012 Jan;88(1):9–13.

26. Wyllie J, Perlman JM, Kattwinkel J, Atkins DL, Chameides L, Goldsmith JP, et al. Part 11: Neonatal resuscitation: 2010 International Consensus on Cardiopulmonary Resuscitation and Emergency Cardiovascular Care Science with Treatment Recommendations. Resuscitation. 2010 Oct;81(Suppl 1):e260–87.

27. Perlman JM, Wyllie J, Kattwinkel J, Atkins DL, Chameides L, Goldsmith JP, et al. Part 11: Neonatal resuscitation: 2010 International Consensus on Cardiopulmonary Resuscitation and Emergency Cardiovascular Care Science With Treatment Recommendations. Circulation. 2010 Oct 19;122(16 Suppl 2):S516–38.

28. Jelin AC, Zlatnik MG, Kuppermann M, Gregorich SE, Nakagawa S, Clyman R. Clamp late and maintain perfusion (CLAMP) policy: delayed cord clamping in preterm infants. J Matern-Fetal Neonatal Med Off J Eur Assoc Perinat Med Fed Asia Ocean Perinat Soc Int Soc Perinat Obstet. 2016 Jun;29(11):1705–9.

29. Arca G, Botet F, Palacio M, Carbonell-Estrany X. Timing of umbilical cord clamping: new thoughts on an old discussion. J Matern-Fetal Neonatal Med Off J Eur Assoc Perinat Med Fed Asia Ocean Perinat Soc Int Soc Perinat Obstet. 2010 Nov;23(11):1274–85.

30. Raju TNK, Singhal N. Optimal timing for clamping the umbilical cord after birth. Clin Perinatol. 2012 Dec;39(4):889–900.

31. Duley L, Batey N. Optimal timing of umbilical cord clamping for term and preterm babies. Early Hum Dev. 2013 Nov;89(11):905–8.

32. Raju TNK. Timing of umbilical cord clamping after birth for optimizing placental transfusion. Curr Opin Pediatr. 2013 Apr;25(2):180–7.

33. Backes CH, Rivera B, Haque U, Copeland K, Hutchon D, Smith CV. Placental transfusion strategies in extremely preterm infants: the next piece of the puzzle. J Neonatal Perinatal Med. 2014;7(4):257–67. doi:10.3233/NPM-14814034. Review. PubMed PMID: 25468622.

34. Kim AJH, Warren JB. Optimal Timing of Umbilical Cord Clamping: Is the Debate Settled? Part 1 of 2: History, Rationale, Influencing Factors, and Concerns. NeoReviews. 2015 May 1;16(5):e263–9.

35. Kim AJH, Warren JB. Optimal Timing of Umbilical Cord Clamping: Is the Debate Settled? Part 2 of 2: Evidence in Preterm and Term Infants, Alternatives, and Unanswered Questions. NeoReviews. 2015 May 1;16(5):e270–7.

36. Eichenbaum-Pikser G, Zasloff JS. Delayed clamping of the umbilical cord: a review with implications for practice. J Midwifery Womens Health. 2009 Aug;54(4):321–6.

37. Katheria AC, Lakshminrusimha S, Rabe H, McAdams R, Mercer JS. Placental transfusion: a review. J Perinatol Off J Calif Perinat Assoc. 2017 Feb;37(2):105–11.

38. Farrar D, Airey R, Law GR, Tuffnell D, Cattle B, Duley L. Measuring placental transfusion for term births: weighing babies with cord intact. BJOG Int J Obstet Gynaecol. 2011 Jan;118(1):70–5.

39. Katheria AC, Brown MK, Rich W, Arnell K. Providing a Placental Transfusion in Newborns Who Need Resuscitation. Front Pediatr. 2017;5:1.

40. Rabe H, Diaz-Rossello JL, Duley L, Dowswell T. Effect of timing of umbilical cord clamping and other strategies to influence placental transfusion at preterm birth on maternal and infant outcomes. Cochrane Database Syst Rev. 2012;8:CD003248.

41. McDonald SJ, Middleton P, Dowswell T, Morris PS. Effect of timing of umbilical cord clamping of term infants on maternal and neonatal outcomes. Cochrane Database Syst Rev. 2013;7:CD004074.

42. Niermeyer S. A physiologic approach to cord clamping: Clinical issues. Matern Health Neonatol Perinatol. 2015;1:21.

43. Rabe H, Jewison A, Alvarez RF, Crook D, Stilton D, Bradley R, et al. Milking compared with delayed cord clamping to increase placental transfusion in preterm neonates: a randomized controlled trial. Obstet Gynecol. 2011 Feb;117(2 Pt 1):205–11.

44. Hosono S, Mugishima H, Fujita H, Hosono A, Minato M, Okada T, et al. Umbilical cord milking reduces the need for red cell transfusions and improves neonatal adaptation in infants born at less than 29 weeks' gestation: a randomised controlled trial. Arch Dis Child Fetal Neonatal Ed. 2008 Jan;93(1):F14–9.

45. Upadhyay A, Gothwal S, Parihar R, Garg A, Gupta A, Chawla D, et al. Effect of umbilical cord milking in term and near term infants: randomized control trial. Am J Obstet Gynecol. 2013 Feb;208(2):120.e1-6.

46. Laptook AR, Salhab W, Bhaskar B. Neonatal Research Network. Admission temperature of low birth weight infants: predictors and associated morbidities. Pediatrics. 2007 Mar;119(3):e643–9.

47. Costeloe K, Hennessy E, Gibson AT, Marlow N, Wilkinson AR. The EPICure study: outcomes to discharge from hospital for infants born at the threshold of viability. Pediatrics. 2000 Oct;106(4):659–71.

48. Bhatt DR, White R, Martin G, Van Marter LJ, Finer N, Goldsmith JP, et al. Transitional hypothermia in preterm newborns. J Perinatol Off J Calif Perinat Assoc. 2007 Dec;27(Suppl 2):S45–7.

49. Boo N-Y, Guat-Sim Cheah I. Malaysian National Neonatal Registry. Admission hypothermia among VLBW infants in Malaysian NICUs. J Trop Pediatr. 2013 Dec;59(6):447–52.

50. Chang H-Y, Sung Y-H, Wang S-M, Lung H-L, Chang J-H, Hsu C-H, et al. Short- and Long-Term Outcomes in Very Low Birth Weight Infants with Admission Hypothermia. PloS One. 2015;10(7):e0131976.

51. Mathur NB, Krishnamurthy S, Mishra TK. Evaluation of WHO classification of hypothermia in sick extramural neonates as predictor of fatality. J Trop Pediatr. 2005 Dec;51(6):341–5.

52. Raman S, Shahla A. Temperature drop in normal term newborn infants born at the University Hospital, Kuala Lumpur. Aust N Z J Obstet Gynaecol. 1992 May;32(2):117–9.

53. Watkinson M. Temperature control of premature infants in the delivery room. Clin Perinatol. 2006 Mar;33(1):43–53, vi.

54. Szymankiewicz M. Thermoregulation and maintenance of appropriate temperature in newborns. Ginekol Pol. 2003 Nov;74(11):1487–97.

55. Belsches TC, Tilly AE, Miller TR, Kambeyanda RH, Leadford A, Manasyan A, et al. Randomized trial of plastic bags to prevent term neonatal hypothermia in a resource-poor setting. Pediatrics. 2013 Sep;132(3):e656–61.

56. Oatley HK, Blencowe H, Lawn JE. The effect of coverings, including plastic bags and wraps, on mortality and morbidity in preterm and full-term neonates. J Perinatol. 2016 May;36(S1):S83–9.

57. L'Herault J, Petroff L, Jeffrey J. The effectiveness of a thermal mattress in stabilizing and maintaining body temperature during the transport of very low-birth weight newborns. Appl Nurs Res ANR. 2001 Nov;14(4):210–9.

58. Mathew B, Lakshminrusimha S, Sengupta S, Carrion V. Randomized controlled trial of vinyl bags versus thermal mattress to prevent hypothermia in extremely low-gestational-age infants. Am J Perinatol. 2013 Apr;30(4):317–22.

59. Laptook AR, Watkinson M. Temperature management in the delivery room. Semin Fetal Neonatal Med. 2008 Dec;13(6):383–91.

60. Meyer MP, Hou D, Ishrar NN, Dito I, te Pas AB. Initial respiratory support with cold, dry gas versus heated humidified gas and admission temperature of preterm infants. J Pediatr. 2015 Feb;166(2):245–250.e1.

61. te Pas AB, Lopriore E, Dito I, Morley CJ, Walther FJ. Humidified and heated air during stabilization at birth improves temperature in preterm infants. Pediatrics. 2010 Jun;125(6):e1427–32.

62. Marín Gabriel MA, Llana Martín I, López Escobar A, Fernández Villalba E, Romero Blanco I, Touza Pol P. Randomized controlled trial of early skin-to-

skin contact: effects on the mother and the newborn. Acta Paediatr Oslo Nor 1992. 2010 Nov;99(11):1630–4.

63. Bergman NJ, Linley LL, Fawcus SR. Randomized controlled trial of skin-to-skin contact from birth versus conventional incubator for physiological stabilization in 1200- to 2199-gram newborns. Acta Paediatr Oslo Nor 1992. 2004 Jun;93(6):779–85.

64. Lenclen R, Mazraani M, Jugie M, Couderc S, Hoenn E, Carbajal R, et al. Use of a polyethylene bag: a way to improve the thermal environment of the premature newborn at the delivery room. Arch Pédiatrie Organe Off Sociéte Fr Pédiatrie. 2002 Mar;9(3):238–44.

65. Doglioni N, Cavallin F, Mardegan V, Palatron S, Filippone M, Vecchiato L, et al. Total body polyethylene wraps for preventing hypothermia in preterm infants: a randomized trial. J Pediatr. 2014 Aug;165(2):261–266.e1.

66. Leadford AE, Warren JB, Manasyan A, Chomba E, Salas AA, Schelonka R, et al. Plastic bags for prevention of hypothermia in preterm and low birth weight infants. Pediatrics. 2013 Jul;132(1):e128–34.

67. Chantaroj S, Techasatid W. Effect of polyethylene bag to prevent heat loss in preterm infants at birth: a randomized controlled trial. J Med Assoc Thail Chotmaihet Thangphaet. 2011 Dec;94(Suppl 7):S32–7.

68. Trevisanuto D, Doglioni N, Cavallin F, Parotto M, Micaglio M, Zanardo V. Heat loss prevention in very preterm infants in delivery rooms: a prospective, randomized, controlled trial of polyethylene caps. J Pediatr. 2010 Jun;156(6):914–917, 917.e1.

69. Vohra S, Roberts RS, Zhang B, Janes M, Schmidt B. Heat Loss Prevention (HeLP) in the delivery room: A randomized controlled trial of polyethylene occlusive skin wrapping in very preterm infants. J Pediatr. 2004 Dec;145(6):750–3.

70. Vohra S, Frent G, Campbell V, Abbott M, Whyte R. Effect of polyethylene occlusive skin wrapping on heat loss in very low birth weight infants at delivery: a randomized trial. J Pediatr. 1999 May;134(5):547–51.

71. Yeh TF, Voora S, Lilien LD, Matwynshyn J, Srinivasan G, Pildes RS. Oxygen consumption and insensible water loss in premature infants in single-versus double-walled incubators. J Pediatr. 1980 Dec;97(6):967–71.

72. Bansal SC, Nimbalkar SM. Updated Neonatal Resuscitation Guidelines 2015 Major Changes. Indian Pediatr. 2016 May 8;53(5):403–8.

73. McCall EM, Alderdice F, Halliday HL, Jenkins JG, Vohra S. Interventions to prevent hypothermia at birth in preterm and/or low birthweight infants. Cochrane Database Syst Rev. 2010;3:CD004210.

74. Sweet DG, Carnielli V, Greisen G, Hallman M, Ozek E, Plavka R, et al. European consensus guidelines on the management of neonatal respiratory distress syndrome in preterm infants–2013 update. Neonatology. 2013; 103(4):353–68.

75. Sweet DG, Carnielli V, Greisen G, Hallman M, Ozek E, Plavka R, et al. European Consensus Guidelines on the Management of Respiratory Distress Syndrome - 2016 Update. Neonatology. 2017;111(2):107–25.

76. Deschmann E, Norman M. Oxygen-saturation targets in extremely preterm infants. Acta Paediatr Oslo Nor 1992. 2017 Jun;106(6):1014.

77. Polin RA, Bateman D. Oxygen-saturation targets in preterm infants. N Engl J Med. 2013 May 30;368(22):2141–2.

78. Kattwinkel J, Perlman JM, Aziz K, Colby C, Fairchild K, Gallagher J, et al. Part 15: neonatal resuscitation: 2010 American Heart Association Guidelines for Cardiopulmonary Resuscitation and Emergency Cardiovascular Care. Circulation. 2010 Nov 2;122(18 Suppl 3):S909–19.

79. Kattwinkel J, Perlman JM, Aziz K, Colby C, Fairchild K, Gallagher J, et al. Neonatal resuscitation: 2010 American Heart Association Guidelines for Cardiopulmonary Resuscitation and Emergency Cardiovascular Care. Pediatrics. 2010 Nov;126(5):e1400–13.

80. DeBoer S, Seaver M. End-tidal CO2 verification of endotracheal tube placement in neonates. Neonatal Netw NN. 2004 Jun;23(3):29–38.

81. Sly PD, Drew JH. Air leak in neonatal respiratory distress syndrome. Anaesth Intensive Care. 1984 Feb;12(1):41–5.

82. Lindner W, Högel J, Pohlandt F. Sustained pressure-controlled inflation or intermittent mandatory ventilation in preterm infants in the delivery room? A randomized, controlled trial on initial respiratory support via nasopharyngeal tube. Acta Paediatr Oslo Nor 1992. 2005 Mar;94(3):303–9.

83. te Pas AB, Walther FJ. A randomized, controlled trial of delivery-room respiratory management in very preterm infants. Pediatrics. 2007 Aug;120(2):322–9.

84. Harling AE, Beresford MW, Vince GS, Bates M, Yoxall CW. Does sustained lung inflation at resuscitation reduce lung injury in the preterm infant? Arch Dis Child Fetal Neonatal Ed. 2005 Sep;90(5):F406–10.

85. Lista G, Boni L, Scopesi F, Mosca F, Trevisanuto D, Messner H, et al. Sustained lung inflation at birth for preterm infants: a randomized clinical trial. Pediatrics. 2015 Feb;135(2):e457–64.

86. Vali P, Mathew B, Lakshminrusimha S. Neonatal resuscitation: evolving strategies. Matern Health Neonatol Perinatol. 2015 Jan;1

87. Morley CJ, Davis PG, Doyle LW, Brion LP, Hascoet J-M, Carlin JB, et al. Nasal CPAP or intubation at birth for very preterm infants. N Engl J Med. 2008 Feb 14;358(7):700–8.

88. SUPPORT Study Group of the Eunice Kennedy Shriver NICHD Neonatal Research Network, Finer NN, Carlo WA, Walsh MC, Rich W, Gantz MG, et al. Early CPAP versus surfactant in extremely preterm infants. N Engl J Med. 2010 May 27;362(21):1970–9.

89. Rojas MA, Lozano JM, Rojas MX, Laughon M, Bose CL, Rondon MA, et al. Very early surfactant without mandatory ventilation in premature infants treated with early continuous positive airway pressure: a randomized, controlled trial. Pediatrics. 2009 Jan;123(1):137–42.

90. Kandraju H, Murki S, Subramanian S, Gaddam P, Deorari A, Kumar P. Early routine versus late selective surfactant in preterm neonates with respiratory distress syndrome on nasal continuous positive airway pressure: a randomized controlled trial. Neonatology. 2013;103(2):148–54.

91. Rojas-Reyes MX, Morley CJ, Soll R. Prophylactic versus selective use of surfactant in preventing morbidity and mortality in preterm infants. Cochrane Database Syst Rev. 2012;3:CD000510.

92. Morley CJ. Volume-limited and volume-targeted ventilation. Clin Perinatol. 2012 Sep;39(3):513–23.

93. Miller JD, Carlo WA. Safety and effectiveness of permissive hypercapnia in the preterm infant. Curr Opin Pediatr. 2007 Apr;19(2):142–4.

94. Ryu J, Haddad G, Carlo WA. Clinical effectiveness and safety of permissive hypercapnia. Clin Perinatol. 2012 Sep;39(3):603–12.

95. Davis PG, Morley CJ, Owen LS. Non-invasive respiratory support of preterm neonates with respiratory distress: continuous positive airway pressure and nasal intermittent positive pressure ventilation. Semin Fetal Neonatal Med. 2009 Feb;14(1):14–20.

96. Thome UH, Ambalavanan N. Permissive hypercapnia to decrease lung injury in ventilated preterm neonates. Semin Fetal Neonatal Med. 2009 Feb;14(1):21–7.

97. Hummler H, Schulze A. New and alternative modes of mechanical ventilation in neonates. Semin Fetal Neonatal Med. 2009 Feb;14(1):42–8.

98. Guven S, Bozdag S, Saner H, Cetinkaya M, Yazar AS, Erguven M. Early neonatal outcomes of volume guaranteed ventilation in preterm infants with respiratory distress syndrome. J Matern Fetal Neonatal Med. 2013 Mar 1;26(4):396–401.

99. Özkan H, Duman N, Kumral A, Gülcan H. Synchronized ventilation of very-low-birth-weight infants; report of 6 years' experience. J Matern Fetal Neonatal Med. 2004 Apr 1;15(4):261–5.

100. Dani C, Lista G, Pratesi S, Boni L, Agosti M, Biban P, et al. Sustained lung inflation in the delivery room in preterm infants at high risk of respiratory distress syndrome (SLI STUDY): study protocol for a randomized controlled trial. Trials. 2013;14:67.

101. Lista G, Fontana P, Castoldi F, Cavigioli F, Dani C. Does sustained lung inflation at birth improve outcome of preterm infants at risk for respiratory distress syndrome? Neonatology. 2011;99(1):45–50.

102. Richmond S, Wyllie J. European Resuscitation Council Guidelines for Resuscitation 2010 Section 7. Resuscitation of babies at birth. Resuscitation. 2010 Oct;81(10):1389–99.

103. Rawat M, Chandrasekharan PK, Williams A, Gugino S, Koenigsknecht C, Swartz D, et al. Oxygen saturation index and severity of hypoxic respiratory failure. Neonatology. 2015;107(3):161–6.

104. Thomas NJ, Shaffer ML, Willson DF, Shih M-C, Curley MAQ. Defining acute lung disease in children with the oxygenation saturation index. Pediatr Crit Care Med J Soc Crit Care Med World Fed Pediatr Intensive Crit Care Soc. 2010 Jan;11(1):12–7.

105. Leone TA, Finer NN, Rich W. Delivery room respiratory management of the term and preterm infant. Clin Perinatol. 2012 Sep;39(3):431–40.

106. Wheeler K, Klingenberg C, McCallion N, Morley CJ, Davis PG. Volume-targeted versus pressure-limited ventilation in the neonate. Cochrane Database Syst Rev. 2010 Nov 10;11:CD003666.

107. Lemyre B, Laughon M, Bose C, Davis PG. Early nasal intermittent positive pressure ventilation (NIPPV) versus early nasal continuous positive airway pressure (NCPAP) for preterm infants. Cochrane Database Syst Rev. 2016 15;12:CD005384.

108. Lemyre B, Davis PG, De Paoli AG, Kirpalani H. Nasal intermittent positive pressure ventilation (NIPPV) versus nasal continuous positive airway pressure (NCPAP) for preterm neonates after extubation. Cochrane Database Syst Rev. 2017 01;2:CD003212.

109. Jobe AH, Bancalari E. Bronchopulmonary dysplasia. Am J Respir Crit Care Med. 2001 Jun;163(7):1723–9.

110. Ardell S, Pfister RH, Soll R. Animal derived surfactant extract versus protein free synthetic surfactant for the prevention and treatment of respiratory distress syndrome. Cochrane Database Syst Rev. 2015 Aug 24;8:CD000144.

111. Pfister RH, Soll RF, Wiswell T. Protein containing synthetic surfactant versus animal derived surfactant extract for the prevention and treatment of respiratory distress syndrome. Cochrane Database Syst Rev. 2007 Oct 17;4:CD006069.

112. Bahadue FL, Soll R. Early versus delayed selective surfactant treatment for neonatal respiratory distress syndrome. Cochrane Database Syst Rev. 2012 Nov 14;11:CD001456.

113. Dani C, Corsini I, Bertini G, Fontanelli G, Pratesi S, Rubaltelli FF. The INSURE method in preterm infants of less than 30 weeks' gestation. J Matern-Fetal Neonatal Med Off J Eur Assoc Perinat Med Fed Asia Ocean Perinat Soc Int Soc Perinat Obstet. 2010 Sep;23(9):1024–9.

114. Dani C, Bertini G, Pezzati M, Cecchi A, Caviglioli C, Rubaltelli FF. Early extubation and nasal continuous positive airway pressure after surfactant treatment for respiratory distress syndrome among preterm infants <30 weeks' gestation. Pediatrics. 2004 Jun;113(6):e560–3.

115. Polin RA, Carlo WA. Committee on Fetus and Newborn, American Academy of Pediatrics. Surfactant replacement therapy for preterm and term neonates with respiratory distress. Pediatrics. 2014 Jan;133(1):156–63.

116. Stevens TP, Harrington EW, Blennow M. Soll RF. Early surfactant administration with brief ventilation vs. selective surfactant and continued mechanical ventilation for preterm infants with or at risk for respiratory distress syndrome. Cochrane Database Syst Rev. 2007;4:CD003063.

117. Herting E. Less invasive surfactant administration (LISA) - ways to deliver surfactant in spontaneously breathing infants. Early Hum Dev. 2013 Nov;89(11):875–80.

118. Göpel W, Kribs A, Härtel C, Avenarius S, Teig N, Groneck P, et al. Less invasive surfactant administration is associated with improved pulmonary outcomes in spontaneously breathing preterm infants. Acta Paediatr Oslo Nor 1992. 2015 Mar;104(3):241–6.

119. Göpel W, Kribs A, Ziegler A, Laux R, Hoehn T, Wieg C, et al. Avoidance of mechanical ventilation by surfactant treatment of spontaneously breathing preterm infants (AMV): an open-label, randomised, controlled trial. Lancet Lond Engl. 2011 Nov 5;378(9803):1627–34.

120. Flidel-Rimon O, Shinwell ES. Respiratory Distress in the Term and Near-term Infant. NeoReviews. 2005 Jun 1;6(6):e289–97.

121. Reuter S, Moser C, Baack M. Respiratory distress in the newborn. Pediatr Rev. 2014 Oct;35(10):417–428; quiz 429.

122. Conway-Orgel M. Management of hypotension in the very low-birth-weight infant during the golden hour. Adv Neonatal Care Off J Natl Assoc Neonatal Nurses. 2010 Oct;10(5):241-245; quiz 246-247.

123. Bhat BV, Plakkal N. Management of Shock in Neonates. Indian J Pediatr. 2015 Oct;82(10):923–9.

124. Kluckow M, Evans N. Relationship between blood pressure and cardiac output in preterm infants requiring mechanical ventilation. J Pediatr. 1996 Oct;129(4):506–12.

125. Pladys P, Wodey E, Beuchée A, Branger B, Bétrémieux P. Left ventricle output and mean arterial blood pressure in preterm infants during the 1st day of life. Eur J Pediatr. 1999 Oct;158(10):817–24.

126. Groves AM, Kuschel CA, Knight DB, Skinner JR. Relationship between blood pressure and blood flow in newborn preterm infants. Arch Dis Child Fetal Neonatal Ed. 2008 Jan;93(1):F29–32.

127. Okorie ON, Dellinger P. Lactate: biomarker and potential therapeutic target. Crit Care Clin. 2011 Apr;27(2):299–326.

128. Kalish BT. Management of Neonatal Hypotension. Neonatal Netw NN. 2017 Jan 1;36(1):40–7.

129. Ballabh P. Pathogenesis and prevention of intraventricular hemorrhage. Clin Perinatol. 2014 Mar;41(1):47–67.

130. Schmidt B, Davis P, Moddemann D, Ohlsson A, Roberts RS, Saigal S, et al. Long-Term Effects of Indomethacin Prophylaxis in Extremely-Low-Birth-Weight Infants. N Engl J Med. 2001 Jun 28;344(26):1966–72.

131. Fowlie PW, Davis PG, McGuire W. Prophylactic intravenous indomethacin for preventing mortality and morbidity in preterm infants. Cochrane Database Syst Rev. 2010 Jul 7;7:CD000174.

132. Clyman RI, Saha S, Jobe A, Oh W. Indomethacin Prophylaxis for Preterm Infants: the Impact of Two Multicentered Randomized Controlled Trials on Clinical Practice. J Pediatr. 2007 Jan;150(1):46–50.e2.

133. Kluckow M, Seri I, Evans N. Functional echocardiography: an emerging clinical tool for the neonatologist. J Pediatr. 2007 Feb;150(2):125–30.

134. Kluckow M, Seri I, Evans N. Echocardiography and the neonatologist. Pediatr Cardiol. 2008 Nov;29(6):1043–7.

135. Fugelseth D. Measuring superior vena cava flow as part of echocardiography examinations performed by neonatologists. Acta Paediatr Oslo Nor 1992. 2017 Jan;106(1):5–6.

136. McGovern M, Miletin J. A review of superior vena cava flow measurement in the neonate by functional echocardiography. Acta Paediatr Oslo Nor 1992. 2017 Jan;106(1):22–9.

137. Ficial B, Finnemore AE, Cox DJ, Broadhouse KM, Price AN, Durighel G, et al. Validation Study of the Accuracy of Echocardiographic Measurements of Systemic Blood Flow Volume in Newborn Infants. J Am Soc Echocardiogr. 2013 Dec;26(12):1365–71.

138. Kumagai T, Higuchi R, Higa A, Tsuno Y, Hiramatsu C, Sugimoto T, et al. Correlation between echocardiographic superior vena cava flow and short-term outcome in infants with asphyxia. Early Hum Dev. 2013 May;89(5):307–10.

139. Jain A, McNamara PJ. Persistent pulmonary hypertension of the newborn: Advances in diagnosis and treatment. Semin Fetal Neonatal Med. 2015 Aug; 20(4):262–71.

140. D'Alto M, Romeo E, Argiento P, Di Salvo G, Badagliacca R, Cirillo AP, et al. Pulmonary arterial hypertension: the key role of echocardiography. Echocardiogr Mt Kisco N. 2015 Jan;32(Suppl 1):S23–37.

141. Sharma V, Berkelhamer S, Lakshminrusimha S. Persistent pulmonary hypertension of the newborn. Matern Health Neonatol Perinatol. 2015;1:14.

142. Bendapudi P, Rao GG, Greenough A. Diagnosis and management of persistent pulmonary hypertension of the newborn. Paediatr Respir Rev. 2015 Jun;16(3):157–61.

143. Nair J, Lakshminrusimha S. Update on PPHN: mechanisms and treatment. Semin Perinatol. 2014 Mar;38(2):78–91.

144. WHO | Baby-Friendly Hospital Initiative [Internet]. WHO. [cited 2016 Jul 14]. Available from: http://www.who.int/nutrition/publications/infantfeeding/bfhi_trainingcourse/en/

145. Aggarwal R, Deorari AK, Paul VK. Fluid and electrolyte management in term and preterm neonates. Indian J Pediatr. 2001 Dec;68(12):1139–42.

146. Chawla D, Agarwal R, Deorari AK, Paul VK. Fluid and electrolyte management in term and preterm neonates. Indian J Pediatr. 2008 Mar; 75(3):255–9.

147. Bell EF, Acarregui MJ. Restricted versus liberal water intake for preventing morbidity and mortality in preterm infants. Cochrane Database Syst Rev. 2014;12:CD000503.

148. Shaffer SG, Weismann DN. Fluid requirements in the preterm infant. Clin Perinatol. 1992 Mar;19(1):233–50.

149. Civardi E, Tzialla C, Garofoli F, Mazzucchelli I, Bollani L, Stronati M. Nutritional needs of premature infants. J Matern Fetal Neonatal Med. 2011 Oct 1; 24(sup1):27–9.

150. Ziegler EE, Carlson SJ. Early nutrition of very low birth weight infants. J Matern Fetal Neonatal Med. 2009 Jan 1;22(3):191–7.

151. Adamkin DH, Radmacher PG. Current trends and future challenges in neonatal parenteral nutrition. J Neonatal-Perinat Med. 2014 Jan 1;7(3):157–64.

152. te Braake FWJ, van den Akker CHP, Riedijk MA, van Goudoever JB. Parenteral amino acid and energy administration to premature infants in early life. Semin Fetal Neonatal Med. 2007 Feb;12(1):11–8.

153. Poindexter BB, Langer JC, Dusick AM, Ehrenkranz RA. National Institute of Child Health and Human Development Neonatal Research Network. Early provision of parenteral amino acids in extremely low birth weight infants: relation to growth and neurodevelopmental outcome. J Pediatr. 2006 Mar;148(3):300–5.

154. Trivedi A, Sinn JKH. Early versus late administration of amino acids in preterm infants receiving parenteral nutrition. Cochrane Database Syst Rev. 2013;7:CD008771.

155. Khanam S, Khan J, Sharma D, Chawla D, Murki S. Nutritional bundle to improve growth outcomes among very low birth weight infants. J Matern-Fetal Neonatal Med Off J Eur Assoc Perinat Med Fed Asia Ocean Perinat Soc Int Soc Perinat Obstet. 2015;28(15):1851–5.

156. Chabra S. Management of Gastroschisis: Prenatal, Perinatal, and Neonatal. NeoReviews. 2006 Aug 1;7(8):e419–27.

157. Sharma D, Farahbakhsh N, Shastri S, Sharma P. Intrauterine growth restriction – part 2. J Matern Fetal Neonatal Med. 2016 Mar 15;0(0):1–12.

158. Dani C, Poggi C. Nutrition and bronchopulmonary dysplasia. J Matern Fetal Neonatal Med. 2012 Oct 1;25(sup3):37–40.

159. Zhou W, Yu J, Wu Y, Zhang H. Hypoglycemia incidence and risk factors assessment in hospitalized neonates. J Matern-Fetal Neonatal Med Off J Eur Assoc Perinat Med Fed Asia Ocean Perinat Soc Int Soc Perinat Obstet. 2015 Mar;28(4):422–5.

160. Staffler A, Klemme M, Mola-Schenzle E, Mittal R, Schulze A, Flemmer AW. Very low birth weight preterm infants are at risk for hypoglycemia once on total enteral nutrition. J Matern Fetal Neonatal Med. 2013 Sep 1;26(13):1337–41.

161. Adamkin DH. Neonatal hypoglycemia. Curr Opin Pediatr. 2016 Apr;28(2): 150–5.

162. Thompson-Branch A, Havranek T. Neonatal Hypoglycemia. Pediatr Rev. 2017 Apr;38(4):147–57.

163. Committee on Fetus and Newborn, Adamkin DH. Postnatal glucose homeostasis in late-preterm and term infants. Pediatrics. 2011 Mar;127(3): 575–579.

164. Adamkin DH. Neonatal hypoglycemia. Semin Fetal Neonatal Med. 2017 Feb; 22(1):36–41.

165. Weston PJ, Harris DL, Battin M, Brown J, Hegarty JE, Harding JE. Oral dextrose gel for the treatment of hypoglycaemia in newborn infants. Cochrane Database Syst Rev. 2016 May 4;5:CD011027.

166. Beardsall K, Vanhaesebrouck S, Ogilvy-Stuart AL, Vanhole C, Palmer CR, van Weissenbruch M, et al. Early insulin therapy in very-low-birth-weight infants. N Engl J Med. 2008 Oct 30;359(18):1873–84.

167. Lozano R, Naghavi M, Foreman K, Lim S, Shibuya K, Aboyans V, et al. Global and regional mortality from 235 causes of death for 20 age groups in 1990 and 2010: a systematic analysis for the Global Burden of Disease Study 2010. Lancet. 2012 Dec 15;380(9859):2095–128.

168. Rajaratnam JK, Marcus JR, Flaxman AD, Wang H, Levin-Rector A, Dwyer L, et al. Neonatal, postneonatal, childhood, and under-5 mortality for 187 countries, 1970-2010: a systematic analysis of progress towards Millennium Development Goal 4. Lancet. 2010 Jun 5;375(9730):1988–2008.

169. Wang H, Liddell CA, Coates MM, Mooney MD, Levitz CE, Schumacher AE, et al. Global, regional, and national levels of neonatal, infant, and under-5 mortality during 1990-2013: a systematic analysis for the Global Burden of Disease Study 2013. Lancet. 2014 Sep 13;384(9947):957–79.

170. Sharma D, Kumar C, Pandita A, Pratap OT, Dasi T, Murki S. Bacteriological profile and clinical predictors of ESBL neonatal sepsis. J Matern-Fetal Neonatal Med Off J Eur Assoc Perinat Med Fed Asia Ocean Perinat Soc Int Soc Perinat Obstet. 2016 Feb;29(4):567–70.

171. Camacho-Gonzalez A, Spearman PW, Stoll BJ. Neonatal infectious diseases: evaluation of neonatal sepsis. Pediatr Clin North Am. 2013 Apr;60(2):367–89.

172. Sharma D, Sharma P, Soni P, Gupta B. Ralstonia picketti neonatal sepsis: a case report. BMC Res Notes. 2017 Jan 7;10(1):28.

173. Sharma D, Patel A, Soni P, Sharma P, Gupta B. Empedobacter brevis Meningitis in a Neonate: A Very Rare Case of Neonatal Meningitis and Literature Review. Case Rep Pediatr. 2016;2016:7609602.

174. Sharma D, Patel A, Soni P, Shastri S, Singh R. Leminorella sepsis in very low birth weight neonate as cause of neonatal mortality. J Matern-Fetal Neonatal Med Off J Eur Assoc Perinat Med Fed Asia Ocean Perinat Soc Int Soc Perinat Obstet. 2016 Jun;29:1–3.

175. Sharma D, Dasi T, Murki S, Oleti TP. Kluyvera ascorbata sepsis in an extremely low birth weight infant. Indian J Med Microbiol. 2015 Sep;33(3):437–9.

176. Sharma D, Shastri S. Lactoferrin and neonatology - role in neonatal sepsis and necrotizing enterocolitis: present, past and future. J Matern-Fetal Neonatal Med Off J Eur Assoc Perinat Med Fed Asia Ocean Perinat Soc Int Soc Perinat Obstet. 2016 Mar;29(5):763–70.

177. Kirpal H, Gathwala G, Chaudhary U, Sharma D. Prophylactic fluconazole in very low birth weight infants admitted to neonatal intensive care unit: randomized controlled trial. J Matern-Fetal Neonatal Med Off J Eur Assoc Perinat Med Fed Asia Ocean Perinat Soc Int Soc Perinat Obstet. 2016 Feb;29(4):624–8.

178. Sharma DK, Gathwala G, Shastri S. Chlorhexidine- A novel intervention to decrease the nursery stay and antibiotic exposure duration- randomized trial. J Matern-Fetal Neonatal Med Off J Eur Assoc Perinat Med Fed Asia Ocean Perinat Soc Int Soc Perinat Obstet. 2014 Dec;1:1–21.

179. Sharma D, Gathwala G. Impact of chlorhexidine cleansing of the umbilical cord on cord separation time and neonatal mortality in comparison to dry cord care - a nursery-based randomized controlled trial. J Matern-Fetal Neonatal Med Off J Eur Assoc Perinat Med Fed Asia Ocean Perinat Soc Int Soc Perinat Obstet. 2014 Aug;27(12):1262–5.

180. Gathwala G, Sharma D, Bhakhri B. kiran. Effect of topical application of chlorhexidine for umbilical cord care in comparison with conventional dry cord care on the risk of neonatal sepsis: a randomized controlled trial. J Trop Pediatr. 2013 Jun;59(3):209–13.

181. Shepherd EG, Kelly TJ, Vinsel JA, Cunningham DJ, Keels E, Beauseau W, et al. Significant Reduction of Central-Line Associated Bloodstream Infections in a Network of Diverse Neonatal Nurseries. J Pediatr. 2015 Jul;167(1):41-46.e1-3.

182. Walz JM, Ellison RT, Mack DA, Flaherty HM, McIlwaine JK, Whyte KG, et al. The bundle "plus": the effect of a multidisciplinary team approach to eradicate central line-associated bloodstream infections. Anesth Analg. 2015 Apr;120(4):868–76.

183. Fisher D, Cochran KM, Provost LP, Patterson J, Bristol T, Metzguer K, et al. Reducing central line-associated bloodstream infections in North Carolina NICUs. Pediatrics. 2013 Dec;132(6):e1664–71.

184. Taylor JE, McDonald SJ, Tan K. Prevention of central venous catheter-related infection in the neonatal unit: a literature review. J Matern Fetal Neonatal Med. 2015 Jul 3;28(10):1224–30.

185. Benitz WE, Gould JB, Druzin ML. Risk factors for early-onset group B streptococcal sepsis: estimation of odds ratios by critical literature review. Pediatrics. 1999 Jun;103(6):e77.

186. Lee SYR, Leung CW. Histological chorioamnionitis - implication for bacterial colonization, laboratory markers of infection, and early onset sepsis in very-low-birth-weight neonates. J Matern-Fetal Neonatal Med Off J Eur Assoc Perinat Med Fed Asia Ocean Perinat Soc Int Soc Perinat Obstet. 2012 Apr;25(4):364–8.

187. Yallapragada SG, Mestan KK, Ernst LM. The Placenta as a Diagnostic Tool for the Neonatologist. NeoReviews. 2016 Mar 1;17(3):e131–43.

188. Queiros da Mota V, Prodhom G, Yan P, Hohlfheld P, Greub G, Rouleau C. Correlation between placental bacterial culture results and histological chorioamnionitis: a prospective study on 376 placentas. J Clin Pathol. 2013 Mar;66(3):243–8.

189. Lamba M, Sharma R, Sharma D, Choudhary M, Maheshwari RK. Bacteriological spectrum and antimicrobial susceptibility pattern of neonatal septicaemia in a tertiary care hospital of North India. J Matern-Fetal Neonatal Med Off J Eur Assoc Perinat Med Fed Asia Ocean Perinat Soc Int Soc Perinat Obstet. 2016 Dec;29(24):3993–8.

190. Bauserman MS, Laughon MM, Hornik CP, Smith PB, Benjamin DK, Clark RH, et al. Group B Streptococcus and Escherichia coli infections in the intensive care nursery in the era of intrapartum antibiotic prophylaxis. Pediatr Infect Dis J. 2013 Mar;32(3):208–12.

191. Schrag SJ, Farley MM, Petit S, Reingold A, Weston EJ, Pondo T, et al. Epidemiology of Invasive Early-Onset Neonatal Sepsis, 2005 to 2014. Pediatrics. 2016 Dec;138(6).

192. Stoll BJ, Hansen NI, Sánchez PJ, Faix RG, Poindexter BB, Van Meurs KP, et al. Early onset neonatal sepsis: the burden of group B Streptococcal and E. coli disease continues. Pediatrics. 2011 May;127(5):817–26.

193. Verani JR, McGee L, Schrag SJ, Division of Bacterial Diseases, National Center for Immunization and Respiratory Diseases, Centers for Disease Control and Prevention (CDC). Prevention of perinatal group B streptococcal disease–revised guidelines from CDC, 2010. MMWR Recomm Rep Morb Mortal Wkly Rep Recomm Rep. 2010 Nov 19;59(RR-10):1–36.

194. Brady MT, Polin RA. Prevention and management of infants with suspected or proven neonatal sepsis. Pediatrics. 2013 Jul;132(1):166–8.

195. Polin RA. Committee on Fetus and Newborn. Management of neonates with suspected or proven early-onset bacterial sepsis. Pediatrics. 2012 May;129(5):1006–15.

196. Gerdes JS. Diagnosis and management of bacterial infections in the neonate. Pediatr Clin North Am. 2004 Aug;51(4):939–959, viii–ix.

197. Gerdes JS, Polin R. Early diagnosis and treatment of neonatal sepsis. Indian J Pediatr. 1998 Feb;65(1):63–78.

198. Riskin A, Aloni Y, Kugelman A, Toropine A, Said W, Bader D. Evaluation and Management of Newborns with Suspected Early-Onset Sepsis: Comparison of Two Approaches and Suggestion for Guidelines. Am J Perinatol. 2017 Mar;34(4):315–22.

199. Sharma D, Farahbakhsh N, Shastri S, Sharma P. Biomarkers for diagnosis of neonatal sepsis: a literature review. J Matern-Fetal Neonatal Med Off J Eur Assoc Perinat Med Fed Asia Ocean Perinat Soc Int Soc Perinat Obstet. 2017 May;7:1–14.

200. Cleminson J, Austin N, McGuire W. Prophylactic systemic antifungal agents to prevent mortality and morbidity in very low birth weight infants. Cochrane Database Syst Rev. 2015;10:CD003850.

201. Ericson JE, Benjamin DK. Fluconazole prophylaxis for prevention of invasive candidiasis in infants. Curr Opin Pediatr. 2014 Apr;26(2):151–6.

202. Hope WW, Castagnola E, Groll AH, Roilides E, Akova M, Arendrup MC, et al. ESCMID* guideline for the diagnosis and management of Candida diseases 2012: prevention and management of invasive infections in neonates and children caused by Candida spp. Clin Microbiol Infect Off Publ Eur Soc Clin Microbiol Infect Dis. 2012 Dec;18(Suppl 7):38–52.

203. Kimberlin DW, Baley J. Committee on infectious diseases, Committee on fetus and newborn. Guidance on management of asymptomatic neonates born to women with active genital herpes lesions. Pediatrics. 2013 Feb;131(2):e635–46.

204. James SH, Kimberlin DW. Neonatal herpes simplex virus infection: epidemiology and treatment. Clin Perinatol. 2015 Mar;42(1):47–59, viii.

205. Waggoner-Fountain LA, Grossman LB. Herpes Simplex Virus. Pediatr Rev. 2004 Mar 1;25(3):86–93.

206. Policy & Guidelines | National AIDS Control Organization | MoHFW | GoI [Internet]. [cited 2017 Jul 4]. Available from: http://naco.gov.in/documents/policy-guidelines

207. Neu N, Duchon J, Zachariah P. TORCH infections. Clin Perinatol. 2015 Mar;42(1):77–103, viii.

208. Cotten CM. Antibiotic stewardship: reassessment of guidelines for management of neonatal sepsis. Clin Perinatol. 2015 Mar;42(1):195–206, x.

209. Crnich CJ, Jump R, Trautner B, Sloane PD, Mody L. Optimizing Antibiotic Stewardship in Nursing Homes: A Narrative Review and Recommendations for Improvement. Drugs Aging. 2015 Sep;32(9):699–716.

210. Gangat MA, Hsu JJ. Antibiotic stewardship: a focus on ambulatory care. S D Med J S D State Med Assoc. 2015;Spec No:44–8.

211. Azra Haider B, Bhutta ZA. Birth asphyxia in developing countries: current status and public health implications. Curr Probl Pediatr Adolesc Health Care. 2006 Jun;36(5):178–88.

212. Costello AM, Manandhar DS. Perinatal asphyxia in less developed countries. Arch Dis Child Fetal Neonatal Ed. 1994 Jul;71(1):F1–3.

213. Azzopardi DV, Strohm B, Edwards AD, Dyet L, Halliday HL, Juszczak E, et al. Moderate hypothermia to treat perinatal asphyxial encephalopathy. N Engl J Med. 2009 Oct 1;361(14):1349–58.

214. Shankaran S, Laptook AR, Ehrenkranz RA, Tyson JE, McDonald SA, Donovan EF, et al. Whole-body hypothermia for neonates with hypoxic-ischemic encephalopathy. N Engl J Med. 2005 Oct 13;353(15):1574–84.

215. Shankaran S. Therapeutic Hypothermia for Neonatal Encephalopathy. Curr Treat Options Neurol. 2012 Dec;14(6):608–19.

216. Shankaran S. Hypoxic-ischemic encephalopathy and novel strategies for neuroprotection. Clin Perinatol. 2012 Dec;39(4):919–29.

217. Shankaran S. Current status of hypothermia for hypoxemic ischemia of the newborn. Indian J Pediatr. 2014 Jun;81(6):578–84.

218. Shankaran S, Laptook A, Wright LL, Ehrenkranz RA, Donovan EF, Fanaroff AA, et al. Whole-body hypothermia for neonatal encephalopathy: animal observations as a basis for a randomized, controlled pilot study in term infants. Pediatrics. 2002 Aug;110(2 Pt 1):377–85.

219. Shankaran S, Laptook AR. Hypothermia as a treatment for birth asphyxia. Clin Obstet Gynecol. 2007 Sep;50(3):624–35.

220. da Silva S, Hennebert N, Denis R, Wayenberg JL. Clinical value of a single postnatal lactate measurement after intrapartum asphyxia. Acta Paediatr Oslo Nor 1992. 2000 Mar;89(3):320–3.

221. Shah S, Tracy M, Smyth J. Postnatal lactate as an early predictor of short-term outcome after intrapartum asphyxia. J Perinatol Off J Calif Perinat Assoc. 2004 Jan;24(1):16–20.

222. Chiang M-C, Lien R, Chu S-M, Yang P-H, Lin J-J, Hsu J-F, et al. Serum Lactate, Brain Magnetic Resonance Imaging and Outcome of Neonatal Hypoxic Ischemic Encephalopathy after Therapeutic Hypothermia. Pediatr Neonatol. 2016 Feb 1;57(1):35–40.

223. Manley BJ, Owen LS, Hooper SB, Jacobs SE, Cheong JLY, Doyle LW, et al. Towards evidence-based resuscitation of the newborn infant. The Lancet. 2017 Apr 22;389(10079):1639–48.

224. Committee on Fetus and Newborn, Papile L-A, Baley JE, Benitz W, Cummings J, Carlo WA, et al. Hypothermia and neonatal encephalopathy. Pediatrics. 2014 Jun;133(6):1146–50.

225. Tagin MA, Woolcott CG, Vincer MJ, Whyte RK, Stinson DA. Hypothermia for neonatal hypoxic ischemic encephalopathy: an updated systematic review and meta-analysis. Arch Pediatr Adolesc Med. 2012 Jun 1;166(6):558–66.

226. Filippi L, Catarzi S, Gozzini E, Fiorini P, Falchi M, Pisano T, et al. Hypothermia for neonatal hypoxic-ischemic encephalopathy: may an early amplitude-integrated EEG improve the selection of candidates for cooling? J Matern-Fetal Neonatal Med Off J Eur Assoc Perinat Med Fed Asia Ocean Perinat Soc Int Soc Perinat Obstet. 2012 Nov;25(11):2171–6.

227. Youn Y-A, Kim JH, Yum S-K, Moon C-J, Lee I-G, Sung IK. The hospital outcomes compared between the early and late hypothermia-treated groups in neonates. J Matern Fetal Neonatal Med. 2016 Jul 17;29(14):2288–92.

228. Shankaran S, Pappas A, McDonald SA, Vohr BR, Hintz SR, Yolton K, et al. Childhood outcomes after hypothermia for neonatal encephalopathy. N Engl J Med. 2012 May 31;366(22):2085–92.

229. Jacobs SE, Berg M, Hunt R, Tarnow-Mordi WO, Inder TE, Davis PG. Cooling for newborns with hypoxic ischaemic encephalopathy. Cochrane Database Syst Rev. 2013;1:CD003311.

230. Sarkar S, Barks JD. Systemic complications and hypothermia. Semin Fetal Neonatal Med. 2010 Oct;15(5):270–5.

231. Alamo L, Vial Y, Gengler C, Meuli R. Imaging findings of bronchial atresia in fetuses, neonates and infants. Pediatr Radiol. 2016 Mar;46(3):383–90.

232. Vellanki H, Antunes M, Locke RG, McGreevy T, Mackley A, Eubanks JJ, et al. Decreased incidence of pneumothorax in VLBW infants after increased monitoring of tidal volumes. Pediatrics. 2012 Nov;130(5):e1352–8.

233. Boo N-Y, Cheah IG-S, Registry MNN. Risk factors associated with pneumothorax in Malaysian neonatal intensive care units. J Paediatr Child Health. 2011 Apr;47(4):183–90.

234. Miller JD, Carlo WA. Pulmonary complications of mechanical ventilation in neonates. Clin Perinatol. 2008 Mar;35(1):273–281, x–xi.

235. Raju U, Sondhi V, Patnaik SK. Meconium Aspiration Syndrome: An Insight. Med J Armed Forces India. 2010 Apr;66(2):152–7.

236. Murki S, Kumar P. Blood exchange transfusion for infants with severe neonatal hyperbilirubinemia. Semin Perinatol. 2011 Jun;35(3):175–84.

237. Doyle KJ, Bradshaw WT. Sixty golden minutes. Neonatal Netw NN. 2012 Oct;31(5):289–94.

238. Kooi EMW, Verhagen EA, Elting JWJ, Czosnyka M, Austin T, Wong FY, et al. Measuring cerebrovascular autoregulation in preterm infants using near-infrared spectroscopy: an overview of the literature. Expert Rev Neurother. 2017 Jun;29:1–18.

239. Beck J, Loron G, Masson C, Poli-Merol M-L, Guyot E, Guillot C, et al. Monitoring Cerebral and Renal Oxygenation Status during Neonatal Digestive Surgeries Using Near Infrared Spectroscopy. Front Pediatr. 2017;5:140.

240. Votava-Smith JK, Statile CJ, Taylor MD. King EC. Nelson DP, et al. Impaired cerebral autoregulation in preoperative newborn infants with congenital heart disease. J Thorac Cardiovasc Surg: Pratt JM; 2017 May 23.

241. Sood BG, McLaughlin K, Cortez J. Near-infrared spectroscopy: applications in neonates. Semin Fetal Neonatal Med. 2015 Jun;20(3):164–72.

242. Pichler G, Cheung P-Y, Aziz K, Urlesberger B, Schmölzer GM. How to monitor the brain during immediate neonatal transition and resuscitation? A systematic qualitative review of the literature. Neonatology. 2014;105(3):205–10.

243. Pellicer A, Greisen G, Benders M, Claris O, Dempsey E, Fumagalli M, et al. The SafeBoosC phase II randomised clinical trial: a treatment guideline for targeted near-infrared-derived cerebral tissue oxygenation versus standard treatment in extremely preterm infants. Neonatology. 2013;104(3):171–8.

244. Winckworth LC, Raj R, Draper L, Leith W. Antenatal counselling: documentation and recall. J Paediatr Child Health. 2013 May;49(5):422–3.

245. Moreno Hernando J, Thió Lluch M, Salguero García E, Rite Gracia S, Fernández Lorenzo JR, Echaniz Urcelay I, et al. [Recommendations for neonatal transport]. An Pediatr Barc Spain 2003. 2013 Aug;79(2):117.e1-7.

246. Rathod D, Adhisivam B, Bhat BV. Transport of sick neonates to a tertiary care hospital, South India: condition at arrival and outcome. Trop Doct. 2015 Apr;45(2):96–9.

247. Kumar PP, Kumar CD, Shaik F, Yadav S, Dusa S, Venkatlakshmi A. Transported neonates by a specialist team - how STABLE are they. Indian J Pediatr. 2011 Jul;78(7):860–2.

10

The timing of umbilical cord clamping at birth: physiological considerations

Stuart B. Hooper[1,2*], Corinna Binder-Heschl[1], Graeme R. Polglase[1,2], Andrew W. Gill[3], Martin Kluckow[4], Euan M. Wallace[1,2], Douglas Blank[1,5] and Arjan B. te Pas[6]

Abstract

While it is now recognized that umbilical cord clamping (UCC) at birth is not necessarily an innocuous act, there is still much confusion concerning the potential benefits and harms of this common procedure. It is most commonly assumed that delaying UCC will automatically result in a time-dependent net placental-to-infant blood transfusion, irrespective of the infant's physiological state. Whether or not this occurs, will likely depend on the infant's physiological state and not on the amount of time that has elapsed between birth and umbilical cord clamping (UCC). However, we believe that this is an overly simplistic view of what can occur during delayed UCC and ignores the benefits associated with maintaining the infant's venous return and cardiac output during transition. Recent experimental evidence and observations in humans have provided compelling evidence to demonstrate that time is not a major factor influencing placental-to-infant blood transfusion after birth. Indeed, there are many factors that influence blood flow in the umbilical vessels after birth, which depending on the dominating factors could potentially result in infant-to-placental blood transfusion. The most dominant factors that influence umbilical artery and venous blood flows after birth are lung aeration, spontaneous inspirations, crying and uterine contractions. It is still not entirely clear whether gravity differentially alters umbilical artery and venous flows, although the available data suggests that its influence, if present, is minimal. While there is much support for delaying UCC at birth, much of the debate has focused on a time-based approach, which we believe is misguided. While a time-based approach is much easier and convenient for the caregiver, ignoring the infant's physiology during delayed UCC can potentially be counter-productive for the infant.

Keywords: Delayed umbilical cord clamping, Birth, Neonatal cardiovascular transition, Umbilical artery flow, Umbilical venous flow

Background

The transition from fetal to newborn life represents one of the greatest physiological challenges that any human will encounter. Once the umbilical cord is clamped, infants must clear their airways of liquid to allow the onset of pulmonary gas exchange and the cardiovascular system must undergo a major structural and functional re-organisation [1]. Although it is well recognized that the cardiovascular transition at birth is triggered by lung aeration [2, 3], the question of how umbilical cord clamping (UCC) influences this relationship is unclear

[1]. It is widely assumed that UCC at birth is an innocuous act, but many have argued that this assumption is false and, if done too early, can deprive the infant of vital blood volume during early newborn life [4, 5]. The aim of this review is to discuss the physiology of umbilical cord clamping and the circumstances that would facilitate placental transfusion if UCC is delayed.

At birth, lung aeration triggers a functional re-organisation of the infant's circulation, largely by stimulating an increase in pulmonary blood flow (PBF) [1]. From a teleological perspective, linking these physiological events is logical. As lung aeration can only occur after birth and is a pre-requisite for newborn survival, it is an ideal trigger for initiating the physiological changes that underpin the transition to newborn life. In this context, when trying to

* Correspondence: stuart.hooper@monash.edu
[1]The Ritchie Centre, Hudson Institute for Medical Research, Melbourne, Australia
[2]Department of Obstetrics and Gynaecology, Monash University, Melbourne, Australia
Full list of author information is available at the end of the article

understand and devise strategies that assist the infant in making the best possible transition to newborn life, it is important to understand the central role that lung aeration plays in this process. Indeed, neonatologists have long recognized that, at birth, ventilation is the key to newborn resuscitation. It not only increases oxygenation, but also increases the infant's heart rate and cardiac function by stimulating an increase in PBF [3]. An increase in PBF restores the preload required to maintain cardiac output after birth (Fig. 1), which is lost upon umbilical cord clamping (UCC) [6, 7]. In view of the central role that lung aeration plays in the cardiovascular transition at birth, it is also likely to have a major impact on placental to infant blood transfusion when UCC is delayed. However, until recently all arguments about delayed UCC have simply focused on the time that UCC should be delayed with little or no reference to the infant's transitional physiology [5]. In this review, we will argue that there is little or no justification for delaying UCC for a set period of time after birth and will discuss physiological factors that may provide a more rational determinant for when UCC should occur after birth.

A historical perspective

It has long been recognized that UCC is not just a symbolic separation of the infant from the mother, but can have a major impact on the infant's well-being after birth. Indeed, the argument of when the umbilical cord should be clamped extends back centuries, at least to Aristotle in 300 BC. In 1801, Erasmus Darwin suggested that, *'Another thing very injurious to the child, is the tying and cutting of the navel string too soon; which should always be left till the child has not only repeatedly breathed but till all pulsation in the cord ceases. As otherwise the child is much weaker than it ought to be'* [8]. In this commentary, Darwin highlights the link between breathing and the timing of UCC, indicating that he considered the two events to be closely linked and to impact on the infant's well being. However, the debate about the timing of UCC at birth has largely overlooked the impact that pulmonary ventilation may have in this process.

Until recently, the benefits of delayed UCC at birth were thought to only involve placental-to-infant blood transfusion. This debate was sparked by a series of studies demonstrating a time dependent "transfusion" of blood into the infant if UCC is delayed for up to 3 mins after birth [9–11]. However, in view of recent studies (see below), it is now time to question whether this concept is an overly simplistic view of the factors controlling blood flow between the placenta and infant immediately after birth. These early studies used ^{125}I-labeled albumen to measure blood volumes in infants that had their cords clamped at different times after birth [9, 11]. However, as we now know that blood flow in the umbilical arteries and veins during delayed UCC is regulated by a complex interplay of physiological factors, mostly respiratory [12], it is hard to envisage how a time-dependent increase in blood volume could be so consistently achieved.

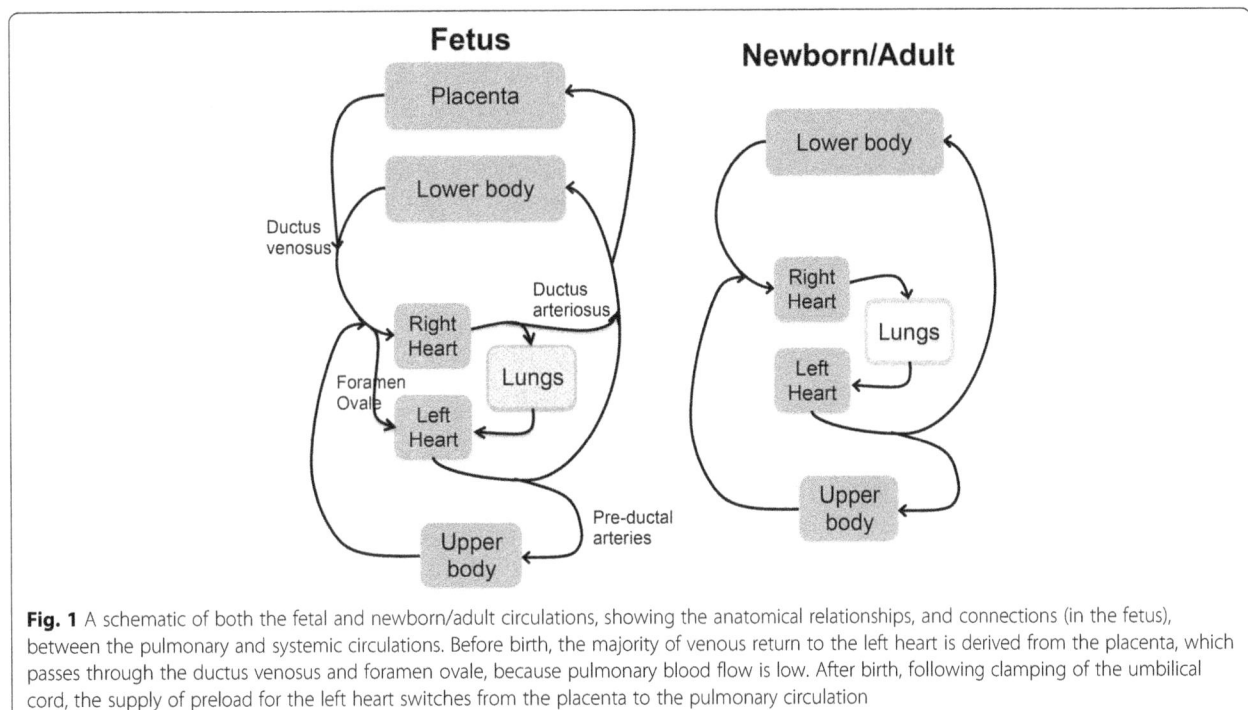

Fig. 1 A schematic of both the fetal and newborn/adult circulations, showing the anatomical relationships, and connections (in the fetus), between the pulmonary and systemic circulations. Before birth, the majority of venous return to the left heart is derived from the placenta, which passes through the ductus venosus and foramen ovale, because pulmonary blood flow is low. After birth, following clamping of the umbilical cord, the supply of preload for the left heart switches from the placenta to the pulmonary circulation

Measurements of increasing infant weight have provided additional evidence supporting the concept of placental-to-infant blood transfusion [13], but there is still considerable uncertainty as to the factors that influence this transfer and whether time is incidental or a significant factor [1].

Recent studies have now begun to investigate the many factors that may influence blood flow in the umbilical arteries and veins during delayed UCC and while there is the potential for placental-to-infant blood transfer, there is also a risk of infant-to-placenta blood transfer [12]. Thus, with regard to making recommendations about the timing of UCC, we need to better understand the factors regulating blood flow in the umbilical vessels after birth and identify the factors that influence the distribution of blood between the placenta and infant at this time. This must also include a better understanding of the physiology underpinning the cardiovascular transition at birth.

The cardiovascular transition at birth: the effect of UCC before lung aeration

Before birth, blood flow through the lungs is low as the majority of blood exiting the right ventricle by-passes the lungs and enters the thoracic aorta via the ductus arteriosus (DA) [6, 7, 14]. As a result, pulmonary venous return is also low and only provides a small proportion of the preload required to maintain left ventricular output in the fetus (Fig. 1). Instead, much of the preload for the left ventricle during fetal life is derived from umbilical venous return [6, 7, 14]. This blood flows from the umbilical vein, via the ductus venosus, inferior vena cava and through the foramen ovale to directly enter the left atrium [14]. The preferential streaming of well-oxygenated umbilical venous blood through the ductus venosus and foramen ovale into the left atrium, gives rise to higher oxygenation levels in fetal preductal (vs postductal) arteries [14].

While the fetal circulatory arrangement allows a relatively direct flow of oxygenated blood from the placenta into the left atrium, which is analogous to flow between the lungs and left atrium in adults (Fig. 1), UCC at birth can severely disrupt venous return and cardiac output [6, 7]. Indeed, UCC causes venous return to decrease by 30–50 %, which reduces preload and cardiac output by a similar amount [6, 7]. At the same time, total peripheral resistance increases with the loss of the low resistance placental circulation, which causes a rapid increase (30 % within 4 heart beats; Fig. 2) in arterial blood pressure [6, 15, 16]. No doubt this increase in afterload contributes to the decrease in cardiac output, which is reflected by both a decrease in stroke volume and a decrease in heart rate [6, 7] (Fig. 3). With regard to the latter, it is important to recognize that the low heart rates commonly observed at birth [17], even in normal term infants, may result from a loss of preload caused by UCC rather than from an acute hypoxic episode. Indeed, a recent study in rabbits has shown that ventilation with 100 % nitrogen also increases PBF and heart rate after birth [18]. Thus, an increase in oxygen is unlikely to be the only stimulus for the increase in heart rate at birth, which also likely involves an increase in PBF via an increase in preload [1].

While the precise mechanisms by which lung aeration stimulates the increase in PBF at birth are still unclear [19], a recent imaging study has shown that lung aeration and the increase in PBF are not spatially related [20]. This study showed that partial lung aeration caused a global increase in PBF, leading to a large ventilation/perfusion mismatch in unaerated regions of the lung (Fig. 4). A follow up study showed that this global increase in PBF in response to partial lung aeration also occurs following ventilation with 100 % nitrogen [18]. These unexpected findings suggest that the dominant mechanisms involved are different to the mechanisms regulating regional PBF in the adult and that while

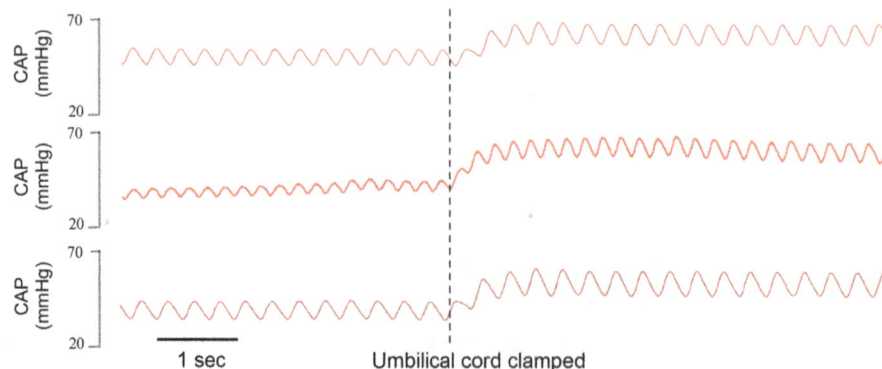

Fig. 2 Effect of umbilical cord clamping (dotted line) on carotid arterial blood pressure (CAP) in three lambs. CAP increases by ~30 % in 4–5 heart beats [6]

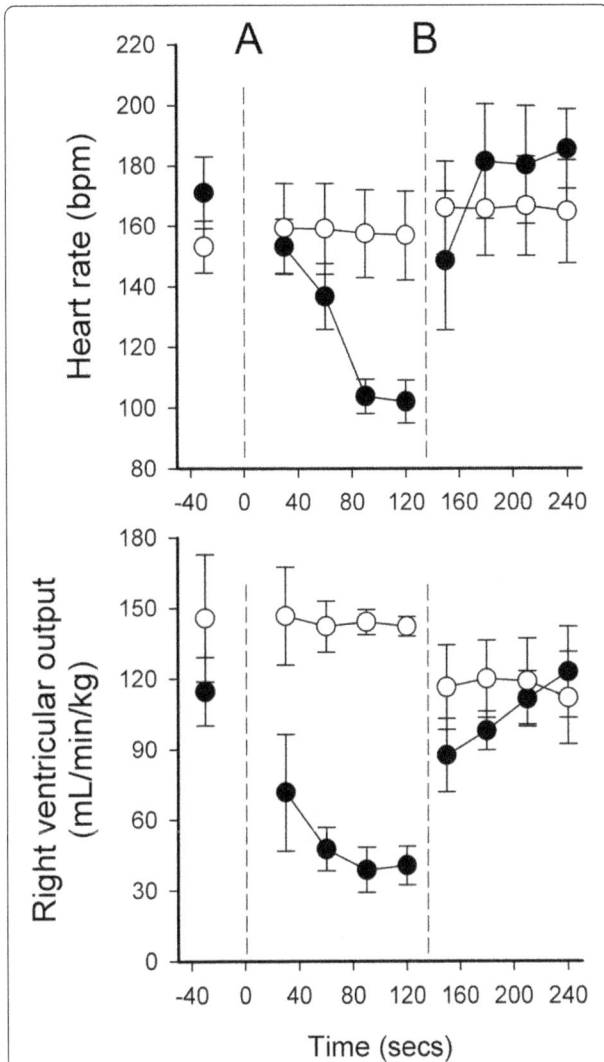

Fig. 3 Heart rate and right ventricular output measured in newborn lambs that either had their umbilical cords clamped 1–2 mins before ventilation was commenced (clamp first; closed circles) or were ventilated and pulmonary blood flow allowed to increase before their cords were clamped (vent first; open circles). The broken line (**a**) indicates either when cord clamping occurred in the clamp first group or ventilation commenced in the vent first group. The broken line (**b**), indicates when either clamping occurred in the vent first group or when ventilation commenced in the clamp first group. Data were obtained from [6] and redrawn

oxygen must play a role [21], other mechanisms are also involved. Nevertheless, as PBF becomes the sole source of preload for the left ventricle after birth, PBF must increase shortly after UCC to replace umbilical venous return as the primary source of preload for the left ventricle [6]. As such, if there is a delay between UCC and the onset of lung aeration, the infant will not only be exposed to hypoxia, due to a lack of gas exchange, but also to a prolonged period of reduced or restricted cardiac output. As the primary physiological defense

mechanism that is invoked during hypoxia is an increase and redistribution of cardiac output [22–24], this period of reduced cardiac output puts the infant at high risk of hypoxic/ischemic injury. On the other hand, if ventilation onset coincides with or immediately follows UCC, any reduction in cardiac output is likely to be brief and greatly reduced.

It is also important to consider how the infant's physiology responds to UCC and the sudden reduction in cardiac output combined with a rapid (over 4 heart beats; Fig. 2) increase in arterial blood pressure (afterload) [6]. As the cerebral circulation is pressure passive over this time frame, this increase in pressure leads to an increase in cerebral blood flow in lambs. However, as cardiac output is also decreased, after ~60 s arterial blood pressure and cerebral blood flow also decrease before stabilizing (after ~2mins), presumably due to a baroreceptor mediated peripheral vasoconstriction [6]. Then after ventilation onset, the sudden increase in PBF restores left ventricular preload and increases cardiac output, leading to a second rapid increase in arterial blood pressure and cerebral blood flow (Fig. 3); increases in cardiac output have also been observed in human infants at birth [25, 26]. The net result of UCC followed by lung aeration after a brief delay (1–2 mins), are large fluctuations in arterial pressure and cerebral blood flow [6]. It is also interesting that right ventricular output rapidly increases with cardiac output following lung aeration, suggesting that left-to-right shunting through the foramen ovale may contribute to right ventricular preload at this time (Fig. 3).

Another consideration with regard to the impact of UCC at birth and the associated reduction in cardiac output, is the question of how PBF increases so rapidly and to such a large extent when right and left ventricular output are initially both low. The answer is partly due to the redirection of right ventricular output through the lungs, rather than through the DA, as pulmonary vascular resistance (PVR) decreases [6, 7, 14]. In addition, because UCC greatly increases peripheral vascular resistance, the decrease in PVR makes the lungs a lower resistance pathway for blood flow compared to the systemic circulation. As a result, blood flow through the DA reverses, leading to left-to-right shunting of blood from the aorta into the pulmonary artery, which makes a significant contribution to the increase in PBF [7]. While the net flow is left-to-right, instantaneous flow is bi-directional at different times throughout the cardiac cycle [7, 27]. This is because the pressure waves emanating from the left and right ventricles reach the pulmonary and aortic ends of the DA at different times after the onset of systole. During early systole, right ventricular contraction produces a pressure gradient across the DA that leads initially to right-to-left flow across the DA. However, as the pressure wave emanating from the left ventricle reaches the DA-aortic junction, the

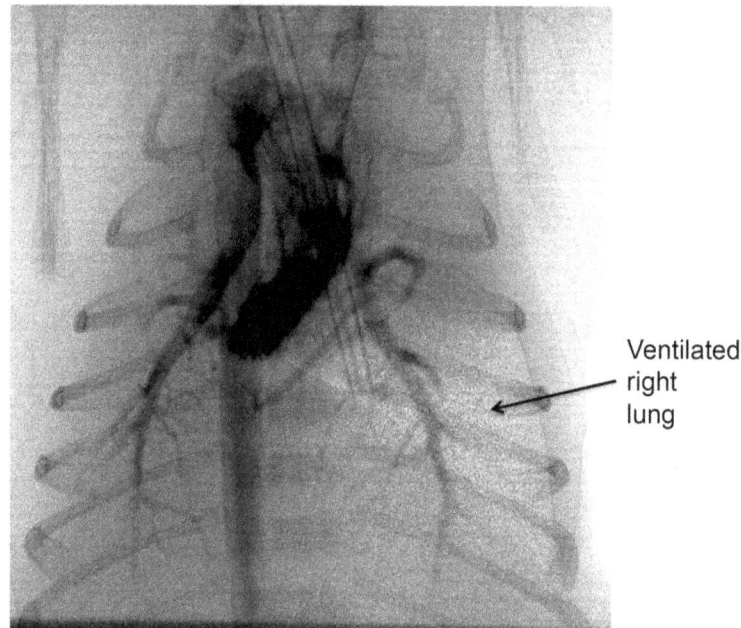

Fig. 4 A combined angiographic and phase contrast X-ray image of a near term (30 days) rabbit kitten that was delivered by caesarean section and received unilateral ventilation of the right lung. Blood flow, as shown by the contrast agent in the pulmonary vessels, increases similarly in both the aerated right lung and the unaerated left lung

pressure gradient reverses, which produces left-to-right flow through the DA that is sustained throughout most of diastole. Interestingly, the net left-to-right flow through the DA leads to a partial left ventricle-lung-left ventricle short circuit [7]. Presumably this allows the two ventricles time (while the DA closes) to gradually balance their outputs after birth, which ensures that the left ventricle is not deprived of preload during this transitional period.

Cardiovascular transition at birth: the effect of UCC after lung aeration

As the source of preload for the left ventricle must switch from umbilical venous return to pulmonary venous return after birth (Fig. 1), to avoid the loss of preload and reduction in cardiac output caused by UCC, it is logical to aerate the lungs and allow PBF to increase before UCC [1, 6, 28]. In this situation, the preload source can immediately switch from the umbilical circulation to the pulmonary circulation with little or no reduction in supply. As a result, there is no reduction in cardiac output and interestingly the normal increase in arterial blood pressure caused by UCC is greatly mitigated [6]. This is because there is an almost instantaneous reversal of blood flow though the DA, which changes from entirely right-to-left to mostly left-to-right following UCC [6, 7]. This indicates that the low resistance pulmonary circulation instantly becomes an alternative route for systemic blood flows and thereby greatly reduces the instantaneous increase in afterload caused by UCC.

Following lung aeration and before UCC, it would appear that there is a competitive interplay between blood flows entering the pulmonary and placental circulations. This is because, while the DA is patent, flow exiting the right and left ventricles can either enter the pulmonary circulation or continue down the aorta and enter the placental circulation (Fig. 1). Clearly the determining factor as to which circulation dominates will depend on the resistance in each circulation. At least initially, flow through the placental circulation appears to dominate as, while right-to-left DA flow is reduced following ventilation onset, no left-to-right flow occurs until after UCC [6]. However, as UCC occurred after only 2–3mins of positive pressure ventilation in that study and it takes up to 10 mins for PBF to peak (and PVR to reach a minimum) following ventilation onset [7, 29], it is possible that the pulmonary circulation dominates after longer periods of ventilation; we have recently observed this in lambs (unpublished observations). This effect may occur sooner and to a greater extent under conditions where the decrease in PVR is enhanced, for example if the infant makes deep inspiratory efforts [27], or when placental vascular resistance is increased, perhaps due to uterine contractions (see below). The logical extension to this concept is the suggestion that the re-direction of both right and left (via the DA) ventricular output into the pulmonary circulation, contributes to the reduction in umbilical artery blood flow after birth and to the eventual closure of these vessels (Fig. 1). In any event, these considerations highlight the fact that flow in the umbilical vessels is likely to be influenced by many interacting factors and whether this results in net placental to infant blood transfusion is not a forgone conclusion.

Factors regulating umbilical blood flows during delayed cord clamping after birth

The concept that net placental to infant blood transfusion occurs if UCC is delayed for a set period of time assumes that umbilical venous flow will exceed umbilical arterial flow during this time. However, until recently, very little was known about the factors determining flow in the umbilical circulation following birth and before UCC. Indeed, it is unclear if flow in the umbilical arteries and vein are influenced by the same factors and to the same extent or are independently regulated, which is highly unlikely. Clearly, if delayed UCC is going to be recommended for clinical practice, it is important to identify the factors that regulate flow in both vessels after birth. This is needed to ensure that factors that promote infant-to-placental blood transfusion are avoided, as clearly this would be counterproductive and detrimental to the infant.

Gravity

While little consideration has been given to the factors determining flows in the umbilical arteries and vein during delayed UCC, there has been much discussion of factors that may influence net placental to infant blood transfusion [4, 30]. In particular, it has been proposed that gravity will assist blood transfusion if the infant is placed below the level of the introitus [10]. However, this assumes that the flows in the umbilical arteries and vein are independent and that gravity will increase flow in the vein but decrease flow in the arteries. We have recently examined this in lambs and found that placing the lamb below the ewe during delayed UCC reduces umbilical artery flow and initiates left-to-right shunting through the DA leading to an increase in PBF (unpublished observations). Logically, the higher pressure-head required for the heart to pump blood through the placenta, due to the vertical height difference between the heart and placenta, makes the lungs a lower resistance option than the placenta. This supports the concept that more blood remains in the infant with each heartbeat. However, placing the lamb below the placenta also reduced umbilical venous flow by a similar amount, indicating that flow into the placenta is a major determinant of flow out of the placenta. As such, unless the resistance of the placental or infant's circulation markedly changes at this time, it is hard to understand how placing the infant below the mother will influence net placental to infant blood transfusion. This is consistent with the findings of a recent clinical trial, which found that placing an infant at the same height or above the introitus does not effect placental to infant blood transfusion, with both groups apparently receiving a similar transfusion of 50–55 mL [31].

Uterine contractions

Another factor proposed to increase placental to infant blood transfusion is uterine contractions. It has been suggested that uterine contractions physically "squeeze" blood out of the placenta and into the infant [9, 30], but this suggestion is not consistent with the changes in umbilical blood flows that occur during labour [32]. While uterine contractions have a major impact on umbilical blood flows, they are primarily thought to cause a pressure-induced, differential reduction in flow in both vessels as well as a reduction in uterine flow [32]. During the contraction, the lower pressure umbilical veins are thought to close earlier than the higher pressure umbilical arteries at the onset of contraction and the venous vessels also open later than the arteries towards the end of the contraction [32]. As such, there is the potential for placental blood accumulation during a contraction. The release of this blood back into the fetal circulation at the end of the contraction is thought to give rise to the small tachycardia that follows a uterine contraction [32].

We have recently examined the effect of oxytocin-induced contractions on umbilical artery and venous blood flows in lambs during delayed UCC (unpublished observations). We found that during the contraction, umbilical venous flow ceased and that while pulsatile flow continued in the umbilical artery, the flow was greatly reduced resulting in retrograde flow during diastole. A similar flow pattern in the umbilical artery has been observed in infants during delayed UCC, although it was unknown whether this flow pattern coincided with a uterine contraction [12]. Uterine contractions were also found to increase arterial blood pressure in lambs, which is consistent with it causing an increase in placental vascular resistance as observed with UCC [6]. Thus, rather than facilitating placental to infant blood transfusion, uterine contractions appear to more closely replicate partial UCC and thereby restrict venous return, reduce cardiac output and increase afterloads. Thus, perhaps the administration of oxytocin-like compounds to mothers immediately after birth, to reduce the risk of post-partum haemorrhage, should be delayed until after UCC.

Spontaneous breathing

The recently published experimental studies on delayed UCC only examined the physiological effects of positive pressure ventilation (PPV) [6], whereas the effects of spontaneous breathing are likely to be different. It is well established that increasing intra-thoracic pressure reduces PBF by increasing PVR and if the pressures are sustained [33, 34], venous return and preload are also reduced, resulting in a reduction in cardiac output. The inhibitory effect of positive airway pressures on PBF also occurs on an inflation-by-inflation basis during PPV. In lambs, when the systolic peak in PBF is in phase with the peak inflation pressure, the amplitude is reduced, whereas when they are out of phase, peak PBF is increased (Fig. 5). The pressure related decrease in PBF is thought to result from alveolar pressurization and expansion causing compression of pulmonary capillaries that lie between adjacent alveoli, in the alveolar walls [34–36]. On the other hand, spontaneous breathing in infants results in a reduction in intra-thoracic pressure, which facilitates venous return and transiently increases both PBF and left-to-right DA shunting [37]. In contrast to positive pressure inflations, when inspiration coincides with systole, peak PBF is increased, which is thought to result from peri-alveolar capillary expansion and a reduction in peri-alveolar tissue pressures [38]. This is caused by lung expansion resulting from chest wall expansion, whereby the expanding forces are projected from the visceral pleura into the alveoli, rather than commencing within the alveoli and expanding out.

Recent studies in infants have shown that spontaneous breathing at birth, particularly deep inspiratory efforts, have a major impact on PBF and blood flow through the DA, which is consistent with a large reduction in PVR during inspiratory efforts [27]. In normal spontaneously breathing infants, the proportion of right-to-left shunting of blood through the DA was found to reduce with time whereas the proportion of left-to-right shunting increased along with an increase in left ventricular output [25, 39]. Large inspiratory efforts associated with crying were found to cause a large increase in left-to-right DA shunting [27].

In view of the finding that spontaneous breathing has a large impact on PBF and DA shunting, it is not surprising that it also influences umbilical venous and arterial blood flows [12]. A recent study in infants has for the first time reported blood flows in the umbilical vessels during delayed UCC and identified some of the factors regulating blood flow between the infant and placenta after birth [12]. As predicted, the flow pattern was not uni-dimensional or uni-directional, with many factors determining blood flow in the cord. Flows continued for longer than previous thought and were found to cease in the umbilical vein before they ceased in the artery in approximately one third of infants; this could result in a net loss of blood from the infant [12]. Umbilical venous flow was very dependent upon the breathing cycle with flow entering the infant predominantly during inspiration and ceasing during expiration as well as during crying. The latter is not surprising as crying causes the abdomen and chest to pressurize and so umbilical venous pressure would have to substantially increase before blood could enter the infant. Similarly, crying was found to greatly reduce umbilical artery flow and in some cases, causes it to briefly cease [12]. In addition, as indicated above, periods of bidirectional flow was observed, which was thought to coincide with uterine contractions. Taken together, these findings clearly demonstrate that blood flow between the placenta and infant after birth is complex, is not unidirectional and is influenced by a number of factors. The dominant factors likely include uterine contractions and whether or not the infant is breathing or crying. Time from birth has little relevance to these factors except that with increasing time there is a higher chance that the infant will have commenced breathing.

Summary

Recent experimental evidence and observations in human infants have provided compelling evidence to

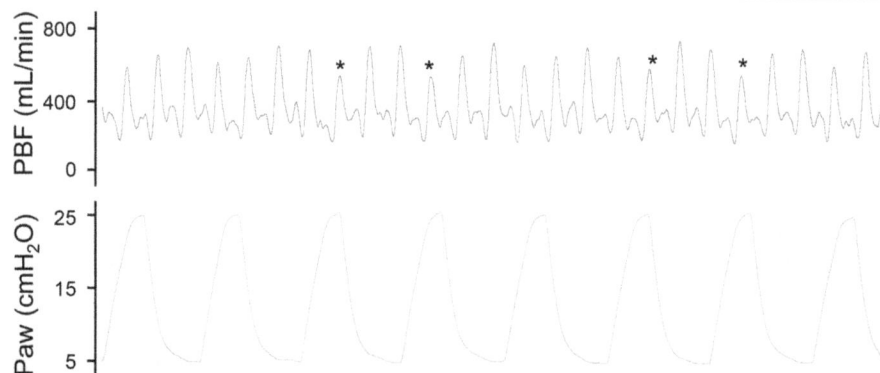

Fig. 5 Simultaneous pulmonary blood flow and airway pressure recordings made in a ventilated newborn lamb. Note that whenever the peak airway pressure coincides with systole, the systolic peak in pulmonary blood flow is reduced, particularly compared with the systolic peaks that coincide with periods when airway pressure is low between inflations. The reductions in pulmonary blood flow result from transient increases in pulmonary vascular resistance caused by the increase in airway pressure. Asterisks indicate good examples of peak pulmonary blood flow reductions coinciding with peak inflation pressures

demonstrate that time is largely incidental and is not a major determining factor of net placental-to-infant blood transfusion after birth. It is also clear, that there are many factors that influence blood flow in the umbilical vessels after birth, which depending on the dominating factors could potentially result in infant-to-placental blood transfusion. Studies investigating factors that influence umbilical artery and venous blood flows before UCC have found that the most dominant factors are lung aeration, spontaneous inspirations, crying and uterine contractions. While it is still not entirely clear whether gravity differentially alters umbilical artery and venous flows, the available data suggests that its influence, if present, is minimal. The physiological consequences of umbilical cord "milking" have not been raised in this review, largely because there is very limited experimental data detailing the physiological effects on the newborn and its circulatory transition at birth. Despite this, numerous trials have been conducted expecting it to increase blood volumes and duplicate the advantages of delayed UCC without really understanding the impact that it will have on the infant's physiology. As such physiological studies on umbilical cord milking are urgently needed.

Conclusions

The debate about when the umbilical cord should be clamped after birth has simply focused on the potential for a time-dependent net placental to infant blood transfusion. However, as there are many factors that influence blood flow in the umbilical arteries and veins immediately after birth, some infants maybe at risk of losing blood volume. If UCC is to be delayed, there is now very good evidence demonstrating that the timing of UCC should be based on the infant's physiology, rather than on a stopwatch. In particular, whether the infant is breathing or not. Aerating the lungs increases PBF, allowing pulmonary venous return to immediately replace umbilical venous return as the primary source of preload, which has the effect of stabilizing the circulation as it transitions after birth.

Abbreviations
DA, Ductus arteriosus; PBF, Pulmonary blood flow; PPV, Positive pressure ventilation; PVR, Pulmonary vascular resistance; UCC, Umbilical cord clamping.

Acknowledgements
The authors would like to acknowledge the continuing discussions and feedback provided by Professors Peter Davis and Colin Morley.

Funding
This research was supported by a NH&MRC Program Grant (606789) and Research Fellowships (GRP: 1026890 and SBH: 545921), a Rebecca L. Cooper Medical Research Foundation Fellowship (GRP), a Eunice Kennedy Shriver National Institute Of Child Health & Human Development of the National Institutes of Health (Award Number R01HD072848), The Financial Markets Foundation for Children and the Victorian Government's Operational Infrastructure Support Program.

Authors' contributions
SH wrote the manuscript and all other authors contributed equally to editing the final submitted version of the manuscript. All authors read and approved the final manuscript.

Authors' information
Not applicable.

Competing interests
The authors declare that they have no competing interests.

Author details
[1]The Ritchie Centre, Hudson Institute for Medical Research, Melbourne, Australia. [2]Department of Obstetrics and Gynaecology, Monash University, Melbourne, Australia. [3]Centre for Neonatal Research and Education, The University of Western Australia, Crawley, WA 6008, Australia. [4]Department of Neonatology, Royal North Shore Hospital and University of Sydney, Sydney, NSW 2065, Australia. [5]Neonatal Services, The Royal Women's Hospital, Melbourne, Australia. [6]Department of Neonatology, Leiden University Medical Centre, Leiden, The Netherlands.

References

1. Hooper SB, Te Pas AB, Lang J, et al. Cardiovascular transition at birth: a physiological sequence. Pediatr Res. 2015;77:608–14. doi:10.1038/pr.2015.21.
2. Rudolph AM. Distribution and regulation of blood flow in the fetal and neonatal lamb. Circ Res. 1985;57:811–21.
3. Hooper SB, Polglase GR, Roehr CC. Cardiopulmonary changes with aeration of the newborn lung. Paediatr Respir Rev. 2015. doi:10.1016/j.prrv.2015.03.003.
4. Niermeyer S, Velaphi S. Promoting physiologic transition at birth: re-examining resuscitation and the timing of cord clamping. Semin Fetal Neonatal Med. 2013;18:385–92. doi:10.1016/j.siny.2013.08.008.
5. McDonald SJ, Middleton P, Dowswell T, Morris PS. Effect of timing of umbilical cord clamping of term infants on maternal and neonatal outcomes. Cochrane Database Syst Rev. 2013;7, CD004074. doi:10.1002/14651858.CD004074.pub3.
6. Bhatt S, Alison B, Wallace EM, et al. Delaying cord clamping until ventilation onset improves cardiovascular function at birth in preterm lambs. J Physiol. 2013;591:2113–26. doi:10.1113/jphysiol.2012.250084.
7. Crossley KJ, Allison BJ, Polglase GR, Morley CJ, Davis PG, Hooper SB. Dynamic changes in the direction of blood flow through the ductus arteriosus at birth. J Physiol. 2009;587:4695–704. doi:10.1113/jphysiol.2009.174870.
8. Darwin E. Zoonomia, or the laws of organic life. 2nd ed. London: J Johnson; 1796. 3rd ed, 1801.
9. Yao AC, Hirvensalo M, Lind J. Placental transfusion-rate and uterine contraction. Lancet. 1968;1:380–3.
10. Yao AC, Lind J. Effect of gravity on placental transfusion. Lancet. 1969;2:505–8.
11. Yao AC, Moinian M, Lind J. Distribution of blood between infant and placenta after birth. Lancet. 1969;2:871–3.
12. Boere I, Roest AA, Wallace E, et al. Umbilical blood flow patterns directly after birth before delayed cord clamping. Arch Dis Child Fetal Neonatal Ed. 2015;100:F121–5. doi:10.1136/archdischild-2014-307144.
13. Farrar D, Airey R, Law GR, Tuffnell D, Cattle B, Duley L. Measuring placental transfusion for term births: weighing babies with cord intact. BJOG. 2011;118:70–5. doi:10.1111/j.1471-0528.2010.02781.x.
14. Rudolph AM. Fetal and neonatal pulmonary circulation. Annu Rev Physiol. 1979;41:383–95.

15. Dawes GS. Fetal and neonatal physiology. Chicago: Year Book Inc; 1968.

16. Iwamoto HS, Teitel DF, Rudolph AM. Effects of lung distension and spontaneous fetal breathing on hemodynamics in sheep. Pediatr Res. 1993; 33:639–44.

17. Dawson JA, Kamlin CO, Wong C, et al. Changes in heart rate in the first minutes after birth. Arch Dis Child Fetal Neonatal Ed. 2010;95:F177–81. doi: 10.1136/adc.2009.169102.

18. Lang JA, Pearson JT, Binder-Heschl C, et al. Increase in pulmonary blood flow at birth; role of oxygen and lung aeration. J Physiol. 2015. doi:10.1113/JP270926.

19. Gao Y, Raj JU. Regulation of the pulmonary circulation in the fetus and newborn. Physiol Rev. 2010;90:1291–335. doi:10.1152/physrev.00032.2009.

20. Lang JA, Pearson JT, Te Pas AB, et al. Ventilation/perfusion mismatch during lung aeration at birth. J Appl Physiol (1985). 2014. doi: 10.1152/japplphysiol. 01358.2013.

21. Morin III FC, Egan EA, Ferguson W, Lundgren CEG. Development of pulmonary vascular response to oxygen. Am J Physiol. 1988;254:H542–6.

22. Cohn HE, Sacks EJ, Heymann MA, Rudolph AM. Cardiovascular responses to hypoxemia and acidemia in fetal lambs. Am J Obstet Gynecol. 1974;120:817–24.

23. Bocking AD, Gagnon R, White SE, Homan J, Milne KM, Richardson BS. Circulatory responses to prolonged hypoxemia in fetal sheep. Am J Obstet Gynecol. 1988;159:1418–24.

24. Bocking AD, White SE, Homan J, Richardson BS. Oxygen consumption is maintained in fetal sheep during prolonged hypoxaemia. J Dev Physiol. 1992;17:169–74.

25. van Vonderen JJ, Roest AA, Siew ML, et al. Noninvasive measurements of hemodynamic transition directly after birth. Pediatr Res. 2014;75:448–52. doi: 10.1038/pr.2013.241.

26. Katheria AC, Wozniak M, Harari D, Arnell K, Petruzzelli D, Finer NN. Measuring cardiac changes using electrical impedance during delayed cord clamping: a feasibility trial. Matern Health Neonatol Perinatol. 2015;1:15. doi: 10.1186/s40748-015-0016-3.

27. van Vonderen JJ, Roest AA, Walther FJ, et al. The influence of crying on the ductus arteriosus shunt and left ventricular output at birth. Neonatology. 2015;107:108–12. doi:10.1159/000368880.

28. Bhatt S, Polglase GR, Wallace EM, Te Pas AB, Hooper SB. Ventilation before umbilical cord clamping improves the physiological transition at birth. Front Pediatr. 2014;2:113. doi:10.3389/fped.2014.00113.

29. Crossley KJ, Morley CJ, Allison BJ, et al. Blood gases and pulmonary blood flow during resuscitation of very preterm lambs treated with antenatal betamethasone and/or Curosurf: effect of positive end-expiratory pressure. Pediatr Res. 2007;62:37–42.

30. Mercer JS, Erickson-Owens DA. Rethinking placental transfusion and cord clamping issues. J Perinat Neonatal Nurs. 2012;26:202–17. doi:10.1097/JPN. 0b013e31825d2d9a. quiz 18–9.

31. Vain NE, Satragno DS, Gorenstein AN, et al. Effect of gravity on volume of placental transfusion: a multicentre, randomised, non-inferiority trial. Lancet. 2014. doi:10.1016/S0140-6736(14)60197-5.

32. Westgate JA, Wibbens B, Bennet L, Wassink G, Parer JT, Gunn AJ. The intrapartum deceleration in center stage: a physiologic approach to the interpretation of fetal heart rate changes in labor. Am J Obstet Gynecol. 2007;197:236 e1–11. doi: 10.1016/j.ajog.2007.03.063.

33. Fuhrman BP, Everitt J, Lock JE. Cardiopulmonary effects of unilateral airway pressure changes in intact infant lambs. J Appl Physiol. 1984;56:1439–48.

34. Hooper SB. Role of luminal volume changes in the increase in pulmonary blood flow at birth in sheep. Exp Physiol. 1998;83:833–42.

35. Polglase GR, Morley CJ, Crossley KJ, et al. Positive end-expiratory pressure differentially alters pulmonary hemodynamics and oxygenation in ventilated, very premature lambs. J Appl Physiol. 2005;99:1453–61.

36. Fuhrman BP, Smith-Wright DL, Kulik TJ, Lock JE. Effects of static and fluctuating airway pressure on intact pulmonary circulation. J Appl Physiol. 1986;60:114–22.

37. van Vonderen JJ, Roest AA, Walther FJ, et al. The influence of crying on the ductus arteriosus shunt and left ventricular output at birth. Neonatology. 2014;107:108–12. doi:10.1159/000368880.

38. Polglase GR, Wallace MJ, Grant DA, Hooper SB. Influence of fetal breathing movements on pulmonary hemodynamics in fetal sheep. Pediatr Res. 2004; 56:932–8.

39. van Vonderen JJ, te Pas AB, Kolster-Bijdevaate C, et al. Non-invasive measurements of ductus arteriosus flow directly after birth. Arch Dis Child Fetal Neonatal Ed. 2014;99:F408–12. doi:10.1136/archdischild-2014-306033.

11

Impact of exposure to cooking fuels on stillbirths, perinatal, very early and late neonatal mortality - a multicenter prospective cohort study in rural communities in India, Pakistan, Kenya, Zambia and Guatemala

Archana B. Patel[1*], Sreelatha Meleth[2], Omrana Pasha[3], Shivaprasad S. Goudar[4], Fabian Esamai[5], Ana L. Garces[6], Elwyn Chomba[7], Elizabeth M. McClure[2], Linda L. Wright[8], Marion Koso-Thomas[8], Janet L. Moore[2], Sarah Saleem[3], Edward A. Liechty[9], Robert L. Goldenberg[10], Richard J. Derman[11], K. Michael Hambidge[12], Waldemar A. Carlo[13] and Patricia L. Hibberd[14]

Abstract

Background: Consequences of exposure to household air pollution (HAP) from biomass fuels used for cooking on neonatal deaths and stillbirths is poorly understood. In a large multi-country observational study, we examined whether exposure to HAP was associated with perinatal mortality (stillbirths from gestation week 20 and deaths through day 7 of life) as well as when the deaths occurred (macerated, non-macerated stillbirths, very early neonatal mortality (day 0–2) and later neonatal mortality (day 3–28).

Questions addressing household fuel use were asked at pregnancy, delivery, and neonatal follow-up visits in a prospective cohort study of pregnant women in rural communities in five low and lower middle income countries participating in the Global Network for Women and Children's Health's Maternal and Newborn Health Registry. The study was conducted between May 2011 and October 2012. Polluting fuels included kerosene, charcoal, coal, wood, straw, crop waste and dung. Clean fuels included electricity, liquefied petroleum gas (LPG), natural gas and biogas.

Results: We studied the outcomes of 65,912 singleton pregnancies, 18 % from households using clean fuels (59 % LPG) and 82 % from households using polluting fuels (86 % wood). Compared to households cooking with clean fuels, there was an increased risk of perinatal mortality among households using polluting fuels (adjusted relative risk (aRR) 1.44, 95 % confidence interval (CI) 1.30-1.61). Exposure to HAP increased the risk of having a macerated stillbirth (adjusted odds ratio (aOR) 1.66, 95%CI 1.23-2.25), non-macerated stillbirth (aOR 1.43, 95 % CI 1.15-1.85) and very early neonatal mortality (aOR 1.82, 95 % CI 1.47-2.22).

Conclusions: Perinatal mortality was associated with exposure to HAP from week 20 of pregnancy through at least day 2 of life. Since pregnancy losses before labor and delivery are difficult to track, the effect of exposure to polluting fuels on global perinatal mortality may have previously been underestimated.

Keywords: Perinatal, Neonatal, Mortality, Cooking fuels, Household air pollution

* Correspondence: dr_apatel@yahoo.com
[1]Lata Medical Research Foundation, Nagpur, Maharashtra 440022, India
Full list of author information is available at the end of the article

Background

As progress continues to be made toward Millennium Development Goal #4 (MDG4), attention increasingly focuses on causes of childhood mortality that have been the most resistant to improvement – particularly neonatal mortality (through day 28 of life) [1–4]. Reducing stillbirths (after week 20 of pregnancy and particularly intrapartum [3, 5]) is not addressed in MDG#4 (which focuses only on babies born alive) but the importance of reducing the burden of stillbirths, many of which may be resuscitatable at birth has been increasingly recognized [6].

Solid fuels and kerosene are used for cooking, heating and lighting by one third of the world's population [7]. Inefficient burning of these fuels results in household air pollution (HAP) that includes particulate matter and toxic chemicals, such as hydrocarbons, oxygenated organic compounds, free radicals and carbon monoxide [8]. HAP is the fourth leading risk factor for the global burden of disease, accounting for 3.5 million premature deaths in adults and children annually [7, 9]. HAP is a recognized risk factor for childhood pneumonia [10] and preterm birth [11], but the role of exposure to HAP on other pregnancy and neonatal outcomes is less clear due to concerns about the quality of evidence in the available observational studies [10]. This information is important as international governments are rolling out improved cookstoves that continue to use solid fuels without evidence on potential perinatal and other health benefits [12]. In addition, while there is a biologic basis for the effects of HAP on the developing fetus, neonate and young infant based on the similar pollutants in tobacco smoke (active and passive smoke exposure) [13–15], it is also unclear whether the effects of tobacco smoking and HAP are additive, synergistic or whether there is no interaction because the effect of one of the exposures (e.g., HAP) overwhelms the other (e.g., tobacco smoke).

The *Eunice Kennedy Shriver* National Institute of Child Health and Human Development's (NICHD's) Global Network (GN) for Women and Children's Health Research supports a Maternal and Newborn Health (MNH) Registry of pregnant women and their babies living in rural communities in low and lower middle income countries. The Registry has focused on documentation of fetal loss after week 20 of pregnancy, accurate and timely measurement of birth, birth weight and early and late neonatal outcomes [16]. It provides an ideal population to address unanswered questions about risk factors for perinatal mortality as well as the timing of fetal loss or neonatal death. Thus our primary objective was to examine whether HAP from cooking with biomass fuels was associated with perinatal mortality (stillbirths from gestation week 20 and deaths through day 7 of life). Secondary objectives were to examine whether HAP exposure was a risk factor for macerated, non-macerated stillbirths, very early neonatal mortality (day 0–2 of life) and mortality from day 3–28 of life. We also address recent issues raised about the use of kerosene as a polluting fuel because of concerns that it has previously inappropriately considered a clean fuel [7].

Methods

Ethics statement

The MNH Registry is an ongoing prospective multicentre cohort study of pregnant women and their babies in 100 rural communities located in Guatemala, 2 states in India, Kenya, Pakistan and Zambia. Pregnant women are recruited as early as possible during pregnancy and followed through day 42 post-partum to obtain details about the pregnancy, labor and delivery and the health of the mother and infant. The study was reviewed and approved at all of the involved institutions' ethics review committees at: The Lata Medical Research Foundation, Nagpur, Maharashtra, India; Aga Khan University, Karachi, Pakistan; JN Medical College, Belgaum, Karnataka, India; Moi University School of Medicine, Eldoret, Kenya; IMSALUD, San Carlos University, Guatemala City, Guatemala; University Teaching Hospital, Lusaka, Zambia; Indiana University School of Medicine, Indianapolis, Indiana; Columbia University, New York, New York; Christiana Care, Newark, Delaware; University of Colorado, Aurora, Colorado; University of Alabama at Birmingham, Birmingham, Alabama; Partners IRB, Massachusetts General Hospital, Boston, Massachusetts and RTI International, Research Triangle Park, North Carolina. The study was registered at ClinicalTrials.gov (NCT01073475). A Data Monitoring Committee appointed by NICHD reviewed the registry data on at least an annual basis.

Pregnant women intending to deliver in the study communities or affiliated hospitals were informed about the study and invited to participate in the MNH Registry. Those who consented signed the IRB approved informed consent form.

Study design, setting and participants

We included pregnant women enrolled in the MNH Registry. We excluded women from households for which there was incomplete information on type of cooking fuel used in the household, multiple gestations, as well as women who had a medical termination of pregnancy or miscarriage before week 20 of pregnancy, and women who had incomplete information on maternal parity or age, or were lost to follow-up (Fig. 1).

Information is obtained at three time points in the registry. On enrolment (before the 20th week of gestation), information on the date of last menstrual period,

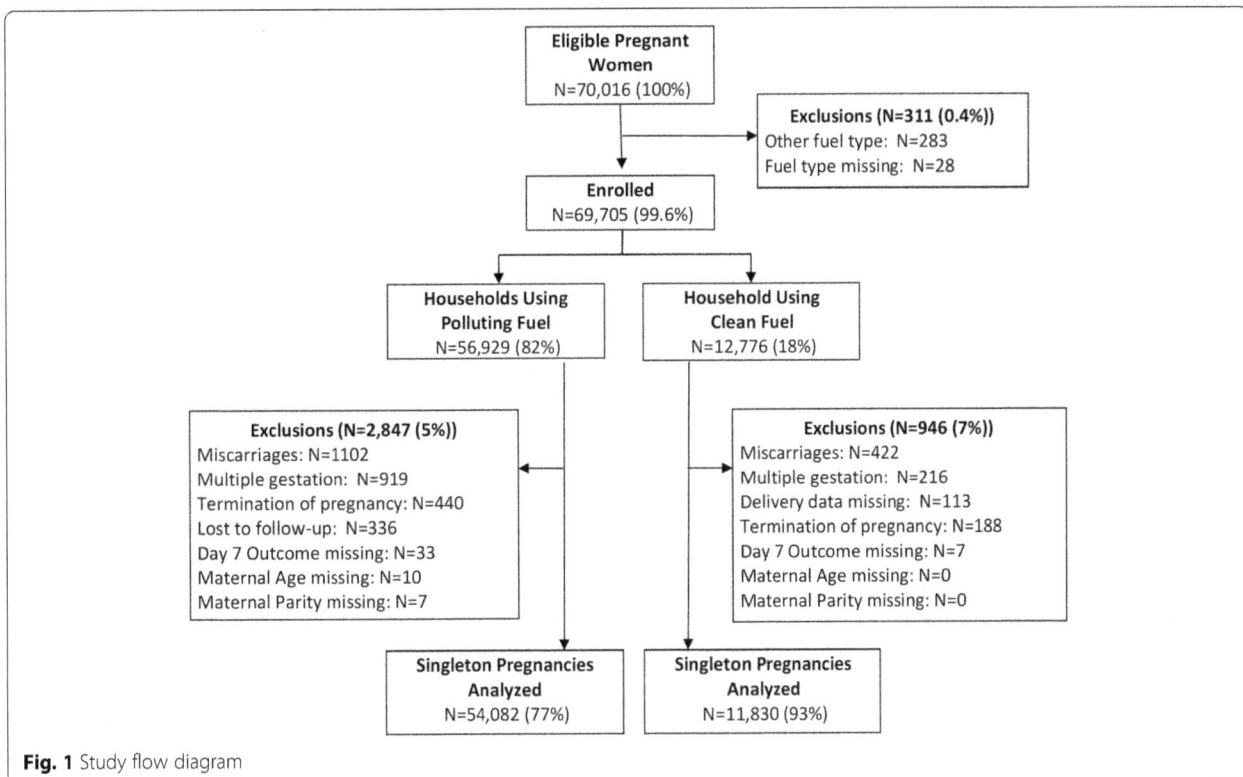

Fig. 1 Study flow diagram

estimated delivery date, age, education, parity, and status of last child is collected. Within 7 days of delivery, information is collected on prenatal care, birth preparedness, complications occurring during pregnancy, details of labor and delivery, including place, mode of delivery, provider, actual birth weight obtained at the time of birth, status of the mother and newborn following delivery, referrals, and treatment provided to the mother and newborn at referral facilities. Interval maternal and newborn health and status is assessed 42 days after birth. Birth weight is recorded for all babies (live born and still births) using locally available scales, calibrated per the local facilities. All study area birth attendants are trained to use and record accurate birth weights as described previously [16].

In May 2011, questions adapted from the Demographic Health Survey's (DHS) Household questionnaire, version 6 [17] on the type of fuel, location used for cooking and tobacco smoking in the household were added to the MNH Registry Questionnaire during the day 42 post-partum visit.

Study variables

Exposures

Households using only electricity, liquefied petroleum gas, natural gas and biogas for cooking in their primary and secondary home (if they moved to a second location during pregnancy) were classified as homes using clean fuels. Households using all other fuels for cooking (kerosene, charcoal, coal, wood, straw, crop waste and dung) were classified as homes using polluting fuels. The location of cooking in the house was classified as in the house (separate kitchen or no separate kitchen), in a separate building or outside.

Outcomes

Primary Perinatal mortality – fetal loss after week 20 of pregnancy through day 7 of life (macerated stillbirths + non-macerated stillbirths + early neonatal mortality (NMR_0-7))/all pregnancies.

Secondary

(i) Macerated stillbirths/all pregnancies
(ii) Non-macerated stillbirths/all pregnancies
(iii) Very early neonatal mortality (NMR_0-2) through day 2 of life/all live births
(iv) Later neonatal mortality (NMR_3-28) from day 3–28 of life/all live births

A stillbirth was defined as birth of a baby after week 20 of gestation that had no signs of life at birth (no gasping, breathing, heart beat or movement). Stillbirths were further classified as macerated (death presumed before onset of labor, based on presence of discoloration and peeling of the skin leaving areas of raw tissue, an unusually soft skull, a dark red or black stained umbilical cord or darkly stained amniotic fluid) vs. non-macerated stillbirth (presumed intrapartum death and no signs of maceration).

Covariates

We collected data on the following covariates: maternal age (<20, ≥20); education (no formal education, any formal education); parity (0, 1–2, ≥ 3); gestational age (preterm (<37 weeks) or term (≥37 weeks) as assessed by last menstrual period, clinical examination, ultrasound, or other method); delivery location (hospital, clinic, home or other location); birth weight using available local scales; infant gender; and household tobacco use (anyone in the household smoking inside the house at least daily, less than daily smoking or no smokers in the household).

Data source

All study data were obtained by trained interviewers who recorded the response on case report forms. The interviewers were unaware of the study hypotheses.

Statistical considerations

Sample size The sample size calculations were based on the assumption that exposure to HAP would increase the risk of perinatal mortality by approximately 1.23 based on the lower 95 % confidence interval of a previously reported odds ratios from a meta-analysis for stillbirths (there are no previously published data for perinatal mortality) and HAP of 1.5 (95 % CI 1.23, 1.85) [18]. Sample size was calculated conservatively and based on the lower level of the reported 95 % CI, although kerosene was classified as a clean fuel in the meta-analysis, so this estimate is conservative. Based on the MNH Registry data for 2010 [16], we assumed a baseline perinatal mortality rate of 32/1000 in the unexposed group. To detect an OR 1.23 (PMR of 37/1000 or greater in the exposed group), significant at alpha = 0.05 (2 sided), with 80 % power, we estimated that we would need to collect outcome data on 61,530 singleton births.

Methods We first estimated population averaged effects of HAP on perinatal mortality using generalized estimating equations (GEE) to control for correlations within clusters. We fitted a modified Poisson regression model with a sandwich error estimation. All relative risks were adjusted for site due to the variability across the sites in the Global Network. Bivariate associations between covariates such as mother's age, mother's education, parity, ante-natal care, birth attendants at the delivery and mortality were evaluated by fitting a regression model that controlled for site and had mortality as the outcome and the covariate of interest as the predictor. We elected not to include low birth weight in the model as a covariate because it may be an intermediate step in the causal pathway between exposure to HAP and perinatal mortality [19–21]. All covariates with significant RRs were included in a final model that had PMR as the outcome and HAP as a predictor.

Since exposure to HAP would have differential effects on the fetus during pregnancy through the first month of life, particularly on macerated stillbirths, non-macerated stillbirths, very neonatal mortality through day 2 of life (NMR_0-2) and later neonatal mortality from day 3–28 of life (NMR_3-28), we also modeled the data using multinomial logistic regression with a 5 level nominal outcome (macerated stillbirth, non-macerated stillbirth, NMR_0-2, NMR_3-28, alive after day 28). The model included exposure to HAP as the predictor and controlled for the same covariates as above. Low birth weight was excluded as explained above. We used the clustered bootstrap method [22] to estimate the variance of the estimates and create 95 % confidence intervals.

Results

Between May 2011 and Oct 2012, we studied 65,912 pregnant women (Fig. 1). Mortality outcomes were available for 65,701 births (99.7 %). There were 1,740 stillbirths (577 macerated and 1,163 non-macerated stillbirths) and 63,961 live births, of which 950 died on or before the second day of life, 275 died between the 3rd and 7th day of life, and 295 died between the 8th and 28th day of life. The distribution of the pregnancy outcomes by geographic location is shown in Fig. 2. Table 1 shows the demographic characteristics of the pregnant women, births and the households including details of the fuels used for cooking. A total of 54,082 (82 %) pregnancies occurred in households using polluting fuel and 11,830 (18 %) in households using clean fuels. The distribution of pregnancies by types of fuel use and geographic location is shown in Fig. 3. LPG was the predominant type of clean fuel (59 %) followed by natural gas (33 %) and wood was the predominant type of polluting fuel (86 %).

The overall perinatal mortality rate was 48/1,000 pregnancies > 20 weeks gestation, ranging from 25/1,000 pregnancies in Guatemala to 90/1,000 pregnancies in Pakistan. Table 2 shows the adjusted and unadjusted relative risks (RR) for exposure to HAP and covariates that were estimated using GEE in a Poisson regression model. The adjusted relative risk for perinatal mortality among babies whose mothers were exposed to HAP vs. clean fuels during pregnancy was 1.44 (95 % CI 1.30, 1.61). Risk factors for perinatal mortality in the multivariate analysis, also adjusted for Global Network site, included cooking with polluting fuel, lack of maternal education (no formal schooling), nulliparity and 3 or

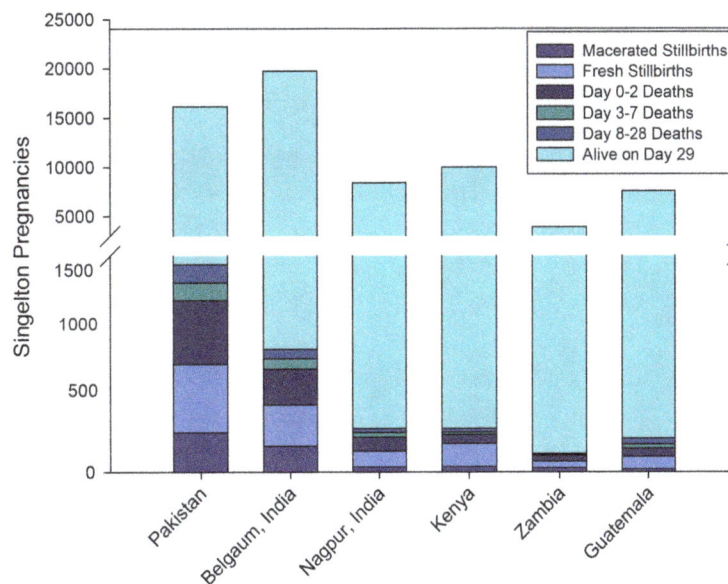

Fig. 2 Pregnancy outcomes by global network site

more prior births, no antenatal care, and male gender. Delivery by nurse or midwife or delivery unattended by a trained birth attendant was associated with lower perinatal mortality compared with delivery by a physician. Presence of anyone in the household who smoked on a daily basis was not associated with perinatal mortality.

Table 3 has the adjusted odds ratios (aOR) estimated using a multinomial logistic regression model. It shows the risk factors for the multi-level mortality variable (macerated and non-macerated stillbirths, very early neonatal deaths on days 0–2 (NMR_0-2) and later neonatal deaths days 3–28 (NMR_3-28) vs. alive on day 29). The aOR for having a macerated stillbirth in mothers exposed to HAP during pregnancy versus not exposed to HAP was 1.66 (95 % CI 1.23, 2.25). The corresponding aOR for having a non-macerated stillbirth was 1.43 (95 % CI 1.15, 1.85), very early neonatal mortality (NMR_0-2) was 1.82 (95 % CI 1.47, 2.22) and later neonatal mortality (NMR_3-28) was 1.28 (95 % CI 0.91, 1.76). Risk factors for having a macerated or non-macerated stillbirth or very early neonatal mortality (NMR_0-2), also adjusted for Global Network site, included cooking with polluting fuel, nulliparity and 3 or more prior births. Delivery by nurse or midwife was associated with lower perinatal mortality compared with delivery by a physician. Lack of formal schooling was associated with having both a macerated and non-macerated stillbirth and surprisingly, lack of antenatal care was only associated with having a non-macerated stillbirth. Male gender was associated with very early neonatal mortality (NMR_0-2) and later neonatal mortality (NMR_3-28), and nulliparity was also associated

with later neonatal mortality. Presence of anyone in the household who smoked on a daily basis was not associated with having a still birth or neonatal death and was not included in the multivariate model.

Discussion

This study shows that in rural populations in five low resource countries, household use of polluting fuels for cooking increases the overall risk of perinatal mortality, after adjusting for maternal education, parity, antenatal visits, delivery location and attendant, and male gender. The important new finding of this research is that when the perinatal period of risk is divided into pre-partum (risk of having a macerated stillbirth), intrapartum (risk of having a non-macerated stillbirth) and postpartum (risk of neonatal death on day 0–2, 3–28 of life), exposure to HAP is associated with both types of stillbirths and early neonatal death through day 2 of life, not later neonatal death. These time periods were chosen for the secondary exploratory analyses (rather than early (day 0–7) and late (day 8–28) neonatal deaths) because there are few deaths after day 2 of life and we wanted to focus on the high mortality period between day 0 and 2 of life. Recognition of the risk of having a macerated fetus after week 20 of gestation is also important, as this outcome is not always recorded and may lead to an underestimate of the impact of exposure to HAP on adverse pregnancy outcomes.

Daily smoking in the household was not an independent predictor of perinatal mortality. It is possible that daily smoking was not an independent predictor of adverse pregnancy and neonatal outcome in our study

Table 1 Demographic characteristics of the study subjects and households

Characteristic	Pakistan	Belgaum, India	Nagpur, India	Kenya	Zambia	Guatemala	Total
Maternal age	16,235	19,728	8,443	9,973	3,876	7,554	65,809
<20	626 (3.9)	1,835 (9.3)	168 (2.0)	2,183 (21.9)	984 (25.4)	1,276 (16.9)	7,072 (10.7)
≥20	15,609 (96.1)	17,893 (90.7)	8,275 (98.0)	7,790 (78.1)	2,892 (74.6)	6,278 (83.1)	58,737 (89.3)
Maternal education	16,239	19,611	8,439	9,974	3,847	7,555	65,665
No formal schooling	13,595 (83.7)	4,464 (22.8)	216 (2.6)	295 (3.0)	422 (11.0)	1,610 (21.3)	20,602 (31.4)
Primary	1,163 (7.2)	5,998 (30.6)	1,414 (16.8)	7,100 (71.2)	2,084 (54.2)	4,769 (63.1)	22,528 (34.3)
Secondary	900 (5.5)	7,278 (37.1)	5,068 (60.1)	2,216 (22.2)	1,275 (33.1)	1,126 (14.9)	17,863 (27.2)
University+	581 (3.6)	1,871 (9.5)	1,741 (20.6)	363 (3.6)	66 (1.7)	50 (0.7)	4,672 (7.1)
Parity	16,238	19,384	8,446	9,976	3,876	7,554	65,474
0	3,412 (21.0)	8,321 (42.9)	4,119 (48.8)	2,498 (25.0)	1,036 (26.7)	2,056 (27.2)	21,442 (32.7)
1-2	5,325 (32.8)	9,746 (50.3)	4,110 (48.7)	4,000 (40.1)	1,455 (37.5)	2,664 (35.3)	27,300 (41.7)
≥3	7,501 (46.2)	1,317 (6.8)	217 (2.6)	3,478 (34.9)	1,385 (35.7)	2,834 (37.5)	16,732 (25.6)
Antenatal care	16,121	19,696	8,426	9,981	3,874	7,529	65,627
Any	14,385 (89.2)	19,689 (100.0)	8,425 (100.0)	9,794 (98.1)	3,856 (99.5)	7,349 (97.6)	63,498 (96.8)
None	1,736 (10.8)	7 (0.0)	1 (0.0)	187 (1.9)	18 (0.5)	180 (2.4)	2,129 (3.2)
Number of antenatal visits	13,557	16,004	8,420	9,794	787	7,349	55,911
1	2,889 (21.3)	954 (6.0)	108 (1.3)	468 (4.8)	124 (15.8)	365 (5.0)	4,908 (8.8)
2	4,617 (34.1)	1,268 (7.9)	84 (1.0)	1,674 (17.1)	148 (18.8)	735 (10.0)	8,526 (15.2)
3	3,359 (24.8)	4,436 (27.7)	502 (6.0)	3,649 (37.3)	269 (34.2)	1,386 (18.9)	13,601 (24.3)
≥4	2,692 (19.9)	9,346 (58.4)	7,726 (91.8)	4,003 (40.9)	246 (31.3)	4,863 (66.2)	28,876 (51.6)
Delivery attendant	16,266	19,755	8,444	9,991	3,881	7,555	65,892
Physician	4,066 (25.0)	11,761 (59.5)	4,963 (58.8)	200 (2.0)	83 (2.1)	2,785 (36.9)	23,858 (36.2)
Nurse/Midwife	4,312 (26.5)	7,055 (35.7)	3,249 (38.5)	3,944 (39.5)	2,067 (53.3)	197 (2.6)	20,824 (31.6)
No skilled birth attendant	7,888 (48.5)	939 (4.8)	232 (2.7)	5,847 (58.5)	1,731 (44.6)	4,573 (60.5)	21,210 (32.2)
Delivery location	16,275	19,755	8,445	9,989	3,881	7,555	65,900
Facility	8,624 (53.0)	18,673 (94.5)	8,186 (96.9)	4,012 (40.2)	2,340 (60.3)	2,960 (39.2)	44,795 (68.0)
Home/Other	7,651 (47.0)	1,082 (5.5)	259 (3.1)	5,977 (59.8)	1,541 (39.7)	4,595 (60.8)	21,105 (32.0)
Infant gender	16,135	19,722	8,390	9,983	3,873	7,551	65,654
Male	8,472 (52.5)	10,335 (52.4)	4,353 (51.9)	5,069 (50.8)	2,038 (52.6)	3,816 (50.5)	34,083 (51.9)
Female	7,663 (47.5)	9,387 (47.6)	4,037 (48.1)	4,914 (49.2)	1,835 (47.4)	3,735 (49.5)	31,571 (48.1)
Fuel used for cooking	16,276	19,755	8,450	9,995	3,881	7,555	65,912
Electricity	50 (0.3)	69 (0.3)	83 (1.0)	6 (0.1)	434 (11.2)	3 (0.0)	645 (1.0)
Liquified petroleum gas	51 (0.3)	3,503 (17.7)	2,837 (33.6)	15 (0.2)	0 (0.0)	576 (7.6)	6,982 (10.6)
Natural gas	3,861 (23.7)	3 (0.0)	16 (0.2)	29 (0.3)	2 (0.1)	27 (0.4)	3,938 (6.0)
Biogas	11 (0.1)	95 (0.5)	123 (1.5)	23 (0.2)	0 (0.0)	5 (0.1)	257 (0.4)
Kerosene	61 (0.4)	198 (1.0)	370 (4.4)	132 (1.3)	6 (0.2)	16 (0.2)	783 (1.2)
Coal	13 (0.1)	3 (0.0)	61 (0.7)	4 (0.0)	0 (0.0)	3 (0.0)	84 (0.1)
Charcoal	3 (0.0)	2 (0.0)	15 (0.2)	733 (7.3)	1,306 (33.7)	0 (0.0)	2,059 (3.1)
Wood	11,968 (73.5)	11,735 (59.4)	4,589 (54.3)	9,033 (90.4)	2,120 (54.6)	6,925 (91.7)	46,370 (70.4)
Straw, etc.	84 (0.5)	369 (1.9)	98 (1.2)	18 (0.2)	1 (0.0)	0 (0.0)	570 (0.9)
Agricultural crop	19 (0.1)	2,398 (12.1)	179 (2.1)	2 (0.0)	0 (0.0)	0 (0.0)	2,598 (3.9)
Animal dung	154 (0.9)	1,380 (7.0)	78 (0.9)	0 (0.0)	0 (0.0)	0 (0.0)	1,612 (2.4)
No food cooked in household/other	1 (0.0)	0 (0.0)	1 (0.0)	0 (0.0)	12 (0.3)	0 (0.0)	14 (0.0)

Table 1 Demographic characteristics of the study subjects and households *(Continued)*

Smoking in primary household	16,272	19,667	8,439	9,993	3,858	7,555	65,784
Daily	5,967 (36.7)	3,446 (17.5)	2,297 (27.2)	905 (9.1)	1,065 (27.6)	123 (1.6)	13,803 (21.0)
Less than daily	259 (1.6)	982 (5.0)	1,681 (19.9)	1,537 (15.4)	232 (6.0)	370 (4.9)	5,061 (7.7)
No smoking	10,046 (61.7)	15,239 (77.5)	4,461 (52.9)	7,551 (75.6)	2,561 (66.4)	7,062 (93.5)	46,920 (71.3)
Cooking location for primary household	16,272	19,666	8,430	9,992	3,858	7,555	65,773
In the house	4,010 (24.6)	19,280 (98.0)	7,768 (92.1)	2,693 (27.0)	860 (22.3)	956 (12.7)	35,567 (54.1)
In a separate building	9,149 (56.2)	284 (1.4)	559 (6.6)	6,930 (69.4)	2,462 (63.8)	3,424 (45.3)	22,808 (34.7)
Outdoors	3,110 (19.1)	100 (0.5)	102 (1.2)	367 (3.7)	519 (13.5)	3,172 (42.0)	7,370 (11.2)
Other	3 (0.0)	2 (0.0)	1 (0.0)	2 (0.0)	17 (0.4)	3 (0.0)	28 (0.0)

because the exposure for most pregnant women in the rural communities studied was likely second hand smoke and exposure of the fetus and young infant to pollutants from second hand smoke would be much lower than the exposure to pollutants from household use of polluting fuel, although both second hand smoke and exposure to HAP has been associated with poor pregnancy outcomes in a prior Global Network study [23]. These different results may have been due to the specific DHS questions that were asked in this study, while the prior Global Network study asked questions adapted from the Global Youth Tobacco Survey, the 2000 US National Health Interview Survey and the Smoke-free Families Screening form. The DHS questions did not include maternal use of smokeless tobacco, which could be a risk factor for stillbirths or other adverse pregnancy outcomes. This is a limitation of our study. In future studies, it will be important to measure urine cotinine to assess actual exposure to tobacco smoke and smokeless tobacco.

Our data on the other independent risk factors for fetal or neonatal death are similar to those reported by others including no formal schooling, nulliparity and 3 or more prior births and no antenatal care visits [24, 25]. Male gender is well recognized as a risk factor particularly for neonatal mortality, [26] associated with the biological survival advantage of girls in the neonatal period. Physician assisted deliveries of women from rural communities is often due to referral of women with high risk conditions to a higher level of care. So the reduced risk of perinatal mortality associated with non-physician delivery attendants may be due to more complicated deliveries being done by physicians.

A major limitation of studies included in Pope et al's meta-analysis [18] is the lack of a clear definition of stillbirth. A strength of this study is the accurate and complete recording of stillbirths (macerated and non-macerated) and timing of neonatal mortality by trained health care workers. However, our study has several limitations. Firstly, almost all published studies examining

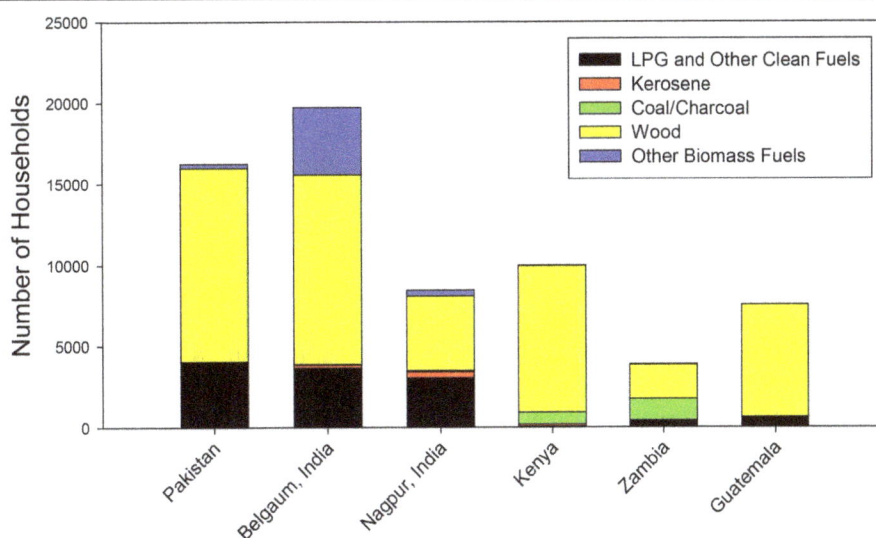

Fig. 3 Fuel use by global network site

Table 2 Risk factors for perinatal mortality

Characteristic	Perinatal mortality (through day 7 of life) N = 3,176 n (%)	Alive on day 8 of life N = 62,736 n (%)	Relative risk adjusted for global network site and community (95 % confidence interval)	Multivariate analysis - adjusted relative risk (95 % confidence interval)
HAP exposure	3,176	62,736		
Polluting fuel	2,683 (84)	51,399 (82)	1.36 (1.25, 1.49)	1.44 (1.30, 1.61)
Clean fuel	493 (16)	11,337 (18)	1.00	1.00
Maternal age	3,172	62,637		
<20	294 (9)	6,778 (11)	1.14 (1.01, 1.29)	1.03 (0.90, 1.18)
≥20	2,878 (91)	55,859 (89)	1.00	1.00
Maternal education	3,168	62,497		
No formal schooling	1,589 (50)	19,013 (30)	1.27 (1.12, 1.45)	1.32 (1.15, 1.52)
Formal schooling	1,579 (50)	43,484 (70)	1.00	1.00
Parity	3,154	62,320		
0	1,079 (34)	20,363 (33)	1.36 (1.25, 1.47)	1.33 (1.21, 1.45)
1-2	1,053 (33)	26,247 (42)	1.00	1.00
≥3	1,022 (32)	15,710 (25)	1.27 (1.16, 1.39)	1.26 (1.13, 1.40)
Antenatal care	3,147	62,480		
Any	2,906 (92)	60,592 (97)	1.00	1.00
None	241 (8)	1,888 (3)	1.49 (1.28, 1.73)	1.35 (1.15, 1.58)
Delivery attendant	3,166	62,726		
Physician	1,236 (39.0)	22,622 (36.1)	1.00	1.00
Nurse/Midwife	861 (27.2)	19,963 (31.8)	0.72 (0.62, 0.83)	0.66 (0.57, 0.77)
No skilled birth attendant	1,069 (33.8)	20,141 (32.1)	0.79 (0.67, 0.95)	0.58 (0.41, 0.80)
Delivery location	3,176	62,724		
Facility	2,108 (66)	42,687 (68)	1.00	1.00
Home/Other	1,068 (34)	20,037 (32)	0.96 (0.83, 1.12)	1.05 (0.77, 1.44)
Infant gender	2,934	62,720		
Male	1,677 (57)	32,406 (52)	1.22 (1.13, 1.32)	1.21 (1.11, 1.31)
Female	1,257 (43)	30,314 (48)	1.00	1.00
Daily smoking in household	3,175	62,721		
Yes	888 (28)	14,547 (23)	1.02 (0.92, 1.13)	
No	2,287 (72)	48,174 (77)	1.00	

the effect of HAP on perinatal mortality [24, 27–31], including ours, have used the type of fuel used for cooking as a proxy for exposure to HAP. We focused on fuels used for cooking, as fuels are rarely used for heating in our Global Network sites, and did not adjust for whether cooking occurred inside or outside the household because where the cooking occurred was confounded by Global Network site. There is also some variation with the way household air pollution is categorized in prior studies, although most compare the relatively homogeneous group of clean fuels with the heterogeneous group of polluting fuels, as we did. Risk of perinatal mortality likely varies by fuel type, in part because pollutants vary by fuel type e.g., kerosene smoke pollutants are quite

different from wood smoke pollutants [24]. Unfortunately, we could not analyze data on kerosene separately because only 1 % of our households used kerosene. We would have also preferred to analyse data on wood smoke and coal/charcoal as additional separate categories, but use of wood as a cooking fuel was confounded with global network location and only 3 % of households used coal/charcoal as a cooking fuel. In future studies, it will be important to measure particulate matter and other pollutants associated with biomass fuels. Secondly, we were only able to control for variables collected for the MNH Registry and specifically, we were not able to adequately control for socioeconomic status, which can be associated with pregnancy outcomes. Biomass fuels,

Table 3 Risk factors for the multilevel mortality variable

Characteristic	Multivariate analysis - adjusted odds ratios (95 % Confidence Interval)				
	Macerated stillbirths	Non-Macerated stillbirths	Early neonatal mortality day 0–2 of life (NMR_0-2)	Later neonatal mortality day 3–28 of life (NMR_3-28)	Alive on day 29 (Reference Group)
HAP exposure					
Polluting fuel	1.66 (1.23, 2.25)	1.43 (1.15, 1.85)	1.82 (1.47, 2.22)	1.28 (0.91, 1.76)	1.00
Clean fuel	1.00	1.00	1.00	1.00	1.00
Maternal age					
<20	0.83 (0.55, 1.13)	1.01 (0.81, 1.24)	1.21 (0.97, 1.48)	1.05 (0.78, 1.42)	1.00
≥20	1.00	1.00	1.00	1.00	1.00
Maternal education					
No formal schooling	1.71 (1.32, 2.22)	1.51 (1.26, 1.81)	1.14 (0.90, 1.44)	1.19 (0.95, 1.47)	1.00
Formal schooling	1.00	1.00	1.00	1.00	1.00
Parity					
0	1.27 (1.03, 1.59)	1.34 (1.13, 1.56)	1.24 (1.05, 1.47)	1.43 (1.17, 1.73)	1.00
1-2	1.00	1.00	1.00	1.00	1.00
≥3	1.30 (1.01, 1.68)	1.39 (1.19, 1.65)	1.22 (1.04, 1.43)	1.11 (0.86, 1.41)	1.00
Antenatal care					
Any	1.00	1.00	1.00	1.00	1.00
None	1.41 (0.99, 2.12)	1.62 (1.23, 2.13)	0.90 (0.68, 1.21)	1.32 (0.85, 1.81)	1.00
Delivery attendant					
Physician	1.00	1.00	1.00	1.00	1.00
Nurse/Midwife	0.69 (0.52, 0.87)	0.65 (0.51, 0.82)	0.68 (0.54, 0.85)	0.87 (0.70, 1.08)	1.00
No skilled birth attendant	0.58 (0.25, 1.03)	0.50 (0.30, 0.80)	0.67 (0.39, 1.00)	0.91 (0.49, 1.67)	1.00
Delivery location					
Facility	1.00	1.00	1.00	1.00	1.00
Home/Other	0.94 (0.49, 2.30)	1.06 (0.70, 1.68)	1.00 (0.72, 1.71)	0.86 (0.48, 1.48)	1.00
Infant gender					
Male	1.08 (0.91, 1.30)	1.13 (0.99, 1.29)	1.39 (1.19, 1.60)	1.18 (1.00, 1.40)	1.00
Female	1.00	1.00	1.00	1.00	1.00

especially fire wood collected from the forests, are used in impoverished rural homes because it is readily available and cheap [32]. The measure of socioeconomic status for this study was level of education and antenatal visits, while we did control for these proxy variables, residual confounding is possible. Although the Global Network has attempted to obtain details of maternal health before and during pregnancy (e.g., pre-pregnancy body mass index), there are limitations to the validity of these data and we are unable to address the impact of maternal conditions and BMI on pregnancy outcomes. Similarly, we do not have valid information on the neonate's nutritional status and cannot address the effect of this confounder on perinatal mortality. Finally, we recognize that since information on exposure to cooking fuels and smoking and confounding variables were collected on day 42 postpartum, there is a potential for recall bias, which is an additional limitation.

The association between polluting fuel and perinatal mortality mediated by LBW is biologically plausible based on studies of the effects of tobacco smoking, outdoor air pollution and animal studies, but the precise mechanisms by which the varying types of HAP cause perinatal mortality and LBW is not clear. We examined the possibility of LBW being a mediator on the causal pathway between HAP and mortality using mediation analysis as follows. We assumed a causal pathway between HAP and PMR and tested to determine whether LBW contributes to the increased PMR in HAP households. In order to do this, we regressed HAP on LBW controlling for site (RR = 1.17 (1.10, 1.24), $p < 0.0001$); we then regressed HAP on PMR while controlling for LBW. The RR for HAP in the model that controls for LBW was attenuated by about 9 % (1.34 to 1.22). If LBW were the only variable on the causal pathway, then introducing LBW into the model with HAP and PMR would explain all of the variability in PMR, LBW would be a significant predictor and HAP would become non-significant in the model. Since the RR is attenuated but still significant, it suggests that some of the increased PMR in HAP households is due to LBW associated with HAP. The mediation effect of LBW on the causal pathway was further tested with Sobel's test. The value of Sobel's z- statistic was 5.08, $p < 0.0001$ confirming that LBW was a mediator in the causal pathway between HAP and PMR. Although the statistical analysis suggests that LBW is probably a mediator on the causal pathway, we do not have any data collected in this study to confirm or deny this. Similarly, preterm, birth defects, and maternal and neonatal complications might be on the causal pathway between exposure to HAP and mortality, or could be confounders. The statistical modelling technique to determine whether a variable is a confounder or a mediator is the same. Since we did not have any data to confirm whether it was one or the other, we decided that it would be better to exclude these variables from the model. Future research should focus on collecting data that will help to clarify these relationships.

Polyaromatic hydrocarbons (PAH) can cross the placenta and reach fetal organs [33–43]. These compounds may interfere with placental development and nutrient and oxygen delivery to the fetus [44, 45]. DNA-adduct levels of PAH in cord blood leukocytes have been linked with decreased birth weight, length, and head circumferences [46, 47]. PAH, metals, and related compounds can induce the production of cytotoxic reactive oxygen species and, ultimately, inflammatory and oxidant stress responses [48, 49]. Ultrafine particles are potent inducers of cellular heme oxygenase-1 expression and deplete intracellular glutathione, both also important in oxidant stress responses [50]. Stress responses and proinflammatory cytokines may also trigger preterm birth [51, 52], although at the maternal fetal interface, not systemically [53]. Carbon monoxide from combustion of any biomass and fossil fuels have been linked with intrauterine growth restriction, possibly as a result of carboxyhemoglobin limiting oxygen delivery to fetal tissue [54]. Early and late neonatal mortality may be caused by neonatal pneumonia.

Conclusions

In September 2010, the United Nations Foundation announced the Global Alliance for Clean Cook Stoves, a new public-private partnership to save lives, empower women, improve livelihoods, and combat climate change by creating a thriving global market for clean and efficient household cooking solutions. The Alliance's '100 by 20' goal calls for 100 million homes to adopt clean, efficient stoves and fuels by 2020. Already there is great urgency to implement improved stoves and fuels and so

there is imminent need to evaluate whether these new stoves actually do save lives [12]. Our study documents that in rural locations in five low and low-middle income countries where use of polluting fuel is widespread, large numbers of pregnant women will need to be studied to determine whether improved cook-stoves and fuels that reduce exposure to HAP also reduces perinatal mortality, LBW and neonatal mortality.

Abbreviations
aOR: Adjusted odds ratio; aRR: Adjusted relative risk; CI: Confidence interval; DHS: Demographic Health Survey; GN: Global Network; HAP: Household air pollution; LBW: Low birth weight; MDG4: Millennium Development Goal #4; MNH: Maternal Newborn Health; NICHD: Eunice Kennedy Shriver National Institute of Child Health and Human Development; NMR_0-2: Very early neonatal mortality day 0–2; NMR_0-7: Early neonatal mortality day 0–7; NMR_3-28: Later neonatal mortality day 3–28; OR: Odds ratio; PAH: Polyaromatic hydrocarbons; PMR: Perinatal mortality rate – deaths from week 20 of gestation through day 7 of life; RR: Relative risk.

Competing interests
The authors declare that they have no competing interests.

Authors' contributions
ABP, SM, LLW, MKT, EMM and PLH developed the protocol with input from OP, SSG, FE, ALG, EC, SS, RLG, RJD, KMH, WAC. ABP, OP, SSG, FE, ALG, EC, and SS oversaw the implementation. ABP and PLH wrote the first draft of the manuscript, with input from SM. SM and JLM conducted the statistical analyses. All authors read and approved the final manuscript.

Author details
[1]Lata Medical Research Foundation, Nagpur, Maharashtra 440022, India. [2]RTI International, Research Triangle Park, North Carolina 27709, USA. [3]Department of Community Health Sciences & Family Medicine, Aga Khan University, Karachi, Pakistan. [4]KLE University's JN Medical College, Belgaum, Karnataka, India. [5]Moi University School of Medicine, Eldoret, Kenya. [6]IMSALUD, San Carlos University, Guatemala City, Guatemala. [7]University Teaching Hospital, Lusaka, Zambia. [8]Center for Research of Mothers and Children, NIH, Rockville, MD 20852, USA. [9]Department of Pediatrics, Indiana University School of Medicine, Indianapolis, IN 46202, USA. [10]Department of Obstetrics/Gynecology, Columbia University, New York, NY 10032, USA. [11]Department of OB-GYN, Christiana Care, Newark, DE 19718, USA. [12]Department of Pediatrics, University of Colorado, Aurora, CO 80045, USA. [13]Department of Pediatrics, University of Alabama at Birmingham, Birmingham, AL 35233, USA. [14]Division of Global Health, Department of Pediatrics, Massachusetts General Hospital, Boston, MA 02114, USA.

References
1. Rajaratnam JK, Marcus JR, Flaxman AD, Wang H, Levin-Rector A, et al. Neonatal, postneonatal, childhood, and under-5 mortality for 187 countries, 1970–2010: a systematic analysis of progress towards Millennium Development Goal 4. Lancet. 2010;375:1988–2008. doi:10.1016/S0140-6736(10)60703-9.
2. Lozano R, Wang H, Foreman KJ, Rajaratnam JK, Naghavi M, et al. Progress towards millennium development goals 4 and 5 on maternal and child mortality: an updated systematic analysis. Lancet. 2011;378:1139–65. doi:10.1016/S0140-6736(11)61337-8.
3. Lawn JE, Lee AC, Kinney M, Sibley L, Carlo WA, et al. Two million intrapartum-related stillbirths and neonatal deaths: where, why, and what can be done? Int J Gynaecol Obstet. 2009;107 Suppl 1: S5-18, S19. doi:10.1016/j.ijgo.2009.07.016.
4. Liu L, Oza S, Hogan D, Perin J, Rudan I, et al. Global, regional, and national causes of child mortality in 2000–13, with projections to inform post-2015 priorities: an updated systematic analysis. Lancet. 2014. doi:10.1016/S0140-6736(14)61698-6.

5. Goldenberg RL, McClure EM, Kodkany B, Wembodinga G, Pasha O, et al. A multi-country study of the "intrapartum stillbirth and early neonatal death indicator" in hospitals in low-resource settings. Int J Gynaecol Obstet. 2013;122:230–3. doi:10.1016/j.ijgo.2013.04.008.

6. Bang A, Bellad R, Gisore P, Hibberd P, Patel A, et al. Implementation and evaluation of the helping babies breathe curriculum in three resource limited settings: does helping babies breathe save lives? a study protocol. BMC Pregnancy Childbirth. 2014;14:116–1471. doi:10.1186/1471-2393-14-116.

7. Gordon SB, Bruce NG, Grigg J, Hibberd PL, Kurmi OP, et al. Respiratory risks from household air pollution in low and middle income countries. Lancet Respir Med. 2014;2:823–60. doi:10.1016/S2213-2600(14)70168-7.

8. World Health Organization. Indoor Air Pollution and Health; 2011. www.who.int/mediacentre/factsheets/fs292/en.

9. Lim SS, Vos T, Flaxman AD, Danaei G, Shibuya K, et al. A comparative risk assessment of burden of disease and injury attributable to 67 risk factors and risk factor clusters in 21 regions, 1990–2010: a systematic analysis for the Global Burden of Disease Study 2010. Lancet. 2012;380:2224–60. doi:10.1016/S0140-6736(12)61766-8.

10. Bruce NG, Dherani MK, Das JK, Balakrishnan K, Adair-Rohani H, et al. Control of household air pollution for child survival: estimates for intervention impacts. BMC Public Health. 2013;13 Suppl 3:S8. doi:10.1186/1471-2458-13-S3-S8.

11. Wylie BJ, Coull BA, Hamer DH, Singh MP, Jack D, et al. Impact of biomass fuels on pregnancy outcomes in central East India. Environ Health. 2014;13:1. doi:10.1186/1476-069X-13-1.

12. Martin WJ, Glass RI, Araj H, Balbus J, Collins FS, et al. Household air pollution in low- and middle-income countries: health risks and research priorities. PLoS Med. 2013;10:e1001455. doi:10.1371/journal.pmed.1001455.

13. Juarez SP, Merlo J. Revisiting the effect of maternal smoking during pregnancy on offspring birthweight: a quasi-experimental sibling analysis in Sweden. PLoS One. 2013;8:e61734. doi:10.1371/journal.pone.0061734.

14. Cnattingius S, Nordstrom ML. Maternal smoking and feto-infant mortality: biological pathways and public health significance. Acta Paediatr. 1996;85:1400–2.

15. Pineles BL, Park E, Samet JM. Systematic review and meta-analysis of miscarriage and maternal exposure to tobacco smoke during pregnancy. Am J Epidemiol. 2014;179:807–23. doi:10.1093/aje/kwt334.

16. Goudar SS, Carlo WA, McClure EM, Pasha O, Patel A, et al. The maternal and newborn health registry study of the global network for Women's and Children's health research. Int J Gynaecol Obstet. 2012;118:190–3. doi:10.1016/j.ijgo.2012.04.022.

17. USAID. DHS Program; 2014. http://www.dhsprogram.com.

18. Pope DP, Mishra V, Thompson L, Siddiqui AR, Rehfuess EA, et al. Risk of low birth weight and stillbirth associated with indoor air pollution from solid fuel use in developing countries. Epidemiol Rev. 2010;32:70–81. doi:10.1093/epirev/mxq005.

19. VanderWeele TJ, Mumford SL, Schisterman EF. Conditioning on intermediates in perinatal epidemiology. Epidemiology. 2012;23:1–9. doi:10.1097/EDE.0b013e31823aca5d.

20. Wilcox AJ, Weinberg CR, Basso O. On the pitfalls of adjusting for gestational age at birth. Am J Epidemiol. 2011;174:1062–8. doi:10.1093/aje/kwr230.

21. Hernandez-Diaz S, Schisterman EF, Hernan MA. The birth weight "paradox" uncovered? Am J Epidemiol. 2006;164:1115–20. doi:10.1093/aje/kwj275.

22. De RM, Worku HM. A warning concerning the estimation of multinomial logistic models with correlated responses in SAS. Comput Methods Programs Biomed. 2012;107:341–6.

23. Kadir MM, McClure EM, Goudar SS, Garces AL, Moore J, et al. Exposure of pregnant women to indoor air pollution: a study from nine low and middle income countries. Acta Obstet Gynecol Scand. 2010;89:540–8. doi:10.3109/00016340903473566.

24. Epstein MB, Bates MN, Arora NK, Balakrishnan K, Jack DW, et al. Household fuels, low birth weight, and neonatal death in India: the separate impacts of biomass, kerosene, and coal. Int J Hyg Environ Health. 2013;216:523–32. doi:10.1016/j.ijheh.2012.12.006.

25. Lakshmi PV, Virdi NK, Sharma A, Tripathy JP, Smith KR, et al. Household air pollution and stillbirths in India: analysis of the DLHS-II National Survey. Environ Res. 2013;121:17–22. doi:10.1016/j.envres.2012.12.004.

26. Jehan I, Harris H, Salat S, Zeb A, Mobeen N, et al. Neonatal mortality, risk factors and causes: a prospective population-based cohort study in urban Pakistan. Bull World Health Organ. 2009;87:130–8.

27. Tielsch JM, Katz J, Thulasiraj RD, Coles CL, Sheeladevi S, et al. Exposure to indoor biomass fuel and tobacco smoke and risk of adverse

reproductive outcomes, mortality, respiratory morbidity and growth among newborn infants in south India. Int J Epidemiol. 2009;38:1351–63. doi:10.1093/ije/dyp286.

28. Boy E, Bruce N, Delgado H. Birth weight and exposure to kitchen wood smoke during pregnancy in rural Guatemala. Environ Health Perspect. 2002;110:109–14.

29. Mavalankar DV, Gray RH, Trivedi CR. Risk factors for preterm and term low birthweight in Ahmedabad, India. Int J Epidemiol. 1992;21:263–72.

30. Mishra V, Dai X, Smith KR, Mika L. Maternal exposure to biomass smoke and reduced birth weight in Zimbabwe. Ann Epidemiol. 2004;14:740–7.

31. Siddiqui AR, Gold EB, Yang X, Lee K, Brown KH, et al. Prenatal exposure to wood fuel smoke and low birth weight. Environ Health Perspect. 2008;116:543–9. doi:10.1289/ehp.10782.

32. Lawn JE, Blencowe H, Oza S, You D, Lee AC, et al. Every Newborn: progress, priorities, and potential beyond survival. Lancet. 2014;384:189–205. doi:10.1016/S0140-6736(14)60496-7.

33. Madhavan ND, Naidu KA. Polycyclic aromatic hydrocarbons in placenta, maternal blood, umbilical cord blood and milk of Indian women. Hum Exp Toxicol. 1995;14:503–6.

34. Rossner Jr P, Milcova A, Libalova H, Novakova Z, Topinka J, et al. Biomarkers of exposure to tobacco smoke and environmental pollutants in mothers and their transplacental transfer to the foetus. Part II. Oxidative damage. Mutat Res. 2009;669:20–6. doi:10.1016/j.mrfmmm.2009.04.010.

35. Sram RJ, Beskid O, Rossnerova A, Rossner P, Lnenickova Z, et al. Environmental exposure to carcinogenic polycyclic aromatic hydrocarbons–the interpretation of cytogenetic analysis by FISH. Toxicol Lett. 2007;172:12–20. doi:10.1016/j.toxlet.2007.05.019.

36. Topinka J, Milcova A, Libalova H, Novakova Z, Rossner Jr P, et al. Biomarkers of exposure to tobacco smoke and environmental pollutants in mothers and their transplacental transfer to the foetus. Part I: bulky DNA adducts. Mutat Res. 2009;669:13–9. doi:10.1016/j.mrfmmm.2009.04.011.

37. Hatch MC, Warburton D, Santella RM. Polycyclic aromatic hydrocarbon-DNA adducts in spontaneously aborted fetal tissue. Carcinogenesis. 1990;11:1673–5.

38. Sanyal MK, Mercan D, Belanger K, Santella RM. DNA adducts in human placenta exposed to ambient environment and passive cigarette smoke during pregnancy. Defects Res A Clin Mol Teratol. 2007;79:289–94. doi:10.1002/bdra.20346.

39. Singh VK, Singh J, Anand M, Kumar P, Patel DK, et al. Comparison of polycyclic aromatic hydrocarbon levels in placental tissues of Indian women with full- and preterm deliveries. Int J Hyg Environ Health. 2008;211:639–47. doi:10.1016/j.ijheh.2007.11.004.

40. Huel G, Girard F, Nessmann C, Godin J, Blot P, et al. Placental aryl hydrocarbon hydroxylase activity and placental calcifications. Toxicology. 1992;71:257–66.

41. Huel G, Godin J, Frery N, Girard F, Moreau T, et al. Aryl hydrocarbon hydroxylase activity in human placenta and threatened preterm delivery. J Expo Anal Environ Epidemiol. 1993;3 Suppl 1:187–99.

42. Huel G, Godin J, Moreau T, Girard F, Sahuquillo J, et al. Aryl hydrocarbon hydroxylase activity in human placenta of passive smokers. Environ Res. 1989;50:173–83.

43. Arnould JP, Verhoest P, Bach V, Libert JP, Belegaud J. Detection of benzo[a]pyrene-DNA adducts in human placenta and umbilical cord blood. Hum Exp Toxicol. 1997;16:716–21.

44. Dejmek J, Selevan SG, Benes I, Solansky I, Sram RJ. Fetal growth and maternal exposure to particulate matter during pregnancy. Environ Health Perspect. 1999;107:475–80.

45. Dejmek J, Solansky I, Benes I, Lenicek J, Sram RJ. The impact of polycyclic aromatic hydrocarbons and fine particles on pregnancy outcome. Environ Health Perspect. 2000;108:1159–64.

46. Perera FP, Rauh V, Tsai WY, Kinney P, Camann D, et al. Effects of transplacental exposure to environmental pollutants on birth outcomes in a multiethnic population. Environ Health Perspect. 2003;111:201–5.

47. Perera FP, Whyatt RM, Jedrychowski W, Rauh V, Manchester D, et al. Recent developments in molecular epidemiology: a study of the effects of environmental polycyclic aromatic hydrocarbons on birth outcomes in Poland. Am J Epidemiol. 1998;147:309–14.

48. Sioutas C, Delfino RJ, Singh M. Exposure assessment for atmospheric ultrafine particles (UFPs) and implications in epidemiologic research. Environ Health Perspect. 2005;113:947–55.

49. Nel AE, Diaz-Sanchez D, Li N. The role of particulate pollutants in pulmonary inflammation and asthma: evidence for the involvement of organic chemicals and oxidative stress. Curr Opin Pulm Med. 2001;7:20–6.

50. Li N, Sioutas C, Cho A, Schmitz D, Misra C, et al. Ultrafine particulate pollutants induce oxidative stress and mitochondrial damage. Environ Health Perspect. 2003;111:455–60.

51. Engel SA, Erichsen HC, Savitz DA, Thorp J, Chanock SJ, et al. Risk of spontaneous preterm birth is associated with common proinflammatory cytokine polymorphisms. Epidemiology. 2005;16:469–77.

52. Keelan JA, Blumenstein M, Helliwell RJ, Sato TA, Marvin KW, et al. Cytokines, prostaglandins and parturition–a review. Placenta. 2003;24 Suppl A:S33-S46.

53. Wei SQ, Fraser W, Luo ZC. Inflammatory cytokines and spontaneous preterm birth in asymptomatic women: a systematic review. Obstet Gynecol. 2010;116:393–401. doi:10.1097/AOG.0b013e3181e6dbc0.

54. Gomez C, Berlin I, Marquis P, Delcroix M. Expired air carbon monoxide concentration in mothers and their spouses above 5 ppm is associated with decreased fetal growth. Prev Med. 2005;40:10–5. doi:10.1016/j.ypmed.2004.04.049.

12

Maternal weight in the postpartum: results from the Delta healthy sprouts trial

Lisa M. Tussing-Humphreys[1]* , Jessica L. Thomson[2], Nefertiti OjiNjideka Hemphill[3], Melissa H. Goodman[2] and Alicia S. Landry[4]

Abstract

Background: Excessive postnatal weight retention may pose a threat to a woman's health and future pregnancies. Women in the Lower Mississippi Delta (LMD) region of Mississippi suffer from among the highest rates of obesity in the U.S. and are more likely to gain an excessive amount of weight during pregnancy. The aim of this study was to determine if LMD women who received a lifestyle enhanced maternal, infant, and early childhood home visiting (MIECHV) curriculum had more favorable weight outcomes through 12-months postpartum compared to women who received a standard MIECHV curriculum.

Methods: Delta Healthy Sprouts was a two-arm, randomized, controlled, comparative impact trial. Pregnant women at least 18 years of age, less than 19 weeks pregnant with a singleton pregnancy, and residing in the LMD region were recruited. On a monthly basis in the participant's home, the control arm (PAT) received the Parents as Teachers curriculum while the experimental arm (PATE) received a lifestyle enhanced Parents as Teachers curriculum. Pre-pregnancy body weight via self-report and maternal body weight at baseline (gestational month 4) and at every subsequent monthly visit through 12 months postpartum was measured. Linear mixed models were used to test for significant treatment, time, and treatment by time effects on postnatal weight outcomes.

Results: Mean postnatal weight losses were 0.8 and 1.1 kg at postnatal month (PM) 6 and PM 12, respectively, for PAT participants. Mean postnatal weight losses for PATE participants were 1.5 and 1.2 kg at PM 6 and PM 12, respectively. Mean weight retention, based on pre-pregnancy weight, were 5.2, 4.0, and 3.6 kg at PM 1, PM 6, and PM 12, respectively, for PAT participants. Mean weight retention for PATE participants were 6.3, 4.5, and 4.0 kg at PM 1, PM 6, and PM 12, respectively. Significant effects were not found for treatment, time, or treatment by time.

Conclusions: An enhanced MIECHV curriculum was not associated with more favorable postpartum weight outcomes when compared to a standard MIECHV curriculum in a cohort of LMD women during the 12 months following the birth of their infant.

Keywords: Postpartum, Body weight, African American women

Background

Pregnancy is a time when a woman intentionally gains weight to support her developing fetus and the pregnancy-related adaptations occurring including growth of the placenta. However, according to the Centers for Disease Control and Prevention, 48% of women in the United States (U.S.) gain an excessive amount of weight with a singleton pregnancy [1]. Specific

weight gain recommendations for singleton pregnancies were put forth by the Institute of Medicine (IOM) in 2009 [2], and are based on a woman's pre-pregnancy body mass index (BMI). The IOM established guidelines given mounting evidence that excessive weight gain in pregnancy can lead to significant transient and long-term health effects for both mother and baby. Specific to the mother's postpartum health, excessive gestational weight gain is a risk factor for excessive postnatal weight retention (> 10 lb) [3], obesity [4], and obesity-related chronic diseases including type 2 diabetes [5]. Excessive postnatal weight retention may pose a threat to reproductive health

* Correspondence: ltussing@uic.edu
[1]Department of Medicine and Cancer Center, University of Illinois at Chicago, 416 West Side Research Office Building, 1747 West Roosevelt Road, Chicago, IL 60608, USA
Full list of author information is available at the end of the article

and future pregnancies by increasing the risk for infertility [6], gestational diabetes [7] and pre-eclampsia [8]. Thus, perinatal lifestyle interventions promoting optimal gestational weight gain and postnatal weight management may have a significant effect on maternal and infant health.

Women of reproductive age in the Lower Mississippi Delta (LMD) region of Mississippi suffer from among the highest rates of obesity in the nation [9]. Furthermore, women residing in this area of the U.S. are likely to gain an excessive amount of weight during pregnancy [10] and have unintended, closely spaced pregnancies [11], both of which are associated with increased risk of obesity [12]. Hence, there is a dire need for perinatal weight management interventions in the LMD region.

Several lifestyle interventions focused on optimizing gestational weight gain have reported promising results [3, 13, 14], although only a few studies have spanned the perinatal period by actively intervening on both gestational weight gain and postnatal weight management [15–19]. Delta Healthy Sprouts was designed to test the impact of a maternal, infant and early childhood (MIECHV) home-visiting curriculum enhanced with a lifestyle recommendations (maternal and infant-related diet and physical activity and maternal weight management) compared to a standard MIECHV curriculum on maternal gestational weight gain and postnatal weight management amongst other infant and maternal health and behavioral outcomes in pregnant women residing in the LMD region [20]. We found that the lifestyle-enhanced MIECHV curriculum was not associated with more favorable gestational weight gain outcomes compared to the standard MIECHV curriculum [21]. Here, we present the 12-month postnatal weight management data for women enrolled in Delta Healthy Sprouts. The goal is to determine if the women who received the lifestyle enhanced MIECHV curriculum had more favorable weight outcomes through 12 months postpartum compared to the women who received the standard MIECHV curriculum.

Methods
Design and recruitment
This was a longitudinal analysis of Delta Healthy Sprouts maternal postnatal weight outcomes through 1 year postpartum. A full description the Delta Healthy Sprouts Trial has been reported previously [20]. Briefly, 82 pregnant women residing in the LMD region were enrolled in their second trimester of pregnancy. Inclusion criteria comprised female gender, 18 years or older, less than 19 gestational weeks with first, second, or third child, singleton pregnancy, and a resident of Washington, Bolivar, or Humphreys County in Mississippi. Women were recruited on a rolling basis between March 2013 and December 2014. Recruitment included active recruitment at local health clinics serving pregnancy

women, publicizing the study in local print media and at local health fairs, referrals from the local health department and Women, Infants, and Children (WIC) staff, and by word of mouth.

The original recruitment goal was 75 women per treatment arm. The sample size of 150 women was based on the following assumptions: 20% attrition rate, 37% of control participants with gestational weight gain within the IOM recommendations, and a 22% difference between treatment arms for gestational weight gain within recommendations. Additionally, assuming an average 12-month postnatal weight loss of 1.5 kg in the PAT arm (SD = 4.7 and 5.4 kg in control and intervention arms, respectively) [22], a postnatal sample size of 120 participants would allow for detection of a 3.8 kg difference in 12-month postnatal weight loss between the two arms. An additional power and sample size calculation for the postnatal primary outcome – child obesity at 1 year of age – also was performed [20]. Recruitment was stopped prior to reaching the goal due to unanticipated difficulties with recruiting pregnant women meeting the study inclusion criteria and lack of resources to further support recruitment activities. All data collection activities concluded in May 2016. Figure 1 illustrates the CONSORT diagram for the study.

Delta Healthy Sprouts was designed to evaluate the impact of the MIECHV Parents as Teachers ® (PAT) curriculum compared with a lifestyle-enhanced PAT curriculum (PATE) on maternal gestational weight gain, postpartum weight management and childhood obesity prevention among other maternal and infant health and behavioral outcomes. PAT is a nationally recognized evidence-based MIECHV program that strives to increase parental knowledge of healthy child development, instill good parenting skills, provide early detection of physical and neurocognitive developmental delays, prevent child abuse, and increase school readiness [23]. Participants in the Delta Healthy Sprouts Trial were randomly assigned to one of the two treatment arms [PAT control (N = 43) or PATE experimental (N = 39)] at approximately 4 months gestation and followed through 12 months postpartum.

The Delta Healthy Sprouts Trial is registered at clinicaltrials.gov (NCT01746394) and was approved by the Institutional Review Board of Delta State University (Cleveland, MS). All women gave their written informed consent prior to study participation.

Interventions
Both arms of the intervention were delivered in the participant's home by trained Parent Educators. Parent Educators were African American, college educated women residing in the target communities. They were trained to deliver both the PAT and the PATE curriculum and to collect data from participants, including

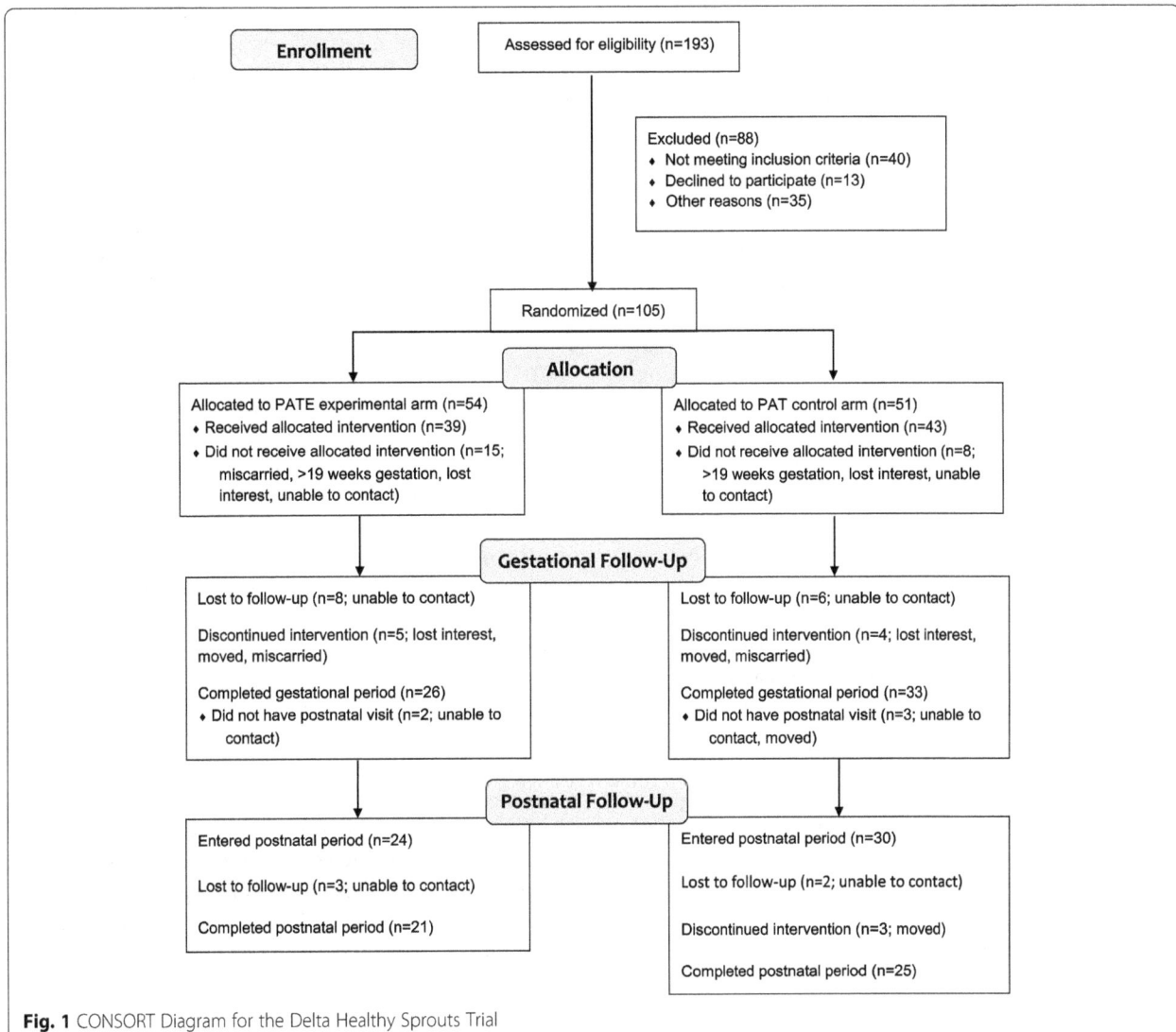

Fig. 1 CONSORT Diagram for the Delta Healthy Sprouts Trial

anthropometrics and dietary intake, by senior research staff members who were certified master trainers for the Nutrition Data System for Research (NDSR) software. Home visits occurred monthly and were approximately 60–90 min in length for the PAT arm and approximately 90–120 min for the PATE arm. Additional details regarding Parent Educator training, study methodology, and lesson plan outlines have been published elsewhere [20].

The PAT arm of the intervention was based on the PAT curriculum that included one-on-one home visits, optional monthly group meetings, developmental screenings, and a resource network for families. Using the PAT model, Parent Educators provided parents with research based information and activities during home visitation. Materials were responsive to parental information requests and were tailored to the age of the child (or gestational age of the fetus in the prenatal period).

The PATE arm of the intervention built upon the PAT curriculum. The curriculum enhancement was guided by the theoretical underpinnings of the social cognitive theory [24] and the transtheoretical model of behavior change [25]. Additionally, the PATE curriculum included foundational elements from the Diabetes Prevention Program and the Infant Feeding Activity and Nutrition Trial. Elements based upon the Diabetes Prevention Program included a culturally sensitive, individualized educational curriculum taught on a one-to-one basis [26]. Elements taken from the Infant Feeding Activity and Nutrition Trial included anticipatory guidance and parenting support principles [27]. Anticipatory guidance involves providing practical, developmentally appropriate, child health information to parents in anticipation of significant physical, emotional, and psychological milestones [28]. Parenting support emphasizes children's psychological and behavioral goals, logical and natural consequences, mutual respect, and encouragement techniques [29].

For the PATE lessons, additional emphasis was placed on educating the women about ways in which they could develop positive eating, physical activity, and other health behaviors in their children, including modeling these behaviors themselves. Specific to the postnatal period, intervention components of the PATE arm included healthy weight management for mom, infant feeding cues, baby tummy time, introduction to solid foods for baby, healthy beverage selections for the family, sitting and screen time for mom and baby, modeling healthy behaviors for the child, creating a healthy home, healthy meal planning and food shopping, and toddler feeding. The entire perinatal lifestyle curriculum is available at: https://www.ars.usda.gov/ARSUserFiles/60000000/DeltaHumanNutritionResearch/DHS%20Lesson%20Plan%20Booklet.pdf.

Postnatal weight management for mothers, including tracking weight gain/loss, was discussed during the postnatal month (PM) 2–11 visits. At PM 2, women in the PATE arm were provided a US Department of Agriculture (USDA) MyPlate for Moms eating plan that was selected to promote 5% weight loss based on their PM 1 body weight while considering caloric needs if the woman was breastfeeding. For PATE participants, mean body weight at PM 1 was 9.3% above pre-pregnancy values. Women were already familiar with the USDA MyPlate eating plan approach given this tool was used to promote optimal gestational weight gain in the prenatal period [20, 21]. At the PM 3–11 visits, Parent Educators reviewed participants' MyPlate diet and physical activity self-monitoring tracking logs, facilitated setting or revising eating and activity goals, and held discussions with participants regarding how to achieve their goals. Other curriculum features specific to maternal weight management included viewing the *How to Create a Great Plate* DVD (Learning Zone, 20 min) in PM 2, *Beverage Basics* DVD in PM 5 (Lemon-Aid Films, 8 min) and *Shop Healthy, Cook Healthy* DVD (Milner-Fenwick Inc., 16 min) in PM 7. At PM 2, 5, 7, and 9, dietary intake data that was collected during the previous month's visit was reviewed with the participant. Parent Educators praised healthy food and beverage choices and discussed methods to amend food selections that were energy dense and nutrient poor. Women who were able to achieve the 5% weight loss goal in PM 3–11 were encouraged to maintain this weight loss through PM 12.

Measures
Anthropometrics
Height at baseline was measured using a portable stadiometer (model 217, seca, Birmingham, UK). Maternal body weight was measured at baseline and every subsequent visit in the gestational and postnatal periods with an electronic scale (model SR241, SR Instruments, Tonawanda, NY). Pre-pregnancy body weight was self-reported. Body mass index was calculated as weight (kg) divided by height (m) squared.

Diet
Self-reported dietary intake data were collected from the participants at the PM 1, 4, 6, 8, and 12 visits via multiple pass 24-h dietary recall using NDSR software. NDSR is a Windows-based dietary analysis program that allows for the calculation of nutrients per ingredient, food, meal, and day in report and analysis formats [30]. Participants' diet quality was calculated using the dietary data collected with NDSR and the Healthy Eating Index-2010 (HEI-2010) which measures adherence to the 2010 Dietary Guidelines for Americans [31].

Physical activity
Self-report postnatal physical activity data were collected from participants at the PM 1, 6, and 12 visits using a modified version of the Pregnancy and Physical Activity Questionnaire [32]. Modifications included small wording changes (e.g., driving or riding in a car vs. driving or riding in a car or bus) and timeframe adjustment (during this month vs. during this trimester) to make the instrument more relevant to this population of rural, Southern women and the Delta Healthy Sprouts Trial design. This 26-item instrument allows for the calculation of physical activity duration, intensity, specific type (i.e., sedentary, light-intensity, moderate-intensity, vigorous-intensity, household/care-giving, occupational, and sports/exercise), and total activity. Moderate and vigorous intensity physical activity responses were combined into a single category, moderate-to-vigorous physical activity (MVPA), because so few women reported time spent in vigorous activity.

Participants also provided information regarding demographic characteristics (e.g., age, marital status, household size, education, employment, household income, insurance, prenatal care), health history, and current health conditions at baseline (approximately 16 weeks gestation). Details regarding other measures and questionnaire data that were collected, but are not relevant to the present paper, have been published elsewhere [20]. All measures and questionnaires were collected or administered by trained research staff (Parent Educators) using laptop computers loaded with relevant software (i.e., Snap Surveys, NDSR) and in the participants' homes.

Statistical analyses
Because maternal postnatal weight control was the primary focus of this paper, analyses were conducted only

for the postnatal cohort (participants who completed the gestational period and had at least one visit in the postnatal period; n = 54). Five participants who completed the gestational period but dropped out of the study prior to the PM 1 visit were excluded from the postnatal cohort. Additionally, one PAT participant who became pregnant again between the PM 1 and PM 2 visits was excluded from the weight control analyses. Similarly, visits occurring after conception for four PATE participants who became pregnant again between the PM 3 and PM 10 visits were excluded from the weight control analyses. Conception dates were determined by inputting participants' reported due dates into an online pregnancy calculator [Pregnancy Calculator, http://www.calculator.net/pregnancy-calculator.html].

Statistical analyses were performed using SAS® software, version 9.4 (SAS Institute Inc., Cary, NC). Descriptive statistics, including means, standard deviations, frequencies, and percentages, were used to summarize participants' demographic characteristics and anthropometric measures. Chi square tests of association or Fisher's exact tests (categorical measures) and two sample t tests (continuous measures) were used to assess differences between PAT and PATE participants' baseline, gestational, and some postnatal characteristics and measures. These tests also were used to assess differences between postnatal period study completers' and non-completers' baseline characteristics. Postnatal period study completers were defined as participants who had their PM 12 visit. Postnatal period study non-completers were defined as participants who had at least one visit in the postnatal period but did not complete the PM 12 visit.

Postnatal weight change was calculated using several methods. First, measured weight at each subsequent postnatal (PM 2 through PM 12) visit was subtracted from the measured weight for the PM 1 visit to obtain a postnatal difference value. Second, these difference values were divided by the PM 1 weight and then multiplied by 100 to obtain a postnatal weight change percentage. Third, self-reported pre-pregnancy weight was subtracted from measured weight at each postnatal (PM 1 through PM 12) visit to obtain a postnatal weight retention value. Fourth, these retention values were divided by the pre-pregnancy weight and then multiplied by 100 to obtain a postnatal weight retention percentage.

Linear mixed models, using maximum likelihood estimation, were used to test for significant treatment, time, and treatment by time (interaction) effects on postnatal weight outcomes. Maximum likelihood estimation is an approach for handling missing data in repeated measures. Treatment (PAT vs. PATE) was modeled as a fixed effect for all outcomes. Postnatal weight outcomes were modeled using a Gaussian (normal) distribution with an identity link function and time (PM1 through PM 12

visits) was modeled as a repeated measure using a variance covariance structure. Least squares means with 95% confidence limits were computed using these models. The first model included treatment, time, and treatment by time as fixed effects. The second model included pre-pregnancy BMI (continuous form) and treatment by BMI as additional covariates. The third model included only treatment as a fixed effect and was restricted to pre-pregnancy and PM 12 body weight data. This third model was run because our original hypothesis stated that the PATE participants would have less pregnancy weight retention at 12 months postnatal [Thomson CCT 2014]. The significance level of the tests was set at 0.05.

Results

Retention rates for the postnatal period for the PAT and PATE treatment arms were 83% (25/30) and 88% (21/24), respectively, and did not differ significantly between treatment arms (p = 0.668). The mean number of postnatal visits were 10.2 and 9.9 (p = 0.717), respectively, for PAT and PATE participants.

Table 1 presents comparisons between treatment arms for baseline socio-demographic characteristics of the postnatal cohort. Significant differences between PAT and PATE participant characteristics at baseline were not found with the exception of percentages receiving SNAP benefits. Significantly more PAT participants (87%) received SNAP benefits as compared to PATE participants (63%). The majority of both PAT and PATE participants were African American (approximately 96% in both groups) and reported single as their relationship status (87% vs. 92%). The mean age in the PAT group was 24.1 years and 23.0 years in the PATE group. Regarding completion status for the postnatal period, significant differences between completers and non-completers were not found for any of the baseline characteristics tested.

Table 2 presents comparisons between treatment arms for pre-pregnancy, pregnancy, and postnatal characteristics of the postnatal cohort. Significant differences between PAT and PATE participant characteristics were not found. Mean pre-pregnancy BMI in both treatment arms was in the overweight range (25.0–29.9 kg/m^2). Mean gestational weight gain was approximately 15 kg in both groups with 53% of PAT participants and 71% of PATE participants gaining above the IOM recommendations for a singleton pregnancy. At the PM 1 visit, mean BMI in the PAT group was 30.4 ± 7.73 kg/m^2 whereas in the PATE group, mean BMI was 31.6 ± 7.77 kg/m^2. Overall, few women initiated and or sustained breastfeeding for more than 1 month. Mean HEI-2010 total score (not reported in table) for PAT participants was 40.2 and 36.4 at PM 6 and 12 while mean HEI-2010 total

Table 1 Delta Healthy Sprouts participant baseline socio-demographic characteristics by treatment arm

Characteristic	PAT (N = 30)		PATE (N = 24)		
	n	%	n	%	P
Race					
African American	29	96.7	23	95.8	1.000
White	1	3.3	1	4.2	
Marital status					
Single[a]	26	86.7	22	91.7	0.682
Married	4	13.3	2	8.3	
Education level					
≤ High school graduate	12	40.0	12	50.0	0.462
≥ Some college/technical	18	60.0	12	50.0	
Employment status					
Full time/part-time	10	33.3	11	45.8	0.608
Unemployed (looking)	12	40.0	7	29.2	
Homemaker/student	8	26.7	6	25.0	
Smoker in household	7	23.3	9	37.5	0.257
Smoker[b]					
Current	1	3.3	1	4.2	0.620
Stopped before pregnancy	1	3.3	0	0.0	
Stopped after became pregnant	1	3.3	0	0.0	
Non	27	90.0	23	95.8	
Medicaid health insurance	30	100.0	24	100.0	0.703
Receiving SNAP	26	86.7	15	62.5	0.039
Receiving WIC	28	93.3	20	83.3	0.389
	Mean	SD	Mean	SD	P
Age (years)	24.1	4.76	23.0	4.96	0.380
Household size	3.6	1.61	4.2	1.52	0.221

PAT Parents as Teachers control treatment, PATE Parents as Teachers Enhanced experimental treatment, SNAP Supplemental Nutrition Assistance Program, WIC Special SNAP for Women, Infants and Children
[a]Included 1 participant who indicated she is divorced
[b]Comparison: non vs. all other responses

Table 2 Delta Healthy Sprouts participant pre-pregnancy, pregnancy and postnatal characteristics by treatment arm

Characteristic	PAT (N = 30)		PATE (N = 24)		
	n	%	n	%	P
Gestational diabetes	0	0.0	0	0.0	NA
Gestational hypertension	5	16.7	2	8.3	0.443
Gestational weight gain[a,b]					
Within IOM recommendations	9	30.0	2	8.3	0.087
Under IOM recommendations	5	16.7	5	20.8	
Above IOM recommendations	16	53.3	17	70.8	
Rate of gestational weight gain[b,c]					
Within IOM recommendations	5	16.7	3	12.5	0.720
Under IOM recommendations	6	20.0	4	16.7	
Above IOM recommendations	19	63.3	17	70.8	
Breastfeeding[d]					
> 1 month	2	6.7	2	8.3	1.000
< 1 month	7	23.3	10	41.7	
Never	21	70.0	12	50.0	
	Mean	SD	Mean	SD	P
Pre-pregnancy weight (kg)	76.4	22.10	80.0	24.78	0.566
Pre-pregnancy BMI	28.6	8.18	29.2	7.72	0.762
Gestational weight gain (kg)[a]	15.3	9.80	14.3	7.19	0.663
Postnatal weight (kg) at PM 1	81.6	22.48	86.4	24.74	0.460
Postnatal BMI at PM 1	30.4	7.73	31.6	7.77	0.577

PAT Parents as Teachers control treatment; PATE, Parents as Teachers Enhanced experimental treatment, NA Not applicable because all participants fall into single category, IOM Institute of Medicine, BMI Body mass index, MVPA Moderate to vigorous physical activity, PM Postnatal month
[a]Based on self-reported pre-pregnancy weight
[b]Comparison = within vs. under and above
[c]Based on measured weight between gestational months 4 and 9
[d]Comparison: > 1 month vs. < 1 month and never

and PM 12, respectively. Significant effects were not found for treatment, time, or treatment by time. These results did not differ (i.e., no treatment effect) when only data for PM 12 were analyzed ($p = 0.852$).

Postnatal weight retention (difference in kg or % body weight from self-reported pre-pregnancy weight) results are presented in Table 4. Mean weight retention for PAT participants was 5.2, 4.0, and 3.6 kg at PM 1, PM 6, and PM 12, respectively. Mean weight retention for PATE participants was 6.3, 4.5, and 4.0 kg at PM 1, PM 6, and PM 12, respectively. Significant effects were not found for treatment, time, or treatment by time. Again, these results did not differ (i.e., no treatment effect) when only data for PM 12 were analyzed ($p = 0.790$).

Pertaining to the results for which pre-pregnancy BMI and its interaction with treatment arm were included as covariates, only pre-pregnancy BMI was significant for the postnatal weight loss outcome models, although its effect was small [slope = 0.1, standard error (SE) = 0.03, $p = 0.002$ for kg difference; slope = 0.1, SE = 0.04,

score for PATE participants was 40.2 and 37.6, respectively, and did not differ between the two groups (Thomson et al., under review). Further, women were well below population-level postpartum physical activity recommendations of 150 min/week [33]. Mean MVPA (not reported in table) for PAT participants was 50 min at both PM 6 and 12 while mean MVPA for PATE participants was 42 and 40 min at PM 6 and 12, respectively, and did not differ between treatment arms. (Thomson et al., accepted, American Journal of Health Promotion).

Postnatal weight loss results (difference in kg or % body weight from PM 1 weight) are presented in Table 3. Mean weight losses for PAT participants were 0.8 and 1.1 kg at PM 6 and PM 12, respectively. Mean weight losses for PATE participants were 1.5 and 1.2 kg at PM 6

Table 3 Delta Healthy Sprouts participant postnatal weight loss by treatment arm and visit (time)

Visit	PAT (n = 29)[a]		PATE (n = 24)[b]		P		
	LSM	95% CL	LSM	95% CL	Arm	Time	Int
Difference (kg) from PM 1 (negative = loss)							
PM 1	0.0	−1.12 1.12	0.0	−1.25 1.25	0.587	0.778	0.980
PM 2	−0.7	−1.83 0.48	−0.5	−1.88 0.78			
PM 3	−1.0	−2.26 0.18	−1.1	−2.49 0.39			
PM 4	−1.0	−2.24 0.26	−1.8	−3.28 −0.32			
PM 5	−0.9	−2.20 0.35	−0.6	−2.09 0.87			
PM 6	−0.8	−2.04 0.40	−1.5	−3.04 0.11			
PM 7	−0.8	−2.03 0.47	−0.8	−2.30 0.75			
PM 8	−1.2	−2.44 0.11	−1.0	−2.47 0.41			
PM 9	−0.9	−2.17 0.38	−0.2	−1.73 1.33			
PM 10	−1.3	−2.58 −0.03	−0.5	−2.05 1.01			
PM 11	−1.2	−2.45 0.04	0.1	−1.54 1.72			
PM 12	−1.1	−2.37 0.12	−1.2	−2.64 0.32			
% difference from PM 1 (negative = loss)							
PM 1	0.0	−1.39 1.39	0.0	−1.56 1.56	0.270	0.665	0.986
PM 2	−0.9	−2.33 0.56	−0.5	−2.22 1.12			
PM 3	−1.5	−3.03 0.03	−1.3	−3.08 0.52			
PM 4	−1.5	−3.10 0.02	−2.2	−4.02 −0.32			
PM 5	−1.5	−3.09 0.10	−0.7	−2.55 1.15			
PM 6	−1.4	−2.88 0.17	−2.0	−3.96 −0.02			
PM 7	−1.3	−2.82 0.29	−1.1	−3.05 0.77			
PM 8	−1.8	−3.38 −0.19	−1.4	−3.22 0.38			
PM 9	−1.3	−2.85 0.34	−0.4	−2.31 1.51			
PM 10	−1.8	−3.36 −0.18	−0.4	−2.36 1.46			
PM 11	−1.6	−3.20 −0.08	0.0	−2.01 2.07			
PM 12	−1.5	−3.04 0.08	−1.2	−3.03 0.68			

PAT Parents as Teachers control treatment, *PATE* Parents as Teachers Enhanced experimental treatment, *LSM* Least squares mean, *CL* Confidence limit, *Int* Interaction, *PM* Postnatal month
[a]Excluded post conception visits for 1 PAT participant who became pregnant again in postnatal period
[b]Excluded post conception visits for 4 PATE participants who became pregnant again in the postnatal period

Table 4 Delta Healthy Sprouts participant postnatal weight retention by treatment arm and visit (time)

Visit	PAT (n = 29)[a]		PATE (n = 24)[b]		P		
	LSM	95% CL	LSM	95% CL	Arm	Time	Int
Difference (kg) from pre-pregnancy weight (positive = retain)							
PM 1	5.2	2.53 7.89	6.3	3.32 9.31	0.390	0.982	1.000
PM 2	4.7	1.94 7.48	5.0	1.84 8.23			
PM 3	3.9	0.94 6.81	5.2	1.72 8.63			
PM 4	3.9	0.88 6.86	3.5	−0.05 7.06			
PM 5	3.9	0.81 6.92	4.7	1.11 8.22			
PM 6	4.0	1.09 6.96	4.5	0.74 8.31			
PM 7	4.0	0.99 6.98	3.9	0.23 7.56			
PM 8	3.5	0.48 6.59	3.7	0.26 7.17			
PM 9	3.6	0.59 6.70	4.4	0.71 8.04			
PM 10	3.2	0.17 6.29	4.3	0.63 7.96			
PM 11	3.6	0.56 6.55	4.7	0.74 8.58			
PM 12	3.6	0.65 6.63	4.0	0.49 7.60			
% difference from pre-pregnancy weight (positive = retain)							
PM 1	7.7	4.47 10.87	9.3	5.71 12.86	0.683	0.649	0.999
PM 2	6.9	3.59 10.22	7.1	3.26 10.91			
PM 3	5.7	2.22 9.23	7.1	2.96 11.22			
PM 4	5.5	1.95 9.10	4.0	−0.23 8.27			
PM 5	5.7	2.09 9.39	5.2	0.97 9.47			
PM 6	5.7	2.17 9.18	4.9	0.36 9.41			
PM 7	5.8	2.18 9.34	4.0	−0.43 8.34			
PM 8	5.0	1.36 8.66	4.0	−0.13 8.13			
PM 9	5.5	1.84 9.15	5.0	0.57 9.33			
PM 10	5.0	1.34 8.65	4.7	0.37 9.13			
PM 11	5.3	1.76 8.91	5.3	0.63 9.99			
PM 12	5.5	1.93 9.08	4.8	0.54 9.04			

PAT Parents as Teachers control treatment, *PATE* Parents as Teachers Enhanced experimental treatment, *LSM* Least squares mean, *CL* Confidence limit, *Int* Interaction, *PM* Postnatal month
[a]Excluded post conception visits for 1 PAT participant who became pregnant again in postnatal period
[b]Excluded post conception visits for 4 PATE participants who became pregnant again in postnatal period

$p = 0.001$ for percent difference). For the postnatal weight retention (kg) model, treatment and its interaction with pre-pregnancy BMI were significant ($p < 0.001$ for both). Specifically, the slope for pre-pregnancy BMI was 0.1 (SE = 0.07) for the PATE treatment arm, while the slope was −0.3 (SE = 0.09) for the PAT treatment arm. That is, for every 1-unit increase in pre-pregnancy BMI, retained weight increased by 0.1 kg for PATE participants, while retained weight decreased by 0.3 kg for PAT participants.

Somewhat similarly, for the postnatal weight retention (percent) model, treatment, pre-pregnancy BMI, and their

interaction term were significant (p = 0.001, < 0.001, and <0.001, respectively). Specifically, the slope for pre-pregnancy BMI was −0.1 (SE = 0.08) for the PATE treatment arm, while the slope was −0.5 (SE = 0.10) for the PAT treatment arm. That is, for every 1-unit increase in pre-pregnancy BMI, retained weight decreased by 0.1% for PATE participants, while retained weight decreased by 0.5% for PAT participants.

Discussion

This paper reports on the treatment effect differences for postnatal weight change and weight retention through 12 months postpartum for women enrolled in the Delta Healthy Sprouts Trial. This trial is one of only a few trials to conduct a maternal weight management intervention targeting both the gestational and postpartum periods in the context of a single intervention [15–19]. Findings from this analysis indicate that participants in the PATE experimental arm did not lose more weight in the postpartum (between PM 1 and PM 12) or retain less weight gained in pregnancy compared to the women in the PAT control arm.

The findings of our study are similar to two other maternal weight management interventions that spanned the perinatal period. In the New Life(style) study conducted by Althuizen and colleagues [17, 34], women received in-person counseling from a midwife to optimize weight gain in the gestational period and one telephone counseling session at 8 weeks postpartum to promote weight loss [34]. They reported no significant effect of the intervention on maternal weight at 1 year postpartum compared to a control group. In the Trial for Reducing Weight Retention in New Moms [19], women randomized to the enhanced care arm received weight loss/behavior change concepts delivered through a single in-person nutrition counseling session and monthly newsletters. There was no difference in weight loss or weight retention between the intervention and standard care group which received information about nutrition guidelines for breastfeeding at 6 months postpartum. However, it is important to highlight that despite similarities in findings, our intervention was longer in duration and more intensive.

In contrast to our study, a perinatal intervention conducted with Taiwanese women [16] reported that women receiving a combined gestational and postpartum weight management intervention retained less weight at 6 months postpartum compared to women receiving only the postpartum intervention or control treatment. In a study conducted by Clasesson and colleagues [15], women receiving weekly weight gain optimization support during pregnancy and every 6 months through 2 years postpartum to promote weight change had significantly greater weight loss compared to a standard care control group. Liu et al. [18] conducted a small pilot study with intervention components comparable to Delta Healthy Sprouts (e.g., used USDA MyPlate for Moms to promote weight management) in a similar population of pregnant Southern, African American women. The gestational intervention involved one face-to face individual meeting and eight group sessions, while the postpartum intervention included one home visit and three telephone-based sessions. At 12 weeks postpartum, 50% of their postnatal cohort was at their pre-pregnancy body weight or lower. However, the authors did not compare these postpartum weight findings against a control group and the sample size of the postnatal cohort was only 14 women.

Several other studies have focused their intervention exclusively on the postpartum period. In a recent systematic review of 11 lifestyle interventions to limit postpartum weight retention [35], seven of the 11 studies were successful at promoting postpartum weight loss. Of the seven successful trials [16, 36–41], six [16, 36–40] incorporated both dietary and physical activity components. Although the dietary components used in these trials were similar to the Delta Healthy Sprouts Trial, there was clearly a greater emphasis placed on increasing postpartum physical activity with some trials including supervised physical activity sessions [36, 38] and the provision of heart rate monitors [36, 41]. The majority of the successful trials also tended to engage with participants on a more frequent basis (i.e., more than monthly). Thus, a greater emphasis on physical activity and more frequent participant contact may have increased the efficacy of our postpartum PATE intervention.

Interestingly, based on our linear mixed models analyses, the PATE treatment appeared more effective in terms of postnatal weight loss for participants with lower pre-pregnancy BMI, while the PAT treatment appeared more effective for participants with higher pre-pregnancy BMI. We also observed that both PATE and PAT treatments appeared more effective in terms of producing a lower percentage of weight retention for participants with higher pre-pregnancy BMI, although the effect was more pronounced in the PAT participants. These findings are difficult to interpret but suggest that the women with pre-pregnancy obesity were more successful with postpartum weight management when it was self-directed vs. through a lifestyle intervention explicitly focusing on postnatal weight management.

Our overall lack of intervention effect could be due to the complexity of our intervention. To promote postpartum weight change in the PATE arm, we recommended following a personalized USDA MyPlate for Moms eating plan designed to produce about a ½ -1 lb of weight loss per week. This approach combined both energy restriction and improving overall diet quality. Leermarkers et al. [39] found a significant effect on postpartum weight loss in a low-intensity intervention that focused exclusively on reducing overall calories. Thus, it is possible that simultaneously targeting multiple dietary behaviors was overwhelming to our participants. Bennett and colleagues [42] have suggested that health literacy may complicate weight management for medically vulnerable populations. He suggests that promoting weight management through easy to understand dietary behavior goals (i.e., reducing sugary beverages) may be more effective for weight management for persons with low health literacy. Although we did not examine health literacy in the context of the Delta Healthy Sprouts Trial, there was relatively low educational attainment in 50% of the PATE and 40% of the PAT women. Thus, future lifestyle interventions targeting this population of pregnant women should consider the health literacy of participants [42].

Phelan and colleagues suggest that the success of an intervention focused on reducing postpartum weight retention is largely dependent on the ability to optimize weight gain in the gestational period [43]. Almost three-fourths of the women in the PATE treatment arm exceeded the IOM recommendations for gestational weight gain. Furthermore, approximately 50% of the women initially enrolled in our trial exceeded the IOM weight gain recommendations in their fourth month of pregnancy [44]. Thus, interventions targeting women earlier in pregnancy (i.e., 6–10 weeks gestation) may allow for more favorable postpartum weight outcomes given that gestational weight gain is a significant predictor of postpartum weight retention [45].

There are strengths and weaknesses in this study. The longitudinal design is one of its greatest strengths given women were followed through 12 months postpartum. Further, the population studied is a strength given that Southern, African American women are at increased risk for obesity and chronic diseases [9]. Our study also was personalized [16], home-based [46], built upon a known national MIECHV program [47], and theory-driven [18], all of which have been cited as salient features for lifestyle interventions targeting pregnant women. A significant limitation of our study was the high level of attrition observed in both PAT and PATE treatment arms (58 and 54%, respectively) from baseline to study end which is higher than dropout reported in similar trials [15–19, 46]. Our small sample size resulting from high attrition may have been a limiting factor in detecting statistically significant differences between the two treatment arms. Additionally, data collection was not blinded and therefore is a potential source of bias. However, having a second set of blinded research staff whose sole purpose was to collect data was not practically, logistically, or financially feasible. Moreover, it is unlikely that bias occurred on the part of the Parent Educators or the participant (e.g., provision of socially desirable responses) given the lack of effect observed in this study. Another limitation was the use of self-report measures, including pre-pregnancy body weight, which could have biased our estimation of gestational weight gain and postpartum weight retention.

Conclusions

Our lifestyle-enhanced MIECHV curriculum was not associated with more favorable postpartum weight outcomes when compared to a standard MIECHV curriculum in a cohort of postpartum LMD African American women. Weight management in the postpartum remains a significant public health concern given that retaining an excessive amount of the weight gained in pregnancy can compromise a woman's future reproductive health [6, 7] and increase her risk for chronic health conditions [4, 5]. Future studies targeting lifestyle behaviors of pregnant and postpartum women in the health disparate LMD region should consider placing a greater emphasis on increasing physical activity, inclusion of simplified dietary messaging to accommodate women with lower levels of health literacy, and increased frequency of contact with participants, particularly in the gestational period.

Acknowledgements

The authors thank Debra Johnson, Donna Ransome, and Sarah Olender for their research support and the mothers who participated in this study.

Funding

This work was supported by the US Department of Agriculture, Agricultural Research Service [Project 6401–5300 003 00D] and in kind support from the Delta Health Alliance. The views expressed are solely those of the authors and do not reflect the official policy or position of the US government.

Authors' contributions

LMT-H participated in the development of the protocol, analytical framework for the study, data interpretation, and writing of the manuscript. JLT had primary responsibility for protocol development, participant screening, enrollment, outcome assessment, and data analysis and interpretation, and contributed to the writing of the manuscript. NOH contributed to data interpretation and the writing of the manuscript. MHG supervised the design and execution of the study, was responsible for enrollment, and contributed to data interpretation and the writing of the manuscript. ASL was responsible for outcome assessment and contributed to data interpretation and the writing of the manuscript. All authors read and approved the final manuscript.

Authors' information

No additional information to disclose.

Competing interests

The authors have no financial or competing interest to declare.

Author details

[1]Department of Medicine and Cancer Center, University of Illinois at Chicago, 416 West Side Research Office Building, 1747 West Roosevelt Road, Chicago, IL 60608, USA. [2]United States Department of Agriculture, Agricultural Research Service, Delta Human Nutrition Research Program, 141 Experiment Station Road, Stoneville, MS 38776, USA. [3]Department of Kinesiology and Nutrition, 484 West Side Research Office Building, 1747 West Roosevelt Road, Chicago, IL 60608, USA. [4]Department of Family and Consumer Sciences, University of Central Arkansas, 201 Donaghey Avenue, McAlister 113, Conway, AR 72035, USA.

References

1. Dosch NC, Guslits EF, Weber MB, Murray SE, Ha B, Coe CL, et al. Maternal obesity affects inflammatory and iron indices in umbilical cord blood. J Pediatr. 2016;172:20–8. PubMed PMID: 26970931

2. Rasmussen KM, Yaktine AL, editors. Weight gain during pregnancy: reexamining the guidelines. Washington (DC): The National Academies Collection: Reports funded by National Institutes of Health; 2009.

3. Vesco KK, Dietz PM, Rizzo J, Stevens VJ, Perrin NA, Bachman DJ, et al. Excessive gestational weight gain and postpartum weight retention among obese women. Obstet Gynecol. 2009;114(5):1069–75. PubMed PMID: 20168109

4. Nohr EA, Vaeth M, Baker JL, Sorensen T, Olsen J, Rasmussen KM. Combined associations of prepregnancy body mass index and gestational weight gain with the outcome of pregnancy. Am J Clin Nutr. 2008;87(6):1750–9. PubMed PMID: 18541565

5. Whiteman VE, Aliyu MH, August EM, McIntosh C, Duan J, Alio AP, et al. Changes in prepregnancy body mass index between pregnancies and risk of gestational and type 2 diabetes. Arch Gynecol Obstet. 2011;284(1):235–40. PubMed PMID: 21544736

6. Endres LK, Straub H, McKinney C, Plunkett B, Minkovitz CS, Schetter CD, et al. Postpartum weight retention risk factors and relationship to obesity at 1 year. Obstet Gynecol. 2015;125(1):144–52. PubMed PMID: 25560116. Pubmed Central PMCID: 4286308

7. Ehrlich SF, Hedderson MM, Feng J, Davenport ER, Gunderson EP, Ferrara A. Change in body mass index between pregnancies and the risk of gestational diabetes in a second pregnancy. Obstet Gynecol. 2011;117(6): 1323–30. PubMed PMID: 21606742. Pubmed Central PMCID: 3222684

8. Hoff GL, Cai J, Okah FA, Dew PC. Pre-pregnancy overweight status between successive pregnancies and pregnancy outcomes. J Women's Health. 2009;18(9):1413–7. PubMed PMID: 19698074

9. Cao C, Pressman EK, Cooper EM, Guillet R, Westerman M, O'Brien KO. Prepregnancy body mass index and gestational weight gain have no negative impact on maternal or neonatal iron status. Reprod Sci. 2016;23(5):613–22. PubMed PMID: 26423600

10. Deputy NP, Sharma AJ, Kim SY. Gestational weight gain - United States, 2012 and 2013. MMWR Morb Mortal Wkly Rep. 2015;64(43):1215–20. PubMed PMID: 26540367. Pubmed Central PMCID: 4862652

11. Shin D, Lee KW, Song WO. Pre-pregnancy weight status is associated with diet quality and nutritional biomarkers during pregnancy. Nutrients. 2016; 8(3):162. PubMed PMID: 26978398. Pubmed Central PMCID: 4808890

12. Davis EM, Babineau DC, Wang X, Zyzanski S, Abrams B, Bodnar LM, et al. Short inter-pregnancy intervals, parity, excessive pregnancy weight gain and risk of maternal obesity. Matern Child Health J. 2014;18(3):554–62. PubMed PMID: 23595566. Pubmed Central PMCID: 3840151

13. Phelan S, Phipps MG, Abrams B, Darroch F, Schaffner A, Wing RR. Randomized trial of a behavioral intervention to prevent excessive gestational weight gain: the fit for delivery study. Am J Clin Nutr. 2011;93(4): 772–9. PubMed PMID: 21310836. Pubmed Central PMCID: 3057546

14. Thangaratinam S, Rogozinska E, Jolly K, Glinkowski S, Roseboom T, Tomlinson JW, et al. Effects of interventions in pregnancy on maternal weight and obstetric outcomes: meta-analysis of randomised evidence. BMJ. 2012;344:e2088. PubMed PMID: 22596383. Pubmed Central PMCID: 3355191

15. Claesson IM, Sydsjo G, Brynhildsen J, Blomberg M, Jeppsson A, Sydsjo A, et al. Weight after childbirth: a 2-year follow-up of obese women in a weight-gain restriction program. Acta Obstet Gynecol Scand. 2011;90(1):103–10. PubMed PMID: 21275923

16. Huang TT, Yeh CY, Tsai YC. A diet and physical activity intervention for preventing weight retention among Taiwanese childbearing women: a randomised controlled trial. Midwifery. 2011;27(2):257–64. PubMed PMID: 19775782

17. Althuizen E, van der Wijden CL, van Mechelen W, Seidell JC, van Poppel MN. The effect of a counselling intervention on weight changes during and after pregnancy: a randomised trial. BJOG : an international journal of obstetrics and gynaecology. 2013;120(1):92–9. PubMed PMID: 23121074

18. Liu J, Wilcox S, Whitaker K, Blake C, Addy C. Preventing excessive weight gain during pregnancy and promoting postpartum weight loss: a pilot lifestyle intervention for overweight and obese African American women. Matern Child Health J. 2015;19(4):840–9. PubMed PMID: 25051907. Pubmed Central PMCID: 4305038

19. Wilkinson SA, van der Pligt P, Gibbons KS, McIntyre HD. Trial for reducing weight retention in new mums: a randomised controlled trial evaluating a low intensity, postpartum weight management programme. Journal of human nutrition and dietetics : the official journal of the British Dietetic Association. 2015;28(Suppl 1):15–28. PubMed PMID: 24267102

20. Thomson JL, Tussing-Humphreys LM, Goodman MH. Delta healthy sprouts: a randomized comparative effectiveness trial to promote maternal weight control and reduce childhood obesity in the Mississippi Delta. Contemporary clinical trials. 2014;38(1):82–91. PubMed PMID: 24685997

21. Thomson JL, Tussing-Humphreys LM, Goodman MH, Olender SE. Gestational weight gain: results from the Delta healthy sprouts comparative impact trial. J Pregnancy. 2016;2016:5703607. PubMed PMID: 27595023. Pubmed Central PMCID: 4993958

22. Witheiss GA, Lovelady CA, West DG, Brouwer RJ, Krause KM, Ostbye T. Diet quality and weight change among overweight and obese postpartum women enrolled in a behavioral intervention program. J Acad Nutr Diet. 2013;113(1): 54–62. PubMed PMID: 23146549. Pubmed Central PMCID: 3529806

23. Recommendations to prevent and control iron deficiency in the United States. Centers for Disease Control and Prevention. MMWR Recommendations and reports : Morbidity and mortality weekly report Recommendations and reports. 1998;47(RR-3):1–29. PubMed PMID: 9563847

24. Bandura A. Human agency in social cognitive theory. The American psychologist. 1989;44(9):1175–84. PubMed PMID: 2782727

25. Prochaska JO, Velicer WF. The transtheoretical model of health behavior change. Am J Health Promot. 1997;12(1):38–48. PubMed PMID: 10170434

26. Knowler WC, Barrett-Connor E, Fowler SE, Hamman RF, Lachin JM, Walker EA, et al. Reduction in the incidence of type 2 diabetes with lifestyle intervention or metformin. N Engl J Med. 2002;346(6):393–403. PubMed PMID: 11832527. Pubmed Central PMCID: 1370926. Epub 2002/02/08. eng

27. Campbell KJ, Lioret S, McNaughton SA, Crawford DA, Salmon J, Ball K, et al. A parent-focused intervention to reduce infant obesity risk behaviors: a randomized trial. Pediatrics. 2013;131(4):652–60. PubMed PMID: 23460688. Epub 2013/03/06. eng

28. Nowak AJ, Casamassimo PS. Using anticipatory guidance to provide early dental intervention. J Am Dent Assoc. 1995;126(8):1156–63. PubMed PMID: 7560574. Epub 1995/08/01. eng

29. Mullis F. Active parenting: an evaluation of two Adlerian parent education programs. J Individ Psychol. 1999;55:359–64.

30. Feskanich D, Sielaff BH, Chong K, Buzzard IM. Computerized collection and analysis of dietary intake information. Comput Methods Prog Biomed. 1989; 30(1):47–57. PubMed PMID: 2582746

31. Guenther PM, Casavale KO, Reedy J, Kirkpatrick SI, Hiza HA, Kuczynski KJ, et al. Update of the healthy eating index: HEI-2010. J Acad Nutr Diet. 2013; 113(4):569–80. PubMed PMID: 23415502. Pubmed Central PMCID: 3810369

32. Chasan-Taber L, Schmidt MD, Roberts DE, Hosmer D, Markenson G, Freedson PS. Development and validation of a pregnancy physical activity questionnaire. Med Sci Sports Exerc. 2004;36(10):1750–60. PubMed PMID: 15595297. Epub 2004/12/15. eng

33. ACOG Committee Opinion No. 650. Physical activity and exercise during pregnancy and the postpartum period. Obstet Gynecol. 2015;126(6):e135–42. PubMed PMID: 26595585

34. Althuizen E, van Poppel MN, Seidell JC, van der Wijden C, van Mechelen W. Design of the new Life(style) study: a randomised controlled trial to optimise maternal weight development during pregnancy. [ISRCTN85313483]. BMC Public Health. 2006;6:168. PubMed PMID: 16800869. Pubmed Central PMCID: 1523339

35. van der Pligt P, Willcox J, Hesketh KD, Ball K, Wilkinson S, Crawford D, et al. Systematic review of lifestyle interventions to limit postpartum weight retention: implications for future opportunities to prevent maternal overweight and obesity following childbirth. Obesity reviews : an official journal of the International Association for the Study of Obesity. 2013;14(10):792–805. PubMed PMID: 23773448

36. Bertz F, Brekke HK, Ellegard L, Rasmussen KM, Wennergren M, Winkvist A. Diet and exercise weight-loss trial in lactating overweight and obese women. Am J Clin Nutr. 2012;96(4):698–705. PubMed PMID: 22952179

37. Colleran HL, Lovelady CA. Use of MyPyramid menu planner for moms in a weight-loss intervention during lactation. J Acad Nutr Diet. 2012;112(4):553–8. PubMed PMID: 22709705

38. Davenport MH, Giroux I, Sopper MM, Mottola MF. Postpartum exercise regardless of intensity improves chronic disease risk factors. Med Sci Sports

Exerc. 2011;43(6):951–8. PubMed PMID: 21085038

39. Leermakers EA, Anglin K, Wing RR. Reducing postpartum weight retention through a correspondence intervention. International journal of obesity and related metabolic disorders : journal of the International Association for the Study of Obesity. 1998;22(11):1103–9. PubMed PMID: 9822949

40. McCrory MA, Nommsen-Rivers LA, Mole PA, Lonnerdal B, Dewey KG. Randomized trial of the short-term effects of dieting compared with dieting plus aerobic exercise on lactation performance. Am J Clin Nutr. 1999;69(5): 959–67. PubMed PMID: 10232637

41. O'Toole ML, Sawicki MA, Artal R. Structured diet and physical activity prevent postpartum weight retention. J Women's Health. 2003;12(10):991–8. PubMed PMID: 14709187

42. Lanpher MG, Askew S, Bennett GG. Health literacy and weight change in a digital health intervention for women: a randomized controlled trial in primary care practice. J Health Commun. 2016;21(Suppl 1):34–42. PubMed PMID: 27043756. Pubmed Central PMCID: 4935541

43. Phelan S, Phipps MG, Abrams B, Darroch F, Grantham K, Schaffner A, et al. Does behavioral intervention in pregnancy reduce postpartum weight retention? Twelve-month outcomes of the fit for delivery randomized trial. Am J Clin Nutr. 2014;99(2):302–11. PubMed PMID: 24284438. Pubmed Central PMCID: 3893723

44. Thomson JL, Tussing-Humphreys LM, Goodman MH, Olender S. Baseline demographic, anthropometric, psychosocial, and behavioral characteristics of rural, southern women in early pregnancy. Matern Child Health J. 2016;20(9):1980–8. PubMed PMID: 27146396

45. Vesco KK, Leo MC, Karanja N, Gillman MW, McEvoy CT, King JC, et al. One-year postpartum outcomes following a weight management intervention in pregnant women with obesity. Obesity. 2016;24(10):2042–9. PubMed PMID: 27670399. Pubmed Central PMCID: 5084910

46. Ostbye T, Krause KM, Lovelady CA, Morey MC, Bastian LA, Peterson BL, et al. Active mothers postpartum: a randomized controlled weight-loss intervention trial. Am J Prev Med. 2009;37(3):173–80. PubMed PMID: 19595557. Pubmed Central PMCID: 2774935

47. Salvy SJ, de la Haye K, Galama T, Goran MI. Home visitation programs: an untapped opportunity for the delivery of early childhood obesity prevention. Obesity reviews : an official journal of the International Association for the Study of Obesity. 2017;18(2):149–63. PubMed PMID: 27911984. Pubmed Central PMCID: 5267322

13

Neonatal mortality and causes of death in Kersa Health and Demographic Surveillance System (Kersa HDSS), Ethiopia, 2008–2013

Nega Assefa[1]* (iD), Yihune Lakew[2], Betelhem Belay[1], Haji Kedir[1], Desalew Zelalem[1], Negga Baraki[1], Melake Damena[1], Lemessa Oljira[1], Wondimye Ashenafi[1] and Melkamu Dedefo[1,3]

Abstract

Background: In the world, Neonatal mortality accounts for 40 % of death of children under the age of 5 years. Majority of neonatal deaths occur in developing countries outside of formal health system, among which death in the first hour of first day of their life constitute the huge bulk. This analysis is intended to estimate neonatal mortality rates and identify the leading causes of death based on the surveillance data over 6 years period in Kersa health and demographic surveillance system (Kersa HDSS) site, Eastern Ethiopia.

Methods: Kersa HDSS is an open dynamic cohort of population established in 2007. The surveillance started after conducting a baseline census followed by population update and events registration on house-to-house visits every 6 months. Data were collected using verbal autopsy (VA) questionnaire from close relatives (usually mothers in this case) and causes of deaths were assigned by 2 to 3 physicians. This analysis was done based on 301 neonatal deaths and 10,934 live births occurred during 2008 to 2013.

Results: The overall neonatal death rate during the study period was 27.5 per 1000 live births. Nearly all neonatal deaths (94 %) occurred at home. More than four-fifth (82.4 %) of the deaths was occurred in the first week of life. More than 80 % of the deaths were due to perinatal causes. Bacterial sepsis of the newborn accounted for 31.2 % followed by birth asphyxia and perinatal respiratory disorder (28.2 %), and prematurity (17.3 %). Higher number of death was observed in Tolla and Bereka sub-districts located at the southern parts of the study site which are away from the main road network.

Conclusion: The overall neonatal mortality over 6 years is the same to the national average (27 per 1000 live births). The leading causes of neonatal death were bacterial sepsis of newborn and birth asphyxia. Community-based skilled health care delivery during birth should be emphasized.

Keywords: Neonatal deaths, Causes of death, Verbal autopsy, Kersa HDSS, Ethiopia

Background

Under 5 mortality remains 1 of the biggest public health concern constituting $7 \cdot 2$ million in 2011, of which $2 \cdot 2$ million were early neonatal, and $0 \cdot 7$ million late neonatal deaths [1]. Neonatal deaths account for 40 % of under 5 mortality [2]. Based on data collected from 193 countries in 2012, the global and Sub-Saharan neonatal mortality rate was 21 and 32 per 1000 live births, respectively.

About 99 % of neonatal deaths were from low and middle income countries, of which 66 % (1.16 million deaths) are in Africa and Southeast Asia [3].

In the same report, the top 5 countries with the greatest number of neonatal deaths were India, Nigeria, Pakistan, China, and Democratic Republic of Congo. According to the 2013 and 2014 report, Ethiopia ranked 6th in neonatal deaths [3, 4]. The 2012-2014 global data indicated that the 3 major causes of neonatal death were preterm birth complications (35 %), neonatal infections (23 %) and intrapartum related complications (23 %).

* Correspondence: negaassefa@yahoo.com
[1]College of Health and Medical Sciences, Haramaya University, P.O.Box 1494, Harar, Ethiopia
Full list of author information is available at the end of the article

These causes account for nearly 80 % of deaths in this age group [3–8].

Majority of the neonatal deaths in developing countries occur outside the formal health system. As a result, many studies on the causes of death of children under the age of 5 excluded neonatal deaths mainly for 2 reasons; 1 is poor reporting on a sign and symptoms that leads to death and the other is the number of cases reported is very small in number. To resolve this, some researchers tried to group neonatal deaths as 'other' childhood or 'perinatal' causes, which has created difficulty to identify causes deaths associated with the neonatal [9]. Recently, several studies have focused exclusively on the use of VA for the newborn deaths, making this an opportune time to assess the current state of knowledge and provide direction for future research efforts [10].

In Ethiopia, due to the absence of vital event registration, most deaths are left undocumented. As the vast majority of deaths occur outside the health system, the ability of health facilities to generate representative statistics is limited in the country [9]. In this regard, the use of verbal autopsy (VA) from health and demographic surveillance system is the most promising interim solution for this problem [11–13].

Reducing under 5 mortality rate by two third was Millennium Development Goal number 5 (MDG-5) that ends in 2015 and Ethiopia is 1 of the countries achieved this goal. However, the rates disaggregated by age showed that neonatal mortality continues to be suspended high with little or no sign of reduction over years [5, 14]. Focusing on under-five mortality in general and neonatal mortality in particular continues to be the focus during Sustainable Development Goal (SDG) period [15].

Consistent to the SDG goals, Ethiopia has also developed a health sector strategic plan to direct its health intervention through 2035. In this plan, the country aspires to be a middle income country averting unnecessary neonatal mortality [16]. Therefore, it is imperative to substantiate with findings on the ground if the country is in the right direction over the years bench marking the end period of MDG.

Hence, information generated using the existing data from Kersa HDSS will help in providing estimate of neonatal mortality and the leading causes of death to support evidence-based decision making at different levels.

Methods

Kersa HDSS Site

The site was established in September 2007 and located at the eastern Hararge of the Oromyia regional state in eastern Ethiopia. The district capital, Kersa, is located 44 km from Harar, west direction. The district has 3 climatic zones with the altitude ranging from 1400 to 3200 meters above sea level (Fig. 1). This surveillance site covers 12 kebeles, the lowest administrative units (2 urban and 10 rural) from 38 randomly selected kebeles (As of January 2015, it is increased to 24 Kebeles). The site started its surveillance on 10,256 households and 52,470 population in 2007 and by 2013, the population has increased to 62,550. In the move to double the size of population and households under surveillance, by 2015, as the number of Kebeles doubled from 12 to 24, the size of the population has increased to 129,000 and the number of households to 27,000. Kersa HDSS is a member of INDEPTH network of Health and Demographic Surveillance System (HDSS) sites in the world [17]. In Kersa HDSS, there are a total of 19 health facilities; including 4 health centers, 10 health posts and 5 clinics. There are 7 research team members, 22 vital events enumerators, 4 verbal autopsy interviewers (VAIs), 5 field supervisors, 2 data managers, and 6 data clerks [18].

Study design and population

Kersa HDSS is an open dynamic cohort study design that longitudinally follow a well-defined entities or primary subjects (individuals, households, and residential units) and all related socio-demographic and health related outcomes within a clearly defined geographic area. The surveillance was started by conducting a baseline census of the population including housing and socio-economic characteristics. Then, population update and events registration on house-to-house visits to register all pregnancy observations and outcomes, deaths, marriage and in-and-out migration has been done every 6 months. Subsequently, any causes of death in the population from registered deaths were identified using Verbal Autopsy (VA) [18].

Verbal autopsy questionnaire

There are 3 verbal autopsy forms (deaths up to 28 completed days of life-neonatal deaths; deaths to children between 4 weeks and 14 years of age; and deaths to persons aged 15 years and above), adopted from the 2007 standardized World Health Organization (WHO) questionnaires [19–21]. The verbal autopsy forms and questionnaire was translated in to Oromefa language for use in the field. The questionnaires were used for collecting information, such as, age, sex, place of death, sign and symptoms observed during the late life period of the deceased. In addition, a short narrative history of the course of disease that leads to death, health services used in the period before death, and documentation of any medical evidence available at the household, including whether a health worker informed the respondent of the cause of death. Particularly, for the neonatal form, the condition of the mother during and after pregnancy and birth was used. The questionnaire also contain the

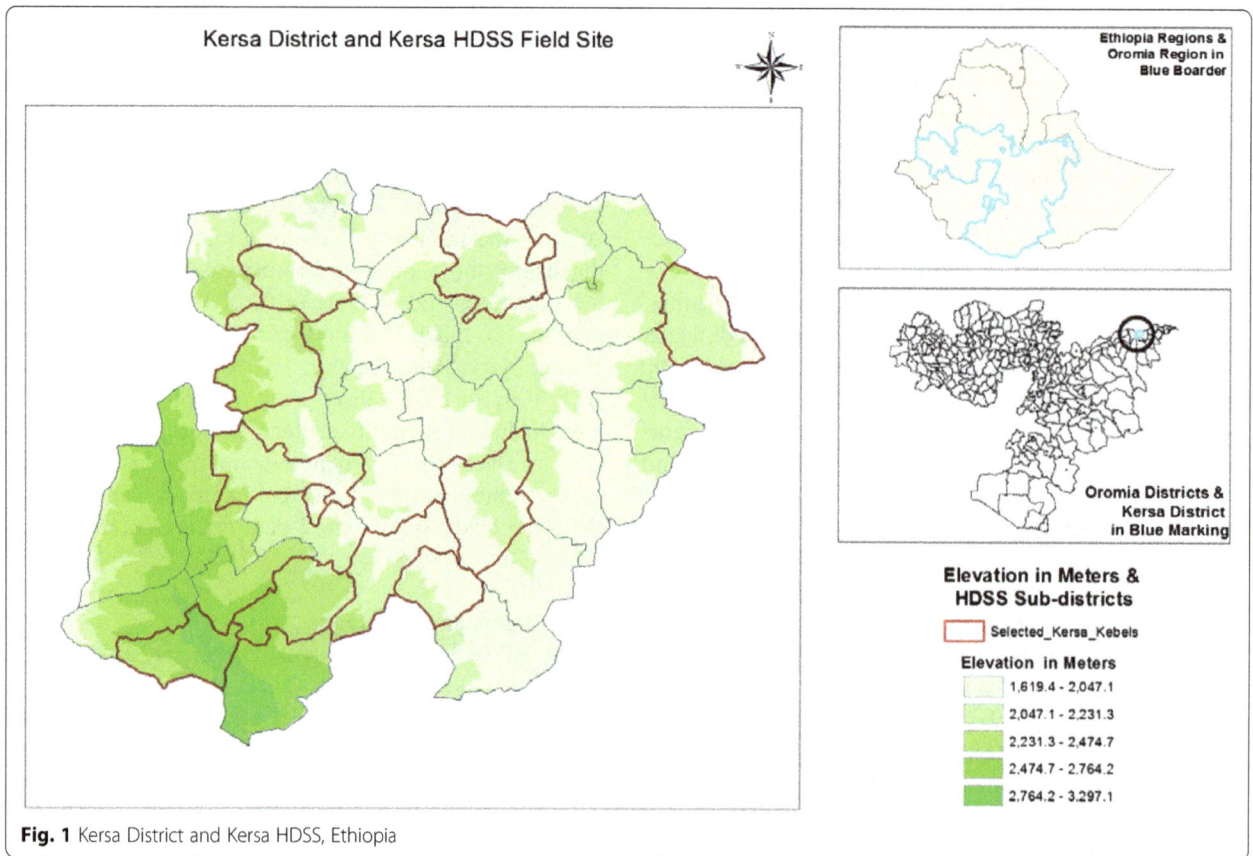

Fig. 1 Kersa District and Kersa HDSS, Ethiopia

symptom duration checklist arranged loosely around anatomical systems and are intended to be as informative as possible in leading a positive diagnosis of probable cause of death, as well as, the confident exclusion of differential diagnoses [18].

VA data collection procedure

The process begins with a report of a death occurring to a resident of the area by the local data collectors. The regular vital event interviewers receive these reports and maintain records of deaths that occur in their working areas using event recording form. The information in the death event recording form is later transferred to death registration book that is kept in the field office for referral purpose. Copy of the recording form with location information is given to the VA interviewer to complete the VA interview after the appropriate mourning period. The vital event interviewers help the VA interviewers to arrange an appointment with the family of the deceased to conduct the VA interview. This was within 1-3 months after a death with due consideration to culturally appropriate mourning periods. On the day of interview, the VA interviewer arrives at the residence of the deceased to conduct the interview with an adult person (with a mother in this case) at the deceased households. When it is difficult to get a reliable respondent, the VA interviewer

arranges an appointment to visit the household on another day when a more informed respondent will be available. Up to 3 attempts were made to conduct an interview if the information given is incomplete after 3 visits, the VA interviewer completes the VA form with the information that is available. A note that the interview is incomplete due to the absence of reliable respondents was made on the form in the 'history of events' section. These events are counted as deaths in the system, although the cause of death will remain unknown. Again, every section of the form was filled in accurately before the form is submitted to the research team for onward processing.

Causes of death assignment

Two physicians, trained in VA diagnosis and coding procedures for the study, assigned codes and titles, up to 3 causes of death (underlying, immediate and contributing factor) independently using information contained in VA forms based on the WHO International Classification of Disease-10 (ICD-10) and VA code system. After checking agreements of physician assigned underlying cause of death based on VA coding discordant cases were sent to the third physician again for independent review and diagnosis. If any of 2 of these 3 physicians assigned an underlying cause of death to the same VA code, this was considered as the final cause of death; otherwise, the causes were labeled as undetermined. In the analysis, 18 cases (6 %) cause of death were not determined based on the 3 physician report.

VA data quality controls

Individuals who have completed at least a high school education and who have been working in the field during the last 1 year was continued to work as VA interviewers. They received 3 days training on the questionnaires, recording, contacting close relatives and data collection procedures. The training curriculum include sessions on discussion of individual symptoms, and their description in local language for easy recognition by the respondents and demonstration of interviewing techniques by research team members. The VA interviewer was informed about new deaths by the resident enumerators and conduct verbal autopsy interviews. Researcher team members coordinate the field activities of all vital events registration and VA interviewers are responsible for making sure that the field operations run smoothly and efficiently and also give supervisory support to events data collectors and VA interviewers. During the course of the fieldwork, supervisors continually visit the sites to check on the progress and sort out problems that may have been encountered by enumerators.

Data management and analysis

Neonatal mortality rate was calculated using the total neonatal death divided by total number of births during the 6 years period. Causes of death were analyzed by some basic socio-demographic characteristics. Tables and graphs were used to summarize and present the data. STATA version 11 software and excel sheet were used for data analysis. Geographic Information System (GIS) mapping is used to plot the extent of death over the map against the sub-district cumulative deaths. Cross tabulations of death events by sex, age and other background characteristics was provided. 95 % confidence interval for neonatal death rate is calculated for sub districts and p-value for 0.05 is taken to determine level of significance.

Ethical approval

Kersa HDSS site has received ethical clearance from the Ethiopian Science and Technology Agency, Ethiopian Public Health Association (EPHA), US Center for Disease Control and Prevention (CDC) and the Health Research Ethics Review Committee (HRERC) of Haramaya University. To capture occurrence of vital events to any family member, head of a family or an eligible adult among the family was interviewed. Therefore, informed verbal consent was obtained from head of the family or eligible adult among the family. This consent procedure was stated in the proposal which was approved by the ethical review committee. To keep confidentiality, data containing personal identifiers of subjects were not shared to third party.

Results

During the period from 2008 to 2013, a total of 301 neonatal deaths were recorded. The lowest proportions of neonatal deaths were observed in 2012 (13.0 %) and in 2013 (13.0 %). The highest proportion of neonatal deaths were seen in 2009 (20.9 %) and in 2010 (20.6 %) (Table 1). As shown in Table 2, the overall neonatal death rate in the study period was 27.5 per 1000 live births.

Over the 6 years period (2008-2013) 61 % of the deceased were male neonates and 39 % were females. Among the deceased neonates, more than four-fifth (82.4 %) of the deaths occurred in the first week of birth and the rest were in the remaining 3 weeks of neonatal period.

Table 1 Demographic characteristics of the deceased by surveillance years, Kersa HDSS site in Ethiopia

Background characteristics	Surveillance years and number of neonatal deaths							
	2008	2009	2010	2011	2012	2013	2008–2013	
	n	n	n	n	n	n	n	Death fraction with 95 % CI
Residence								
Urban	3	3	1	9	0	1	17	5.6 [3.44–8.71]
Rural	44	60	61	42	39	38	284	94.4 [91.29–96.56]
Sex								
Male	28	34	44	32	23	23	184	61.1 [55.53–66.52]
Female	19	29	18	19	16	16	117	38.9 [33.48–44.47]
Age at death								
0–7 days	47	53	52	41	29	26	248	82.4 [77.78–86.39]
8–28 days	0	10	10	10	10	13	53	17.6 [13.61–22.25]
Total	47	63	62	51	39	39	301	

Table 2 Neonatal death rate over the study period between 2008 and 2013, Kersa HDSS in Ethiopia

Surveillance years	Neonatal deaths	Live births	NMR with 95 % CI
2008	47	1616	29.1 [21.7–38.2]
2009	63	1756	35.9 [27.9–45.4]
2010	62	1983	31.3 [24.3–39.6]
2011	51	1549	32.9 [24.9–42.7]
2012	39	1770	22.0 [15.9–29.7]
2013	39	2260	17.3 [12.5–23.3]
2008–2013	301	10,934	27.5 [24.6–30.7]

NMR-Neonatal Mortality Rate

Although it shows persistent decline, the pattern of neonatal and early neonatal death rates over the course of the study period was significantly higher than late neonatal death rates. The late neonatal death rate remains relatively constant over the study period with no declining pattern (Table 2 and Fig. 2).

Over the 6 years period, a statistically significant higher death rate was observed among male newborns compared to female newborns. The gap in male and female newborn deaths was highest in 2010. A decreasing pattern was also documented in both male and female newborn death rates over the study period (Fig. 3).

Of the total neonatal deaths observed during the 6 years period, the vast majority (94.4 %) occurred in rural parts of the study area, and only 17 (5.6 %) were occurred in urban areas. Nearly all neonatal deaths (94 %) occurred at home and the remaining were in hospital and health centers. As depicted in Fig. 4, over the study period, a relatively highest neonatal death rate was recorded in 2 villages of Bereka and Tolla followed by other neighboring villages that are located in southern parts of the study site.

Causes of neonatal deaths

Based on the broad classification of causes of neonatal deaths, more than 80 % of the deaths were due to perinatal causes. Deaths due to circulatory diseases, external causes and gastro-intestinal diseases account for only 1 % of neonatal deaths while 3.3 %, 6 %, and 6.3 % of neonatal deaths were due to infectious or parasitic diseases, undetermined causes and unspecified causes, respectively (Fig. 5).

With regard to the specific causes of neonatal death, bacterial sepsis of the newborn accounts for 31.2 %, while it is closely followed by birth asphyxia and perinatal respiratory disorder (28.2 %), and prematurity (17.3 %). Other causes of deaths are other diseases related to the perinatal period (3.3 %) and acute lower respiratory infection (2.7 %) (Table 3).

As part of neonatal causes, the leading causes of death for early neonatal period (from birth to 7 days) were birth asphyxia and perinatal respiratory disorder (33.1 %), bacterial sepsis of newborn follows (24.2 %) and prematurity (including respiratory distress) (20.2 %) (Table 4). The late neonatal (8-28 days) causes of deaths where dominated by bacterial sepsis of newborn (64.2 %) and acute lower respiratory infection including pneumonia (7.5 %) (Table 5). As indicated in Table 6, over the study period, in most of the Kebeles, the leading causes of neonatal death were bacterial sepsis of newborn, birth asphyxia and prematurity including respiratory distress.

Discussion

The cumulative average neonatal mortality rate was 27 per 1000 live births. This is lower than many of the reports from countries in Africa and other developing countries in Asia like Pakistan and Bangladesh [3, 4, 22–25]. The rate reported by the present study is consistent to the

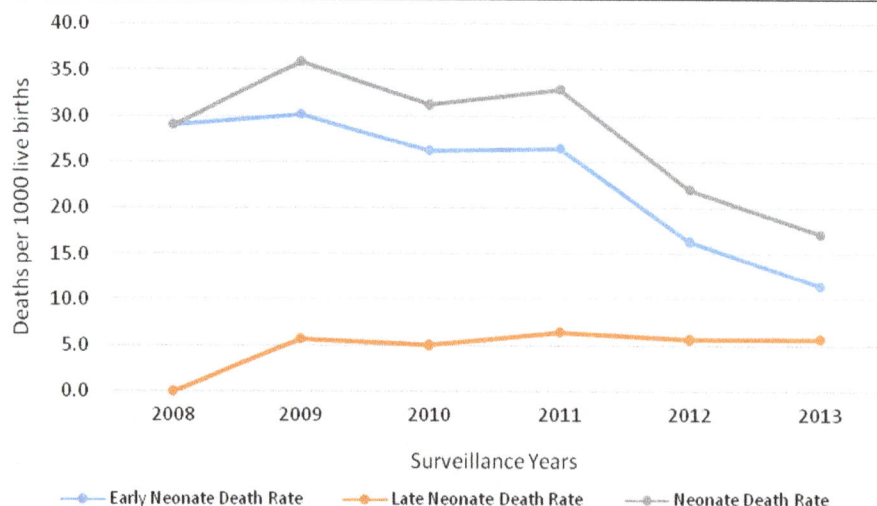

Fig. 2 Pattern of Neonatal death rates over years (2008–2013), Kersa HDSS, Ethiopia

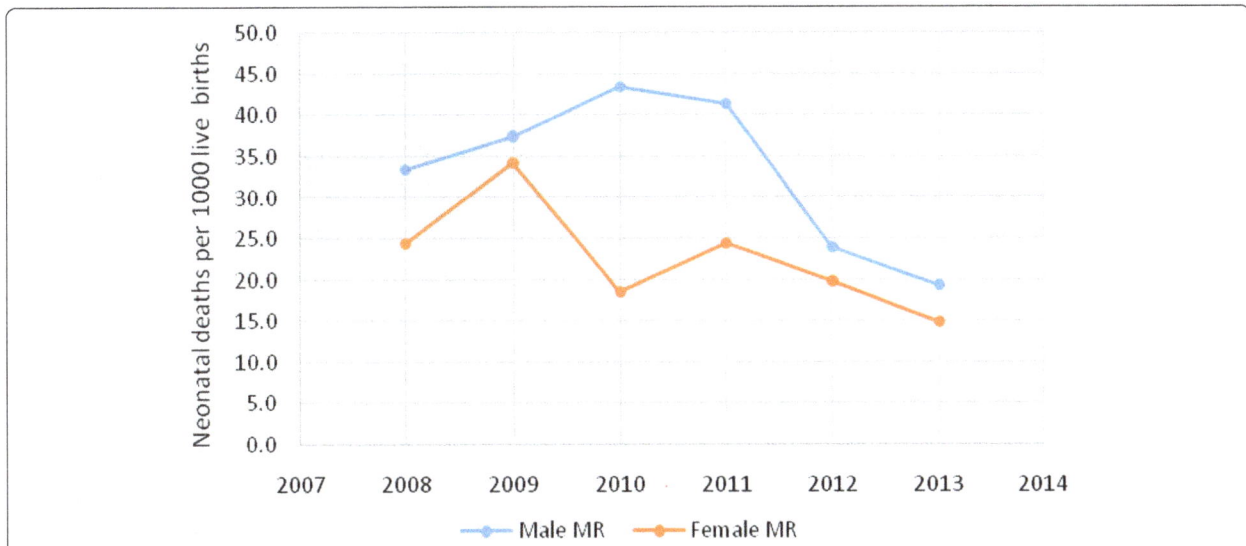

Fig. 3 Difference between male and female neonatal death over the years (2008–2013), Kersa HDSS, Ethiopia

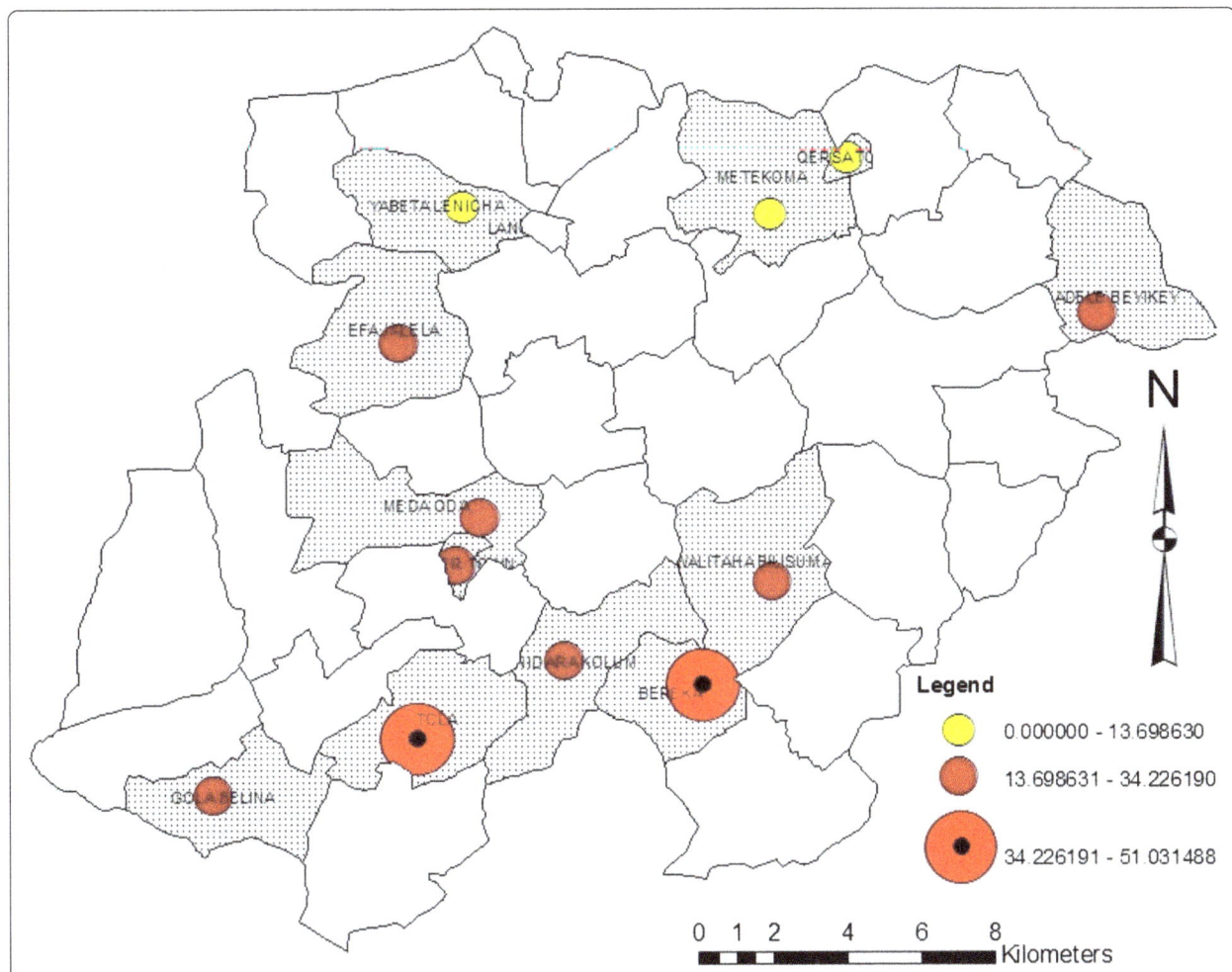

Fig. 4 Sum of 2008–2013 Neonatal death rate distribution in sub-districts of Kersa HDSS, Ethiopia

Causes	%
Perinatal causes	83.4
Unspecified causes	6.3
Undermined causes	6.0
Infectious and parasitic diseases	3.3
Others*	1.0

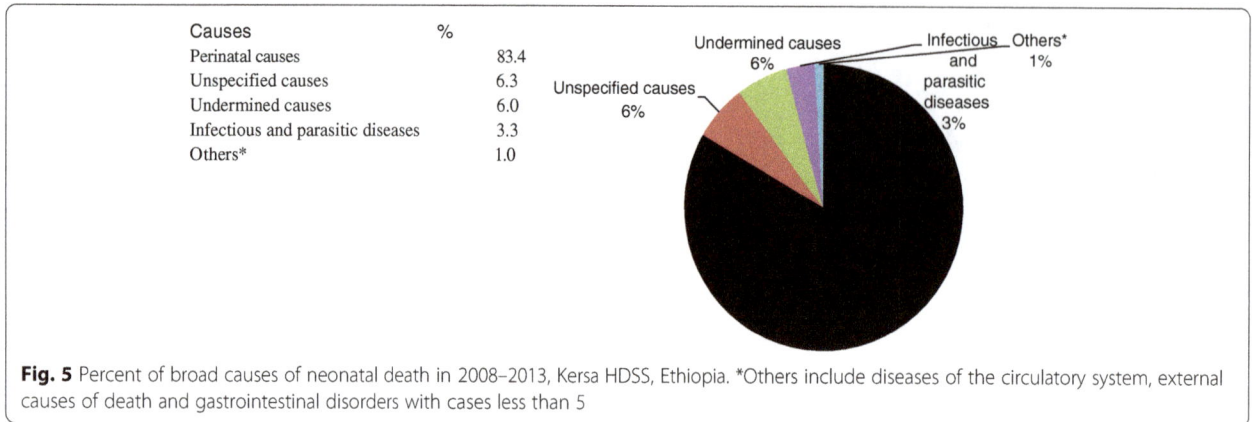

Fig. 5 Percent of broad causes of neonatal death in 2008–2013, Kersa HDSS, Ethiopia. *Others include diseases of the circulatory system, external causes of death and gastrointestinal disorders with cases less than 5

previous study in south west Ethiopia around Bonke district of Gamo Gofa zone [26], however it is lower than the 35.5 per 1000 live births that has been recently reported from southwest Ethiopia around Jimma Zone [27]. The differences in the reports could be attributed to the timing and differences in the settings of the 2 studies. The lower level of neonatal mortality in the present study could be partly explained due to the fact that the present study was conducted on health and demographic surveillance site (HDSS) and the population in such setting could have better awareness about the health issues. The neonatal mortality rate seems to reduce over the study period, however, the level of cumulative average of neonatal mortality observed in this study is nearly what is considered to be high and calls for policy attention [28].

The findings revealed that neonatal deaths observed over 6 years period were mainly males that nearly

accounted for 3 out of 5 neonatal deaths and most deaths occurred at home and among the rural part of the study area. This is in agreement with other reports from elsewhere and in Ethiopia [23, 29]. Consistent to other studies, most of neonatal deaths occurred during the first 7 days of birth [8, 22, 30, 31]. Most neonatal deaths occurred at home and during the first week of life imply that the observed level of neonatal mortality could be attributed to lack of skilled birth assistance as home deliveries are the major place of delivery in the study area [32, 33]. The absence of neonatal Intensive Care Unit (ICU) in the area has also contributed for unabated neonatal mortality.

The study also revealed that sepsis, birth asphyxia and prematurity accounted for three-fourth or more of early neonatal deaths, while sepsis is the commonest cause of late neonatal death, contributing to more than 60 % of neonatal deaths occurring to this age group. These are

Table 3 Specific neonatal causes of death from 2008–2013, Kersa HDSS in Ethiopia

Causes of death	2008–2013	
	Deaths	Cause of death fraction with 95 % CI
Acute lower respiratory infection	8	2.7 [1.24–4.98]
Bacterial sepsis of newborn	94	31.2 [26.18–36–64]
Birth asphyxia and perinatal respiratory disorder	85	28.2 [23.37–33.53]
Other diseases related to the perinatal period	10	3.3 [1.70–5.84]
Prematurity (including respiratory distress)	52	17.3 [13.32–21.86]
Others [a]	15	5.0 [2.92–7.91]
Undetermined cause of death	18	6.0 [3.70–9.11]
Unspecified causes of death	19	6.3 [3.96–9.51]
Total	301	

[a] Birth trauma, congenital malformation, other and unspecified, congenital malformation of nervous system, congestive heart failure, contact with unspecified venomous animal or plant, intestinal infectious diseases including diarrhea, neonatal pneumonia and tetanus neonatorum with cases less than 5

Table 4 Specific early neonatal causes of death from 2008–2013, Kersa HDSS in Ethiopia

Causes of death	2008–2013	
	Deaths	Cause of death fraction with 95 % CI
Bacterial sepsis of newborn	60	24.2 [19.17–29.84]
Birth asphyxia and perinatal respiratory disorder	82	33.1 [27.42–39.10]
Other diseases related to the perinatal period	8	3.2 [1.51–6.03]
Prematurity (including respiratory distress)	50	20.2 [15.52–25.50
Others [a]	17	6.9 [4.18–10.53]
Undetermined causes of death	15	6.0 [3.56–9.56]
Unspecified causes of death	16	6.5 [3.87–10.05]
Total	248	

[a] Acute lower respiration including pneumonia, birth trauma, congenital malformation of the nervous system, contact with unspecified venomous animal, intestinal infectious diseases including diarrhea, neonatal pneumonia and tetanus neonatorum

Table 5 Specific late neonatal causes of death from 2008–2013, Kersa HDSS in Ethiopia

Causes of death	2008–2013	
	Deaths	Cause of death fraction with 95 % CI
Acute lower respiratory infection including pneumonia	4	7.5
Bacterial sepsis of newborn	34	64.2
Birth asphyxia and perinatal respiratory disorder	3	5.7
Congenital malformation, other and unspecified	1	1.9
Congestive heart failure	1	1.9
Other diseases related to the perinatal period	2	3.8
Prematurity (including respiratory distress)	2	3.8
Undetermined causes of death	3	5.7
Unspecified causes of death	3	5.7
Total	53	100.0

consistent to the previous reports on the cause of neonatal mortality [4, 5, 8, 24, 26].

Recently, other studies have indicated that sepsis is the major cause of late neonatal death [5]. Delivery complications are associated with odds of neonatal deaths. The world Health organization estimated the most direct causes of neonatal deaths to be preterm birth, severe infection and asphyxia [34].

Previous research from Bangladesh [25], Tanzania [35] Pakistan [36] and Ethiopia [27] have consistently established that birth asphyxia is 1 of the major causes of death. These findings imply that most of the neonatal deaths are mainly due to lack of access to skilled birth assistance and complications of labor and delivery.

The report also indicted the highest number of deaths in the southern part of the district in Tola and Baraka villages. These villages are away from the main road and their access to health care is limited due to terrain and poor feeding road network. This is an important implication to further focus on community based skilled birth attendants in resource limited setting.

Ethiopia has strived to reach every family with basic health service using a home born strategy referred to as 'Health Extension Program" [37, 38]. The health extension program is designed to provide basic health promotion activities principally to the rural community. Though, the services rendered by this program are sixteen health promotion packages including family planning, antenatal, delivery and postnatal care [39, 40], the toll of neonatal death at the early days of neonatal life persists.

Reports on the rate and cause of neonatal death helps countries to track their performance towards the set national and international targets [15, 16]. Many of the earlier reports are based on estimates of data from clinical setting, which doesn't represent the health condition in the general population. This report is based on a verbal autopsy for the deceased neonates from the ongoing health and demographic surveillance system in the rural Ethiopia; hence it gives a good bench mark to track the performance of SDG and Ethiopian health sector strategic plan in the future.

The verbal autopsy generate information through conversations with family members of the deceased, the VA method uses information on circumstances leading to death, including symptoms and signs during terminal illness to assign causes of death [41–45]. The VA method has been used in different resource constraint countries to develop a viable mid or long-term strategy for improving neonatal mortality. It is a popular and reliable method for community diagnoses of major causes of death in developing countries, where majority of the

Table 6 Neonatal death rates and leading causes per Kebele in the period from 2008–2013, Kersa HDSS site

Study villages	Deaths	LB	NNM rate	Leading causes of death (COD)
Qersa town	5	397	12.6	Bacterial sepsis of newborn
Metekoma	10	730	13.7	Bacterial sepsis of newborn
Yabeta Lencha	8	920	8.7	Bacterial sepsis of newborn
Ifa Jalela	30	1113	27.0	Prematurity including Respiratory Distress (RD)
Mede Oda	23	850	27.1	Bacterial sepsis of newborn and prematurity RD
Weter Town	12	529	22.7	Bacterial sepsis of newborn and birth asphyxia
Handhura Kossum	33	1249	26.4	Bacterial sepsis of newborn and birth asphyxia
Tolla	47	921	51.0	Bacterial sepsis of newborn and birth asphyxia
Gola Belina	23	672	34.2	Bacterial sepsis of newborn and birth asphyxia
Bereka	32	645	49.6	Birth asphyxia
Walteha Bilisuma	29	1378	21.0	Bacterial sepsis of newborn
Adele Key Key	49	1530	32.0	Birth asphyxia

deaths occur at home. It has been demonstrated to produce valid estimates of cause-specific mortality fractions in many settings [11].

Limitations of this method are problem of remembering the state of health condition for someone during the late periods of life that introduce recall bias, the reported health problems might not be exactly the same conditions felt by the deceased that introduce reporting error, and the agreement of physician to diagnose based on reported health condition might introduced misclassification. In order to reduce these errors it was advised to collect the information from close relatives with the best knowledge relatives could remember, in this case from the mother or father of the baby [12, 23, 27, 44, 45].

Conclusion
The cumulative neonatal mortality over 6 year period is 27 per 1000 live birth. Over years it showed a little decline without significant difference between subsequent years. Early neonatal death contributed to majority of the neonatal deaths. Perinatal causes of death; sepsis, birth asphyxia and prematurity accounted for three-fourth or more of early neonatal deaths, while sepsis is the commonest cause of late neonatal death. Increasing access to skilled birth attendant in the community setting through the health extension program by improving the approach to delivery service could avert preventable neonatal deaths.

Abbreviations
CDC, Center for Disease Control and Prevention; EPHA, Ethiopian Public Health Association; GIS, Geographic Information System; HDSS, Health and Demographic Surveillance System; HRERC, Health Research Ethics Review Committee; ICD-10, International Classification of Disease-10; MDG, Millennium Development Goal; SDG, Sustainable Development Goal; VA, Verbal Autopsy; WHO, World Health Organization

Acknowledgments
The authors would like to acknowledge Center for Disease Control and Prevention (CDC), Ethiopian Public Health Association (EPHA) and Haramaya University for supporting Kersa HDSS. We are also thankful for study participants, data collectors and supervisors in the surveillance.

Funding
Kersa HDSS has been supported by the President's Emergency Plan for AIDS Relief (PEPFAR) through US Center for Disease Control and Prevention (CDC), in accordance with the EPHA-CDC Cooperative Agreement GH001039-01.

Authors' contributions
NA, YL, BB, and HK conceptualized the manuscript. NA, YL, BB, and HK and performed the data analysis, made interpretations and drafted the manuscript. NA, YL, BB, HK, LO, MD, NB, WA, DZ and MD reviewed the manuscript and approved the final version.

Competing interests
The authors declare that they have no competing interests.

Disclaimer
The findings and conclusions in this report are those of the authors and do not necessarily represent the official position of the Centers for Disease Control and Prevention/the Agency for Toxic Substances and Disease Registry.

Author details
¹College of Health and Medical Sciences, Haramaya University, P.O.Box 1494, Harar, Ethiopia. ²Ethiopian Public Health Association, Addis Ababa, Ethiopia. ³College of Computing and Informatics, Haramaya University, Harar, Ethiopia.

References
1. Rafael L, Haidong W, Kyle JF, Julie KR, Mohsen N, Jake RM, Laura D, Katherine TL, David P, Charles A, et al. Progress towards Millennium Development Goals 4 and 5 on maternal and child mortality: an updated systematic analysis. Lancet. 2011;378:1139–65.
2. Lawn JE, et al. Health Policy Plan. Lancet. 2012;79(9832):2151–61.
3. UNICEF, WHO, Worldbank, UNFPA. Levels and trends in child mortality report 2012. New York: UNICEF; 2013.
4. UNICEF, WHO, Worldbank, UNFPA. Levels and trends in child mortality report 2013. New York: UNICEF, WHO, Worldbank, and UNFPA; 2014.
5. Liv L, Jonson H, Cousens S, et al. Global, regnal and national causes of child mortality: updated system analysis. 2012.
6. UNICEF. Levels and Trends in Child Mortality- Report 2012. 2012.
7. UNICEF, WHO, BANK TW, Division UNDP. Levels & Trends in Child Mortality. In: Report on Estimates Developed by the UN Inter-agency Group for Child Mortality Estimation. 2011.
8. Bassani D, Jha P. Causes of neonatal and child mortality in India: nationally representative mortality survey. Lancet. 2010;376(9755):1853–60.
9. Lulu K, Berhane Y. The use of simplified verbal autopsy in identifying causes of adult death in a predominantly rural population in Ethiopia. BMC Public Health. 2005;5:58.
10. Kutschera J, Reiterer F, Müller W, Urlesberger B. Neonatology and Pediatric Intensive Care. In: 33 th annual meeting of the Society for Neonatology and Pediatric Intensive Care 2007; 2005 jun 14-16. Hamburg: Z Geburtsh Neonatol; 2007.
11. Begg S, Rao C, Lopez A. Design options for sample-based mortality surveillance. Int J Epidemiol. 2005;34(5):1080–7.
12. Chandramohan D, Maude G, Rodrigues L, Hayes R. Verbal Autopsies for Adult Deaths: Issues in their Development and Validation. Int J Epidemiol. 1994;23:213–22.
13. Velkoff V, Setel P. Sample vital Registration using Verbal Autopsy: A new approach for collecting mortality data. In: International Programs Center Population Division. Atlanta: US Census Bureau; 2005.
14. Liu L, Oza S, Hogan D, Perin J, Rudan I, Lawn JE, Cousens S, Mathers C, Black RE. Global, regional, and national causes of child mortality in 2000–13, with projections to inform post-2015 priorities: an updated systematic analysis. Lancet. 2015;385:430–40.
15. WHO. Towards a monitoring framework with targets and indicators for the health goals of the post-2015 Sustainable Development Goals. Geneva: World Helath Organization; 2015.
16. FMOH-Ethiopia. Envisioning Ethiopia's Path towards Unviersal Helath Coverae Through Strengthning Primary Health Care. Addis Ababa: Federal Minstry of Health; 2015.
17. INDEPTH. Delivering Better Health Information Driving Better Health Policy The Past, The Present and The Future. Acra: Ghana INDEPTH Network; 2014.
18. Assefa N, Oljira L, Baraki N, Demena M, Zelalem D, Ashenafi W, Dedefo M. Profile of Kersa HDSS: the Kersa Health andDemographic Surveillance System. Int J Epidemiol. 2015;1:8.
19. Measure Evaluation. Verbal Autopsy Interviewer's Manual, SAVVY Sample Vital Registration with Verbal Autopsy system. Washington: MEASURE Evaluation project; 2007.
20. WHO. Verbal Autopsy Standards. The 2007 verbal autopsy instrument. Release 1. Geneva: WHO; 2007.
21. WHO. Verbal Autopsy Standards. Ascertaining and attributing cause of death. Geneva: WHO; 2007.
22. Jehan I, Harris H, Salat S, Zeb A, Mobeen N, Pasha O, McClure E, Janet M, Wright L, Goldenberg R. Neonatal mortality, risk factors and causes: a prospective population based cohort study in urban Pakistan. Bull World Health Organ. 2009;130:138.

23. Mekonnen Y, Tensou B, Telake DS, Degefie T, Bekele A. Neonatal mortality in Ethiopia: trends and determinants. BMC Public Health. 2013;13:483.

24. UNICEF, Worldbank WHO, UNFPA. Levels and trends in child mortality report 2011. WHO, Worldbank, and UNFPA: UNICEF; 2012.

25. Chowdhury HR, Thompson S, Ali M, Alam N, Yunus M, Streatfiel PK. Causes of Neonatal Deaths in a Rural Subdistrict of Bangladesh: Implications for Intervention. J HEALTH POPUL NUTR. 2010;28(4):375–82.

26. Yaya Y, Eide KT, Norheim OF, Lindtjørn B. Maternal and Neonatal Mortality in South-West Ethiopia: Estimates and Socio-Economic Inequality. PLoS ONE. 2014;9(4):e96294. doi:96210.91371/journal.pone.0096294.

27. Debelew GT, Afework MF, Yalew AW. Determinants and Causes of Neonatal Mortality in Jimma Zone, Southwest Ethiopia: A Multilevel Analysis of Prospective Follow Up Study. PLoS ONE. 2014;9:e107184. doi:107110.101371/journal.pone.0107184.

28. CSA. Ethiopia Demographic and Health Survey 2011. Addis Ababa: Central Statstics Authority, ICF, International; 2012.

29. Gizaw M, Molla M, Mekonnen W. Trends and risk factors for neonatal mortality in Butajira District, South Central Ethiopia, (1987-2008): a prospective cohort study. BMC Pregnancy Childbirth. 2014;14:64.

30. Khatun F, Rasheed S, Moran AC, Alam AM, Shomik MS, Sultana M, Choudhury N, Bhuiya MI. Causes of neonatal and maternal deaths in Dhaka slums: Implications for service delivery. BMC Public Health. 2012;12:84.

31. Fottrell E, Osrin D, Alcock G, Azad K, Bapat U, Beard J. Cause-specific neonatal mortality: analysis of 3772 neonatal deaths in Nepal, Bangladesh, Malawi and India. Arch Dis Child Fetal Neonatal. 2015;F1:F9.

32. Assefa N, Berhane Y, Worku A. Pregnancy rates and pregnancy loss in Eastern Ethiopia. Acta Obstet Gynecol Scand. 2013.

33. Lee AC, Cousens S, Darmstadt GL, Blencowe H, Pattinson R, Moran NF, Hofmeyr GJ, Haws RA, Bhutta SZ, Lawn JE. Care during labor and birth for the prevention of intrapartum-related neonatal deaths: a systematic review and Delphi estimation of mortality effect. BMC Public Health. 2011;11(3):S10.

34. Lawn JE, Cousens S, Zupan J, Team LNSS. 4 million neonatal deaths: when? Where? Why? Lancet. 2005;365(9462):891–900.

35. Ersdal HL, Mduma E, Svensen E, Perlman J. Birth Asphyxia: A Major Cause of Early Neonatal Mortality in a Tanzanian Rural Hospital. Pediatrics. 2012;129:e1238–43.

36. Jehan I, Harris H, Salat S, Zeb A, Mobeen N, Pasha O, McClure EM, Moore J, Wright LL, Goldenberg RL. Neonatal mortality, risk factors and causes: a prospective population-based cohort study in urban Pakistan. Bull World Health Organ. 2009;87:130–8.

37. Girma S, G/Yohannes A, Kitaw Y, Ye-Ebiyo Y, Seyoum A, Desta H, Teklehaimanot A. Human Resource Development for Health in Ethiopia: Challenges of Achieving the Millennium development Goals. Ethiop J Health Dev. 2007;21(3):216–31.

38. El-Saharty S, Kebede S, Dubusho PO, Siadat B. Improving Health Service Delivery. In: Health, Nutrition and Population (HNP) Discussion Paper. The World Bank. 2009.

39. FMOH. Health and Health related indicator. Planning and Programming Department Federal Ministry of Health: Addis Ababa; 2007.

40. FMoH. Health Extension Program in Ethiopia: Profi le. In: Center HeaE, editor. Addis Ababa: Federal Ministry of Health (ET). 2007.

41. Andreas J, et al. Evaluation of a village-informant riven demographic surveillance system. Demogr Res. 2007;16:8.

42. Mobley C, Boerma J, Titus S, Lohrke B, Shangula K, Black R. Validation study of a verbal autopsy method for causes of childhood mortality in Namibia. J Trop Pediatr. 1996;42:365–9.

43. Quigley M, JRM A WS. Algorithms for verbal autopsies: a validation study in Kenyan children. Bull World Health Organ. 1996;74:147–54.

44. Rodriguez L, Reyes H, Tome P, Ridaura C, Flores S, Guiscafre H. Validation of the verbal autopsy method to ascertain acute respiratory infection as cause of death. Indian J Pediatr. 1998;65:579–84.

45. Setel P, Rao C, Hemed Y, Whiting DR, Yang G, Chandramohan D. Core Verbal Autopsy Procedures with Comparative Validation Results from Two Countries. PLoS Med. 2006;3(8):e268.

14

Risk factors for acute bilirubin encephalopathy on admission to two Myanmar national paediatric hospitals

G. Arnolda[1,2*] (iD), H. M. Nwe[3], D. Trevisanuto[4,5], A. A. Thin[6], A. A. Thein[7], T. Defechereux[8], D. Kumara[1] and L. Moccia[1,4]

Abstract

Background: Jaundice is the commonest neonatal ailment requiring treatment. Untreated, it can lead to acute bilirubin encephalopathy (ABE), chronic bilirubin encephalopathy (CBE) or death. ABE and CBE have been largely eliminated in industrialised countries, but remain a problem of largely undocumented scale in low resource settings.

As part of a quality-improvement intervention in the Neonatal Care Units of two paediatric referral hospitals in Myanmar, hospitals collected de-identified data on each neonate treated on new phototherapy machines over 13–20 months. The information collected included: diagnosis of ABE at hospital presentation; general characteristics such as place of birth, source of referral, and sex; and a selection of suspected causes of jaundice including prematurity, infection, G6PD status, ABO and Rh incompatibility. This information was analysed to identify risk factors for hospital presentation with ABE, using multiple logistic regression.

Results: Data on 251 neonates was recorded over 20 months in Hospital A, and 339 neonates over 13 months in Hospital B; the number of outborn neonates presenting with ABE was 32 (12.7 %) and 72 (21.2 %) respectively. In the merged dataset the final multivariate model identified the following independent risk and protective factors: home birth, $OR_{adj} = 2.3$ (95 % CI: 1.04-5.4); self-referral, $OR_{adj} = 2.6$ (95 % CI: 1.2-6.0); prematurity, $OR_{adj} = 0.40$ (95 % CI: 0.18-0.85); and a significant interaction between hospital and screening status because screening positive for G6PD deficiency was a strong and significant risk factor at Hospital B ($OR_{adj} = 5.9$; 95 % CI: 3.0-11.6), but not Hospital A ($OR_{adj} = 1.1$; 95 % CI: 0.5-2.5).

Conclusion: The study identifies home birth, self-referral and G6PD screening status as important risk factors for presentation with ABE; prematurity was protective, but this is interpreted as an artefact of the study design. As operational research, there is likely to be substantial measurement error in the risk factor data, suggesting that the identified risk factor estimates are robust. Additional interventions are required to ensure prompt referral of jaundiced neonates to treatment facilities, with particular focus on home births and communities with high rates of G6PD deficiency.

Keywords: Neonatal jaundice, Hyperbilirubinaemia, Acute Bilirubin Encephalopathy, Kernicterus, Chronic Bilirubin Encephalopathy

* Correspondence: gaston.arnolda@gmail.com
[1]Thrive Networks, Oakland, CA, USA
[2]School of Public Health & Community Medicine, Faculty of Medicine, University of New South Wales, Wales, NSW, Australia
Full list of author information is available at the end of the article

Background

High levels of unconjugated bilirubin in the neonate can lead to the development of acute bilirubin encephalopathy (ABE) which first presents as lethargy, hypotonia and poor sucking. If untreated this can proceed to hypertonia manifested as backward arching of the neck and back (retrocollis and opisthotonos), and ultimately to apnoea, coma and death [1]. The long term sequelae of bilirubin toxicity, termed chronic bilirubin encephalopathy (CBE), previously 'kernicterus' [2], is characterised by a combination of abnormal motor control, movements and muscle tone, disturbed auditory processing, impairment of upward vertical gaze, and dysplasia of the enamel of deciduous teeth [3].

In high resource settings, the incidence of CBE decreased markedly with the introduction of double volume blood exchange transfusion in the 1940s [4]. The need for exchange transfusion, in turn, has been reduced by the use of phototherapy [5], post-partum administration of anti-D immune globulin G to Rh(D) negative mothers exposed to an Rh(D) positive fetus to prevent maternal Rh (D) alloimunisation that can lead to neonatal haemolytic disease in future pregnancies [6], or immunoglobulin directly to the newborn as treatment for Rh (D) or ABO haemolytic disorders [7].

A variety of estimates of the incidence of CBE in high resource settings suggest that the incidence in the early twenty-first century ranges from 1.0-3.7 per 100,000 live births [8]. The incidence increases with Total Serum Bilirubin [TSB]; of neonates with TSB >428 µmol/L, about 6 % develop CBE, while of neonates with TSB >513 µmol/L, around 14 % develop CBE [8].

In low resource settings, information about the actual incidence of ABE and CBE is sparse. A population estimate is available in a survey of 16,979 people <20 years old in Kolkata, India, which found a prevalence of cerebral palsy [CP] of 283/100,000, with 16.7 % of the CP associated with a history of 'profound jaundice' (i.e., 47 cases of jaundice-related CP per 100,000 live births) [9]; this prevalence of jaundice-related CP is an underestimate of the actual incidence of CBE to the extent that there is excess mortality among children and young people with jaundice-related CP. A separate population estimate derived from a four-month study in a single Baghdad hospital, estimated an incidence of ABE of 1,749/100,000 live births, during a period of severe health system disruption in 2007–08 [10].

Despite our lack of detailed understanding of the mechanism for bilirubin neurotoxicity, experience in industrialised countries makes clear that we have sufficient knowledge and technical capacity to virtually eliminate CBE. A systems-based approach has been recommended in high resource settings, incorporating individual risk assessment and/or pre-discharge TSB, lactation support, close-follow up in the community, and prompt and effective intervention when needed [11]. Improving systems of care in low-resource settings, along similar lines, is feasible.

The data presented in this report were collected in the course of a pilot project to improve care in the Neonatal Care Units (NCUs) at two specialist paediatric referral hospitals in Myanmar. As neonatal jaundice was the most common reason for admission to the target NCUs, and to other NCUs not included in the pilot project, we undertook to collect relevant information as part of program implementation, to better understand the clinical spectrum of jaundiced neonates at admission, to guide project enhancement in the target hospitals, and to inform the future direction of jaundice prevention and treatment programs in Myanmar. These data, while primarily collected for the purpose of planning and project evaluation, were retrospectively examined to identify pre-admission risk factors for admission to hospital with ABE.

Methods

Setting and context

This study was conducted as part of an intervention at two tertiary paediatric referral hospitals in Yangon and Mandalay, Myanmar, hereafter referred to as Hospitals A and B. We chose these institutions because, in late 2011, they were the two most significant national level tertiary paediatric referral hospitals in Myanmar; neither hospital provided birthing facilities, but both had a NCU for neonatal admissions. The data reported here were initially collected for a separate purpose – to monitor and evaluate the intervention. In the current study, we have used that data opportunistically, to identify risk factors for ABE at hospital admission and to guide the design of research and future interventions to encourage earlier hospital presentation of neonates at risk of ABE.

Ethical approval

Data were collected in the process of routine care provision. De-identified data were originally collected for operational purposes, but once a decision to publish was made, retrospective ethics clearance was sought from the Ethical Committee on Medical Research involving Human Subjects, Myanmar Department of Health [approval #14/2014].

Data collection

During the training, both hospitals agreed to collect data on each neonate treated on the LED phototherapy machines donated as part of the intervention, and participated in the specification of the data items for an LED Phototherapy Treatment Register (LPTR). Hospitals were not required to collect information on neonates treated exclusively with conventional fluorescent light phototherapy machines. While the data elements were prospectively defined, we decided to explore risk factors for presentation with ABE retrospectively, so the study is best described as a retrospective cohort.

Individual patient information collected in the LPTR included the following variables: hospital name; date of birth; gender; gestational age; admission weight; place of birth (home/health facility); source of referral (self/health facility); signs of kernicterus, the term routinely used in Myanmar to describe both ABE and CBE, at admission, classified as ABE (Yes/No); previous sibling had received phototherapy (Yes/No); significant bruising (Yes/No); breastfeeding + feeding poorly (Yes/No); other suspected cause of jaundice (sepsis/G6PD/ABO/Rh D/Other/Not stated; multiple selections permitted); date started phototherapy on LED machine; TSB at start of phototherapy; TSB prior to exchange transfusion; and discharge status (discharged [with or without 'kernicterus']/removed by family/transferred/died).

TSB readings were performed in the hospital laboratory at Hospital A. At Hospital B, the overwhelming majority of readings were performed in the NCU on a desktop Bilirubinometer with a maximum of 513 μmol/L; some readings were performed in the hospital laboratory, but we did not record which tests were performed in which location.

At both facilities, G6PD screening was performed using the qualitative methaemoglobin reduction test. Although G6PD deficiency is an X-linked genetic disorder, both hospitals screen all neonates admitted for treatment of jaundice, not just males. At the time of the study, families were expected to pay for the test, but hospitals paid if families could not; clinicians are therefore confident that the vast majority of eligible neonates were screened. While this G6PD screening test is adequate in most situations, it is known to produce false-negative results in neonates with low to moderate levels of G6PD deficiency who are haemolysing, so the test must be repeated 2–4 weeks later to determine actual G6PD deficiency status in neonates who screen negative [12]; delayed repeat testing of screen-negative neonates was not performed at either hospital.

The recording of (suspected) infection/sepsis as a cause of jaundice was at the discretion of the clinician completing the LPTR, and was not subject to pre-agreed diagnostic rules (e.g., laboratory confirmation).

At both facilities, gestation was usually reported as 'post-term,'term', 'preterm' or sometimes as a specified gestational week or range of weeks. The recorded data was used to classify neonates as 'Term' ($\geq$37 weeks') or 'Preterm' (<37 weeks'); where a range of weeks was recorded (e.g., "36-38 weeks'"), classification was based on the midpoint (e.g., 37 weeks').

Analysis

In the first stage of analysis, we simply described the characteristics of the treated neonates in each of the hospitals, with no statistical testing performed. The second stage compared characteristics of two sub-groups of neonates' treated for jaundice: those presenting with ABE, and those not recorded as having ABE at hospital admission. The statistical significance of the difference in proportions was assessed using Fisher's Exact Test for categorical variables, and the Kruskal-Wallis test for a difference in medians in continuous variables. These comparison were performed separately for each hospital.

In the final stage of analysis, we aggregated data from the two hospitals and used multiple logistic regression to assess the joint effect of multiple risk factors, restricted to variables that were not considered to be intervening variables; TSB at presentation and poor feeding at presentation were both excluded for this reason. The analysis followed a pre-specified modelling strategy: [13] all variables statistically significant at $p < 0.20$ in univariate models were screened in the multivariate model and retained if significant at $p = 0.05$; first order interaction terms between significant main effects were assessed and retained if statistically significant; and the fit of the final model was assessed using the area under the ROC curve ('c-statistic') and the Hosmer-Lemeshow Goodness of Fit test. Analysis was undertaken in SAS v9.4.

Results

Individual patient data was collected for 251 neonates treated on LED phototherapy machines, over 20 consecutive months, at Hospital A (from December 2011 to July 2013, inclusive), and for 339 neonates treated over 13 *non-consecutive* months at Hospital B (from December 2011 to 30 June 2013, but with no data provided for February 2012, May to July 2012, and for January and February 2013). The average number of neonates treated per complete month was 13/month (Interquartile Range [IQR] of 4–32) at Hospital A, and 30/month (IQR: 11–46) at Hospital B.

Characteristics of treated neonates

Table 1 presents key characteristics of neonates treated with LED phototherapy. Both hospitals report a slight preponderance of male patients (57 % at Hospital A vs 59 % at Hospital B). Home birth and self-referral to hospital were not uncommon, affecting around a quarter of treated patients at each hospital, while phototherapy prior to hospital admission was relatively rare (11 % at both hospitals). The hospitals differed in two important ways: Hospital A had a lower proportion of infants admitted weighing <2,500 g (27 %) than Hospital B (42 %); and the reported incidence of ABE at admission was lower at Hospital A (13 %) than Hospital B (21 %).

Table 2 shows relevant information at the start of phototherapy treatment. The median age at the start of phototherapy was 3 days (IQR: 2–5 days) at both hospitals, and

Table 1 Characteristics of LED phototherapy patients

	Hospital A	Hospital B
	n = 251	n = 339
Percentage male: n (%)[a]	142 (56.6 %)	195 (58.9 %)
Place of birth: n (%)		
Home: n (%)	78 (31.1 %)	88 (26.0 %)
Hospital/Clinic: n (%)	160 (63.7 %)	237 (69.9 %)
Other/Not stated: n (%)	13 (5.2 %)	14 (4.1 %)
Source of referral: n (%)		
Home: n (%)	54 (21.5 %)	90 (26.6 %)
Hospital: n (%)	40 (15.9 %)	212 (62.5 %)
Clinic: n (%)	103 (41.0 %)	12 (3.5 %)
Other/Not stated: n (%)	54 (21.5 %)	25 (7.4 %)
Phototherapy elsewhere, prior to admission: n (%)	28 (11.2 %)	34 (11.0 %)
Admission weight (g)[c]: Median (IQR)	2,800 (2,400-3,200)	2,600 (1,940-3,040)
< 1,000 g: n (%)	2 (0.8 %)	2 (0.6 %)
1,000-1,499 g: n (%)	5 (2.0 %)	29 (8.8 %)
1,500-2,499 g: n (%)	61 (24.5 %)	107 (32.5 %)
2,500 g +: n (%)	181 (72.7 %)	191 (58.1 %)
ABE[d] noted at admission		
No: n (%)	219 (87.3 %)	267 (78.8 %)
Yes: n (%)	32 (12.7 %)	72 (21.2 %)

n number, IQR Interquartile range (25th percentile – 75th percentile)
[a]Gender missing for 8 records at Hospital B
[b]Phototherapy elsewhere, prior to admission missing for 31 records at Hospital B
[c]Admission weight missing for two records at Hospital A, and 10 records at Hospital B
[d]The term 'kernicterus' is routinely used in both hospitals – this has been re-classified as ABE

Table 2 Information available at the start of LED phototherapy

	Hospital A	Hospital B
	n = 251	n = 339
At start of phototherapy		
Age (days): Median (IQR)	3.0 (2.0-5.0)	3.0 (2.0-5.0)
TSB (μmol/L)[a]: Median (IQR)	311 (224–445)	325 (234–473)
Risk factors for hyperbilirubinaemia		
Preterm (<37 weeks')[c]: n (%)	38 (15.3 %)	85 (25.5 %)
Previous sibling treated: n (%)	1 (0.4 %)	66 (19.5 %)
Significant bruising: n (%)	2 (0.8 %)	9 (2.7 %)
Breastfeeding and feeding poorly: n (%)	25 (10.0 %)	Unclear
Suspected cause (multiple selections permitted)		
Suspected infection: n (%)	158 (63.0 %)	183 (54.0 %)
G6PD deficiency[d]: n (%)	91 (36.3 %)	58 (17.1 %)
ABO incompatibility: n (%)	43 (17.1 %)	52 (15.3 %)
Rhesus incompatibility: n (%)	4 (1.6 %)	2 (0.6 %)
Not specified: n (%)	14 (5.6 %)	32 (9.4 %)

n number, IQR Interquartile range (25th percentile – 75th percentile)
[a]TSB at admission missing for 31 records at Hospital A, and seven records at Hospital B
[c]Gestation at admission missing for one record at Hospital A, and six records at Hospital B
[d]Screening test performed, and assessed as screen positive

Table 3 Outcomes of neonates treated with LED phototherapy

	Hospital A	Hospital B
	n = 251	n = 339
Exchange transfusions[a]		
n (%)	38 (15.3 %)	88 (26.0 %)
TSB (μmol/L) at ET: Median (IQR)[b]	474 (416–539)	500 (475–513)
Duration of treatment (days): Median (IQR)[c]	2.0 (1.0-2.0)	1.0 (1.0-2.0)
Discharge status		
Discharged: n (%)	221 (88.1 %)	276 (81.4 %)
Removed by family: n (%)	3 (1.2 %)	8 (2.4 %)
Died: n (%)	18 (7.2 %)	38 (11.2 %)
Transferred to other hospital: n (%)	0 (0.0 %)	2 (0.6 %)
CBE[d]: n (%)	5 (2.0 %)	5 (1.5 %)
Not stated: n (%)	4 (1.6 %)	10 (3.0 %)

n number, IQR Interquartile range (25th percentile – 75th percentile)
[a]At Hospital A, data missing on exchange transfusion status of three records
[b]TSB at ET missing for 12 transfused neonates at Hospital A and for 42 transfused neonates at Hospital B; note that most readings at Hospital B were performed on equipment with a maximum reading of 513 μmol/L
[c]Duration of treatment unavailable for 22 records at Hospital A and 84 records at Hospital B
[d]'Kernicterus' is the term routinely used in both hospitals; in this situation it is assumed to refer to CBE

median TSB at the start of phototherapy was also similar (311 μmol/L at Hospital A vs 325 μmol/L at Hospital B). Both prematurity and previous sibling treated with phototherapy were less common among treated neonates at Hospital A (15 and 0.4 % respectively) than at Hospital B (26 and 19 %). Significant bruising was rarely recorded in both hospitals, while breastfeeding and feeding poorly was reported in 10 % of treated neonates in Hospital A, but not reported in Hospital B. Infection was the commonest suspected cause of jaundice (63 in Hospital A and 54 % in Hospital B), followed by G6PD deficiency (36 and 17 %) and ABO incompatibility (17 and 15 %); Rhesus incompatibility was rarely recorded (2 and 1 %).

Table 3 shows key outcomes for treated neonates. The rate of Exchange Transfusion among treated neonates was high in Hospital A (15 %) and markedly higher in Hospital B (26 %). Mortality was also high (7 % at Hospital A vs 11 % at Hospital B). At each facility, 5 infants were noted to have been discharged with CBE, representing around 2 % of treated infants.

Comparing characteristics of neonates with and without ABE at admission

Table 4 compares neonates presenting with and without ABE for age at admission to hospital and TSB at admission. At both hospitals, neonates admitted with ABE had a statistically significantly higher median TSB at admission (694 vs 291 μmol/L at Hospital A, and 496 vs 287 μmol/L at Hospital B; both with $p < 0.0001$). At both hospitals, the median age of neonates admitted with ABE was 4 days, in comparison to 3 days for jaundiced neonates admitted without ABE ($p = 0.27$ at Hospital A, and $p = 0.10$ at Hospital B).

Table 5 shows the discharge status of neonates with and without ABE at admission. ABE at hospital presentation was the key predictor of poor outcome at both hospitals. At Hospital A, 15 of 32 (47 %) neonates with ABE at presentation died, and an additional five (16 %) survived with CBE; this compares to three deaths and no CBE at discharge among the 219 neonates who did not have ABE at admission (1.4 %). At Hospital B, 18 of 72 neonates (25 %) admitted with ABE died, and an additional 5 neonates (7 %) survived with kernicterus; this compares to 20 deaths (7 %) and no survivors with kernicterus among neonates admitted without ABE.

Table 5 also compares neonates with and without ABE at admission for a variety of risk factors for jaundice, and suspected causes of jaundice. At Hospital A, the only statistically significant univariate risk factors for presentation with ABE were home birth and direct referral from home (both $p < 0.0001$). At Hospital B, home birth and self-referral were again significant, and screening positive for G6PD deficiency was also a risk, while preterm birth was protective ($p < 0.0001$ for all factors).

Multivariate regression model

In the merged dataset the final multivariate model (n = 582 after exclusion of 8 records without data on prematurity) identified the following independent risk and protective factors: home birth, $OR_{adj} = 2.3$ (95 % CI: 1.04-5.4); self-referral, $OR_{adj} = 2.6$ (95 % CI: 1.2-6.0); prematurity, $OR_{adj} = 0.40$ (95 % CI: 0.18-0.85); and a significant interaction between hospital and screening status because screening positive for G6PD deficiency was a strong and significant risk factor at Hospital B ($OR_{adj} = 5.9$; 95 % CI: 3.0-11.6), but not at Hospital A ($OR_{adj} = 1.1$; 95 % CI: 0.5-2.5).

Discussion

In 2002, the American National Quality Forum defined "Death or serious disability (kernicterus) associated with failure to identify and treat hyperbilirubinemia in neonates" as a serious reportable event [14], reflecting its belief that kernicterus should be a 'never-event' that can be entirely avoided. The weak systems of perinatal care that are typical in low resource settings, however, create additional challenges on the path to making kernicterus a 'never-event'. The reality in low resource settings is that neonates frequently arrive in paediatric emergency rooms with signs of ABE. Numerous studies have demonstrated higher risks of ABE or kernicterus among outborn neonates in low resource settings [15–18]; the current study seeks to add to this, by identifying specific risk factors which lead to these outborn neonates being admitted with established signs of ABE.

Risks and protective factors for admission with ABE in the current study

Home-birth or self-referral

Home born and self-referred neonates are substantially overlapping groups, with 80 % of home births and only 3 % of facility births being self-referred, so it was surprising that both were retained in the final model. We are aware of one study that examined home birth and found no study reporting on self-referral as risk factors for presentation with ABE: a Baghdad study during a period of severe health system disruption found that home birth was not a significant risk factor for CBE or death (OR = 1.2; 95 % CI: 0.6-2.5); the study did not report risk of ABE at presentation [10].

It is unclear that something intrinsic to place of birth would make urban or peri-urban home birth a risk factor for presentation with ABE, so it seems more plausible that home birth is a proxy for other factors. Plausible factors include: characteristics of mothers that give birth at home (e.g., racial differences correlated with both genetic risk and socio-economic status); characteristics of the

Table 4 Age and TSB at admission of neonates with and without ABE at admission

	Hospital A					Hospital B				
	ABE at admission (n = 32)		No ABE at admission (n = 219)		p-value	ABE at admission (n = 72)		No ABE at admission (n = 267)		p-value
	n	Median [IQR]	n	Median [IQR]		n	Median [IQR]	n	Median [IQR]	
Age at start of phototherapy (days)	32	4.0 (2.0-5.0)	219	3.0 (2.0-5.0)	0.27	72	4.0 (2.0-5.5)	267	3.0 (2.0-5.0)	0.10
Total serum bilirubin at admission[a](μmol/L)	28	694 (581–795)	192	291 (211–401)	<0.0001	69	496 (475–513)	263	287 (210–393)	<0.0001

n number, IQR Interquartile range (25th percentile – 75th percentile)
[a]The majority of readings at Hospital B were performed on equipment with a maximum reading of 513 μmol/L

Table 5 Selected characteristics and outcomes of neonates with and without ABE at admission

		Hospital A						Hospital B					
		ABE at admission (n = 32)		No ABE at admission (n = 219)		p-value	ABE at admission (n = 72)		No ABE at admission (n = 267)		P-value
		n	%	n	%		n	%	n	%	
Demographic	Male[a]	17	53.1	125	57.1	0.71	45	62.5	150	57.9	0.50
	Home birth	22	68.8	56	25.6	<0.0001	38	52.8	50	18.7	<0.0001
	Referred from home	16	50.0	38	17.4	0.0001	40	55.6	50	18.7	<0.0001
Selected risk factors for hyperbilirubinaemia	Preterm (<37 weeks')[b]	3	9.4	35	16.1	0.43	6	8.3	79	30.3	<0.0001
	Previous sibling	0	0.0	1	0.5	1.0	15	20.8	51	19.1	0.74
	Significant bruising	1	3.1	1	0.5	0.24	3	4.2	6	2.3	0.41
Previous phototherapy		2	6.3	26	11.9	0.55	9	12.5	25	10.6	0.67
Suspected cause (multiple selections permitted)	Suspected infection	23	71.9	135	61.6	0.32	34	47.2	149	55.8	0.23
	G6PD deficiency[c]	14	43.8	77	35.2	0.43	29	40.3	29	10.9	<0.0001
	ABO incompatibility	3	9.4	40	18.3	0.31	8	11.1	44	16.5	0.36
	Rhesus incompatibility	0	0.0	4	1.8	1.0	0	0.0	2	0.8	1.0
	Other/Not specified	3	9.4	11	5.0	0.40	4	5.6	28	10.5	0.26
Discharge Status	Died	15	46.9	3	1.4	<0.0001	18	25.0	20	7.5	<0.0001
	Lived, with ABE	5	15.6	0	0.0		5	6.9	0	0.0	
	All other discharge	12	37.5	216	98.6		49	68.1	247	92.5	

n number, IQR Interquartile range (25th percentile – 75th percentile)
[a]Gender missing for 8 records at Hospital B (none of whom had ABE at presentation)
[b]Gestation missing for two records at Hospital A, and six records at Hospital B (none of the eight had ABE at presentation)
[c]Screening test performed, and assessed as screen positive

accoucher (e.g., Traditional Birth Attendants vs midwives) and/or characteristics of the quality of care (e.g., high rates of asphyxia, lower rates of provision of high quality post-partum education about signs requiring referral to hospital); characteristics of the post-partum follow-up (e.g., less frequent follow-up of home births); and persistence of barriers to facility access for both delivery and care of the sick neonate (e.g., physical, attitudinal, or financial). Self-referral, on the other hand, may be a proxy for inaccessibility of facility-based care and/or delayed access for other reasons. The fact that both factors remain significant in the final model, despite substantial overlap, suggests a complex interplay of factors resulting in late presentation.

While it is clear from the prevalence of ABE at admission that *late* presentation is important, it is not clear from our data that age at start of phototherapy is associated with ABE at presentation. Age at presentation was measured crudely in the current study (in days rather than hours, for practical reasons) and that this introduced random error which results in a bias towards statistically non-significant findings, despite the fact that neonates with ABE presented at a median of 4 days, compared to a median of 3 days for neonates without ABE. It is plausible that 'late' presentation may need to be defined in terms of disease progression, as well as in chronological terms.

G6PD deficiency

G6PD deficiency has been identified as suspected cause of ABE at admission in about a third of the babies in two Nigerian case series of neonates with ABE [15, 19], slightly lower than the rate found in neonates with ABE at Hospitals A and B (44 and 40 % respectively). The prevalence of G6PD deficiency in Myanmar is estimated at 6.1 % [20], somewhat higher than the median of 3.95 % (IQR: 3.4 %- 7.9 %) in 184 countries for which there are estimates [21], but substantially lower than the 16.9 % estimated in Nigeria [20]. On the face of it, one would therefore expect Nigerian studies to have a higher prevalence of neonates with ABE that screen positive for G6PD deficiency. A separate Nigerian case control study found that 67-75 % of neonates with ABE screened positive for G6PD deficiency, in comparison to only 17-22 % of neonates without ABE (range provided as some neonates not screened) [18]. In the current study, G6PD deficiency was only a risk factor for ABE at Hospital B (40 % in neonates with ABE vs 11 % in neonates without ABE). It is unclear why G6PD deficiency was not a risk factor in Hospital A: Hospital A had a higher overall rate of G6PD deficiency (36 % vs 17 % in Hospital B) and a lower overall rate of ABE at presentation (13 % vs 21 %); one possibility is that there are differences in the distribution of local genetic variants causing G6PD deficiency which are in turn related to the incidence of ABE.

Prematurity

Several facility-based studies have noted that premature or low birth weight babies have *lower* rates of ABE at presentation: a Nigerian study found that 14 % of cases with ABE weighed <2,500 g in comparison to 37 % of controls admitted to the nursery for any reason ($p = 0.01$) [15]; a separate Nigerian study found that 22 % of cases with ABE weighted ≤2,500 g, in comparison to 42 % of clinically jaundiced neonates admitted to the nursery ($p = 0.46$) [18]; and a Bangladeshi study found that 11 % of neonates that presented with or developed ABE during the study were preterm, in comparison to 21 % of neonates admitted to the nursery with jaundice or who developed jaundice during their stay ($p = 0.55$) [22].

Conversely, low gestation has long been identified as an epidemiological risk factor for kernicterus. For example, a classic 1950–54 study estimated the incidence of kernicterus by gestation among neonates admitted to the newborn units and surviving to 48 h: ≤30 weeks 10,100/100,000 admitted survivors; 31–32 weeks 5,700/100,000; 33–34 weeks 3,200/100,000; 35–36 weeks 1,100/100,000; and ≥37 weeks 800/100,000 admitted survivors [23]. Given this long established risk-factor status, the apparent protective role of low gestation found in the current study, and in the other studies reported above, is interpreted as an artefact arising from the use of controls admitted to the neonatal nursery. The term neonates in these studies are drawn from a pool at extremely high risk of ABE, whereas the preterm neonates are all likely to be routinely admitted and often receive prophylactic phototherapy, simultaneously preventing the development of ABE.

Other risk factors for ABE

Rh (D) isoimmunisation

The incidence of kernicterus in Greece prior to the introduction of exchange transfusion or phototherapy has been estimated at 40/100,000 live births among neonates affected by Rh haemolytic disease [24], while a recent modelling study estimated that roughly one third of ABE cases were caused by Rh disease [21]. In Myanmar, the prevalence of Rh negative blood group prevalence is estimated at 0.8 %, substantially lower than the median of 3.7 % (IQR: 3.5 %-10.0 %) for 138 countries with a neonatal mortality rate above 5/1,000 live births [21]. This low prevalence in Myanmar results in few neonates with ABE due to Rh (D) incompatibility, despite the lack of systematic screening and prophylaxis to prevent Rh (D) isoimmunisation.

Sepsis

It has been noted that sepsis can increase the risk of severe hyperbilirubinaemia and or bilirubin neurotoxicity by altering the binding affinity of albumin [25], and that sepsis can result in acute, severe hyperbilirubinaemia [26]. Investigation of this factor in the current study was hampered by the lack of a firm definition, or laboratory confirmation. At Hospital A, 63 % of treated neonates had 'suspected sepsis' recorded as a cause while at Hospital B the figure was slightly lower at 54 %; infection/sepsis was not a statistically significant predictor of ABE at presentation in either hospital. The literature on the role of sepsis as a risk factor for ABE in low resource settings is limited: a Nigerian study attributed sepsis as the cause of ABE in 43 % of cases but did not give the rate of sepsis in a control series [15].

Limitations

The current study was conducted as operational research, resulting in a number of limitations. First, the cohort studied represents neonates treated on LED phototherapy. Participating clinicians state that most infants were treated on the LED machines, and those that were not tended to have lower TSB. Any bias is therefore likely to be small and, if there is bias, it is likely to result in a compressed patient spectrum towards higher risk infants, shrinking risk estimates towards the null.

Second, there were a number of measurement-related limitations: ABE was not formally defined, but relied on the clinical judgement of experienced clinicians at each facility, leaving open the possibility of under- or over-diagnosis of ABE; age at admission was measured in days rather than hours; there was no delayed re-test of neonates that received a negative G6PD screening result; there were no strict definitions of sepsis as a suspected cause of jaundice; different hospitals may have different proclivities to record particular risk factors (e.g., previous sibling treated with phototherapy and significant bruising); and the in-unit desktop Bilirubinometer at Hospital B, used for the majority of TSB readings, was restricted to an upper limit of 513 μmol/L. All of these limitations result in misclassification of risk factors for ABE, or of ABE itself, and this misclassification necessarily results in a bias towards the null (i.e., OR = 1.0). Care should therefore be taken not to over-interpret *non-significant* findings, but statistically significant risk factors can be considered to be robust estimates, possibly with the risk factor status diminished due to misclassification errors.

Conclusions and next steps

This study demonstrates that home birth and self-referral to a paediatric hospital and, in one hospital screening positive for G6PD deficiency, are significant risk factors for paediatric hospital admission of jaundiced neonates with ABE in Myanmar. Additional information is required to identify possible points at which it is feasible to intervene,

Risk factors for acute bilirubin encephalopathy on admission to two Myanmar national...

145

to reduce clinically late presentation of outborn neonates with ABE.

Prospective case–control studies have been initiated to identify in more detail the barriers to timely presentation of jaundiced neonates. Depending on the findings of these case–control studies, a range of interventions are possible. Examples of possible interventions include: general information for the community (e.g., to ensure that mothballs are removed from the home environment of neonates to prevent triggering G6PD deficiency); training and information to be distributed by healthcare providers (public and private) to ensure new mothers and their families can identify jaundice, and are aware of the need to self-refer quickly if a baby becomes jaundiced in the first 72 h, or if severe jaundice appears rapidly at any time thereafter; home visits by nurses/midwives in the first week of life, in line with national policy, could be optimally-timed, targeting home-births; training of staff at primary healthcare settings to identify and rapidly transfer babies at risk of exchange transfusion, and development of protocols to ensure rapid transfer of these neonates; and provision of TSB testing equipment and high quality phototherapy equipment to lower level facilities. While the provision of TSB screening equipment to home visit staff is not currently feasible due to cost, new systems such as 'Bilistick' costing €150 for the prototype and a few cents per test have been found to be highly accurate [27], raising the possibility that screening can be undertaken at lower levels in the health care system.

Given the many demands on health systems in low-resource settings, it is important to prioritise interventions with a goal of achieving optimal results from any given resource input. The data presented in this report, represent a first step in the process of identifying the interventions required to address the mortality and morbidity associated with ABE in Myanmar, as part of the process of intervening to reduce that mortality and morbidity.

Abbreviations

ABE: Acute Bilirubin Encephalopathy; BOL: Breath of Life Program; CI: Confidence Interval; CP: Cerebral palsy; CBE: Chronic Bilirubin Encephalopathy; INGO: International Non-Governmental Organization; MTTS: Medical Technology Transfer Services, Hanoi, Viet Nam; NCU: Neonatal Care Unit; NS: Not statistically significant; OR: Odds Ratio; OR$_{adj}$: Adjusted Odds Ratio; TSB: Total Serum Bilirubin.

Competing interests

The authors declare that they have no competing interests.

Authors' contribution

GA led the study design, analysis and drafting of the manuscript. HN, DT and LM conceived of the study, and played significant advisory roles in its design and in drafting of the manuscript; additionally, LM coordinated study implementation and HN oversaw in-hospital data collection. AA Thin contributed to the design and oversaw in-hospital data collection. DT and DK oversaw overall data collection and entry, and played significant advisory roles in drafting the manuscript. All authors read and approved the final manuscript.

Acknowledgments

The funding for the pilot project described in this study was provided in a fund matching agreement between three partners: the Archdioceses of Trento, Italy, and the Autonomous Province of Trento, Italy; donors to Amici della Neonatologia Trentina, an INGO headquartered in Trento, Italy; and Eric Hemel and Barbara Morgen, donors to Thrive Networks, an INGO headquartered in Oakland, California, USA.

The pilot project was implemented by the Breath of Life Program, Thrive Networks, which supported the involvement of some of the authors as employees [DK], consultants [GA, LM] and volunteers [DT, TD]. Other authors [HN, AA Thin, AA Thein] were financially supported by the Myanmar Ministry of Health, in their roles as Hospital Clinicians. Data was collected by many hospital staff. We gratefully acknowledge the contribution of donors and staff who, together, made this work possible.

Author details

[1]Thrive Networks, Oakland, CA, USA. [2]School of Public Health & Community Medicine, Faculty of Medicine, University of New South Wales, Wales, NSW, Australia. [3]Department of Paediatrics, University of Medicine (1), Yangon, Myanmar. [4]Amici della Neonatologia Trentina, Trento, Italy. [5]Children and Women's Health Department, Medical School University of Padua, Padua, Italy. [6]Mandalay Children's Hospital (300), Mandalay, Myanmar. [7]Department of Neonatology, University of Medicine (1), Yangon, Myanmar. [8]Department of Surgery, Liege University Hospital, Liege, Belgium.

References

1. Maisels MJ. Neonatal hyperbilirubinemia and kernicterus - not gone but sometimes forgotten. Early Hum Dev. 2009;85(11):727–32.
2. AAP. Management of hyperbilirubinemia in the newborn infant 35 or more weeks of gestation. Pediatrics. 2004;114:297–316.
3. Shapiro SM. Chronic bilirubin encephalopathy: diagnosis and outcome. Semin Fetal Neonatal Med. 2010;15(3):157–63.
4. Murki S, Kumar P. Blood exchange transfusion for infants with severe neonatal hyperbilirubinemia. Semin Perinatol. 2011;35(3):175–84.
5. Brown AK, Kim MH, Wu PY, Bryla DA. Efficacy of phototherapy in prevention and management of neonatal hyperbilirubinemia. Pediatrics. 1985;75(2 Pt 2):393–400.
6. Crowther CA, Middleton P, McBain RD. Anti-D administration in pregnancy for preventing Rhesus alloimmunisation. Cochrane Database Syst Rev 2013;(2):CD000020. DOI: 10.1002/14651858.CD000020.pub2.
7. Gottstein R, Cooke RWI. Systematic review of intravenous immunoglobulin in haemolytic disease of the newborn. Arch Dis Child Fetal Neonatal Ed. 2003;88(1):F6–F10.
8. Bhutani VK, Johnson L. Kernicterus in the 21st century: frequently asked questions. J Perinatol. 2009;29 Suppl 1:S20–24.
9. Banerjee TK, Hazra A, Biswas A, Ray J, Roy T, Raut DK, et al. Neurological disorders in children and adolescents. Indian J Pediatr. 2009;76(2):139–46.
10. Hameed NN, Na' Ma AM, Vilms R, Bhutani VK. Severe neonatal hyperbilirubinemia and adverse short-term consequences in Baghdad. Iraq Neonatology. 2011;100(1):57–63.
11. Bhutani VK, Maisels MJ, Stark AR, Buonocore G. Management of jaundice and prevention of severe neonatal hyperbilirubinemia in infants > or = 35 weeks gestation. Neonatology. 2008;94(1):63–7.
12. Beutler E. G6PD Deficiency. Blood. 1994;84(11):3613–36.
13. Hosmer DW, Lemeshow S. Applied Logistic Regression. 2nd ed. New York: Wiley; 2000.
14. National Quality Forum. Serious Reportable Events in Healthcare, 2006 Update: A Consensus Report. Washington, DC: National Quality Forum; 2007.
15. Adebami OJ. Factors associated with the incidence of acute bilirubin encephalopathy in Nigerian population. J Pediatr Neurol. 2011;9(3):347–53.
16. Owa JA, Ogunlesi TA. Why we are still doing so many exchange blood transfusion for neonatal jaundice in Nigeria. World J Pediatr. 2009;5:2.
17. Eneh A, Oruamabo R. Neonatal jaundice in a special care baby unit (SCBU) in port Harcourt, Nigeria: a prospective study. Port Harcourt Med J. 2008;2(2):110–7.
18. Slusher TM, Vreman HJ, McLaren DW, Lewison LJ, Brown AK, Stevenson DK. Glucose-6-phosphate dehydrogenase deficiency and carboxyhemoglobin concentrations associated with bilirubin-related morbidity and death in Nigerian infants. J Pediatr. 1995;126(1):102–8.

19. Ogunlesi TA, Dedeke IO, Adekanmbi AF, Fetuga MB, Ogunfowora OB. The incidence and outcome of bilirubin encephalopathy in Nigeria: a bi-centre study. Niger J Med. 2007;16(4):354–9.

20. Howes RE, Piel FB, Patil AP, Nyangiri OA, Gething PW, Dewi M, et al. G6PD deficiency prevalence and estimates of affected populations in malaria endemic countries: a geostatistical model-based map. PLoS Med. 2012;9(11), e1001339.

21. Bhutani VK, Zipursky A, Blencowe H, Khanna R, Sgro M, Ebbesen F, et al. Neonatal hyperbilirubinemia and Rhesus disease of the newborn: incidence and impairment estimates for 2010 at regional and global levels. Pediatr Res. 2013;74 Suppl 1:86–100.

22. Rasul CH, Hasan MA, Yasmin F. Outcome of neonatal hyperbilirubinemia in a tertiary care hospital in Bangladesh. MJMS. 2010;17(2):40.

23. Crosse VM, Meyer TC, Gerrard JW. Kernicterus and prematurity. Arch Dis Child. 1955;30(154):501–8.

24. Valaes T, Koliopoulos C, Koltsidopoulos A. The impact of phototherapy in the management of neonatal hyperbilirubinemia: comparison of historical cohorts. Acta Paediatr. 1996;85(3):273–6.

25. Watchko JF, Tiribelli C. Bilirubin-induced neurologic damage–mechanisms and management approaches. N Engl J Med. 2013;369(21):2021–30.

26. Maisels MJ, Bhutani VK, Bogen D, Newman TB, Stark AR, Watchko JF. Hyperbilirubinemia in the newborn infant ≥35 Weeks' gestation: an update with clarifications. Pediatrics. 2009;124(4):1193–8.

27. Coda Zabetta CD, Iskander IF, Greco C, Bellarosa C, Demarini S, Tiribelli C, et al. Bilistick: a low-cost point-of-care system to measure total plasma bilirubin. Neonatology. 2013;103(3):177–81.

15

Factors associated with cesarean delivery rates: a single-institution experience

Spencer McClelland[1], Naomi Gorfinkle[2], Alan A. Arslan[3], Maria Teresa Benedetto-Anzai[1], Teresa Cheon[1] and Yuzuru Anzai[1*]

Abstract

Background: The aim of this study was to identify factors associated with variability in Cesarean delivery (CD) rates amongst providers at a single institution.

Methods: A retrospective cohort analysis was carried out on all births at NYU Langone Medical Center from 2005–2013. Data was collected for subjects and linked to diagnosis codes for singleton and twin deliveries. Descriptive characteristics were generated for all deliveries, and inferential analysis was performed including multiple covariates for singleton deliveries in the 2010–2013 cohort, including both univariate and multivariate regression analyses to identify factors associated with higher CD rates.

Results: 37,692 deliveries were identified at our institution during the study period, performed by 88 unique providers. The mean CD rate was 29.6%, with a range for individual physicians from 9.9% to 75.6%. In multivariate regression analysis, CD rate was directly correlated with average patient age, physician male gender, proportion of high-risk deliveries, and Maternal-Fetal Medicine specialty, and it was inversely correlated with total number of deliveries by physician and forceps delivery rate. There was no significant difference in CD rates between group and solo practices. Within the same group practice, each member's CD rate was strongly correlated with the average CD rate of the group.

Conclusion: Our study demonstrates the wide range of CD rates for providers practicing within the same institution and reiterates the association of CD rates with patient age, high-risk pregnancy, and provider volume. Among operative vaginal deliveries, forceps delivery rate was associated with lower CD rates whereas vacuum delivery rate was not. Despite these findings, practice patterns within individual practices appear to contribute significantly to the wide range of CD rates.

Keywords: Cesarean delivery, Cesarean section, Reduction, Forceps, Provider volume

Background

Cesarean delivery (CD) is the most commonly performed major surgery in the United States, accounting for approximately one third of all deliveries [1]. The CD rate had been increasing steadily in recent years, although the national rate has remained stable for the past three years [2]. Compared to vaginal deliveries, CDs are associated with higher maternal morbidity and mortality and can lead to significant complications in future pregnancies [3–5]. While CDs carry clear maternal risks, many studies have failed to show any clear benefits, particularly with regard to neonatal outcomes that would favor CD over vaginal delivery. In light of this evidence, there is growing concern regarding the rising CD rates in United States.

CD rates vary significantly by geographic location and between hospitals, with reported hospital rates ranging from 7.1 to 69.9% [6]. A number of factors have been identified that contribute to this variability, such as regional differences in operative vaginal delivery rates, practice models, (e.g., use of laborists), and medico-legal environments [6–8]. Studies have also been published demonstrating a marked variation in CD rates between providers within an institution, which argues against regional differences being the only—or even the dominant—factor determining CD rates [9, 10].

* Correspondence: yuzuru.anzai@nyumc.org
[1]NYU Langone Medical Center, Department of Obstetrics and Gynecology, 800 2nd Avenue, Suite 815, New York, NY 10017, USA
Full list of author information is available at the end of the article

Recent publications by the Eunice Kennedy Shriver National Institute of Child Health and Human Development (NICHD), Society for Maternal-Fetal Medicine, and American College of Obstetricians and Gynecologists have cast attention on the rise in CD rates, with a goal of modifying practices and factors that lead to non-indicated CDs. Although certain conditions requiring CD are non-modifiable (e.g. complete placenta previa, cord prolapse) and others are strongly influenced by standards of care and common practice (e.g. malpresentation), these represent a relatively small proportion of the cited indications for CD in the U.S. The two most common indications for CD are labor arrest and non-reassuring fetal status. The criteria for diagnosing these conditions are often subjective, and variation in rates of these diagnoses are believed to contribute to the significant variation in CD rates [3–5]. The above publications have also identified use of operative vaginal delivery as a factor influencing CD rates, with the continued observation that the waning use of operative vaginal deliveries has resulted in decreasing opportunities for training, creating a vicious cycle that will result in fewer and fewer physicians becoming proficient in operative vaginal deliveries.

Among the major academic medical centers in New York City for 2011, CD rates ranged from 25.3 to 38.8% [11]. During this period, the published CD rate at NYU Langone Medical Center was 27.7%, placing our institution at the lower end of the spectrum. In this study, we analyzed the CD rates within our single institution from 2005 to 2013 for all providers, with the goal of demonstrating our intra-hospital range in CD rates and identifying factors that may have contributed to variation.

Methods

This retrospective study of deliveries at NYU Langone Medical Center from 2005 to 2013 was approved and received exempt status by the Institutional Review Board. Virtually all patients either had private insurance or were self-pay. Deliveries were almost always performed by private attending physicians who independently dictate management decisions, including the mode of delivery.

Data in this study were extracted from several sources. For deliveries from 2010 to 2013, the data was extracted from the Clinical Database Resource Manager of the University HealthSystem Consortium (UHC). UHC is a data aggregator that collects information from over 200 University and University–affiliated hospitals. It stores clinical information such as diagnosis and procedure codes, as well as information on patient demographics, complications, and readmissions. It has been validated in prior studies with regard to its fidelity to other available databases and has been used in many publications [12]. We extracted data for subjects linked to the diagnosis

codes V270 (Singleton Deliveries) and V272 (Twin deliveries). We excluded multiple gestations higher than twins because these accounted for very few deliveries and were almost always delivered by Cesarean section.

Extracted data included patients' age, race, mode of delivery (Normal Vaginal Delivery, Cesarean Delivery, Forceps Delivery, Vacuum Delivery), delivering physician code, and presence or absence of multiple medical and obstetric co-morbidities. The modes of delivery were stratified by using codes for the delivering physicians, and CD rates and operative vaginal delivery rates for the different physicians were calculated. We linked the physician codes to classify gender, place of residency training, year of completion of residency, practice, and type of practice model.

In our institution, the physicians are either solo practitioners, who are on call on their own and cover the majority of deliveries for their own patients, or belong to group practices, where responsibility for patients is shared and call coverage is split between the members of the practice. Nineteen physicians are solo practitioners and 69 physicians are part of group practices (9 groups in total).

For the deliveries from 2005–2009, we obtained data from NYU Langone Medical Center's administrative records. This database contains information for all deliveries including mode of delivery(CD, spontaneous vaginal delivery or operative vaginal delivery), physician code, and whether the patient received a blood transfusion. This database is more limited than the UHC database, and does not include data such as patient age or race, number of gestation, or medical and obstetric co-morbidities.

For this reason, our analysis was performed in two parts. Descriptive statistics were analyzed for both cohorts, inclusive of all deliveries from 2005–2013. These included total number of deliveries (by type), mean rates of different delivery types for the hospital, and CD rates for different providers. Mean hospital length of stay, cost of hospitalization per patient, and blood transfusion rates were also calculated for each physician.

Inferential analysis was performed on singleton deliveries from the 2010–2013 cohort only, to more accurately analyze the influence of different factors on the CD rates of individual providers. Univariate analysis was performed using Chi-square test for categorical variables, and ANOVA test for continuous variables. Correlation analysis was carried out to calculate Pearson correlation coefficients (r), followed by multivariate regression analysis to identify variables that were independently associated with CD rates. Multivariate regression analysis was carried out using a stepwise backward elimination approach to identify the most significant variables influencing CD rates. Variables included in the initial multivariate model were: average patient age, physician years since completion of residency, physician gender, total number of deliveries, forceps rate, vacuum rate, specialty (MFM, non-MFM), provider (specific provider or practice), proportion of high-risk deliveries by provider, and practice model (solo, group) [13]. The statistical analyses were performed using IBM SPSS Statistics for Windows, Version 21.0. (Armonk, NY: IBM Corp.).

The intraclass correlation coefficient (ICC) was calculated using two-way random effects model. The ICC is commonly used to quantify the degree to which individuals (in our case, OB providers) resemble each other in terms of a quantitative trait (in our case, singleton CD rate). High ICCs suggest a strong within-provider correlation (or high reliability) of CD rate from year to year, while small ICCs indicate that observations are similar across providers, suggesting no group or clustering effect [14]. As a rule of thumb, ICC values less than 0.5 are indicative of poor reliability, values between 0.5 and 0.75 indicate moderate reliability, values between 0.75 and 0.9 indicate good reliability, and values greater than 0.90 indicate excellent reliability [15].

Providers with fewer than 30 deliveries per year were excluded from this study. When physicians perform very few deliveries, their apparent CD rates may not be an accurate representation of their true CD rate, as a result of a small sample size. They may appear to have an artificially high or low CD rate, which would skew our statistical analysis.

A final key assumption for our analysis was the use of a physician's total singleton CD rate as the dependent variable, rather than the primary CD rate, low-risk CD rate, or other rates. To support this decision, we performed preliminary correlation analyses of individual physicians' CD rates, which are discussed in the Results section below.

Results

From 2005–2013, 88 providers were included in our analysis, with a total of 37,692 deliveries performed between them at our institution. 57 providers were female and 31 were male. The providers trained at a variety of programs and completed residency from 1975 up until 2013. Fourteen providers were identified as MFM subspecialists, and 74 providers were identified as general Obstetrics and Gynecology specialists. The mean patient age was 32.9 +/– 1.4 years. 67% of patients identified as White, 5.0% as Black, 13.7% as Asian, and 13.4% other.

From 2005–2013, the mean CD rate was 29.6%, with an individual range by provider by year of 9.9 to 75.6%. From 2010–2013, there were 385 twin deliveries, with a mean twin CD rate of 73.2%. The mean operative

vaginal delivery rate was 5.2%, with an individual provider range of 0 to 22.4%. The mean forceps rate was 1.8% and the mean vacuum rate was 3.4% (Table 1). For the entire hospital, the mean length of stay per patient was 2.8 days, and the mean cost per patient of hospitalization was $6498.73.

Singleton CD rate was very strongly correlated with overall CD rate ($r = 0.993$), singleton primary CD rate ($r = 0.941$), and singleton CD rate excluding non-modifiable indications such as malpresentation, abnormal placentation, and cord prolapse ($r = 0.984$). Twin deliveries were an extremely small proportion of the overall deliveries and did not contribute significantly to any provider's CD rate. Given the above, twins were excluded from our inferential analysis, and singleton CD rate was used for all subsequent descriptive and inferential statistical analyses.

To account for factors known to influence CD rates, we separated the deliveries into low-risk and high-risk deliveries. "High-risk" deliveries were those associated with the following diagnoses, as used in multiple similar database-derived studies: advanced maternal age, malpresentation, previous Cesarean delivery, placenta previa, preeclampsia and hypertension, obesity, preterm delivery, thyroid disease, asthma, fetal-placental problems, amniotic infection, maternal fever, and cord prolapse [16–20]. Providers' individual low-risk and high-risk CD singleton CD rates were strongly correlated ($r = 0.62$, $p <0.0001$) [21]. High-risk deliveries constitute the majority of deliveries at our institution at 55.9%, with a range from 30.0 to 77.4% by provider. In light of these facts, we included high-risk deliveries in our analyses, in order to accurately reflect the case-mix at our institution, and to ensure our findings would be generalizable to and pertinent to similar academic institutions.

Providers who were identified as MFM specialists had a significantly higher CD rate than other providers (41.8% vs 29.9%, $p <0.0001$). Male providers had a higher mean CD rate than female providers (33.6% vs 29.9%, $p = 0.002$).

With regard to practice model, the mean CD rate was 33.0% and 31.0% for solo and group practices, and this difference was not statistically significant (solo vs group, $p = 0.13$). Within the group practices, the CD rates ranged by practice from 10.2 to 65.6%. The CD rates of the individual providers within those practices ranged from 9.9 to 75.6%. Among the group practices, the average CD rate of each physician was strongly correlated with their practice's CD rate ($r = 0.72$, $p < 0.0001$).

The intraclass correlation coefficient (ICC) for the CD rates among the providers was 0.76 ($p = 0.0001$), suggesting that there was good reliability within providers' personal rates over time, and a much higher rate of variability between providers. In other words,

Table 1 Delivery statistics by year, 2005-2013

Year	All deliveries	Cesarean deliveries	Cesarean delivery rate, mean %	Cesarean delivery rate, range	Twin deliveries	Twin Cesarean delivery rate	Operative vaginal delivery rate	Forceps vaginal delivery rate	Vacuum vaginal delivery rate
2005	3627	1111	30.6%	10.8–49.4%	N/A	N/A	6.0%	N/A	N/A
2006	3720	1148	30.9%	14.8–55.2%	N/A	N/A	4.9%	N/A	N/A
2007	4318	1375	31.8%	16.4–62.2%	N/A	N/A	4.8%	N/A	N/A
2008	4477	1389	31.0%	11.8–65.6%	N/A	N/A	4.8%	N/A	N/A
2009	4332	1270	29.3%	15.1–55.3%	N/A	N/A	4.0%	N/A	N/A
2010	4373	1254	28.7%	12.7–50.8%	103	69.9%	4.2%	1.6%	2.6%
2011	4331	1245	28.7%	11.5–66.0%	98	74.5%	4.6%	1.6%	3.6%
2012	4019	1113	27.7%	10.2–75.6%	108	75.0%	5.6%	1.9%	4.5%
2013	4495	1233	27.4%	9.9–65.8%	76	73.7%	5.5%	2.2%	2.7%
Total	37692	11138	29.6%	9.9–75.6%	385	73.2%	5.2%	1.8%	3.4%

each provider's CD rate remained relatively constant during the period we analyzed, and the wide range of CD rates observed in our institution was therefore primarily a function of differences between providers.

On univariate correlation analysis, singleton CD rate was directly correlated with the following provider characteristics: mean patient age, years since completion of residency, and proportion of high-risk deliveries. It was inversely correlated with the following provider characteristics: total number of deliveries, operative vaginal delivery rate, and forceps rate. Singleton CD rate was also directly correlated with mean hospital length of stay and cost per patient, but not with the rate of blood transfusions (Table 2).

In the multivariate regression analysis, singleton CD rate remained positively associated with mean patient age, physician male gender, proportion of high-risk deliveries, and MFM specialty, and negatively associated with forceps rate and total number of deliveries (Table 3).

Discussion

CD is associated with both higher maternal mortality and higher morbidity, namely hemorrhage, infectious morbidity, and the need for emergent hysterectomy, and these risks are even higher when comparing post-labor CD to scheduled CD. CD also brings with it the potential for complications in future pregnancies, such as the need for repeat CDs, or the possibility of abnormal placentation (previa, accreta). It is also associated with increased costs to both patients and hospitals. Despite these downsides, there is not demonstrated improvement in neonatal outcomes [22, 23]. Many private insurance companies provide higher reimbursement rates for CD than for either spontaneous vaginal delivery or operative vaginal delivery, both of which can require significantly more investment of time and skill on behalf of an individual provider. And although CD rates are a

national quality measure when applied to hospitals, the same is not true of individual physicians, who are neither rewarded for low CD rates nor penalized for high CD rates [24].

It is widely known, even to the general public, that CD rates differ among practitioners. However, there have been few publications regarding the variation of CD rates among individual physicians practicing in the same setting [25, 26]. Therefore, it is important to analyze the factors affecting individual variation in CD rates in order to better address the national goal of reducing the CD rate, particularly non-indicated Cesarean deliveries.

There exists a wide range of CD rates among the providers and practices in our study. The ICC for the CD rates among the individual providers was 0.76, suggesting good inter-observer reproducibility, i.e., the rates within individual providers are more similar than the rates between individual providers. Within group practices, the CD rates of the individual providers were strongly correlated with the mean practice rate. This may suggest that there are factors within individual practices that encourage or discourage trends in CD, such as similarities in prenatal counseling, management of labor, thresholds for CD, and operative delivery skills, as well as similarity in patient populations and risk factors.

We identified several factors that were independently associated with higher CD rates. Increasing patient age is a known risk factor for CD, and providers with higher average patient ages had higher CD rates [27].

Providers who had higher numbers of deliveries had lower CD rates. This is consistent with prior publications regarding the effect of provider volume on clinical outcomes in other fields, and it also supports the findings of Clapp et al., who demonstrated a similar phenomenon with regard to provider volume and CD rates [28, 29]. This finding is plausible insofar as physicians who perform more deliveries may be more comfortable managing labor

Table 2 Pearson correlations between selected characteristics and singleton CD rate

	Singleton CD rate	Patient age	Total deliveries, n	Singleton operative vaginal delivery rate	Forceps rate	Vacuum rate	Blood transfusion rate	Hospital length of stay	Cost per patient	Years since graduation	Specialty (MFM)	Proportion of high-risk deliveries
Singleton CD rate	1	0.30[b]	−0.39[b]	−0.24[b]	−0.30[b]	−0.04	0.13	0.45[b]	0.41[b]	0.30[b]	0.34[b]	0.50[b]
Patient age		1	−0.28[b]	−0.09	0.03	−0.03	0.11	0.07	0.09	−0.16[a]	−0.03	0.57[b]
Total deliveries, n			1	−0.02	0.40[b]	0.05	−0.21[b]	−0.24[b]	−0.26[b]	0.07	−0.13	−0.29[b]
Singleton operative vaginal delivery rate				1	0.61[b]	0.50[b]	0.10	0.01	0.03	−0.02	−0.06	−0.05
Forceps rate					1	−0.04	−0.07	−0.17[a]	−0.14	0.07	−0.13	−0.12
Vacuum rate						1	0.09	0.17[a]	0.12	0.01	−0.03	−0.07
Blood transfusion rate							1	0.19[a]	0.33[b]	0.10	0.16[a]	0.17[a]
Hospital length of stay								1	0.79[b]	0.21[b]	0.38[b]	0.27[b]
Cost per patient									1	0.20[b]	0.38[b]	0.37[b]
Years since graduation										1	0.31[b]	0.10
Specialty (MFM)											1	0.34[b]
Proportion of high-risk deliveries												1

[a]Correlation is significant at the 0.05 level (2-tailed)
[b]Correlation is significant at the 0.01 level (2-tailed)

Table 3 Multivariate linear regression modeling[a] of factors influencing singleton CD rate

Factor	Standardized Beta	P-value
Physician gender (males vs. females)	0.369	0.0001
Patient age	0.301	0.0004
Proportion of high-risk deliveries	0.210	0.01
Specialty (MFM vs. non-MFM)	0.147	0.027
Forceps rate	−0.240	0.0003
Total number of deliveries	−0.209	0.003

[a]Multivariate linear regression model using step-wise backward elimination procedure. The variables included in the initial multivariate model included: average patient age, years since completion of residency, physician gender (male, female), total number of deliveries, forceps rate, vacuum rate, specialty (MFM, non-MFM), provider (specific provider or practice), practice model (solo, group), and proportion of high-risk deliveries (percent). The following factors were removed by the model since they met the criteria for removal ($p > 0.05$) in order of removal (practice model, vacuum rate, provider, and years since completion of residency)

and have different thresholds for performing CDs compared to providers who practice less frequently. As the above authors point out, this also represents a potentially modifiable factor for providers and hospitals seeking to reduce CD rates.

Male providers had higher CD rates than female providers, and this remained true on multivariate regression analysis. This may be due to the specific providers within our institution and may not be generalizable in other practice settings.

Providers with higher operative vaginal delivery rates had lower CD rates. This observation is consistent with prior studies and with ACOG recommendations regarding the importance of training in operative vaginal delivery [30]. It is also in agreement with the recent publication by Fitzwater et al. which showed increased CD rate in nulliparous women in the second stage of labor in conjunction with the decreasing operative vaginal delivery rate [31]. It is important to note that higher forceps rates were significantly associated with lower CD rates, while higher vacuum rates were not. In keeping with this finding, there seems to be a consensus among experts in operative vaginal delivery that the risk of failure is higher with vacuum than with forceps deliveries [32]. This relationship has implications for resident education, as training residents in vacuum deliveries may not be as effective in lowering CD rates as would training them in forceps deliveries. Given the decreasing frequency with which forceps are practiced, it may be worth considering limiting the teaching of forceps deliveries to those physicians who will practice obstetrics in the future, as recently suggested by Barth [33].

Providers with higher proportions of high-risk deliveries had higher CD rates, which is an expected finding. Providers who identified as MFM subspecialists had higher CD rates, and this was true on both univariate

and multivariate analysis, and was independent of the effect of proportion of high-risk deliveries. While it is possible that the higher CD rates for MFM providers are related to management of high-risk pregnancies, several points argue against this explanation. First, the existing literature is clear that very few high-risk conditions warrant choosing CD as mode of delivery preferentially over induction and vaginal delivery at the point at which delivery is indicated [4, 5]. Second, many of the most common high-risk conditions (particularly preeclampsia and PPROM) are managed by both generalist and MFM providers, and even when MFM providers act as consultants, the delivering provider is often the patient's primary physician (i.e. original generalist provider), which should reduce the observed difference. Lastly, high-risk conditions that mandate CD over vaginal delivery (maternal contraindications to vaginal delivery, fetal malformations, etc.) are rare and unlikely to explain the differential we observed in CD rates. We therefore do not have a strong explanation for this finding, other than individual provider practice.

One additional finding in our study was the role of practice model. Solo providers are ones who manage their patients in their own practice and deliver the majority of their own patients. Group practices share prenatal care responsibilities and divide labor and delivery call responsibilities based on shifts. Based on these categories, we found that there was no statistically significant difference in CD rates between solo providers and group practices. This runs counter to some speculation, particularly in the lay press, that solo providers are prone to higher CD rates than group practices because of fatigue and a desire to expedite delivery of their patients in order to limit their time in the hospital. In addition, the high correlation of CD rates among physicians in the same group practices suggests a possible effect of similar labor management style and protocols regarding CD.

To the best of our knowledge, this is one of few studies examining the characteristics of individual physicians and their influence on CD rates. There are several strengths to this study. First, there is a large sample size, both in terms of number of providers and number of deliveries. Second, the single-institution nature allows us to analyze physician factors in a homogenous practicing environment, potentially correcting for variations in hospital factors (infrastructure, ancillary services, medico-legal context, etc.) that may lead to variations between institutions. Lastly, we were able to analyze many important covariates, including controlling for high-risk conditions so as to demonstrate the influence of other factors in a mixed low-risk and high-risk population.

This study is not without limitations. While we were able to control for obesity and preterm delivery, the retrospective nature limited our ability to collect certain covariates like body mass index, parity, and gestational age at delivery in more detail. Also, as we were using two separate databases, we were only able to perform inferential statistics on one half of our total cohort. Additionally, we are not able to account for the effect of differences in prenatal care by the different providers, particularly with regard to significant risk factors for CD, such as maternal weight gain.

Despite these limitations, we believe our findings add to national and international conversations regarding CD by shedding light on certain potentially modifiable factors. The range of CD rates observed in the providers in a single institution, both among MFM subspecialists and generalists, was wide. Although we were able to identify several factors associated with higher CD rates, these are unlikely to explain the extremely high rates observed in some providers. Our findings reinforce the influence of patient age on CD risk, as well as the more newly identified effect of provider volume on CD rates. Our findings also emphasize once again the importance of skills in forceps-assisted vaginal deliveries as a means of reducing CD rates, over and above the utility of vacuum-assisted vaginal deliveries, a finding that continues to have important implications for the training of residents.

Conclusions

There remains great variability between providers practicing at the same institution with regard to CD rates. This variability is related to many factors, including patient variables like age and high-risk pregnancy, but also provider variables, such as volume of practice, rate of forceps deliveries, and MFM specialty. These findings reinforce the need for addressing efforts to reduce CD rates at the institution level by focusing on potentially modifiable provider factors that may drive higher CD rates.

Abbreviations
CD: Cesarean delivery; ICC: Intraclass correlation coefficient; MFM: Maternal-Fetal Medicine

Acknowledgments
Not applicable.

Funding
not applicable.

Authors' contributions
SM, NG, and YA performed data collection. AA performed data analysis. SM, YA, AA, MTB, and TC wrote the manuscript. All authors read and approved the final manuscript.

Competing interests
The authors declare that they have no competing interests.

Author details
[1]NYU Langone Medical Center, Department of Obstetrics and Gynecology, 800 2nd Avenue, Suite 815, New York, NY 10017, USA. [2]Johns Hopkins University School of Medicine, 4 South Broadway, Baltimore, MD 21231, USA. [3]NYU Langone Medical Center, Division of Epidemiology, Departments of Obstetrics and Gynecology, Environmental Medicine, and Population Health, 650 First Ave, Rm. 532, New York, NY 10016, USA.

References
1. Martin JA, Hamilton BE, Osterman MJK, et al. Births: final data for 2013. National vital statistics reports; vol 64 no 1. Hyattsville: National Center for Health Statistics; 2015.
2. Changes in Cesarean Delivery Rates by Gestational Age: United States, 1996–2011. http://www.cdc.gov/nchs/data/databriefs/db124.pdf. Accessed 12 Apr 2017.
3. Caughey AB, Cahill AG, Guise JM, Rouse DJ. Safe prevention of the primary cesarean delivery. Am J Obstet Gynecol. 2014;210(3):179–93.
4. Spong CY, Berghella V, Wenstrom KD, Mercer BM, Saade GR. Preventing the first cesarean delivery: summary of a joint Eunice Kennedy Shriver national institute of child health and human development, society for maternal-fetal medicine, and american college of obstetricians and gynecologists workshop. Obstet Gynecol. 2012;120(5):1181–93.
5. American College of Obstetricians and Gynecologists, Society for Maternal-Fetal Medicine, Caughey AB, Cahill AG, Guise JM, Rouse DJ. Safe prevention of the primary cesarean delivery. Am J Obstet Gynecol. 2014;210(3):179–93.
6. Kozhimannil KB, Law MR, Virnig BA. Cesarean delivery rates vary tenfold among US hospitals: reducing variation may address quality and cost issues. Health Aff. 2013;32:527–35.
7. O'Callaghan M, MacLennan A. Cesarean delivery and cerebral palsy: a systematic review and meta-analysis. Obstet Gynecol. 2013;122(6):1169–75.
8. Localio AR, Lawthers AG, Bengtson JM, Hebert LE, Weaver SL, Brennan TA, Landis JR. Relationship between malpractice claims and cesarean delivery. JAMA. 1993;269(3):366–73.
9. Goyert GL, Bottoms SF, Treadwell MC, Nehra PC. The physician factor in cesarean birth rates. N Engl J Med. 1989;320(11):706–9.
10. Demott RK, Sandmire HF. The green Bay cesarean section study: I. The physician factor as a determinant of cesarean birth rates. Am J Obstet Gynecol. 1990;162(6):1593–9.
11. New York State Department of Health. Hospital Maternity-Related Procedures and Practices Statistics. Available at: http://www.health.ny.gov/statistics/facilities/hospital/maternity/. Accessed 12 Apr 2017.
12. Sutton JM, Hayes AJ, Wilson GC, Quillin 3rd RC, Wima K, Hohmann S, et al. Validation of the university HealthSystem consortium administrative dataset: concordance and discordance with patient-level institutional data. J Surg Res. 2014;190(2):484–90. doi:10.1016/j.jss.2014.03.044.
13. Janevic T, Loftfield E, Savitz DA, Bradley E, Illuzzi J, Lipkind H. Disparities in cesarean delivery by ethnicity and nativity in New York city. Matern Child Health J. 2014;18(1):250–7.
14. Killip S, Mahfoud Z, Pearce K. What is an intracluster correlation coefficient? crucial concepts for primary care researchers. Ann Fam Med. 2004;2(3):204–8.
15. Portney LG, Watkins MP. Foundations of clinical research: applications to practice. New Jersey: Prentice Hall; 2000.
16. Maso G, et al. Risk-adjusted operative delivery rates and maternal-neonatal outcomes as measures of quality assessment in obstetric care: a multicenter prospective study. BMC Pregnancy Childbirth. 2015;15:20.
17. Bailit JL. Measuring the quality of inpatient obstetrical care. Obstet Gynecol Surv. 2007;62:207–13.
18. Bailit JL, Srinivas SK. Where should I have my baby? Am J Obstet Gynecol. 2012;207:1–2/23.
19. Bailit JL. Measurement is just the beginning. Am J Obstet Gynecol. 2013;208:427–8.
20. Gregory KD, Korst LM, Gornbein JA, Platt LD. Using administrative data to identify indications for elective primary cesarean delivery. Health Serv Res. 2002;37(5):1387–401.
21. Evans JD. Straightforward statistics for the behavioral sciences. Pacific Grove: Brooks/Cole Publishing; 1996.
22. Watson WJ, George RJ, Welter S, et al. High-risk obstetric patients. Maternal morbidity after cesareans. J Reprod Med. 1997;42(5):267–70.
23. Maternal Morbidity for Vaginal and Cesarean Deliveries. National Vital Statistics Reports, Vol. 64 No. 4, May 20, 2015. Centers for Disease Control and Prevention. 2015.

24. Specifications Manual for Joint Commission National Quality Measures. https://manual.jointcommission.org/releases/TJC2014A1/MIF0167.html. Accessed 12 Apr 2017.

25. Main EK. New perinatal quality measures from the National Quality Forum, the Joint Commission and the Leapfrog Group. Curr Opin Obstet Gynecol. 2009;21(6):532–40.

26. Reducing Unnecessary C-Section Births. The Opinionator: The New York Times. http://opinionator.blogs.nytimes.com/2016/01/19/arsdarian-cutting-the-number-of-c-section-births/?_r=0. Accessed 12 Apr 2017.

27. Peipert JF, Bracken MB. Maternal age: an independent risk factor for cesarean delivery. Obstet Gynecol. 1993;81(2):200–5.

28. Boyd LR, Novetsky AP, Curtin JP. Effect of surgical volume on route of hysterectomy and short-term morbidity. Obstet Gynecol. 2010;116:909–15.

29. Clapp MA, Melamed A, Robinson JN, Shah N, Little SE. Obstetrician volume as a potentially modifiable risk factor for cesarean delivery. Obstet Gynecol. 2014;124(4):697–703.

30. Practice Bulletin 154: Operative Vaginal Delivery. American College of Obstetrics and Gynecology. Obstet Gynecol. 2016; 127 (5): e56-65.

31. Fitzwater JL, Owen J, Ankumah N-A, Campbell SB, Biggio JR, Szychowski JM. Edwards RF Nulliparous Women in the Second Stage of Labor. Obstet Gynecol. 2015;126(1):81–6.

32. Yeomans ER. Operative vaginal delivery. Obstet Gynecol. 2010;115(3):645–53.

33. Barth Jr WJ. Persistent occiput posterior. Obstet Gynecol. 2015;125(3):69.

Newborn intensive care survivors: a review and a plan for collaboration in Texas

Alice Gong[1*], Yvette R. Johnson[2], Judith Livingston[1], Kathleen Matula[1] and Andrea F. Duncan[3]

Abstract

Background: Neonatal intensive care is a remarkable success story with dramatic improvements in survival rates for preterm newborns. Significant efforts and resources are invested to improve mortality and morbidity but much remains to be learned about the short and long-term effects of neonatal intensive care unit (NICU) interventions. Published guidelines recommend that infants discharged from the NICU be in an organized follow-up program that tracks medical and neurodevelopmental outcomes. Yet, there are no standardized guidelines for provision of follow-up services for high-risk infants.

The National Institute of Child Health and Human Development Neonatal Research Network and the Vermont Oxford Network have made strides toward standardizing practices and conducting outcomes research, but only include a subset of developmental follow-up programs with a focus on extremely preterm infants. Several studies have been conducted to gain a better understanding of current practices in developmental follow-up. Some of the major themes in these studies are the lack of personnel and funding to provide comprehensive follow-up care; feeding difficulties as a primary issue for NICU survivors, families, and programs; wide variability in referral and follow-up care practices; and calls for standardized, systematic developmental surveillance to improve outcomes.

Findings: We convened a one day summit to discuss developmental follow-up practices in Texas involving four academic and three nonacademic centers. All seven centers described variable age and weight criteria for follow-up of NICU patients and a unique set of developmental practices, including duration of follow-up, types and timing of developmental assessments administered, education and communication with families and other health care providers, and referrals for services. Needs identified by the centers focused on two main themes: resources and comprehensive care. Participants identified key challenges for developmental follow-up, generated recommendations to address these challenges, and outlined components of a quality program.

Conclusions: The long-term goal is to ensure that all children maximize their potential; a goal supported through quality, comprehensive developmental follow-up care and outcomes research to continuously improve evidence-based practices. We aim to contribute to this goal through a statewide working group collaborating on research to standardize practices and inform policies that truly benefit children and their families.

Keywords: Preterm birth, Developmental follow-up, Standardized practice, Collaboration, Outcomes research

Introduction

Neonatal intensive care is a remarkable success story. Survival rates of infants weighing <800 grams increased from 0 % in 1943–1945 to 34 % in 1987–1988 and 70 % in 1994 [1]. In the early 1980s, preterm newborns <28 weeks gestation had a 90 % mortality rate. Recently the Eunice Kennedy Shriver National Institute of Child Health and Development (NICHD) Neonatal Research Network (NRN) reported survival of 65 % and 56 % survival without severe impairment in infants <27 weeks gestation [2].

Extraordinary advances in obstetric and neonatal care have resulted in tremendous gains for the premature infant. The efforts and resources invested to achieve such gains come at a significant cost. The financial cost alone of neonatal intensive care has been estimated at $3,400 per hospital day [3]. Preterm births cost the U.S. health care system more than $26.2 billion in 2005 [4].

* Correspondence: gong@uthscsa.edu
[1]Department of Pediatrics, The University of Texas Health Science Center at San Antonio, 7703 Floyd Curl Dr. San Antonio, Texas 78229, USA
Full list of author information is available at the end of the article

The substantial investment in neonatal care has resulted in improved mortality and morbidity outcomes of preterm infants. However, the significant decrease in mortality and short-term morbidities has not had a proportionate effect on long-term neurodevelopmental outcomes. Rigorous long-term outcome studies evaluating the impact of neonatal care and perinatal interventions have informed our understanding of their impact on long-term outcomes and helped to refine the care that has resulted in improved outcomes. Research on perinatal interventions, such as studies supported by NICHD, demonstrate the impact of obstetric and neonatal care on long-term outcomes of neonatal intensive care unit (NICU) survivors. Several key examples include findings that show: (1) Apgar scores do not predict cerebral palsy [5]; (2) the clear benefits of antenatal corticosteroids in reducing the risk of life-threatening morbidities including respiratory distress syndrome and intraventricular hemorrhage (IVH), balanced against studies demonstrating lack of benefit and possible harm from repeated courses [6]; (3) lack of benefit of antenatal treatment with magnesium sulfate on school-age outcomes [7]; (4) improved childhood outcomes following hypothermia for neonatal encephalopathy [8] and (5) benefit of early caffeine administration among preterm infants <1250 grams at birth and reduction of bronchopulmonary dysplasia (BPD) and improved long-term developmental outcomes [9].

The value of follow-up is also emphasized by studies isolating factors that impact long-term outcomes. For example, certain morbidities (e.g. IVH, necrotizing enterocolitis [NEC], BPD, retinopathy of prematurity [ROP]) have been identified that adversely affect outcomes whereas certain psychosocial factors (e.g. higher maternal and paternal IQ and socioeconomic status) positively impact child developmental outcomes and loss to follow-up [10–14]. Guillén, et al. [15] conducted a systematic review to assess center variation in rates of neurodevelopmental impairment (NDI) at 18–24 months corrected age among extremely low-birth-weight (ELBW) or extremely low-gestational-age (ELGA) infants. NDI was defined as the presence of at least one of the following: a mental developmental index score two standard deviations below the mean on the Bayley Scales of Infant Development-Second Edition®; cerebral palsy (nonprogressive motor impairment characterized by abnormal muscle tone in at least one extremity and a decreased range or control of movements); visual impairment (visual acuity of less than 20/200 unilaterally or bilaterally or blindness); or significant hearing impairment (hearing loss requiring amplification). NDI and follow-up rates were reported for 34,185 infants from 20 publications involving 24 cohorts. Follow-up rates ranged from 71–100 % and higher rates of NDI correlated with loss to follow-up rates, suggesting the healthier children may not be followed [15].

Van der Pal-de Bruin et al. [16] reported on a Dutch cohort of 1,338 infants born <32 weeks gestation or very low birth weight (<1500 grams; VLBW) for whom data was longitudinally collected from birth through age 19 years. Follow-up data were captured for 74 % participants still alive at age 19 years. Outcomes assessed included physical, cognitive, behavioral, quality of life measures, and impact of disabilities. Study participants demonstrated significant developmental impairment over time. However, major disabilities were unchanged as children aged but minor disabilities increased [16]. A German study of 148 children with birth weights <1000 grams analyzed the relationship between perinatal risk factors, social parameters, and neurodevelopmental outcomes at 10–13 years. Results indicated that regardless of brain compromises, neurodevelopmental outcomes between 10–13 years of age were better among children from more educated mothers: low maternal education was the strongest factor associated with a decreased composite intelligence quotient (IQ) [14].

The NICHD has recommended follow-up for all ELBW infants to assess growth, neurologic status, behavior, language, socioeconomic status, and family resources [17]. The American Academy of Pediatrics (AAP) Committee on The Fetus and Newborn's 2008 guidelines for hospital discharge of high risk neonates, state that "most high-risk infants should be enrolled in a follow-up clinic that specializes in the neurodevelopmental assessment of high-risk infants" and that "standardized assessments should be performed in the follow-up clinic at specific ages through early childhood" [18]. Furthermore, guidelines published by the AAP and American College of Obstetrics and Gynecology [19] recommend that infants discharged from the NICU be in an organized follow-up program that tracks and records medical and neurodevelopmental outcomes for analysis later; this follow-up is an essential component of level 3 and level 4 services. Data from multiple follow-up studies indicate that perinatal therapeutic interventions may dramatically alter later growth and development and there is increased recognition of the potential disconnect between perinatal and long-term outcomes [1, 17]. Yet there are no standardized guidelines for provision of follow-up services for high-risk infants and inadequate support for follow-up programs [18, 20]. However, there are initiatives designed to reach this goal such as the MedImmune and National Initiative for Children's Healthcare Quality's toolkit for follow-up of premature infants up to 12 months chronological age [21].

Review of practices in developmental follow-up

Several U.S. studies have been conducted to gain a better understanding of current practices in developmental follow-up, including online surveys of follow-up programs associated with academic and private practice based follow-up programs [20, 22]; retrospective analysis of referral data from California Children's Services [23]; and analysis of programs associated with the NICHD NRN [1]. Follow-up practices in states such as Rhode Island [24], as well as in other countries, such as Australia [25, 26] and Canada [27-30], have also been described. Some of the major cross-cutting themes in these studies are the lack of personnel and funding to provide comprehensive follow-up care, the significant feeding difficulties among NICU survivors, wide variability in referral and follow-up practices, and calls for standardized, systematic developmental surveillance to improve outcomes.

The need for developmental follow-up and outcome studies is recognized by leaders and organizations concerned about the impact of preterm birth. The NICHD NRN and Vermont Oxford Network (VON), a non-profit organization that maintains a database on medical interventions and outcomes for preterm infants at member institutions worldwide [31], are working toward standardizing practices and conducting outcomes research. However, these organizations only include a subset of developmental follow-up programs.

We, too, are concerned about the need for standardized practices and outcomes research and sought to have a better understanding of perspectives on developmental follow-up practices in Texas through a focused dialogue with stakeholders. Texas is a large state with multiple academic and private developmental follow-up programs. In 2012, the total number of live births in Texas was 382,438 and 8.3 % of newborns were low birth weight (<2500 grams) [32]. Among Texas mothers, 42.3 % were unmarried, only 62.6 % received prenatal care in the first trimester of pregnancy with 53.8 % of births covered by Medicaid [32]. In 2013, the preterm birth rate in Texas was 12.3 % (compared with the U.S. rate of 9.6 %), with higher rates for Blacks and Hispanics compared to Whites [33]. Sixteen percent of Texas women, ages 18–24, had less than a high school education as compared to 13 % of U.S. women. For women ages 25 and over, 18.3 % as compared to 13.4 % of U.S. women did not have a high school diploma [34]. These data underscore the many challenges to ensuring a healthy start for Texas newborns, particularly those born premature.

Developmental follow-up of high-risk infants in Texas exemplifies the problems nationally as they relate to socioeconomic factors that impact developmental and behavioral outcomes. These risk factors include maternal education, adolescent pregnancy, poverty, and race/ethnicity. Hoffman et al. [35] found that premature infants born to adolescent mothers, who are less educated, single, and of Hispanic or African American race/ethnicity are at significantly higher risk for adverse behavioral outcomes and cognitive impairment at 18–22 months corrected age. Using the Bayley Scales of Infant and Toddler Development, Third Edition® (BSITD III),

premature infants of adolescent mothers have lower composite language scores of <85 (56 % vs. 49 %, $p = 0.07$). These infants are also significantly more likely to have unstable housing, be under state supervision, and have multiple rehospitalizations compared to similar premature infants born to older, better-educated mothers. Using the Brief Infant Social Emotional Assessment (BITSEA), premature infants of adolescent mothers had higher scores of behavioral and social problems compared to premature infants of adult mothers (mean 14.8 vs. 12.1, $p < 0.001$). These findings underscore the need to include premature infants and their families in a comprehensive follow-up program that includes care coordination and education to ensure optimal outcomes [35].

Findings

First annual summit on follow-up practices in Texas

On February 20, 2015, we convened a one-day summit to discuss follow-up practices in Texas among centers offering care for children and families affected by preterm birth. Our objective was to initiate dialogue about NICU follow-up best practices and explore the feasibility of creating a working group focused on long-term follow-up of high-risk NICU survivors. An email invitation was sent to nine Texas follow-up programs and, of these, four academic and three non-academic programs participated. Representatives from the NICHD, Texas Department of Assistive and Rehabilitative Services' Early Childhood Intervention (ECI) program, and Hand to Hold, a family advocacy group for NICU survivors, also participated in the meeting.

Prior to the meeting, follow-up program directors were asked to present information about the following: (1) patient population; (2) a list of personnel who perform developmental, behavioral, and psychological testing; (3) follow-up practices; (4) the names of developmental tests administered; (5) the age and schedule of testing; (6) the processes for reporting results; (7) the procedure for referrals and interventions; (8) the duration of tracking; (9) the interface with neonatology and primary care colleagues; (10) the experience with impact of follow-up; (11) the perceived needs of follow-up practice; and (12) a perspective on feasibility of a statewide collaboration.

Center reports

Across the seven centers, there was significant variability in follow-up practices (Table 1), although not all reported on every item listed above. Age and weight criteria for NICU patients were different at all centers as was the annual census. However, a common feature among centers was that they operated with a small, part-time staff. All seven of the centers described a unique set of developmental practices, including duration of follow-up, types and timing of developmental assessments administered,

Table 1 Select data from seven NEON follow-up centers

Patient population	2 centers ≤ 1500 g or < 32 weeks
	1 center ≤ 1500 g or ≤ 32 weeks
	1 center < 1500 g
	1 center < 800 g
	1 center < 27 weeks, in any research study or other at team discretion
	1 center – extended list of NICU graduates
	Annual census ranged from 200 (private center) to 5,200 (private center with three hospital systems)
	84 % was highest percentage of Medicaid NICU patients
Personnel	3 academic and 1 private center were supervised by neonatologists; 1 academic and 2 private centers were supervised by developmental pediatricians
	All 7 centers had small, often part-time staff
	5 centers "borrowed" staff from hospital NICU
	3 academic centers used physicians-in-training
	Types of non-physician professional staff involved in follow-up included: advanced nurse practitioner, nurse, social worker, physical therapist, occupational therapist, speech therapist (needed most for feeding therapy), audiologist, dietician, nutritionist, lactation consultant, psychometrician, and case manager.
Duration of follow-up	2 years up to 22 years, although the majority of centers reported following patients for 5 years or less.
Communications with families	2 centers reported providing verbal and written feedback to parents about testing at the time of the visit
	4 centers reported providing feedback to the parents at the time of the visit, as well as mailing written reports to parents and primary care providers after clinic visits
	1 center did not include communications in the report
Communications with providers	1 academic center and 2 private centers reported providing updates and maintaining on-going communications with their neonatology groups. The academic center and one of the two private centers reported trying to engage with community pediatricians and include them in meetings or on a committee, while the other private center reported functioning as a de facto medical home. A third private center commented, "We let the pediatricians drive."

education and communication with families and other health care providers, and referrals for subspecialty services. Despite the variation in assessments performed, all centers used the BSITD-III at some point. Only two of the centers administered the scales at the same age (18–24 months post-menstrual age) and one of these two centers outsourced the testing separate from the clinic visit while the other administered the scales at the time of the clinic visit. Most centers are correcting for gestational age up until age two; this process is generally well accepted [17]. Due to increased survival of the most immature and fragile infants, centers discussed whether two years of correcting for gestational age is still appropriate; however there are no data to guide a change in practice.

General comments about the impact of follow-up were that it allows care coordination and continuity with the NICU and helps eliminate fragmentation in systems of care. Follow-up facilitates early identification of growth and feeding problems and earlier referrals to subspecialty care and rehabilitative services. Earlier referral helps to ensure children receive needed subspecialty medical care and frequent and longitudinal provision of information to families about their children's developmental status. This aids in the prevention of developmental delay and secondary social, emotional, or behavioral problems.

Ultimately, follow-up improves developmental outcomes. One optimal goal articulated was to provide follow-up through school age to assess and improve school readiness and school performance.

Needs identified by the centers focused on two main themes: resources and comprehensive multidisciplinary care. In terms of resources, centers reported needing funding to support infrastructure and research. Adequate resources would support the centers' vision to provide comprehensive acute and well-baby care at least through transition to primary care providers. A comprehensive care follow-up program would adhere to and effectively implement established best practice guidelines (Table 2).

Key follow-up challenges identified

Summit participants discussed a number of systemic challenges for NICU survivors. Among these, length of stay (LOS) with urgency to discharge babies from the NICU is a major issue. Hospitals, insurers, families, and society may be unaware that an adequate support structure both during the NICU stay and during transition home is vital to ensure safe discharge.

Feeding challenges in the NICU have a major impact on LOS. NICU discharges are frequently focused on infant weight gain and achievement of full oral feedings

Table 2 Components of a quality comprehensive care NICU follow-up program

Personnel	• A multidisciplinary team with adequate staffing from physicians, psychologists, nurses, social workers, physical, occupational, speech, and respiratory therapists, nutritionists, lactation consultants, case managers, and ECI collaborators
	• Support for case management and home visits
Practices	• A standardized manual of operations
	• Processes to engage effectively with neonatologists, community pediatricians, and other primary care providers including data sharing linkages
	• Mechanisms for tracking during and after clinic discharge, including follow-up at school age, adolescence, and adulthood
	• Databases for tracking and research
Programs	• Family support groups
	• Organized educational program for outreach to families, providers, and community
	• Website with resources for families, providers, and community
Facilities	• Appropriate clinic space

that are not always sustained after discharge. This issue becomes a major problem for NICU survivors and their families as ability to feed the infant then becomes stressful. It is well recognized that breast milk is the best source of nutrition, providing protective immunities, growth hormones, and other elements tailored to the newborn's needs [36, 37]. Low birth weight infants fed predominately with mothers' own milk had better outcomes and less viral infections up to 8 months of life [38]. Exclusive breastfeeding is ideal; however, this presents many challenges for VLBW infants and their mothers [39]. NICUs need to change many practices in order to help families achieve optimal feeding goals after discharge. Many mothers forego their desire to breastfeed in order to get the baby home sooner since bottle-feeding is perceived as easier and faster [40]. Frequent post-discharge feeding issues include: mothers unable to breastfeed directly and resorting to continued pumping and feeding from bottles; babies not thriving, development of oral aversion, and feeding refusal; primary care providers changing to formulas that are inadequate for the growing premature infant or difficult to access in the outpatient setting and adding medications inconsistent with current guidelines.

All NICU survivors are at risk for neurodevelopmental deficits but, due to resource limitations, follow-up clinics are usually reserved for those who are sickest and have the most need. Some clinics are open to all who seek services but indigent populations, for a variety of reasons, often do not present to these clinics. The challenge for most developmental follow-up programs is ensuring long-term follow-up of all who are at risk, not just the sickest premature infants. Organized follow-up of all at-

risk children is extremely important, as preterm children remain at risk for severe behavioral and cognitive deficits at school-age, even in the absence of early global deficits [41] and more subtle harbingers of these later deficits may present in very early life [42]. Lack of organized follow-up of all at-risk children and the resulting delay in early recognition of abnormalities may result in a missed opportunity for interventions aimed at improving modifiable outcomes. Limited budgets and resources encountered by many follow-up programs present a significant challenge to casting "a wider net" to include a representative population of premature infants at risk.

Families often face barriers to receiving follow-up services. Delays in first follow-up appointments because of staffing shortages or other systemic problems impact families' access and use of follow-up services. When a follow-up program is funded exclusively through patient revenue, it negatively impacts follow-up rates [20]. Lack of insurance or inadequate insurance coverage and high co-pays for mental health services prevent children from receiving neurodevelopmental testing. From the parent's perspective, one of the greatest values of developmental testing is the opportunity to learn about growth and development and tools and strategies to aid their child's development. Parents of all socioeconomic levels are capable of learning to interact responsively with their children. Trials of parenting interventions in early childhood have demonstrated improvement in behavioral problems and responsivity [43]. Further, in a study of an intervention aimed at improving parental responsivity, VLBW children showed greater gains after the intervention than their term-born counterparts [44]. Given the tools and education, they can do the work to preserve and protect the care initiated in the NICU to help their children survive and thrive.

Follow-up programs are charged with identifying the need for therapy services among a population at high risk for delay. The tools used by most programs are not screeners; they are full assessments that identify delays warranting intervention. Screening has little purpose in an inherently high-risk population and is not effective in identifying subtle impairments [45]. Screening instruments are likely to under-identify infants in need of services, in part because they rely on parent report. Parental report may be unreliable if the questions are misunderstood or the parent has not attended to the child's skills in all areas of development. One major challenge when referring a child to ECI is that Texas ECI programs are mandated to use only a customized version of the Battelle Developmental Inventory™ [46], and cannot accept results from any other developmental assessment. In many instances, assessments offered by follow-up programs should be accepted because these are based upon lengthy administrations of standardized clinical assessments, along with neuromotor exams provided by highly qualified professionals. This would save the ECI programs time and expense of performing a redundant service. Texas ECI is underfunded with an annual allocation of $400 per child as of February 2015. To finance operations, ECI is currently billing Medicaid and managed care organizations.

Recommendations for statewide collaboration

Two overarching recommendations were made at the meeting as steps toward achieving quality comprehensive follow-up care in Texas: (1) create a statewide database and (2) establish uniform, evidence-based guidelines for developmental follow-up. Consensus should be reached about which populations, outcome variables, and long-term outcomes to track, as well as duration of follow-up. Data could also be used for benchmarking and linking immediate and long-term outcomes, collaborative statewide quality improvement initiatives, and standardizing protocols for ECI and Women, Infant, and Children (WIC) programs. Perhaps most importantly, levels of care for follow-up need to be established as not all NICU survivors will need every test and service.

Table 3 NEON recommendations for achieving quality comprehensive follow-up care

Systems	• Develop guidelines to determine levels of post-NICU discharge care based upon current knowledge and to update levels as data is acquired.
	• Start a database with meaningful, de-identified data that can be shared.
	• Choose common data points to gather from all units and build incrementally.
	• Educate hospitals, insurers, and society that time in the NICU is treatment as maturity is important for survival.
	• Work toward establishing universal nutrition guidelines for NICU and beyond.
	• Build consensus that breast milk is best.
	• Develop more family friendly NICUs.
	• Gather data to support that formula-fed premature infants need post-discharge preterm formula for the length of time determined by the medical specialist following the child.
	• Engage state and national professional organizations to promote support for quality comprehensive follow-up care, including advocacy to ensure ECI has adequate resources to provide timely and appropriate early intervention services.
	• Advocate at the state level for ECI acceptance of a referral for services based upon a comprehensive developmental evaluation by an appropriate professional.
	• Educate policy makers and insurers to change the culture away from waiting for a problem to occur to a prevention orientation, especially in vulnerable populations.
	• Educate WIC on post-menstrual age versus chronological age and dietary issues.
Families	• Provide support to families by focusing on children's progress and what families are doing well, rather than just their deficits.
	• Empower parents.
	• Give educational information in multiple modalities addressing the needs of the adult learner (e.g. web-based resources, handouts, information videos, "just-in-time" educational or interactive tools). Information should be varied and repetitive to enhance learning and overall impact.
	• Help parents learn how to engage with health care professionals.
	• Provide education that time in the NICU is a treatment and impacts brain development.
	• Facilitate appropriate discharge with training and preparation for parents.
	• Provide education to families on how to breastfeed and use a breast pump and ensure the best kind of pump is immediately available.
	• For formula-fed infants, ensure families know how to mix formula correctly.
	• Arrange initial follow-up visits (and link with ECI) before NICU discharge.
	• Continue Post-discharge support with outpatient care, home visits, and phone calls.
	• Set up Life Line for families to call for guidance and assistance finding resources and family support groups such as Hand to Hold.
	• Create a Text for Baby for preterm babies modeled on the program for term babies.
	• Keep in mind what matters to families, e.g. will my child go to kindergarten with the rest of the children?
	• Teach parents about the role of early intervention to decrease the stigma.
Providers	• Educate neonatologists about why follow-up is part of the NICU continuum of care.
	• Educate community pediatricians that follow-up supports, not supplants, their work.
	• Educate community pediatricians caring for NICU survivors about existing guidelines.
	• Educate providers to help ensure they are helping families use evidence-based, developmentally appropriate feeding practices.

A proposal was made to create a database and establish guidelines through the formation of a statewide consortium of high-risk providers to share data on best practices, outcomes, and protocols. The consortium could also partner with the VON, Texas Pediatric Society, Texas Association for Infant Mental Health, Texas Society for Clinical Social Work, and other groups. To this end and in deliberations after the February meeting, the group named itself the Neonatal Evaluation and Outcomes Network (NEON) and began the process to develop infrastructure to function. Given the current milieu and challenges in follow-up, the meeting participants outlined a series of recommendations that might be pursued by the network, organized thematically in three areas (Table 3).

Discussion

Many NICU graduates have survived multi-organ disease such as IVH, BPD, ROP, and NEC and have lifelong complications from them. We frequently send them out of the NICU to be cared for by overwhelmed families and over-burdened primary care providers who do not have the time to provide a proper medical home. As we learn more about the devastating changes happening to fragile children during a period of great vulnerability in the NICU, we need to continue to research the consequences of care and how to help these children develop to their full potential.

There are many unanswered questions. As scientists, are we doing our due diligence if we are not tracking the outcomes of NICU survivors? What are the long-term consequences of NICU interventions? What are the unintended consequences of interventions on NICU survivors and their families? What are the factors that affect outcomes and how do these impact disease mechanisms and processes of resiliency? In Texas, are there disparities in referral, based on maternal race or ethnicity, similar to what was reported in California [23]? If so, what are the causes and how can these be addressed?

The Colorado Department of Public Health and Environment convened a stakeholder summit in 2012 to "optimize the health and developmental outcomes of premature and high risk infants and their families by sharing best practices and systems of care that support the transition home from the NICU and hospital to the medical home and supportive community-based services" [47]. The multidisciplinary groups participating came to many of the same conclusions as the Texas summit. With the growing awareness of the needs of the NICU survivor, it is time to link collaboratives and develop national databases in order to answer some of the key questions.

Conclusion

"I am delighted to approve the legislation authorizing the creation of a National Institute of Child Health and Human Development. . . . The future health of our Nation rests on the care of our children and the development of our knowledge of the medical and biological sciences. . . . Research in recent years has established beyond question that adult behavior, intelligence, and motivation are established by the experience and patterns of response developed in the formative years of life. . ."

President John F. Kennedy, signing HR 11099, Public Law 87–838 (76 Stat. 1072), on October 17, 1962 [48].

The long-term goal of the NEON group is to ensure that all Texas infants reach their full potential. This goal is supported through quality, comprehensive developmental follow-up care and outcomes research to continuously improve evidence-based practices. We aim to reach this goal through collaboration and research for practice standardization and policy information that truly benefits Texas children and their families.

Abbreviations

AAP: American Academy of Pediatrics; BITSEA: Brief Infant Social Emotional Assessment; BPD: Bronchopulmonary Dysplasia; BSITD: Bayley Scales of Infant and Toddler Development; ECI: Early Childhood Intervention; ELBW: Extremely Low-Birth-Weight; ELGA: Extremely Low-Gestational-Age; IQ: Intelligence Quotient; IVH: Intraventricular Hemorrhage; LOS: Length of Stay; NDI: Neurodevelopmental Impairment; NEC: Necrotizing; NEON: Neonatal Evaluation and Outcomes Network; NICHD: National Institutes of Child Health and Development; NICU: Neonatal Intensive Care Unit; NRN: Neonatal Research Network; ROP: Retinopathy of Prematurity; VLBW: Very Low Birth Weight; VON: Vermont Oxford Network; WIC: Women, Infants, and Children.

Competing interests

The authors have no competing financial interests. The authors have no non-financial competing interests, neither political, personal, religious, ideological, academic, intellectual, commercial, or otherwise.

Authors' contributions

AG conceived the idea for the Texas summit, organized and presented at the meeting, drafted, and supervised editing of the manuscript. YJ attended and presented at the meeting and contributed to writing the manuscript. JL participated in the meeting, synthesized reports from the Texas centers for use in the manuscript, and contributed to writing and editing the manuscript. KM attended and presented at the meeting and contributed to editing the manuscript. AD attended and presented at the meeting and contributed to editing the manuscript. All authors read and approved the final manuscript.

Authors' information

AG is Professor of Pediatrics in the Division of Neonatology, Department of Pediatrics at the University of Texas Health Science Center at San Antonio, with 30 years of experience as an academic Neonatologist. She recently was named the medical director of the Premiere program, a NICU follow-program that was developed by Dr. Marilyn Escobedo and Dr. Rajam Ramamurthy. She is the Rita and William Head Distinguished Professor of Environmental and Developmental Neonatology.

YJ is an attending Neonatologist with the Fort Worth Pediatrix Medical Group at Cook Children's Hospital, and is currently the Medical Director of the NICU graduate Early Support and care Transition (N.E.S.T.) developmental follow-up clinic. YJ has over 15 years' experience with neonatal developmental follow-up, clinical outcomes research, and perinatal quality improvement initiatives. She previously served as a site Follow-up Principal Investigator for The NICHD Neonatal Research Network and is currently serving as a team member for the VON NICQ Next QI project "Brain Savers" group to prevent brain injury in premature infants after birth.

JL is an instructor and master certified health education specialist in the Department of Pediatrics at The University of Texas Health Science Center at

San Antonio, with 30 years of experience working collaboratively on public health initiatives. She is currently involved in the second phase of the Texas Pulse Oximetry Project, an education and quality improvement initiative to ensure critical congenital heart disease newborn screening for all newborns in Texas.

KM is a Clinical Assistant Professor in the Department of Pediatrics at the University of Texas Health Science Center at San Antonio. She has worked for the past 16 years in a clinic assessing high-risk infants' development and for 10 years as part of a diagnostic team assessing young children's intelligence, achievement, and behavior including Autism Spectrum Disorder. Prior work involved developing standardized assessments for a major test publisher.

AD is Associate Professor of Pediatrics, Division of Neonatology and Department of Pediatrics at the University of Texas at Houston Medical School. She is an academic neonatologist whose research has focused on long-term outcomes in the areas of executive functioning, neuroimaging, cognition and language in extremely preterm children. She is the medical director of the High Risk Infant Clinic and is the Principal Investigator for Neurodevelopmental Follow-up for the UT Houston site of the Eunice Kennedy Shriver National Institute of Child Health and Development Neonatal Research Network.

Acknowledgments

We gratefully acknowledge the following individuals for their contributions and participation in the summit and their dedication to the developmental follow-up of preterm newborns:
Ma Teresa Ambat, MD, Texas Tech University Health Sciences Center - Paul L Foster School of Medicine; Christine Aune, MD, Pediatrix Medical Group-San Antonio; Sara Baker RN, BSN, University of Texas Health Science Center at San Antonio (UTHSCSA); Marcia Berretta, LCSW, Baylor College of Medicine, Texas Children's Hospital; Jenny Carr, CCRN, NNP-BC, Driscoll Children's Hospital-Corpus Christi; Silvia Castaneda RN, MSN, University Hospital/UTHSCSA; Wanda Daniels RN, MSN, UTHSCSA; Marilyn Escobedo, MD, The University of Oklahoma Health Science Center; Mario Fierro, MD, Pediatrix Medical Group-San Antonio; Jeremy Goodman, MBA-HCA, Driscoll Children's Hospital-Corpus Christi; Erika Goyer, Hand to Hold; Mary Sue King PT, DPT, University Hospital-San Antonio; Carol Maupin-Macias, OTR, Texas Department of Assistive and Rehabilitative Services' Early Childhood Intervention-Austin; Lisa McGill-Vargas, MD, UTHSCSA; Carolyn McLerran RN, MSN, UTHSCSA; Jennifer Palarczyk, DO, UTHSCSA; Alicia Quim, University Hospital/UTHSCSA; Amy Quinn, MD, UTHSCSA; Rajam Ramamurthy, MD, UTHSCSA; Steven Seidner, MD, UTHSCSA; Melissa Svoboda, MD, Children's Hospital of San Antonio; Robert Voigt, MD, Baylor College of Medicine, Texas Children's Hospital.

Author details
[1]Department of Pediatrics, The University of Texas Health Science Center at San Antonio, 7703 Floyd Curl Dr. San Antonio, Texas 78229, USA. [2]Cook Children's Hospital, 1500 Cooper St., Dodson Specialty Building, 2nd Floor, Fort Worth, TX 76104, USA. [3]The University of Texas Health Science Center-Houston, 6431 Fannin St., Houston, Texas 77030, USA.

References

1. Vohr BR, O'Shea M, Wright LL. Longitudinal multicenter follow-up of high risk infants: Why, who, when and what to assess. Sem in Perinatal. 2003;27(4):333–42.
2. Rysavy MA, Li L, Bell EF, et al. for the Eunice Kennedy Shriver National Institute of Child Health and Human Development Neonatal Research Network. Between-Hospital Variation in Treatment and Outcomes in Extremely Preterm Infants. N Engl J M. 2015;372(19):1801–11.
3. Tyson JE, Parikh NA, Langer J, et al. for the National Institute of Child Health and Human Development Neonatal Research Network. Intensive care for extreme prematurity — moving beyond gestational age. N Engl J M. 2008;356(16):1672–81.
4. Institute of Medicine, Board of Health Policy, Committee on Understanding Premature Birth and Assuring Healthy Outcomes. Preterm Birth: Causes, Consequences, and Prevention. Berham R, Butler AS, eds. Washington, DC: National Academies Press; 2007.
5. Nelson KB, Ellenberg JH. Apgar scores as predictors of chronic neurologic disability. Pediatrics. 1981;68(1):36–44.
6. Wapner RJ, Sorokin Y, Mele L, et al. for the National Institute of Child Health and Human Development Maternal-Fetal Medicine Units Network. Long-term outcomes after repeated doses of antenatal corticosteroids. N Engl J M. 2007;357(12):1190–8.
7. Doyle LW, Anderson PJ, Haslam R, et al. for the Australasian Collaborative Trial of Magnesium Sulphate (ACTOMgSO4) Study Group. School-age outcomes of very preterm infants after antenatal treatment with magnesium sulfate vs placebo. JAMA. 2014;312(11):1105–13.
8. Shankaran S, Pappas A, McDonald SA, et al. for the Eunice Kennedy Shriver NICHD Neonatal Research Network. Childhood outcomes after hypothermia for neonatal encephalopathy. N Engl J M. 2012;366(22):2085–92.
9. Schmidt B, Roberts R, Millar D, Kirpalani H. Evidence-based neonatal drug therapy for prevention of bronchopulmonary dysplasia in very-low-birth-weight infants. Neonatology. 2008;93:284–7.
10. McCrea HJ, Ment LR. The diagnosis, management and postnatal prevention of intraventricular hemorrhage in the Preterm Neonate. Clin Perinatol. 2008;35(4):777–vii.
11. Shah TA, Meinzen-Derer J, Gratton T, et al. Hospital and neurodevelopmental outcomes of extremely-low-birth-weight infants with necrotizing enterocolitis and spontaneous intestinal perforation. J Perinatol. 2012;32(7):552–8.
12. Ronkainen E, Dunder T, Peltoniemi O. New BPD predicts lung function at school age: follow-up study and meta-analysis. Pediatr Pulmonol. 2015. doi:10.1002/ppul.23153.
13. O'Connor AR, Spencer R. Birch EE/ Predicting long-term visual outcome in children with birth weight under 1001 g. JAAPOS. 2007;11:541–5.
14. Voss W, Jungmann T, Wachtendorf M, Neubauer AP. Long-term cognitive outcomes of extremely-low-birth-weight infants: The influence of the maternal educational background. Acta Pædiatr. 2012;101(5):569–73.
15. Guillén U, DeMauro S, Ma L, et al. Relationship between attrition and neurodevelopmental impairment rates in extremely preterm infants at 18 to 24 months. Arch Pediatr Adoles Med. 2012;166(2):178–84.
16. van der Pal-de Bruin KM, van der Pal SM, Verloove-Vanhorick SP, Walther FJ. Profiling the preterm or VLBW born adolescent; implications of the Dutch POPS cohort follow-up studies. Early Hum Dev. 2015;91:97–102.
17. Vohr BR, Wright LL, Hack M, et al. Follow-up care of high-risk infants. Pediatrics. 2004; 114 (5 Part 2): Supplement: 1377–97.
18. American Academy of Pediatrics, Committee on Fetus and Newborn. Hospital discharge of the high-risk neonate. Pediatrics. 2008;122(5):1119–26.
19. American Academy of Pediatrics, Committee on Fetus and Newborn and American College of Obstetrics and Gynecology, Committee on Obstetric Practice. Guidelines for Perinatal Care. Riley LE, Stark AR, Kilpatrick SJ, Papile LA, eds. Elk Grove Village, IL: American Academy of Pediatrics and Washington, DC: American College of Obstetrics and Gynecology; 2012
20. Bockli K, Andrews B, Pellerite M, Meadow W. Trends and challenges in United States neonatal intensive care units follow-up clinics. J Perinatol. 2014;34:71–4.
21. MedImmune and National Initiative for Children's Healthcare Quality. Toolkit for the follow-up care of the premature infant https://www.preemietoolkit.com/index.aspx. Accessed 17 September 2015.
22. Kuppala VS, Tabangin M, Haberman B, et al. Current state of high-risk infant follow-up care in the United States: results of a national survey of academic follow-up programs. J Perinatol. 2012;32:293–8.
23. Hintz SR, Gould JB, Bennett MV, et al. Referral of very low birth weight infants to high-risk follow-up at neonatal intensive care unit discharge varies widely across California. J Pediatr. 2015;166(2):289–95.
24. Vohr BR, Stevens B, Tucker R. 35 years of neonatal follow-up in Rhode Island. Medicine & Health Rhode Island. 2010;93(5):151–3.
25. Doyle LW, Anderson PJ, Battin M, et al. Long term follow up of high risk children: Who, why and how? BMC Pediatrics. 2014;14(279):1–15.
26. Walker K, Holland AJA, Halliday R, Badawi N. Which high-risk infants should we follow-up and how should we do it? J Paediatr Child Health. 2012;48:789–93.
27. Lee S, McMillan D, Sale J, et al. Variations in practice and outcomes in the Canadian NICU network: 1996–1997. Pediatrics. 2000;106(5):1070–9.
28. Sauve R, Lee SK. Neonatal follow-up programs and follow-up studies: Historical and current perspectives. Paediatr Child Health. 2006;11(5):267–70.
29. Ballantyne M, Benzies K, Rosenbaum P, Lodha A. Mothers' and health care providers' perspectives of the barriers and facilitators to attendance at Canadian neonatal follow-up programs. Child: Care, health, and development (pp. 1–12). John Wiley & Sons; 2014

30.   Ballantyne M, Stevens B, Guttmann A, et al. Transition to neonatal follow-up programs: Is attendance problem? J Perinat Neo Nursing. 2012;26(1):90–8.

31.   Horbar JD, Soll RF, Edwards WH. The Vermont Oxford Network: A community of practice. Clin Perinatol. 2010;37(1):29–47.

32.   Texas Department of State Health Services, Center of Health Statistics. Texas Health Data. 2015. http://healthdata.dshs.texas.gov/HealthFactsProfiles. Accessed 17 September 2015.

33.   March of Dimes. Premature Birth Report Card. 2014. http://www.marchofdimes.org/materials/premature-birth-report-card-texas.pdf. Accessed 17 September 2015.

34   U.S. Census Bureau. Educational attainment (2013 ACS, S1501). http://factfinder.census.gov/faces/nav/jsf/pages/index.xhtml. Accessed 17 September 2015.

35.   Hoffman L, Bann C, Higgins RH, Vohr B. Developmental outcomes of extremely preterm infants born to adolescent mothers. Pediatrics. 2015;135:1082–92.

36.   Vohr BR, Poindexter BB, Dusick AM, et al. Persistent beneficial effects of breast milk ingested in the neonatal intensive care unit on outcomes of extremely low birth weight infants at 30 months of age. Pediatrics. 2007;120:e953–9.

37.   Ballard O, Morrow AL. Human milk composition: Nutrients and bioactive factors. Pediatr Clin North Am. 2013;60(1):49–74.

38.   Dritsakou K, Liosis G, Valsami G, et al. Improved outcomes of feeding low birth weight infants with predominately raw human milk versus donor banked milk and formula. J Mat-Fet Neo Med. 2015;24(4):1–8.

39.   Meier PP, Engstrom JL, Patel AL, et al. Improving the use of human milk during and after the NICU stay. Clin Perinatol. 2012;37(1):217–45.

40.   Maia C, Brandão R, Roncalli Â, Maranhão H. Length of stay in a neonatal intensive care unit and its association with low rates of exclusive breastfeeding in very low birth weight infants. J Mat-Fet Neo Med. 2011;24(6):774–7.

41   Scott MN, Taylor G, Fristad MA, et al. Behavior disorders in extremely preterm/extremely low birth weight children in kindergarten. Dev Behav Pediatr. 2012;33(3):202–13.

42.   Spittle AJ, Treyvaud K, Doyle, et al. Early emergence of behavior and social-emotional problems in very preterm infants. J Am Acad Child Adolesc Psych. 2009;48(9):909–18.

43.   Gardner FI, Shaw DS, Dishion TJ, et al. Randomized prevention trial for early conduct problems: Effects on proactive parenting and links to toddler disruptive behavior. J Fam Psychol. 2007;21(3):398–406.

44.   Landry SH, Smith KE, Swank PR. Responsive parenting: Establishing early foundations for social, communication, and independent problem-solving skills. Dev Psychol. 2006;42(4):627–42.

45.   Johnson S, Marlow N. Developmental screen or developmental testing? Early Hum Dev. 2006;82:173–83.

46.   Newborg J, Stock JR, Wnek L, et al. Battelle Developmental Inventory. Allen, Tex: DLM; 1988.

47.   Key Stakeholder Colorado Premature Infant And Follow Up Meeting: Assuring Premature Infant Follow Up through a Medical Home. Summary and Report (10-24-12). http://www.specialkids-specialcare.org/wpcontent/uploads/2011/09/KeyStakeholderCOPrematureInfantSummitFollowUpReport2012.pdf. KeyStakeholderCOPrematureInfantSummitFollowUpReport2012.pdf. Accessed 17 September 2015.

48.   Raju TNK, Bock R, Alexander D. Renaming of the National Institute of Child Health and Human Development in honor of Mrs. Eunice Kennedy Shriver. Pediatrics. 2008;122(4):e948–9.

17

A half century of electronic fetal monitoring and bioethics: silence speaks louder than words

Thomas P. Sartwelle[1], James C. Johnston[2,3*] and Berna Arda[4]

Abstract

Bioethics abolished the prevailing Hippocratic tenet instructing physicians to make treatment decisions, replacing it with autonomy through informed consent. Informed consent allows the patient to choose treatment after options are explained by the physician. The appearance of bioethics in 1970 coincided with the introduction of electronic fetal monitoring (EFM), which evolved to become the fetal surveillance modality of choice for virtually all women in labor. Autonomy rapidly pervaded all medical procedures, but there was a clear exemption for EFM. Even today, EFM remains immune to the doctrine of informed consent despite continually mounting evidence which proves the procedure is nothing more than myth, illusion and junk science that subjects mothers and babies alike to increased risks of morbidity and mortality. And ethicists have remained utterly silent through a half century of EFM misuse. Our article explores this egregious ethical failure by reviewing EFM's lack of clinical efficacy, discussing the EFM related harm to mothers and babies, and focusing on the reasons that this obstetrical procedure eluded the revolutionary change from the Hippocratic tradition to autonomy through informed consent.

Keywords: Medical ethics, Cerebral palsy, Electronic fetal monitoring, Medical malpractice

Background

"Declare the past, diagnose the present, foretell the future. As to diseases, make a habit of two things—to help and not to harm." From the book *Epidemics I*

Fifty years ago electronic fetal monitoring (EFM) became an overnight sensation when first introduced into labor suites. Declared to be the long awaited cerebral palsy (CP) cure [1], EFM, in a very short time, was virtually the sole monitoring method used in the industrialized world, the *raison d'etre* of fetal surveillance in labor [2–5]. And today EFM remains obstetrics' *deus ex machine* [6] despite overwhelming and damning scientific evidence that EFM theory is nothing more than myth and wishful thinking [7–18] and despite evidence that CP is caused chiefly by prenatal factors operating before

* Correspondence: johnston@GlobalNeurology.com
[2]1150 N Loop 1604 W, Ste 108-625, San Antonio, TX 98110, USA
[3]Global Neurology Consultants, Auckland, New Zealand
Full list of author information is available at the end of the article

labor begins, that CP is not preventable by any response to EFM patterns, that EFM has never reduced the rate of CP in 50 years of intense use and supposed improvement [4–13, 15–31], and that EFM use has and is today causing more harm to mothers and babies that it has ever helped [5, 8, 9, 12, 13, 17].

At almost the same instant that EFM became a clinical sensation, bioethics, a word coined in the 1960s, became a recognized entity, linking scientific advances to human values [32]. The foundation of bioethics was autonomy—a person's right to choose or refuse medical treatment based on informed consent—replacing the centuries-old deontology based on the Hippocratic tradition of benign paternalism—the physician's duty is to choose the treatment for the patient [32–35].

Linking EFM use with the new bioethics should have been a seamless affair following Thomas Kuhn's six stages of scientific revolution resulting in his now famous paradigm shift from the old to the new [36]. And while this shift to the new bioethics indeed occurred in most medical arenas [32–35], it failed utterly with EFM and obstetrics. Today obstetrical EFM use without mothers' informed consent is the epitome of medical paternalism. The cause of this momentous failure was the confluence of three powerful influences that even the brilliant Kuhn failed to see on the horizon.

Throughout EFM's rise to deus ex machina and its evasion of autonomy-informed consent, the clinical evidence against EFM rose up like a mammoth volcanic ocean island, plain for all to see [5–31]. And while a few clinicians were bold enough to challenge the EFM medical establishment that insisted on continued EFM use despite the evidence of harm, evidence that should have provoked bioethical outrage, the bioethics community's silence was deafening and remains so today. The question is, why the silence?

And just as important a question is, could bioethics, having no enforcement mechanisms other than words, forced the EFM establishment to recognize autonomy-informed consent and rescued those mothers who believed in EFM's magic powers only because they were never told the truth about EFM? The answer is yes. As will be demonstrated, bioethical silence is louder that its words, but if words had at least been spoken and written bioethics could have changed forever the EFM dynamic just as Kuhn foretold.

In the beginning

"To help and not to harm" has been an integral part of medicine from the very first attempts to organize medicine into books and explain theories of disease and the moral, ethical wisdom associated with healing and healers [32]. The thought is perhaps more familiar when written, "first do no harm," and while both phrases have obscure origins, they have been repeated as part of the Hippocratic tradition by many Western physician commentators and teachers throughout the centuries [32–34, 37]. Repeated not only in writings and lectures, but also formalized in various ethics codes like Percival's Code, the codes of early medical societies, the first AMA Code in 1847, and just about all subsequent ethics codes of Western-oriented medical societies [32]. It is curious, however, why it was necessary to warn physicians not to harm their patients when the idea of helping patients is dominant. The idea of doing no harm, however, becomes apparent when the second Hippocratic medical principle is considered—it is the physician who must decide what is best for the patient according to the physician's ability and judgment [32–34].

Thus, Western ethics through the ages was dominated by Hippocratic medical paternalism—physician-centered medicine [38]. Oliver Wendell Holmes, addressing an 1871 medical school graduating class, advised the physicians to conform to the Hippocratic tradition and conceal almost everything from patients, saying that the patient had no right to the truth [38]. In the 1930s, when a patient asked the physician a question during an examination, the physician "slapped her face, saying, 'I'll ask the questions here. I'll do the talking.'" [38] In 1944, President Roosevelt's physicians did not reveal to him their diagnosis of elevated blood pressure and congestive heart failure diagnoses, a year before a stroke took his life [39]. In 1961, a published study revealed that 88% of U.S. physicians surveyed did not tell the truth to terminally ill cancer patients [33, 38]. And it was not until 1981 that AMA revised its Principles of Medical Ethics to revise the previously accepted Hippocratic-approved lying to patients, mandating that physicians were required to deal honestly with patients and colleagues [33].

This was the state of the centuries-old medical ethics milieu in 1960, when, amid unimagined breakthroughs in science, medicine, and technology, medical inventors worked to perfect an electronic fetal monitor that could, so they believed, predict fetal distress and prevent cerebral palsy [1, 2]. It was a milieu in which physicians were viewed by themselves and the public as being superior to patients and most others in knowledge and insight. Physicians were authoritarian, determining what was in the patients' best interests, even if the patients did not agree [34].

Deus ex machina

Thus, in 1970, when EFM was introduced into clinical practice [2], obstetricians were comfortable operating in the Hippocratic sphere in which they made all medical decisions without input from patients. There was, therefore, no necessity to inform patients that EFM was totally experimental and had never been proven in even one clinical trial [5–17]. Nor was there any necessity to advise patients that the very foundational theories undergirding EFM—fetal heart rate reflected past and present fetal brain function and oxygen deprivation in labor was the sole cause of CP—were unscientific myths handed down from generation to generation and untested by modern medicine [4, 5, 7–13, 15–18, 20–28]. Rather, obstetricians throughout the industrialized world accepted the new monitor as the machine that would, as its proponents assured the world, reduce by half intrapartum deaths, mental retardation, and CP [1]. There was no necessity for informed consent, because that concept is a product of bioethics, which, in 1970, had only just emerged as a deontology that would eventually overtake the Hippocratic tradition [32–34]. While simple consent—the patient may say "yes" or "no" to a surgery—was a legal concept [38, 40], true informed consent, the product of bioethics and autonomy [33–35], lay in the future. Thus, when it came to employing the new EFM, obstetricians continued in the Hippocratic physician-is-dominant tradition. And, unfortunately, as will be seen, obstetricians and EFM have continued in the Hippocratic tradition despite the fact that overwhelming evidence demonstrates EFM use has done more harm than good for mothers and babies during the last 50 years.

A new deontology

Immanuel Kant is credited with the development of deontological ethical theory, a result of enlightenment rationalism and liberal political philosophy, the central focus of which is the individual's liberties and rights [33]. This liberal political philosophy bypassed Western medicine, however, until after World War II, when a series of disclosures, beginning with the Nuremburg trials and disclosure of wartime medical experiments, began to focus attention on medical research conducted without patients' consent [33, 34, 41]. The Tuskegee syphilis study, plutonium injections by Manhattan Project doctors, radioactive iodine trials, and a host of other human experiments, 22 of which were exposed in Henry Beecher's 1966 groundbreaking whistleblower exposé, shocked the public [41]. The common denominator of these medical experiments was that meaningful consent was never obtained from the patients [38, 41].

These experiments and their public exposure, along with other societal upheavals in the 1950s and '60s, caused physicians, scientists, philosophers, religious and legal scholars, and other disciplines, to come together to focus on the moral, ethical, and philosophical ambiguities presented by the dizzying array of worldwide scientific medical advances [32–35, 38]. This new discipline, said to have been born around 1970 [32–34], soon took on a new name—bioethics.

This new deontology, based on duty, was dominated by one overwhelming theme—autonomy—respect for the individual and individual self-rule, a duty, fidelity, and faithfulness of one human being to another [34], such that the individual patient could meaningfully choose her medical treatment based on knowledge of the choices available inputted by the physician. And while the term "informed consent" had been used before bioethics was born, from 1970 on, that term was inculcated with new meaning, becoming synonymous with autonomy and driving medicine's focus away from Hippocratic physician-centered medicine to patient-centered medicine, where it remains today [32–34, 38]. Closely associated with this first bioethics principle are two duties—non-maleficence—do not impose unnecessary harm or risk of harm—and beneficence—dedication to the patient's welfare, a positive medical goal different in substantial degree from merely avoiding harm [32–35, 38].

While there are still many controversies over the exact meaning and reach of these and other bioethical duties and obligations, it is clear that medicine's primary bioethical, moral duty is to enable patients to make their own medical decisions, perhaps even wrong in the physician's judgment, decisions based on relevant, current information provided by the physician [32–35, 38]. And while it is assumed that a given number of patients will not want the burden of deciding, that does not diminish the physician's duty to provide the information to all patients—in other words, meaningful, informed consent is a moral imperative [33, 34]. This imperative and much of bioethics was, of course, the antithesis of the Hippocratic traditions that had dominated medicine for centuries, yet bioethical thinking became dominant in medicine in only a few short years. A paradigm shift occurred in almost all aspects of medicine, save and except one—electronic fetal monitoring.

The revolution

Science is always progressing. New theories become settled science and old theories disappear. Ptolemy's math was impeccable. His calculations were subject to multiple proofs by scholars for well over a thousand years. The conclusion was the same—the earth was the center of the universe. Not so, said Copernicus. Geocentricity was a myth. Real-world cosmology was heliocentric—the sun was the center of the universe. There were few believers. The myth had stood the test of time. One hundred years later, Galileo confirmed the new cosmology with a telescope.

The Copernican revolution was Thomas Kuhn's prime example of how science is driven to change [36]. In normal periods of science, a paradigm exists by which certain anomalies can be solved. But a crisis in science arises when confidence is lost in a paradigm's ability to solve particularly worrisome anomalies, and thus a scientific revolution occurs by which an existing paradigm is superseded by a rival.

Before Kuhn, there was little to explain how science changes. There was, however, a conception of scientific change as a smooth, flowing addition of new truths to the stock of old truths and an occasional correction of past errors. According to Kuhn's theory, science is not uniform, but has normal and revolutionary or extraordinary phases, which he referred to as the puzzle-solving power of the competing ideas. But these competing theories, according to Kuhn, are generally incommensurable, because they share very little commonality [36]. And so it was that Kuhn's scientific revolution perfectly presaged the medical ethics revolution from the Hippocratic paradigm to the bioethics paradigm.

As we have seen, the bioethics paradigm shift occurred when the Hippocratic ethics was found inadequate to solve the exposés related to medical human experimentation without consent, as well as other patient centering problems [32–35, 38]. The change from Hippocratic ethics to bioethics was extremely rapid when compared to

Kuhn's Copernican revolution and other examples of scientific paradigm shift, but the paradigm shift to bioethics did indeed follow Kuhn's theory. Autonomy replaced physician-centered medicine, hospital ethics committees were created, institutional review boards were appointed, and many other dynamic changes occurred in the practice of medicine and the field of medical scientific research [33–35]. But while many things changed, at least one thing stayed the same—electronic fetal monitoring, an experimental machine, is still used today without the informed consent of mothers and with no explanation of the conflict of interest physicians have with respect to continued EFM use despite a half-century of uncontradicted proof that EFM does more harm than good.

Is EFM really experimental?

EFM began clinical life with only a few detractors questioning its basic premise [42]—the conventional but unproven wisdom that CP and neurologic birth maladies were caused by birth asphyxia, hypoxia, and cerebral ischemia, which were reflected in out-of-norm fetal heart rate that, if stopped in time—by C-section or instrumented delivery—would prevent CP and birth maladies [4, 5, 7–11]. Most physicians simply accepted EFM inventors' claims and promises, even though EFM inventors skipped the rigors of the scientific method and the crucible of randomized clinical trials, and introduced EFM with no instruction manual, with unrealistic efficacy expectations, and no clearly defined parameters for use [43]. As EFM accelerated in use to 85% of births in the United States [5], more and more vehement criticism appeared following its first clinical use. Criticism completely ignored by most physicians and their birth related professional organizations (BRPOs) worldwide as well as ethicists [5, 7–9, 25].

When EFM was subjected to 12 clinical trials versus auscultation beginning in 1976, EFM showed no benefit, but only a dramatic increase in C-sections due to EFM's 99% false-positive rate [7, 11, 19, 26–29]. In the 1970s, critics wrote that EFM use is unjustified by any evidence [44, 45]. In the 1980s, critics wrote that EFM is increasing unnecessary C-sections [46], and the procedure should be abandoned [46]. In the 1990s, critics wrote that because of EFM and medical malpractice liability concerns, United States obstetricians were performing cesarean sections at a rate much higher than anywhere else in the world; [47] EFM is nothing but a disappointing story, and the hoped-for EFM benefit has not been realized; [48] EFM promised much but achieved little because fetal heart rate changes reflect neurologic insult earlier in pregnancy, not intrapartum events; [49] and no data exists that intervention based on any EFM patterns has reduced CP [49]. By the turn of the century, the critics became even more vocal as the evidence proved CP was not caused by birth events and EFM

was not in any manner efficacious, but indeed harmful, primarily because it triggered unnecessary C-sections with the attendant morbidity and mortality: tests leading to unnecessary abdominal surgery in 99% of cases is absurd; [17] EFM has done more harm than good to mothers and babies; [17] EFM has had no effect on perinatal mortality or neurologic morbidity; [26] EFM interpretation is subjective, difficult to standardize, and poorly reproducible; [6] after almost 50 years, there is no consensus on EFM pattern interpretation and management; [3] EFM as a screening tool for absence of harm is no better than tossing a coin; [12] EFM overall caused more harm than good; [12] there is a growing consensus in the maternal-fetal medicine community that it is time to start over with EFM and establish a common language, standard interpretation and management principles [43]. In 2014, the authors of *Neonatal Encephalopathy and Neurologic Outcome, Second Edition*, published by ACOG and American Academy of Pediatrics, and assisted by an international array of Task Force consultants, conceded EFM defeat after a concerted 50-year effort to make EFM predict asphyxia, hypoxia, ischemia, acidemia, CP, and neurologic injury: "There are no long-term benefits of EFM as currently used" [21] (at 88); "no evidence exists demonstrating that electronic FHR monitoring reduces the rate of neonatal encephalopathy" [21] (at 92); "there is no evidence in the current literature to support the ability of practitioners to predict neonatal neurologic injury, cerebral palsy, or stillbirth using EFM" [21] (at 91); "cesarean delivery as an obstetrical intervention to reduce neonatal encephalopathy and cerebral palsy has been considered unsuccessful" [21] (at 104). This Task Force report was endorsed not only by ACOG and AAP, but also by 11 other worldwide birth-related organizations from Australia, New Zealand, Japan, Canada, and the United States [21].

Even today, efforts to make EFM heel to command have failed once more. EFM assisted by ST-segment analysis did not improve perinatal outcomes or decrease C-section rates [50], which are now 33% in the United States [51] and even higher in other parts of the world [5]. And more voices are calling on BRPOs to condemn EFM use in both labor rooms and in CP-EFM worldwide litigation because it is junk science [5, 7–13, 15–17, 19, 25, 43, 52]. Other voices are calling to reduce the C-section rate recognized to be caused in large part by defensive medicine and EFM's 99% false positive rate [12, 53, 54], which subjects mothers and babies to unnecessary morbidity and mortality risks from not only the immediate surgery but from subsequent sequela [5, 8, 9, 12, 13, 17]. And other voices are citing increasing evidence that C-sections are exposing babies to the specter of subsequent lifelong chronic diseases and neuropsychiatric disorders [55–58].

A practical, common sense definition of experimental medical procedures would be that until the published, peer-reviewed medical evidence regarding risks, benefits, and overall safety and efficacy demonstrate that the procedure has a beneficial effect on healthcare outcomes, the procedure is experimental. It is without question that the unrefuted evidence over five decades has proven EFM is unsafe, un-efficacious, and has no beneficial effect on healthcare outcomes. Just the opposite. EFM does little good, but considerable harm. Thus, it is unfathomable that the ACOG-AAP Task Force [21] and individual practitioners in many countries continue to call for EFM use in every labor [2, 59–61].

Why?

Vincible ignorance

It is no longer a secret why BRPOs, medical societies, and individual physicians and hospitals ignored the 50-year EFM volcano erupting with undeniable, unrefuted evidence that EFM is junk science and causes harm to mothers and babies. The secret has been exposed in government studies [62, 63], medical journals [4, 7, 9, 11, 12, 15, 16, 19, 23, 43, 47, 53, 54], legal journals [5, 25, 64–67], newspaper and popular magazine articles [68, 69] since at least 1979: obstetrical defensive medicine. Physicians and hospitals use EFM because they believe it protects them from trial lawyers and CP lawsuits. This concept of EFM providing malpractice protection is, and always has been, another birth myth, as has been pointed out in the medical and legal literature for many years [5, 8, 25, 52, 64–66]. But, like the other birth myths, the truth would destroy the collective obstetrical illusions handed down from generation to generation. But clinging to obstetrical illusions and myths is merely practicing nineteenth century medicine, which was based on whim, personal belief, and bias, rather than evidence-based, scientific-based medicine. It also violates every past and current concept in bioethics, especially the heart and soul of bioethics—autonomy.

So the question arises, why did bioethics issue an ethical pass to EFM? How did virtually all of medicine succumb to Kuhn's paradigm shift from Hippocratic ethics to bioethics in just a few decades, while EFM continues to be used without informed consent, continues to cause harm without discernible benefits, and all without raising any concern or alarm from the bioethics community? Who issued EFM the ethics pass?

In plain sight

Although it is impossible to determine the moment that paternalism died and autonomy was born, we can isolate one period in early EFM history when autonomy was recognized as dominant over paternalistic EFM use. That dominance quickly faded, however, because of influences unforeseen and unaccounted for by contemporary scholars—trial lawyers, medical malpractice lawsuits, and defensive medicine.

In the 1970s, NIH organized consensus-development Task Forces to address recent developments in medical research and practice [62]. One Task Force on predictors of intrapartum fetal distress was composed of physicians, sociologists, lawyers, and ethicists, among others. The Task Force's 1979 report was subsequently published in three prominent journals [62]. With respect to EFM, the Task Force recommended, because there was no evidence of EFM efficacy, that mothers be informed, during the course of prenatal care and again on admission to the labor suite, about EFM limitations and risks [62]. This Task Force's EFM bioethical recommendation was followed by the International Federation of Gynecology and Obstetrics and Family Health International (FIGO) in 1986 in their Guidelines for Fetal Monitoring Use: "Mothers should have the opportunity to discuss the use of electronic fetal heart rate monitoring during antepartum care and again upon admission to hospital in labor, so that they are able to give or to withhold informed consent." [70].

But informed consent never happened. With these two exceptions, EFM medical literature and BRPOs are completely silent regarding when, how, and what to tell mothers about EFM's limitations and risks and, as the evidence increased in later years, about EFM's morbidity and mortality, current and future. There is also complete silence in the bioethical literature urging BRPOs and physicians to make EFM informed consent a duty. The EFM informed consent issue did not escape the nursing, midwife, and legal literature [65, 66, 71, 72], and, in fact, is still discussed today [67, 73, 74]. But these voices have been ignored by obstetricians and ethicists alike.

Murphy's law and paradigm shifts

Kuhn started challenging the scholarly community with his revolutionary science, paradigms, and puzzle-solving in his 1962 book, *The Structure of Scientific Revolutions* [36]. While Kuhn's revolution model perfectly presaged the coming bioethical paradigm shift, a retrospective view reveals that Kuhn, his proponents, and critics alike overlooked a paradigm shift taking place under their feet—trial lawyers, medical malpractice, and defensive medicine.

In the 1960s, for reasons still debated today, there was a sudden, dramatic rise in the frequency and severity of medical malpractice lawsuits and claims, which accelerated rapidly to unprecedented levels, precipitating the first of many medical malpractice-insurance coverage crises early in the 1970s [5, 8, 9, 25]. Obstetrics was a particular target because, until EFM, the only evidence of fetal heart rate during labor had been the obstetrician's recollection. With EFM, there was a permanent paper tracing that trial lawyers' courtroom experts could interpret years and even decades after a birth and, of course, inevitably find the precise moment the inattentive or ignorant attending physician should have performed a C-section to save what the courtroom experts said was a neurologically perfect infant from lifelong crippling injuries. EFM, nobly conceived, met Murphy's Law, and for 50 years has been the trial lawyer's weapon to extract billions from physicians and hospitals the world over, even as the evidence mounted that EFM did not predict CP and CP was not caused primarily by asphyxia, anoxia, hypoxia, or ischemia during birth. On the other hand, physicians, new at the litigation game, ironically adopted the trial lawyers' preferred weapon, EFM, as their sole CP-lawsuit defense [5, 8, 9, 25]. But over the past half-century, physicians worldwide have lost the CP-EFM battle to the trial lawyers for a variety of reasons [5, 8, 9, 25] and are now engulfed in an epidemic explosion of malpractice lawsuits, especially CP-EFM neurologic impairment birth-injury lawsuits [5, 7–11, 15, 25].

The result of the initial trial lawyers versus doctors litigation battle was defensive medicine—prophylactic medicine of little use to the patient, administered primarily for the protection of doctors and hospitals from trial lawyers and lawsuits [5, 7–11, 23, 25]. And while most defensive medicine received considerable criticism from bioethicists, economists, and some clinicians as being medically and ethically questionable, not to mention costly to society [75–78], the EFM criticism, as we have seen, came only from a small number of clinicians and scholars, and even they never addressed the bioethical issue of physicians violating patient autonomy by EFM use without informed consent. Ethicists defaulted in the EFM debate by their overwhelming silence. The use of a scientifically bankrupt machine solely to protect healthcare providers from trial lawyers and lawsuits when the machine is known to be harming mothers and babies is an egregious conflict of interest and outrageous endorsement of obstetrical defensive medicine—post-modern ethical relativism solely to benefit healthcare providers—and is undeniable proof that evidence-based standard of care and bioethical principles are nothing more than empty rhetoric [79, 80].

A part of bioethical morality requires that patients be allowed autonomy and that in the treatment process the physician refrain from harm to the extent practical. But the third principle—beneficence—requires more than avoiding harm. It requires positive steps to benefit the patient, steps that balance benefits, risks, costs, and other patient goals to produce the most optimum results possible [33, 34]. In other words, beneficence requires the physician to favor the patient's interest over the physician's self-interest [33, 34]. This obligation is fidelity. It results in a fiduciary relationship between patient and physician [33, 34]. In daily practice, this fiduciary relationship is often challenged by potential divided loyalties—conflicts of interest—to the physician's colleagues,

institutions, third parties, funding sources, and the physician's self-protection interests [33, 34]. Conflicts of interest have received enormous attention, primarily due to perceived conflicts in commercial, manufacturing, and financial relationships [33, 34]. However, the EFM conflict of interest—using a device that actually causes harm to patients primarily to protect doctors and hospitals from CP lawsuits—is enormously more compromising than gifts, trips, and money, because it has been and is hidden from public view and because the EFM device is fraudulently presented to mothers as a safety device necessary for a healthy baby. Fidelity could not possibly be more compromised.

Ethicists' silence on a woman's right to EFM truth and her right to choose what happens to her body and to her baby has spoken more loudly than words ever could.

Conclusion - *POST TENEBRAS LUX*

Law and bioethics are separate, distinct entities. Law is more structured, concerning itself with rules that stabilize society's social institutions and structures. Law concentrates on the criminal and civil penalties to be brought to bear on miscreants who fail to conform [33, 34]. Bioethics, on the other hand, are conceived of as moral rules and ideals—how one ought to act toward others—some aspirational and some even unobtainable. How seriously these moral rules must be taken is still in dispute among the ethical legalists and ethical antinomianists [33, 34], but neither extreme in that debate contradicts the fact that ethical rules are essentially unenforceable save for the mild, occasional organizational enforcement and perhaps occasional licensing rebuke.

But perhaps bioethics' unenforceability is actually an illusion. After all, at the dawn of bioethics there was no enforceability other than words and public exposure of medical procedures that most agreed were morally wrong and dismissive of individual autonomy. Bioethics changed the entirety of medicine and the Hippocratic tradition that had ruled for centuries. Words were the only weapons needed. So the question arises, can words still be used to change the EFM bioethics? Said another way, can bioethics shed light in the darkness of 50 years of EFM paternalism? It would be a far better thing to voluntarily come to the light of EFM autonomy-informed consent now, rather than being forced into the light tomorrow by the trial lawyers.

Abbreviations
BRPO: Birth related professional organizations; CP: Cerebral palsy; EFM: Electronic fetal monitoring

Acknowledgements
Not applicable.

Funding

The authors received no financial support for the research, authorship or publication of this article.

Authors' contributions

All authors contributed to the research, drafting, reviewing and editing of this paper. All authors read and approved the final manuscript.

Competing interests

The authors declare that they have no competing interests.

Author details

[1]Deans and Lyons, LLP, Houston, TX, USA. [2]1150 N Loop 1604 W, Ste 108-625, San Antonio, TX 98110, USA. [3]Global Neurology Consultants, Auckland, New Zealand. [4]Department of Medical Ethics, University of Ankara, Ankara, Turkey.

References

1. Quilligan EJ, Paul RH. Fetal monitoring: is it worth it? Obstet Gynecol. 1975; 45(1):96–100.

2. Freeman RK, Garite TJ, Nageotte MP, Miller LA. Fetal heat rate monitoring. 4th ed. Philadelphia: Lippincott Williams & Wilkins; 2012.

3. Parer JT. Personalities, politics, and territorial tiffs: a half century of fetal heart rate monitoring. Am J Obstet Gynecol. 2011;204(6):548–50.

4. Jenkins HML. Thirty years of electronic intrapartum fetal heart rate monitoring: discussion paper. J Royal Soc Med. 1989;82:210–4.

5. Sartwelle TP. Electronic fetal monitoring: a bridge too far. J Legal Med. 2012; 33:313–79.

6. Greene MF. Obstetricians still await a *deus ex machina*. New Engl J Med. 2006;355(21):2247–8.

7. MacLennan AH, Thompson SC, Gecz J. Cerebral palsy – causes, pathways, and the role of genetic variants. Am J Obstet Gynecol. 2015;213(6):779–88.

8. Sartwelle TP, Johnston JC. Neonatal encephalopathy 2015: opportunity lost and words unspoken. J Maternal-Fetal & Neonatal Med. 2016;29(9):1372–5.

9. Sartwelle TP, Johnston JC. Cerebral palsy litigation: change course or abandon ship. J Child Neurol. 2015;30(7):828–41.

10. Donn SM, Chiswick ML, Fanaroff JM. Medico-legal implications of hypoxic-ischemic birth injury. Semin Fetal Neonatal Med. 2014;19(5):317–21.

11. Badawi N, Keogh JM. Causal pathways in cerebral palsy. J Pediatrics and Child Health. 2013;49:58.

12. Constantine MM, Saade GR. The first caesarean: role of "fetal distress" diagnosis. Semin Perinatol. 2012;36:379–83.

13. Grimes DA, Peipert JF. Electronic fetal monitoring as a public health screening program: the arithmetic of failure. Obstet Gynecol. 2010;116(6): 1397–400.

14. Khalil A, O'Brien P. Fetal heart rate monitoring—is it a waste of time? Obstet & Gynecol Of India. 2006;56(6):481–5.

15. MacLennan A, Hankins G, Speer N. Only an expert witness can prevent cerebral palsy. Obstet Gynecol. 2006;8(1):28–30.

16. MacLennan A, Nelson KB, Hankins G, Speer N. Who will deliver our grandchildren? JAMA. 2005;294(13):1688–90.

17. Clark S, Hankins G. Temporal and demographic trends in cerebral palsy—facts and fiction. Am J Obstet & Gynecol. 2003;188:628–32.

18. Beller FK. The cerebral palsy story: a catastrophic misunderstanding in obstetrics. Obstet Gynecol Survey. 1995;50:83–6.

19. Nelson KB, Blair E. Prenatal factors in singletons with cerebral palsy born at or near term. New Eng. J. Med. 2015;373(10):946–53.

20. Blair E, Nelson KB. Fetal growth restriction and risk of cerebral palsy in singletons born after at least 35 weeks' gestation. Am J Obstet Gynecol. 2015;212(4):520e1–7.

21. Am Coll Obstet & Gynecol & Am Acad. Pediatricians, neonatal encephalopathy and neurologic outcome. (2nd ed.) (2014).

22. Ellenberg JH, Nelson KB. The association of cerebral palsy with birth asphyxia: a definitional quagmire. Devel Med & Child Neuro. 2013;55:210–6.

23. MacLennan AH. A 'no fault' cerebral palsy pension scheme would benefit all Australians. Aust NZ J Obstet Gynecol. 2011;52(6):479 84.

24. Obladen M. Lame from birth: early concepts of cerebral palsy. J Child Neuro. 2011;26(2):248–56.

25. Sartwelle TP. Defending a neurologic birth injury: asphyxia neonatorum redux. J Legal Med. 2009;30(2):181–247.

26. Graham EM, Peterson SM, Christo DK, et al. Intrapartum electronic fetal heart rate monitoring and the prevention of perinatal brain injury. Obstet Gynecol. 2006;108(3):656–66.

27. Am. Coll. Obstet. & Gynecol. & Am. Acad. Pediatricians, neonatal encephalopathy and cerebral palsy: defining the pathogenesis and pathophysiology (2003).

28. MacLennan AH. A template for defining a causal relation between acute intrapartum events and cerebral palsy: international consensus statement. Br Med J. 1999;319:1054–9.

29. Nelson KB, Dambrosia J, Ting TY, Grether JK. Uncertain value of electronic fetal monitoring in predicting cerebral palsy. New Engl. J. Med. 1996; 334(10):613–8.

30. Scheller JM, Nelson KB. Does cesarean delivery prevent cerebral palsy or other neurologic problems of childhood? Obstet Gynecol. 1994;83:624–30.

31. Friedman EA. The obstetrician's dilemma: how much fetal monitoring and cesarean section is enough? New Engl. J. Med. 1986;315(10):641–3.

32. Jonsen AR. A short history of medical ethics. New York: Oxford University Press; 2000.

33. Veatch RM. The basics of bioethics. 3rd ed. New Jersey: Pearson Education Inc; 2012.

34. Beauchamp TL, Childress JF. Principles of biomedical ethics. 7th ed. New York: Oxford University Press; 2013.

35. Jecker NS, Jonsen AR, Pearlman RA. Bioethics. 3rd ed. Sudbury: Jones & Bartlett Learning LLC; 2012.

36. Kuhn TS. The structure of scientific revolutions, 50th anniversary edition with an introductory essay by Ian hacking. 4th ed. Chicago: The University of Chicago Press; 2012.

37. Smith CM. Origin and uses of Primum non Nocere—above all do no harm! J Clin Pharmacology. 2005;45:371–7.

38. Laine C, Davidoff F. Patient-centered medicine. JAMA. 1996;275(2):152–6.

39. Baron RJ. Professional self-regulation in a changing world. JAMA. 2015; 313(18):1807–8.

40. Chervenak J, McCullough LB, Chervenak FA. Surgery without consent or miscommunication? A new look at a landmark case. Am. J. Obstet. & Gynecol. 2015;212(5):586–90.

41. Beecher HK. Ethics and clinical research. New Eng. J. Med. 1966;274(24): 1354–60.

42. Benson RC, Schubeck F, Deutschberger J, et al. Fetal heart rate as a predictor of fetal distress: a report from the collaborative project. Obstet Gynecol. 1968;32:259–66.

43. Clark SL, Nageotte MP, Garite TJ, et al. Intrapartum management of category II fetal heart rate tracings: toward standardization of care. Am J Obstet & Gynecol. 2013;209(2):89–97.

44. Banta HD, Thacker SB. Assessing the costs and benefits of electronic fetal monitoring. Obstet Gynecol Surv. 1979;34:627–42.

45. Illingworth RS. Why blame the obstetrician: a review. Brit Med J. 1979; 1(6166):797–801.

46. Thacker SB. The efficacy of intrapartum electronic fetal monitoring. Am J Obstet Gynecol. 1987;156(1):24–30.

47. Manuel BM. Professional liability—a no-fault solution. New Eng. J. Med. 1990;322(9):627–30.

48. Freeman R. Intrapartum fetal monitoring—a disappointing story. New Eng. J. Med. 1990;322(9):624–6.

49. MacDonald D. Cerebral palsy and intra-partum fetal monitoring. New Engl. J. Med. 1996;334(10):659–60.

50. Belfort MA, Saade GR, Thom E, et al. A randomized trial of intrapartum fetal ECG ST-segment analysis. New Engl J Med. 2015;373(7):632–41.

51. Osterman MJK, Kochanek KD, MaDorman MF, et al. Annual summary of vital statistics: 2012-2013. Pediatrics. 2015;135(6):1115–25.

52. Maso G, Piccoli M, DeSeta F, et al. Intrapartum fetal heart monitoring interpretation in labour: a critical appraisal. Minerva Ginecol. 2015;67:65–79.

53. Spong CY, Berghella V, Wenstrom KD, et al. Preventing the first cesarean delivery: summary of a joint Eunice Kennedy Shriver National Institute of Child Health and Human Development, Society for Maternal Fetal Medicine, and American College of Obstetrics and Gynecology Workshop. Obstet Gynecol. 2012;120:1181–93.

54. American College Obstetricians & Gynecologists and Society for Maternal Fetal Medicine. Safe prevention of the primary cesarean section. Am J Obstet Gynecol. 2014;123:179–93.

55. Sevelsted A, Stokholm J, Bonnelykke K, et al. Cesarean section and chronic immune disorders. Pediatrics. 2015;135(1):e92–8.

56. Friedrich MJ. Unraveling the influence of gut microbes on the mind. JAMA. 2015;313(17):1699–701.

57. Borre YE, O'Keeffe GW, Clarke G, et al. Microbiota and neurodevelopmental windows: implications for brain disorders. Trends Mol Med. 2014;20(9):509–18.

58. Neu J. The pre- and early postnatal microbiome: relevance to subsequent health and disease. Neo Reviews. 2013;13(12):e-592–e599.

59. Ayres-de-Campos D. Why is intrapartum foetal monitoring necessary—impact on outcomes and interventions. Best Pract Res Clin Obstet Gynecol 2016;30:3–8.

60. Nageotte MP. Fetal heart monitoring. Sem Fetal Neo Med. 2015;20(3):144–8.

61. Berkowitz RL, D'Alton ME, Goldberg JD, et al. The case for an electronic fetal heart rate monitoring credentialing examination. Am J Obstet Gynecol. 2014;210(3):204–7.

62. Zuspan FP, Quilligan EJ, Iams JD, et al. NICHD consensus development task force report: predictors of intrapartum fetal distress—the role of electronic fetal monitoring. J Pediatrics. 1979;95(6):1026–30. *See also* Zuspan FP, Quilligan EJ, Iams JD, et al. Predictors of intrapartum fetal distress: The role of electronic fetal monitoring, Report of the National Institute of Child Health and Human Development Consensus Development Task Force. Am. J. Obstet. Gynecol. 1979; 135(3):287-291; Zuspan FP, Quilligan EJ, Iams JD et al. NICHD consensus development Task Force report. Predictors of intrapartum fetal stress: the role of electronic fetal monitoring. J. Reproductive Med. For Obstet. and Gynecol. 1979; 23(4): 207-212

63. Comm. Study Med. Prof'l Liab. & Delivery Obstetrical Care, Inst. Med., Div. Health Promotions & Disease Prevention, 1 Med. Prof. Liability & Delivery Ob. Care 73-91 (1989).

64. Lent M. The medical and legal risk of the electronic fetal monitor. Stan L Rev. 1999;51(4):807–37.

65. Gilfix MG. Electronic fetal monitoring: physician liability and informed consent. Am J Law and Med. 1984;10:1–48.

66. Rhoden NK. Informed consent in obstetrics: some special problems. Western New Eng L Rev. 1987;99(1):67–88.

67. Abrams JR. The illusion of autonomy in women's medical decision-making. Fla State Univ L Rev. 2015;42(1):1–45.

68. Wolfberg A. The future of fetal monitoring. Rev Obstet Gynecol. 2012;5(3/4): e132–6. https://doi.org/10.3909/riog0197. acknowledging that EFM is "plagued by false positive results and other technical limitations," but will continue to be used with "novel metrics" in the coming years

69. Berlatsky N. The most common childbirth practice in America is unnecessary and dangerous. New Republic Aug. 2015. Available at http://www.newrepublic.com/article/122532/most-common-childbirth-practice-us-unnecessary-dangerous. Accessed 12 Sept 2017.

70. International Federation of Gynaecology and Obstetrics and Family Health International, Guidelines for the use of fetal monitoring. Int J Gynaecol Obstet. 1987; 25:159-167. Available at http://www.ctgutbildning.se/course/referencer//referenser/FIGO%20CTG%20Guidelines.pdf. Accessed 12 Sept 2017.

71. Wood SH. Should women be given a choice about fetal assessment in labor? MCN Am J Matern Child Nurs. 2003;28(5):292–8.

72. Heelan L. Fetal monitoring: creating a culture of safety with informed consent. J Perinat Educ. 2013;22(3):156–65.

73. Grady C. Enduring and emerging challenges of informed consent. New Eng J Med. 2015;372(9):855–62.

74. Schenker Y, Meisel A. Informed consent in clinical care. JAMA. 2011;305(11): 1130–1.

75. Anderson RE. Billions for defense: the pervasive nature of defensive medicine. Arch Inter Med. 1999;159:2399–402.

76. DeVille K. Act first and look up the law afterward? Medical malpractice and the ethics of defensive medicine. Theoretical Medicine and Bioethics. 1998; 19(6):569–89.

77. Kachalia A, Mello MM. Defensive medicine—legally necessary but ethically wrong? JAMA Intern Med. 2014;173(12):1056–7.

78. Studdert DM, Mello MM, Sage WM, et al. Defensive medicine among high risk specialist physicians in a volatile malpractice environment. JAMA. 2005; 293(2):2609–17.

79. Sartwelle TP, Johnston JC, Arda B. Myths, fables and fairy tales: a half century of electronic fetal monitoring. Surg J. 2015; https://doi.org/10.1055/s-0035-1567880

80. Sartwelle TP, Johnston JC. Cerebral palsy and electronic fetal monitoring: rearranging the Titanic's deck chairs. J Child and Dev Disord. 2016;2(2:5):1–10.

18

Delayed cord clamping during elective cesarean deliveries: results of a pilot safety trial

Caroline J. Chantry[1]*(iD), Aubrey Blanton[2], Véronique Taché[2], Laurel Finta[2] and Daniel Tancredi[1]

Abstract

Background: Delayed cord clamping (DCC) results in decreased iron deficiency in infancy. The American College of Obstetrics and Gynecology has called for research on the optimal time to clamp the cord during cesarean deliveries (CD). Our objective was to conduct a pilot trial examining the safety of delayed cord clamping (DCC) for maternal-infant dyads during elective cesarean delivery (CD).

Methods: We enrolled 39 dyads [23 at 90 s, 16 at 120 s; (DCC Pilot)] between 10/2013 and 9/2014. We abstracted data from the electronic medical record (EMR) for historical controls (HC) birthing between 1/2012–6/2013 for whom DCC was not performed ($n = 112$).

Results: Available data for 37 mothers and 30 infants compared to HC revealed 174 (95% CI: 61–286) mL lower mean estimated maternal blood loss [(EBL) mean (SD) mL]: DCC Pilot 691(218) vs. HC 864(442), $p = 0.003$ and lower incidence of maternal transfusions, DCC Pilot 2.7% vs. HC 18.8%, $p = 0.016$. There was no significant between group difference between DCC Pilot and HC in other a priori definitions of excess maternal blood loss: a) EBL > 800 ml, 21. 6% vs. 38.8%, $p = 0.07$ or b) post-op hgb/pre-op hgb < 80%, 16.7% vs. 20.6%, $p = 0.81$. There were also no statistically significant between group differences in rates of NICU admission DCC Pilot 8.1% vs. HC 7.1%, $p = 1.0$., but there was a higher rate of newborn cold stress or hypothermia ≤36.2 °C in study subjects, DCC Pilot 27.0% vs. HC 11.9%, $p = 0.038$.Prevalence of newborn anemia was decreased [DCC pilot 3.3% (1 of 30) vs. HC 40.0% (4 of 10 infants with data), $p = 0.012$. No infants were polycythemic.

Conclusions: These pilot data suggest cord clamping can be delayed to 120 s during elective CD without increased risk of excessive maternal blood loss. More aggressive prevention of infant heat loss may be warranted. A randomized trial to evaluate long-term maternal and infant outcomes is indicated.

Keywords: Delayed cord clamping, Elective cesarean delivery, Safety pilot, Maternal blood loss, Newborn

Background

Iron deficiency is globally the most common nutrient deficiency and is the only such deficiency with significant prevalence in industrialized countries [1]. The most recently published analysis of national data reports the prevalence (± SE) of iron deficiency in US children aged 12–23 months of age at 15.1 (± 1.7) % [2] Iron is essential for normal neuronal development and pre-anemic iron deficiency in infants and young children is associated with poorer neurodevelopment [3, 4]. Prevention of iron deficiency is therefore important to optimize development, and doing so at birth with delayed cord clamping (DCC) is an inexpensive, safe and effective option [5–8]. A commentary in Evidence Based Medicine makes the compelling case that our current practice of early cord clamping unnecessarily increases infant risk for iron deficiency and subsequent poorer neurodevelopmental outcomes [9]. A randomized trial in Sweden documented DCC to successfully reduce an already low prevalence of iron deficiency anemia [10].

* Correspondence: cjchantry@ucdavis.edu
[1]Department of Pediatrics, University of California Davis Medical Center, 2516 Stockton Blvd, Sacramento, CA 95817, USA
Full list of author information is available at the end of the article

There is limited evidence, however, regarding outcomes of DCC in cesarean deliveries (CD). No studies to our knowledge have analyzed maternal or infant outcomes for term cesarean deliveries separately from vaginal deliveries. Further, there are different definitions of 'delayed cord clamping' with some experts recommending a delay of at least 2 min [5] The American College of Obstetrics and Gynecology identified the timing of umbilical cord clamping after CD vs. vaginal births as an especially important area for future research [11]. They also noted a paucity of data to support or refute the benefit of DCC for term infants in resource rich settings. To begin addressing these gaps, our objective was to perform a pilot safety trial of DCC during cesarean delivery (CD) of term infants to determine if longer intervals (90 and 120 s) relates to poorer maternal and/or newborn outcomes vs. historical controls. Our primary outcome was maternal blood loss and we hypothesized that the time to cord clamping can be safely increased from immediate clamping, to 2 min in CD without causing an increase in adverse outcomes including excessive maternal blood loss, moderate or severe neonatal hypothermia, polycythemia or neonatal ICU admission for respiratory distress. We chose a target of 2 min as the World Health Organization (WHO) recommends a delay of 1–3 min in both vaginal and cesarean deliveries [12] with some experts recommending a minimum of 2 min [5] and it is the time by which most (approximately 55%) of the placental blood has been transfused into the infant.

Methods

Study subjects and design

After study approval by the Institutional Review Board at the University of California Davis Medical Center (UCDMC), a convenience sample of dyads undergoing elective CD at term was recruited. Inclusion criteria included women ≥18 years of age with a singleton pregnancy scheduled for an elective CD at ≥37 weeks gestation. Dyads were excluded if mother or infant were medically unstable, or the mother had poorly controlled diabetes mellitus, multiple gestations, or there were known fetal anomalies and/or severe fetal growth restriction. Whenever possible, written consent of the father of the child was obtained in addition to that of the mother.

Operating room procedures included presence of the research assistant in order to alert obstetric, nursing, anesthetic and neonatology staff that the dyad was enrolled in the DCC study. Immediately upon delivery of the infant (at which time the clock began timing delay) and before cord clamp, anesthesiology began administration of IV oxytocin at a rate of 20 mU/min and the infant was dried, placed on the operating table (warmed underneath the sterile drapes by a 'bear hugger') between the mothers' legs and covered with a sterile blanket and hat.

The research assistant notified the team when 90 s (or 120 s for the subsequent arm) had elapsed. After cord clamp, cord traction was applied along with manual uterine pressure to express the placenta. If intraoperative blood loss was clinically deemed excessive, or the infant or mother was clinically unstable (e.g. no spontaneous respirations by 10 s) the obstetricians were to clamp the cord immediately upon this assessment and the time to clamp recorded.

Recruitment was continued until there were 15 dyads with complete data at 90 s delay, with an interim analysis and review by the Data Safety and Monitoring Board [(DSMB) consisting of 3 members - a statistician, perinatologist and neonatologist] was performed. After review of interim results in comparison with Historical Controls (HC), the DSMB recommended proceeding with recruitment for the 120 s arm, with modification of the protocol to include: a) a specific time to take the infant's temperature (which was specified at 15 min of age), rather than the clinical protocol being utilized which specifies the newborn temperature will be taken rectally 'within 30 min of birth'; b) recording operating room temperature; c) specific protocol for prevention of heat loss. While the drying and covering with dry blanket and hat had been previously employed, the addition of a warm, dry blanket was added.

Historical controls (HC) were collected via de-identified EMR data by the information technologists for the time period from January 2012–July 2013 when the EMR template for infant delivery first included a discrete section for DCC (yes/no and if yes, length of time of delay). During this period, non-immediate clamping was utilized per physician discretion; recorded time of those with delay ranged from 30 to 120 s, but was not always recorded. HC group consisted of those with immediate clamping ($n = 112$). Data were excluded from HC for those without a specified 'no DCC'.A delay of 30 s or longer was considered DCC per EMR template.

The primary outcome was maternal blood loss measured by the anesthesiologist's visually estimated blood loss (EBL). Excessive blood loss was a priori defined as 1 or more of the following: a) EBL > 800 mL, (per standard institutional practice at the time); b) > 20% difference between pre- and post-operative hemoglobin levels; c) need for a transfusion; d) need for maternal ICU admission for hemodynamic instability (HC data not available for comparison). Maternal blood loss was also measured quantitatively (QBL), via changing suction canisters after the amniotic fluid was suctioned and calculating wet vs. dry weight of surgical drapes and sponges; these data, however, were not available for comparison in HC data. The QBL measurement was not yet implemented clinically at the time of the study and was therefore protocolized by one of the study's authors (LF) and performed jointly by the head OR nurse and attending obstetrician. If multiple postoperative hemoglobin levels were performed, that closest to 24 h after birth was utilized.

Newborn outcomes were secondary and included the prevalence of: a) neonatal cold stress or hypothermia (≤36.2 °C) on admission; (36.2 °C was chosen as the cut-off as temperatures at or below this indicates routine screening for hypoglycemia per institutional protocol); b) newborn hemoglobin levels determined by venipuncture at 12 h (0–24) of age; c) incidence of newborn anemia or polycythemia (hgb < 14.5 or > 22.5 g/dL) [13]. Hospital protocol was to measure temperatures rectally, however mothers are encouraged to place their healthy infants skin-to-skin in the operating room, and if the infant was skin-to-skin at the time the temperature was taken, an axillary temperature was recorded.

Other measured outcomes included: a) neonatal ICU admission for respiratory distress; and b) phototherapy treatment during the first 2 weeks of life (birth hospitalization or otherwise), in the absence of evidence of hemolysis, as determined by chart review and a follow-up telephone call at 2 weeks. The latter outcomes could not be compared to the HC group as data on reason for NICU admission or on treatment with phototherapy were not available in the de-identified data. Rates of NICU admission for any cause during the first 5 days were therefore compared. This trial was registered at clinicaltrials.gov, NCT02229162.

Statistical analysis

We enrolled until there were 15 subjects per group with complete data in order to gather preliminary data and to estimate and compare the means and variances between the groups and with data from historical controls. Data were entered into REDCap [14]. A sample size of 12 has been proposed for pilot studies as appropriate for early phase trials when comparing normally distributed outcomes [15]. We chose 15 per group to achieve suitable precision in estimating means and proportions. For group means that have approximately normal sampling distributions, our sample size permits sufficient precision such that 90% confidence intervals (CI) would have half widths less than 0.5 standard deviations (SD) and that estimates of between-group differences in means would have a 90% CI half width of 0.62 SD. For less frequent binomial outcomes, the exact 90% confidence interval for the true probability of a successful outcome in case all 15 of 15 subjects have a successful outcome would be (0.818, 1.00). If the true probability of success is 0.986 or higher, we would have at least an 80% chance of observing successes in all 15 subjects.

Statistical significance testing was conducted using Fisher Exact Test for binary outcomes and with oneway ANOVA for continuous outcomes in SAS. SAS PROC GLIMMIX with robust variance estimation was used to protect inferences against heteroscedacity (varying variance) and with the HC3 adjustment to protect against small-sample biases. Differences in means/incidence from the reference group (HC without DCC) were estimated with 95% CI, using the same robust variance estimation procedures for differences in means of continuous outcomes and using Agresti-Min unconditional exact 95% CI for risk differences for binary outcomes [16, 17] via SAS PROC FREQ using the RISKDIFF(Method = FMScore) option on the EXACT statement, to base the Agresti-Min 95% CI on the Farrington-Manning score statistic.

Finally, in addition to comparing the DCC pilot vs. the HC groups, we compared outcomes between the 90 s and 120 s DCC pilot groups to evaluate for differences between the two durations of delay.

Results
Study subjects

Study recruitment took place between October 2013 and September 2014 and is diagrammed in Fig. 1. Briefly, a convenience sample of 53 women who met inclusion criteria were approached to participate and a total of 41 consented. Mean (SD) maternal parity and age were 2.7 (1.2) and 32.2 (5.0) respectively.

DCC pilot vs. historical controls (HC)
Maternal blood loss

The primary outcome for the mothers was blood loss during surgery (See Table 1). Mean estimated blood loss (EBL) in the DCC pilot group was 174 mL less (95% CI -61, – 286), compared to the HC group, p = 0.003. There was also a corresponding lesser percentage of mothers in the DCC group receiving transfusions (2.7%) compared to the HC group (18.8%), p = 0.016. There were no statistical between group differences in the other two measures of excess blood loss, EBL > 800 mL or post-operative/pre-operative hgb ratio < 80% (See Table 1).

No mothers in the study required ICU admission for hemodyamic instability.

Infant outcomes

There were few newborn hemoglobin (hgb) results among the HC group, as hemoglobin was not routinely checked historically. Although the DCC pilot group had a mean hgb 0.9 g higher than the HC control group, this was not statistically significant. There was a lower prevalence of anemia in the DCC pilot vs. HC group, 40.07% vs. 3.3%, p = 0.01 (Table 1). No infants in any group were polycythemic.

Mean admission temperatures were not different by group. There were, however, more infants in the DCC pilot group experiencing cold stress or hypothermia

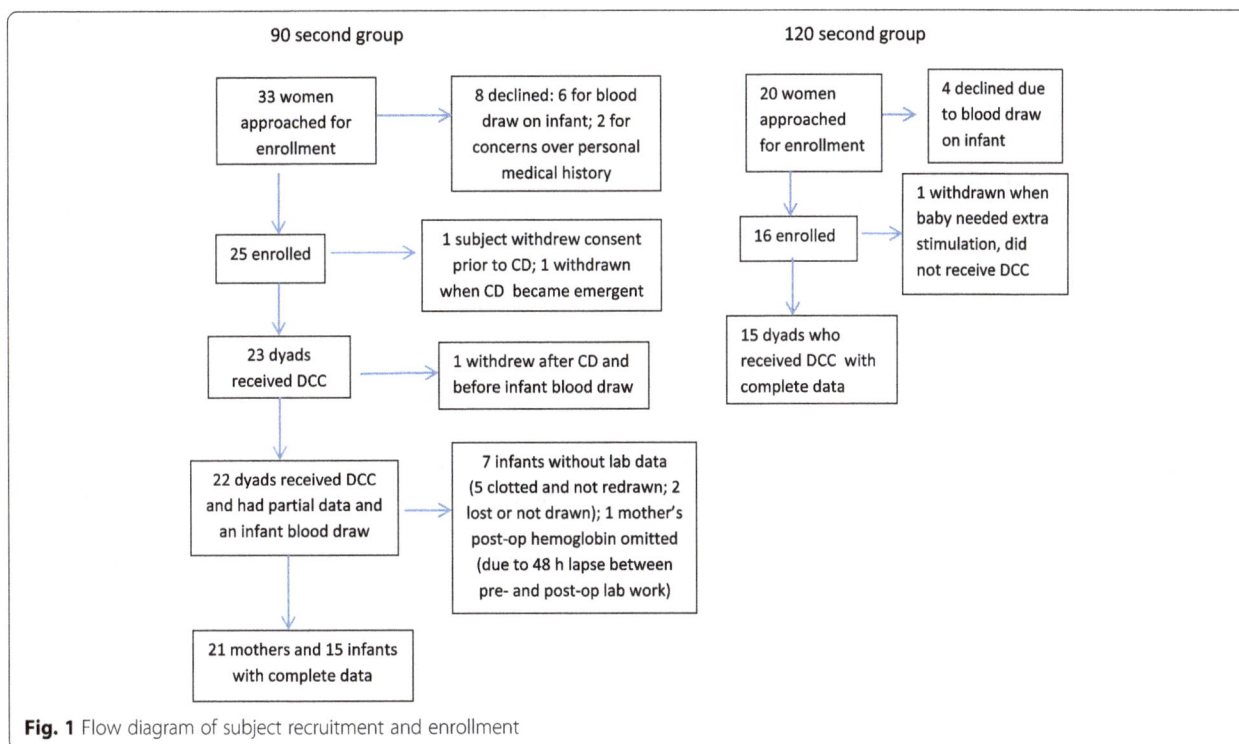

Fig. 1 Flow diagram of subject recruitment and enrollment

(admission temperature ≤ 36.2 °C, 27.0% vs. 11.9%, $p = 0.038$). There was no difference in prevalence of more severe hypothermia of admission temperature < 36.0 °C (data not shown).

Admission to the neonatal ICU occurred in 3 of the DCC pilot group infants (8.1%); all 3 of these were for respiratory distress. We do not have reasons for neonatal ICU admissions in the HC group, but prevalence of ICU admission was nearly identical at 7.1%.

Finally, phototherapy was instituted during the birth hospitalization for only 1 infant that had ABO incompatibility with anti-A antibodies in the DCC pilot group. No infants required readmission for phototherapy. This information was not available for the HC groups.

Table 1 Maternal and Newborn Outcomes for Historical Control and DCC Pilot Groups

Maternal Blood Loss –Indicator	DCC Pilot $n = 39$ Mean (SD)	HC n = 112 Mean (SD)	P value	Difference in Means/Risk (Risk difference expressed as percentage points) (95%CI)
EBL (mL)	691 (218) $n = 38$	864 (442) $n = 103$	0.003	− 174 (− 286, −81)
Maternal Excess Blood Loss Indicator % yes (n/total)	% yes (n/total)	% yes (n/total)		
EBL > 800 mL	21.6% (8/37)	38.8% (40/103)	0.074	−17.2 (−2.0,32.3)
PostOp/PreOp Hgb < 80%	16.7% (6/36)	20.6% (20/97)	0.81	−4.0 (−17.6, 13.5)
PostOp transfusion	2.7% (1/37)	18.8% (21/112)	0.016	−16.0 (−25.2,-6.9)
Newborn outcomes				
Mean (SD)				
Newborn Hemoglobin (mg/dL)	16.8(2.0) $n = 30$	15.9(3.8) n = 10	0.35	0.8 (−1.8, 3.5)
Admission temperature (°C)	36.6(0.4) $n = 37$	36.7(0.4) $n = 109$	0.08	−0.1 (− 0.3, 0.02)
% yes (n/total)				
Anemia (Hgb < 14.5 g/dL)	3.3% (1/30)	40.0% (4/10)	0.010	−36.7 (−69.2,-5.9)
Cold stress /moderate hypothermia (temp ≤36.2 °C)	27.0% (10/37)	11.9% (13/109)	0.038	15.1 (−0.02,32.6)
NICU admission	8.1% (3/37)	7.1% 8/112	1.0	1.0 (−15.7,7.9)

DCC 90s vs. DCC 120 s

The only statistically significant difference between the two pilot groups of 90 s ($n = 23$) vs. 120 s ($n = 16$) was in EBL, which was 752 (207) mL for the 90 s group vs. 600 (206) mL for the 120 s group, $p = 0.04$. There was a corresponding greater percentage of mothers in the 90 s group which experienced greater than 20% drop in hgb, (24% vs. 7%), but this was not statistically significant ($p = 0.16$); nor was the greater percentage of mothers in the 90 s group with EBL > 800 mL, 27% vs. 13%, $p = 0.32$.

Interestingly, quantitatively measured blood loss (QBL) in the DCC pilot groups was significantly higher than the EBL; QBL [mean (SD)] was 1056 (507) and 1050 (484) mL for 90 and 120 s vs. EBL of 752 mL (207) and 600 mL (206) respectively, paired t-test $p = 0.02$ and < 0.001. Also, QBL did not corroborate the finding of statistically significantly greater EBL in the 90 vs. 120 s DCC group. Quantitatively measured blood loss was not available in historical controls.

There were no statistically significant differences in any of the newborn outcomes between the 90 and 120 s DCC groups.

Discussion

The primary outcome results of this pilot safety trial are reassuring. Maternal blood loss, using multiple measurement techniques, was not significantly increased from a clinical or statistical standpoint, in the DCC pilot group compared to the HC group. In fact, two of the measures -EBL and percent of mothers requiring transfusion- actually indicated *lower* blood loss in the DCC Pilot vs. the HC group. These findings support our hypothesis that cord clamping can be safely increased to 2 min in CD without increased maternal blood loss. Similar findings were observed in the 3-arm trial in Argentina [18] (immediate vs. 1 or 3 min of delay), in which 28–30% of deliveries in each arm were CD with no increased blood loss in delayed vs. immediate clamping; results of CD were not analyzed separately however. Maternal blood loss data were separately reported for CD recently when comparing before vs. after instituting a policy of 30 s delay in cord clamp for premature infants; there was no significant difference in EBL during CD for mothers after policy institution [19]. It is interesting to note they also reported a trend towards *less* of a decrease in hemoglobin in those with clamping at 30 s compared to immediate clamping [mean (95% CI) difference 0.4 (0.0,0.08) gm/dL, $p = 0.05$].

The finding of fewer mothers requiring transfusion in the DCC pilot vs. HC group is important to note and suggests mothers undergoing elective CD may actually benefit from DCC. It is unclear if this was related to greater care of the surgeons to prevent blood loss in the setting of late cord clamping (e.g. more clamping off of

small bleeding vessels), altered response of the uterus to an emptier placenta or receipt of oxytocin during the delay in the 120 s group, or a combination thereof. It is also possible that this could be a chance finding. The Cochrane review did not find a difference in risk of severe postpartum hemorrhage or need for transfusion by use of prophylactic uterotonic before vs. after clamping, [7] but few studies reported timing of use, and those that did typically used intramuscular administration, likely to have less impact than intravenous administration used in our protocol.

We also note that the quantitatively measured blood loss (QBL) in both DCC pilot groups was significantly greater than that estimated by EBL, by 40 and 75% respectively. This discrepancy is even greater than the 30% noted in the literature previously [20] and supports current recommendations to implement quantitative blood loss measures [21–24]. We acknowledge that the difference in EBL between the 90 and 120 s study groups was not corroborated by the QBL. This raises the concern of possible bias in EBL estimates. It may also reflect implementation challenges with accurate measurement of QBL, as this procedure had not yet been implemented clinically at our institution at the time of the study.

Newborn outcomes of anemia, polycythemia, cold stress/hypothermia, and NICU admission were secondary outcomes; of these only the cold stress/hypothermia measure was statistically significantly increased in the DCC pilot vs. HC groups. While it was reassuring that there was not a difference in prevalence of admission temperature < 36 °C, the rate of admission temperature ≤ 36.2 °C (27%) is nevertheless of concern and may be clinically significant. It is possible that other factors may have contributed to hypothermia, e.g. recent practice of placing the infant skin-to-skin in the operating room per maternal preference. In this setting mothers may also be cool and it may be difficult to cover the infant well. Regardless, we believe more aggressive measures to prevent heat loss are warranted, such as use of polyethylene wraps for the infant during delayed clamping, previously documented to decrease hypothermia in premature infants during resuscitation [25]. A recent institutional protocol for DCC in premature infants < 34 weeks successfully utilized polyethylene wraps along with delivery room temperatures of 76–79 °C to prevent hypothermia in both vaginal as well as cesarean deliveries [19].

No infants in any group were polycythemic, and statistically fewer in the intervention groups were anemic, as might be expected. However, a significant limitation of this study is relatively few infants in the HC group had hemoglobin data available for comparison, and therefore those with data may not represent the overall historical term, elective CD group.

Limitations to this study are several and include this being a small, single-center pilot study, which limits generalizability. Our controls are historical, so results may be confounded by temporal trends and they were not matched for maternal characteristics. Also limiting is that we are unable to confirm if the EMR record of DCC in the historical controls is accurate. As noted, there were limitations in the de-identified newborn data we obtained, with few hemoglobin results, and no data available on treatment with phototherapy or cause for NICU admission. Strengths of the study include observation of the time to cord clamp, and objective measures of maternal blood loss in addition to EBL.

Despite the above limitations, our findings suggest that cord clamping can be safely delayed for at least 120 s in elective CD without resulting in excess maternal blood loss and further suggest maternal blood loss may be *decreased* with the protocol utilized. Given the potential benefit of improved iron status on infant neurodevelopmental outcomes and the dearth of data available in this country regarding infant iron status and related outcomes, these results call for a larger, randomized trial of DCC in elective CD evaluating both short- and longer-term outcomes for both members of the dyad. The need for such a trial is particularly compelling with the recent report that delayed cord clamping in Sweden, a high-income country, reduced the number of children with low fine-motor and social skill scores at 4 years of age [26]. An editorial in the same JAMA issue highlighted that since 2000, no randomized trial has documented symptomatic polycythemia in infants [27]. Intuitively, there is reason to think newborn outcomes related to DCC are likely similar to those in vaginal deliveries, but this needs to be confirmed prior to recommending its use. Lastly, it will be important to confirm if this 120 s delay can also improve outcomes for the mother, an intriguing possibility which is suggested by our and other data.

Conclusions

Data from this pilot safety study suggest that delaying cord clamping for 2 min in elective, term cesarean deliveries does not increase risk of excessive maternal blood loss. More aggressive prevention of infant heat loss than utilized in our protocol may be warranted. A randomized trial to evaluate longer term maternal and infant outcomes is indicated.

Abbreviations
C: Centigrade; CD: cesarean delivery; CI: confidence interval; DCC: delayed cord clamping; DSMB: Data Safety and Monitoring Board; EBL: estimated blood loss; EMR: electronic medical record; gm/dL: grams/deciliter; h: hour; HC: historical control; hgb: hemoglobin; ICU: intensive care unit; IQR: interquartile range; IV: intravenous; min: minutes; mL: milliliter; mU: milliunits; OR: operating room; QBL: quantitatively measured blood loss; s: seconds; SD: standard deviation

Acknowledgments
We gratefully acknowledge the families who participated and the nursing staff of the University Birth Suites and Women's Pavilion, University California Davis Medical Center, with special thanks to Barbara Taylor and Brenda Chagolla. We also gratefully acknowledge the Data Safety and Monitoring Board: Drs. Ana-Maria Iosif, Herman Hedriana and Francis Poulain. This study was supported in part by a pilot grant from the UC Davis Center for Healthcare Policy and Research (PI Chantry).

Funding
This study was supported by a grant from the Center for Healthcare Policy and Research, at University of California Davis Medical Center. The de-identified historical control data and Research Electronic Data Capture (REDCap) were provided by the Biomedical Informatics program at the UC Davis Clinical and Translational Science Center supported by grant #UL1000002 from the National Center for Advancing Translational Sciences, a component of the National Institutes of Health (NIH).

Authors' contributions
CC contributed to study design, acquisition, analysis and interpretation of data, and drafting and critical revision of the article. AB contributed to acquisition and analysis of data, and drafting and critical revision of the article. VT contributed to study design, acquisition, analysis and interpretation of data, and critical revision of the article. LF contributed to study design, acquisition of data, and critical revision of the article. DT contributed to study design, analysis and interpretation of data, drafting and critical revision of the article. All authors read and approved the final manuscript.

Competing interests
The authors declare that they have no competing interests.

Author details
[1]Department of Pediatrics, University of California Davis Medical Center, 2516 Stockton Blvd, Sacramento, CA 95817, USA. [2]Obstetrics and Gynecology, University of California Davis Medical Center, Sacramento, CA, USA.

References
1. Iron deficiency anemia. The Challenge. World Health Organization. http://www.who.int/nutrition/topics/ida/en/. Accessed 10 Apr 2018.
2. Gupta PM, Hamner HC, Suchdev PS, Flores-Ayala R, Mei Z. Iron status of toddlers, nonpregnant females, and pregnant females in the United States. Am J Clin Nutr. 2017;106(Suppl 6):1640S–6S. https://doi.org/10.3945/ajcn.117.155978. Epub 2017 Oct 25.3.
3. Beard J. Recent evidence from human and animal studies regarding iron status and infant development. J Nutr. 2007;137:524S–30S.
4. McCann JC, Ames BN. An overview of evidence for a causal relation between iron deficiency during development and deficits in cognitive or behavioral function. Am J Clin Nutr. 2007;85:931–45.
5. Hutton EK, Hassan ES. Late vs. early clamping of the umbilical cord in full-term neonates. Systematic review and Mata-analysis of controlled trials. JAMA. 2007;297(11):1241–52.
6. McDonald SJ, Middleton P. Effect of timing of umbilical cord clamping of term infants on maternal and neonatal outcomes. Cochrane Database of Systematic Reviews 2008; Issue 2. Art. No: CD004074.pub2. https://doi.org/10.1002/14651858.CD004074.pub2.
7. McDonald SJ, Middleton P, Dowswell T, Morris PS. Effect of timing of umbilical cord clamping of term infants on maternal and neonatal outcomes. Cochrane Database of Systematic Reviews 2013, Issue 7. Art. No.: CD004074.pub3. https://doi.org/10.1002/14651858.CD004074.pub3.
8. Chaparro CM, Neufeld LM, Tena Alavez G, Eguia-Liz Cedillo R, Dewey KG. Effect of timing of umbilical cord clamping on iron status in Mexican infants. Lancet. 2006;367:1997–2004.
9. Weeks A. Early umbilical cord clamping increases the risk of neonatal anaemia and infant iron deficiency. Evid Based Med. 2012;17(6):179–80.
10. Andersson O, Hellstrom-Westas L, Andersson D, et al. Effect of delayed versus early umbilical cord clamping on neonatal outcomes and iron status at 4 months: a randomised controlled trial. BMJ. 2011;343:1–12.

11. American College of Obstetrics and Gynecology Committee on Obstetric Practice. Committee opinion 543.Timing of umbilical cord clamping after birth. Obstet Gynecol. 2012;120(6):1522–6.

12. World Health Organization. Guideline: delayed umbilical cord clamping for improved maternal and infant health and nutrition outcomes. Geneva: World Health Organization; 2014. http://www.who.int/nutrition/publications/guidelines/cord_clamping/en/. Accessed 3 Feb 2018.

13. The *Harriet Lane handbook*. A manual for pediatric house officers. (Twenty-first edition). Table 14.1 Hughes, H., & Kahl, L. Harriet Lane Service (Johns Hopkins Hospital), 2018. Philadelphia, PA: Elsevier.

14. Agresti A, Min YY. On small-sample confidence intervals for parameters in discrete distributions. Biometrics. 2001;57(3):963–71.

15. Santner TJ, Pradhan V, Senchaudhuri P, Mehta CR, Tamhane A. Small-sample comparisons of confidence intervals for the difference of two independent binomial proportions. Comput Stat Data An. 2007;51(12):5791–9.

16. Harris PA, Taylor R, Thielke R, Payne J, Gonazlea N, Conde JG. Research electronic data capture (REDCap) – a metadata-driven methodology and workflow process for providing translational research informatics support. J Biomed Inform. 2009;42(2):377–81.

17. Julious SA. Sample size of 12 per group rule of thumb for a pilot study. Pharmaceut Statist. 2005;4:287–91.

18. Ceriani Cernadas JM, Guillermo C, Pellegrini L, et al. The effect of timing of cord clamping on neonatal venous hematocrit values and clinical outcome at term: a randomized, controlled trial. Pediatrics. 2006;117:e779–86.

19. Kuo K, Gokhale P, Hackney DN, Ruangkit C, Bhola M, March M. Maternal outcomes following the initiation of an institutional delayed cord clamping protocol: an observational case-control study. J Matern Fetal Neonatal Med. 2017;31(2):1–5.

20. Al Kadri HM, Al Anazi BK, Tamim HM. Visual estimation versus gravimetric measurement of postpartum blood loss: a prospective cohort study. Arch Gynecol Obstet. 2011;283(6):1207–13.

21. Bose P, Regan F, Paterson-Brown S. Improving the accuracy of estimated blood loss at obstetric haemorrhage using clinical reconstructions. BJOG. 2006;113:919–24.

22. Patel A, Goudar SS, Geller SE, et al. Drape estimation vs. visual assessment for estimating postpartum hemorrhage. Int J Gynaecol Obstet. 2006;93(3):220–4.

23. Dildy G, Paine A, George N, Velasco C. Estimating blood loss: can teaching significantly improve visual estimation? Obstet Gynecol. 2004;104(3):601–6.

24. Toledo P, McCarthy RJ, Hewlett BJ, Fitzgerald PC, Wong CA. The accuracy of blood loss estimation after simulated vaginal delivery. Anesth Analg. 2007;105:1736–40.

25. Cordaro T, Phalen AG, Zukowsky K. Hypothermia and occlusive skin wrap in the low birth weight premature infant. An Evidentiary Review NAINR. 2012;12(2):78–85.

26. Andersson O, Lindquist B, Lindgren M, Stjernqvist K, Domellof M, Hellstrom-Westas L. Effect of delayed cord clamping on neurodevelopment at 4 years of age: a randomized clinical trial. JAMA Pediatr. 2015;169(7):631–8.

27. Rabe H, Erickson-Owens DA, Mercer JS. Long-term follow-up of placental transfusion in full-term infants. Editorial JAMA Pediatr. 2015;169(7):623–4.

19

Evaluation of transcutaneous bilirubinometer (DRAEGER JM 103) use in Zimbabwean newborn babies

Gwendoline Lilly Tanyaradzwa Chimhini[1*], Simbarashe Chimhuya[1] and Vasco Chikwasha[2]

Abstract

Background: Acute Bilirubin Encephalopathy in the neonatal period is a major cause of permanent disability. Effective screening and surveillance are essential in the newborn period to enable timely management. Noninvasive transcutaneous bilirubin devices have been successfully used for screening in many settings. We evaluated the accuracy of the Draeger JM 103 (Medical Systems, USA) for estimating serum bilirubin in Zimbabwean newborns.

Methods: Paired transcutaneous (forehead and sternum) and serum bilirubin measurements were compared on 283 infants consecutively recruited between 01 August and 30 November 2015 at Harare Hospital Neonatal Unit. Using serum bilirubin as gold standard, Pearson Correlation Coefficient (r) was calculated for the two transcutaneous measurement sites. Linear regression plots of transcutaneous versus serum estimates were performed. Comparison was made between preterm and term babies. Specificity, sensitivity, positive predictive value and negative predictive value of the JM103 were calculated including ROC curves to assess the accuracy of the diagnostic tests.

Results: Fifty-five percent of the babies were male. Median gestational age was 38 weeks (range 28–42). One hundred and fifteen (41%) were preterm. Median postnatal age was 3 days (range 0–10). Serum bilirubin ranged 85–408 μmol/l, transcutaneous bilirubin sternum; 170–544 μmol/l and forehead; 119–510 μmol/l. Correlation between serum and transcutaneous bilirubin (sternum) was 0.77 and between serum and transcutaneous (forehead) was 0.72. Preterm babies correlation for sternum was 0.77 and forehead was 0.75. Term babies correlation for sternum was 0.76 and forehead was 0.70. The sensitivity for the sternum site was 76%, specificity 90%, Positive Predictive Value of 70 and Negative Predictive Value 92. Sensitivity for forehead site was 62%, specificity 95% with a Positive Predictive Value of 80 and Negative Predictive Value of 90. Bland-Altman plot of serum versus transcutaneous measurements showed agreement between the tests. The ROC curves showed that the accuracy of the two diagnostic tests were good with no significant difference between the two, $p = 0.2954$.

Conclusion: The study demonstrated a strong positive correlation for both sternum and forehead sites with serum bilirubin in this Zimbabwean population of African origin. However, the sternum is a better site for identifying babies with jaundice compared to forehead. The Draeger JM-103 can be used to screening for neonatal jaundice in this population.

Keywords: Zimbabwe, Jaundice, Neonate, Bilirubin, JM-103, Correlation

---

* Correspondence: gwenchimhini@gmail.com
[1]Department of Paediatrics and Child Health, University of
Zimbabwe-College of Health Sciences, Mazoe Street, Box A178 Avondale,
Harare, Zimbabwe
Full list of author information is available at the end of the article

Background

Acute Bilirubin Encephalopathy (ABE), resulting from severe neonatal jaundice, is a cause of permanent disability in children in Zimbabwe. ABE is preventable if diagnosed and treated before serum bilirubin reaches dangerous levels. ABE is a condition that has been virtually eliminated as a cause of cerebral palsy in most developed countries [1].

Effective screening and surveillance are essential to ensure that infants with severe or pathological jaundice are timely identified and correctly managed in the immediate newborn period. Newborn jaundice is known to have cephalo-caudal progression [2]. However visual assessment of jaundice has been shown to correlate poorly with measured serum bilirubin levels [3]. Visual assessment of the skin and sclera, though well documented as inaccurate, is employed where objective means of measurement are unavailable, and is a major reason for inadequate case identification of jaundiced newborns by health workers [3–5]. This is even more difficult in darkly pigmented infants resulting in late referral for care when infants are in an advanced state of bilirubin encephalopathy.

In the majority of babies on our unit phototherapy is initiated empirically upon identification of jaundice before laboratory determination of the actual level of serum bilirubin. In our hospital laboratory determination of total serum bilirubin (TSB) is not always possible due to various health system constraints such as unavailability of testing reagents or machine breakdown. Similar constraints are also experienced at other health institutions in the public sector, particularly in rural areas. Similar problems affect health institutions in most resource limited countries. The majority of hospitals in Zimbabwe, therefore, manage jaundiced infants using visual estimation.

Melanin affects the clinical estimation of jaundice in the newborn [6]. Clinical assessment of jaundice often leads to over or underestimation of jaundice and results in unnecessary blood draws from the baby with resultant maternal anxiety [7, 8]. Blood sampling for the estimation of serum bilirubin is one of the commonest tests ordered in the neonatal units and postnatal wards. This is often done by heel prick and is considered painful [8, 9] with potential long-term consequences [9]. Turnaround time for obtaining the laboratory result varies between 2 and 24 h in our hospital. In the event of stock-out of reagents to measure TSB in the hospital laboratory, most parents cannot afford the 20 USD charged by the private laboratories.

Transcutaneous bilirubin (TcB) devices that estimate serum bilirubin noninvasively have been found to reduce the need for blood draws from neonates [7]. The American Academy of Pediatrics recommends the use of TcB devices for the screening of jaundice in infants at more than 35 weeks of gestation [10]. The point of care TcB devices have been in use in the developed countries for a long time. Transcutaneous bilirubinometry was introduced into clinical practice in 1980 by Yamanouchi et al. [11]. The JM103 was first used in 2003 in Japan [12].

In 2004 the American Academy of Paediatrics recommended pre discharge measurement of bilirubin using point of care TcB for babies more than 35 weeks gestational age [13, 14]. These devices, when used prior to the commencement of phototherapy, have been shown to correlate well with TSB levels in both term and preterm infants [6, 15–18]. There are, however, conflicting reports on the use of the JM103 in newborns of African origin. The device has been reported to overestimate bilirubin levels in pigmented African Nigerian and African American newborns [19, 20]. Studies from Malawi indicated that the JM103 could be used to assess jaundiced babies for phototherapy [21]. In Malawi, the JM103 has been used to guide phototherapy in jaundiced newborns [21].

We, therefore, set out to evaluate the accuracy of TcB measurements using the Draeger JM 103 device in assessing jaundice in black Zimbabwean newborns against the diazo method as the gold standard.

Methods

Study design

Analytical Cross Sectional Study.

Table 1 Clinical characteristics of the study participants

Characteristic		Number (n)	Percentage (%)
Gender	Male	155	55
	Female	127	45
Gestational age (weeks)	28–36	115	41
	≥37–42	168	59
Postnatal age at measurement	≤24 h	9	3
	2 days	54	19
	3 days	84	30
	4 days	73	25
	5–10 days	58	21

Table 2 Summary statistics (TSB mean, TcB mean, median)

Variable	Number of patients	Minimum value	Max	Mean	Std Deviation
TSB	283	85	408	186	66,1
TcB Sternum	283	170	544	221	76,7
TcB forehead	283	119	510	212	73,8

Table 3 Pearson correlation coefficient (r) of TcB sternum and TcB forehead

Variable	r	Confidence Interval	p-value
TcB forehead	0.724	0.663–0.775	<0,001
TcB Sternum	0.766	0.714–0.811	<0,001

Study setting

The study was conducted at Harare Central Hospital (Zimbabwe) between 1st August and 30th November 2015. The hospital is the largest teaching and specialist health care center in Zimbabwe. The maternity unit has on average, 1200 deliveries and 400 neonatal admissions per month.

Study subjects

Hospitalized newborns with visible jaundice, where phototherapy had not yet been commenced.

Inclusion Criteria

Jaundiced infants aged 0–10 days before commencement of phototherapy.

Exclusion Criteria

Infants with major congenital abnormalities, severely dehydrated infants with poor peripheral perfusion.

Laboratory tests

Draeger JM103 assessments Paired TcB and TSB measurements were performed on eligible infants. TcB was measured on the forehead and on the sternum using a Draeger JM 103 (Medical Systems, USA). Three TcB measurements were done for each site and an average was taken. The TcB machine was calibrated daily according to the manufacturer's instructions.

TSB estimation

A venous blood draw for TSB was done within 30 min of the TcB measurement. TSB was measured in the laboratory by a photometric technique using diazo methods. The hospital laboratory has two types of analyzers, Dimension Xpand Plus (Siemens, Germany) and Mindary BS 400 (China). TSB measurements were performed using either of these machines. The analyzers are always calibrated daily in the morning as part of the standard operating procedure of the laboratory.

The TcB measurements and TSB were entered onto a log sheet alongside with the following variables: gestational age, gender, age of infant and type of treatment given to patient (phototherapy, exchange transfusion or observe). The patients were managed according to WHO guidelines for management of jaundiced newborn.

Permission to conduct the study was obtained from Harare Hospital Ethics Committee Approval number HCHEC 200515/39. Written Informed consent was obtained from the parents.

Data management and analysis

Data were entered into EPI INFO Version 6.4 and then exported to STATA version 12 for cleaning and analysis.

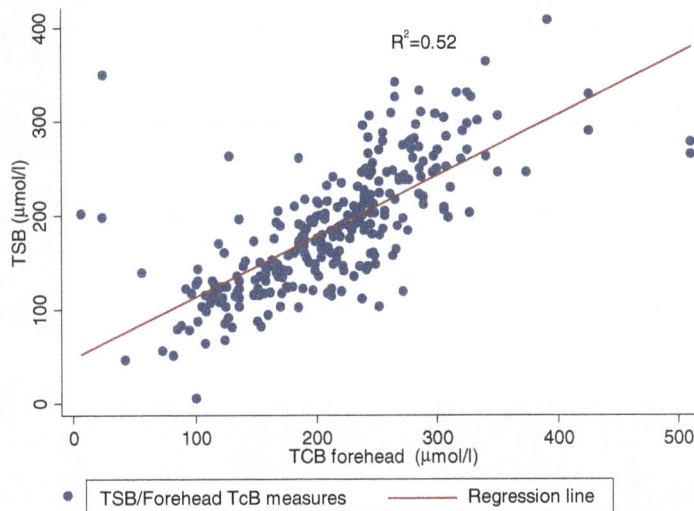

Fig. 1 Linear Regression Plot for Forehead TcB Versus TSB. Linear regression plot showing the relationship between Forehead TcB and TSB. As Forehead TcB concentration increase TSB concentration also increase showing a positive linear relationship with a coefficient of determination, $R^2 = 0.52$

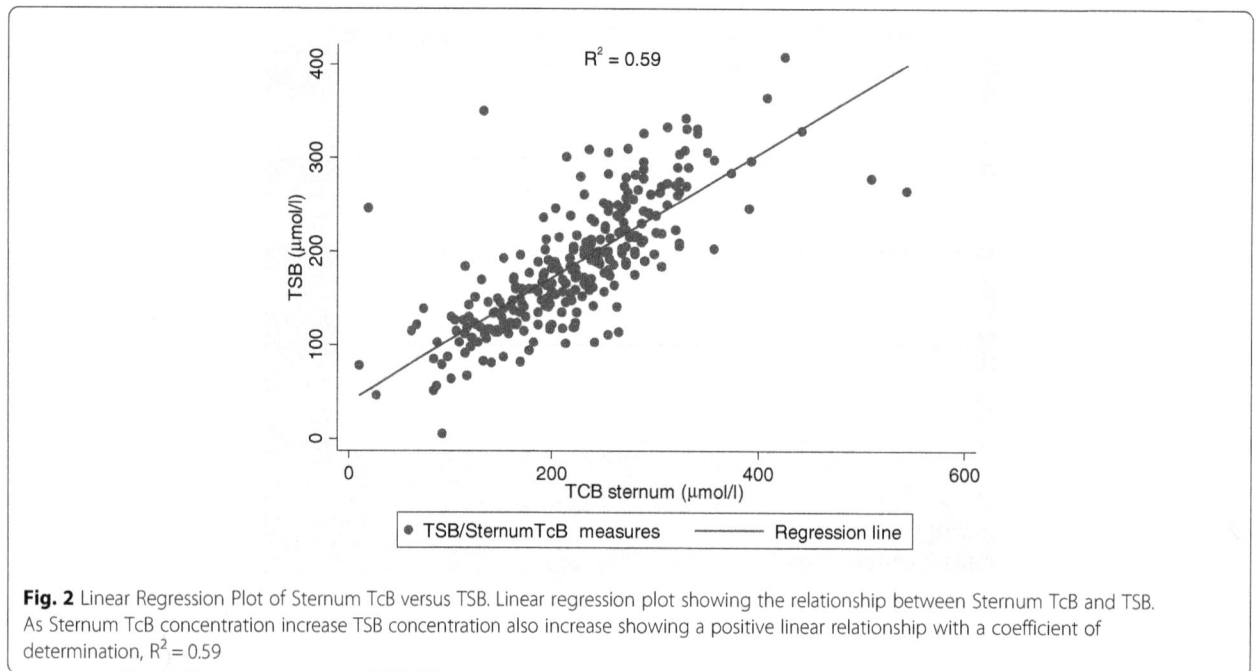

Fig. 2 Linear Regression Plot of Sternum TcB versus TSB. Linear regression plot showing the relationship between Sternum TcB and TSB. As Sternum TcB concentration increase TSB concentration also increase showing a positive linear relationship with a coefficient of determination, $R^2 = 0.59$

The Pearson Correlation Coefficient (r) was calculated for the two TcB measurement sites, forehead and sternum. Linear regression plots of the JM-103 TcB versus TSB estimates were plotted. A comparison was made between the preterm and term babies for the two measured sites. Using the TSB as the gold standard, the specificity and sensitivity of the JM103 TcB measurements were calculated including the positive and negative predictive values. The Bland-Altman plot was used to check for agreement between the TSB and Forehead TcB measures. McNemar's test was used for sensitivity and specificity comparison between the TcB Sternum and TcB Forehead diagnostic tests. The Receiver Operator Characteristic curves were used to access for the accuracy of the two diagnostic tests.

Results

Two hundred and eighty-three newborns were recruited during the study period. Fifty-five percent (55%) were male. The gestational age ranged from 28 to 42 weeks with a median gestational age of 38 weeks [Q1, 34; Q3, 40]. Forty-one percent (41%) were preterm. The median postnatal age was 3 days [Q1,3; Q3, 4, range 1–10 days]. Table 1 shows the clinical characteristics of the study participants.

TSB ranged between 85 and 408 µmol/l. Sternum TcB ranged between 170 and 544 µmol/l and forehead TcB 119–510 µmol/l as shown in Table 2. The correlation between paired serum bilirubin and

sternum TcB was 0.77, and that between the TSB and forehead TcB was 0,72 as shown in Table 3 and Figs 1 and 2. The paired correlation in preterm babies was 0.77 for sternum and 0.75 for forehead. The correlation was 0.76 for sternum and 0.70 for forehead for term babies as shown in Table 4.

Using cut offs for phototherapy according to the WHO guidelines, the sensitivity of the TcB sternum was 76% [95% CI 64–86] and specificity was 90% [95% CI 86–94]. The Positive Predictive Value (PPV) was 70 [90% CI 58–81] and Negative Predictive Value (NPV) was 92 [95% CI 88–96]. The sensitivity for the TcB (forehead) was 62% [95% CI 52–77] and specificity 95% [95% CI 91–97] with a PPV of 80 [95% CI 67–89] and NPV of 90 [95% CI 85–93]. There was no difference in the sensitivity ($p = 0.1799$) and the specificity ($p = 0.0648$) for the two anatomical sites.

Bland-Altman plot of TSB versus TcB forehead showed agreement between the tests. Only 11/283 (3,89%) of the tests were outside the limits of agreement with a mean difference of –26.34 as shown in Fig. 3.

Table 4 Pearson Correlation coefficient (r) of TcB sternum and TcB forehead for term and preterm babies

TcB site	Gestational age	r
Forehead	28–36 weeks	0.7548
	≥37 weeks	0.7048
Sternum	28–36 weeks	0.7691
	≥37 weeks	0.7614

11/283 = 3.89% outside the limits of agreement
Mean difference -26.336
95% limits of agreement (-129.220,76.549)
Averages lie between 44.250 and 399.500

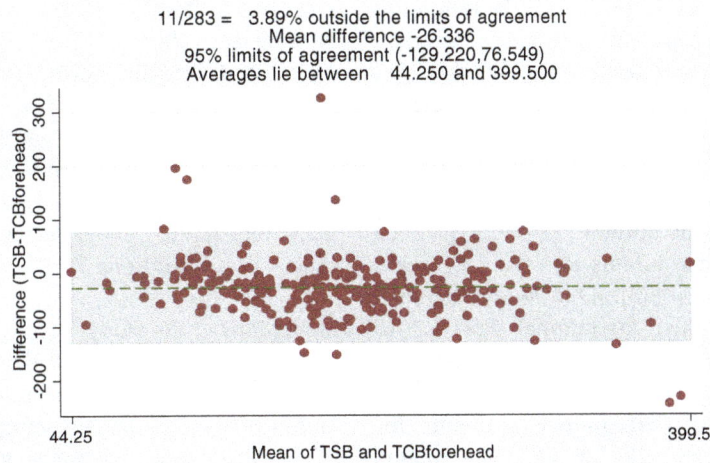

Fig. 3 Bland Altman Plot showing difference between TSB and TcB forehead. The Bland Altman plot shows the agreement between Forehead TcB and TSB measurements. The plot shows that only 3.89% of the points lie outside the limits of agreement

Receiver operator characteristic curves

The accuracy of the two two diagnostic tests were compared using the ROC curves as shown in Fig. 4. The area under the Forehead TcB curve = 0.80 and the area under the Sternum TcB curve = 0.83. The difference was not statistically significant though, $p = 0.2954$. Given the area under the curve for each test, the two anatomical sites can be classified as good at separating babies needing phototherapy and those not in need.

Discussion

The study was performed on newborns in a tertiary neonatal unit of a resource constrained setting. The gestational age ranged from 28 to 42 weeks. There was agreement between transcutaneous bilirubin values and serum bilirubin levels for both sternum and forehead. The study demonstrated a strong correlation between TcB (both sternum and forehead) and TSB in an ethnic Zimbabwean population. There are a number of previous

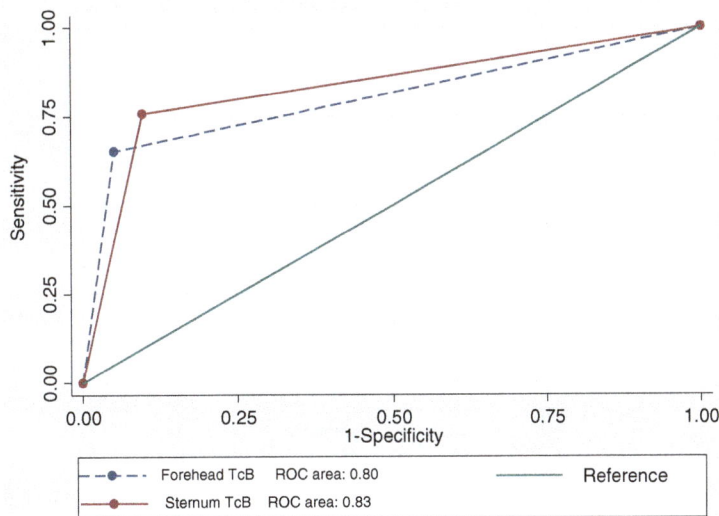

Fig. 4 Receiver Operator Characteristic Curves for Sternum and Forehead TcB. The ROC curve shows the accuracy of Forehead TcB and Sternum TcB. The ROC curves show good accuracy in the two methods in separating babies needing phototherapy and those not in need with no significant difference in the two methods

reports of validation of the Draeger JM103 machine in different populations [6, 15, 16, 18, 19, 21]. In this study, the site of TcB measurement and gestational age were examined. Other studies have examined the postnatal age, severity of illness of the infant, effect of phototherapy on TcB and type of instrument used to measure the TcB [16, 19, 21, 22].

There are huge variations in the number of patients and inclusion criteria in the studies [17–19, 21]. Some studies excluded premature infants less than 35 weeks gestation and sick infants [23]. Our study included sick newborns and included gestational ages 28 to 42 weeks. Several researchers have shown that race has a significant effect on TcB with Caucasian infants having higher TcB values than nonwhite infants for similar TSB concentrations [19, 23, 24]. The infants in our study were all black Zimbabweans.

The forehead is the most frequent site for TcB measurement in clinical practice. In our study, the correlation coefficient for TcB (sternum) was higher than TcB (forehead). However, the difference was not statistically significant. Various studies have shown similar results with better correlation of TSB to TcB (sternum) compared to any other part of the body and TcB (forehead) more likely to under estimate TSB compared to TcB (sternum) as has been found in other studies [6, 19, 22, 23, 25]. The reason for this difference between sternum TcB and forehead TcB is not clear. It has been postulated that the difference could be because the sternum is usually covered whereas the fore head is usually exposed to sunlight ultraviolet rays. Exposure to ultraviolet rays stimulates melanin production. This results in reduction of the basal yellow skin colour, which TcB devices measure [26]. In some studies, gestational age, as well as postnatal age, have been shown to have an effect on TcB. This could be attributed to maturation of skin seen in term babies and changes in albumin binding which occurs with maturity [26]. In the current study, there was a better estimation of TSB by TcB for both anatomical sites in the less than 37 weeks gestation compared to those more than 37 weeks though this was not statistically different [26]. There were very few preterms in the current study and this could probably explain why there was no statistical difference in the correlation coefficients between the term and premature newborns.

There are conflicting reports on the effect of TCB at high serum bilirubin levels. Some reports suggest that TcB results may become less accurate with a tendency to over-estimate TSB at high bilirubin concentrations [17, 27, 28]. Olusanya O. B. reported overestimation of jaundice using the JM 103 TcB machine on Nigerian newborns [20]. Other studies have found a tendency of TcB to under estimate serum bilirubin levels at high concentrations [6, 25, 29]. In the current study, we did not explore the effect of TcB on high concentrations of bilirubin. Generally, normo grams in use are based on total serum bilirubin levels. The gold standard Laboratory methods for measuring bilirubin are not without their own inherent limitations. Rubattelli et al. reported that standard methods of evaluating TSB tended to under estimate serum bilirubin at higher concentrations [30].

Limitations of the study

The study was done on ill newborn babies. We are not sure if the results are reproducible on well babies with jaundice in the outpatient set up.

The gestational age range was wide (28–42 weeks). There might be variations according to gestation. We did not have enough numbers to use narrow gestational age ranges for comparison.

Conclusion

This study established the validity of the Draeger JM103 transcutaneous bilirubinometer in indigenous Zimbabwean newborns. In this population, this noninvasive method of measuring jaundice may be considered as a screening tool for babies who require serum bilirubin and possibly decision to commence phototherapy. Our data support the use of sternum TcB in this population because it had less false negatives. Use of the TcB devices is recommended for decreasing blood sampling during screening for neonatal jaundice. There is a need, however, to establish local nomograms for the cutoff thresholds for treatment based on TcB rather than TSB levels. Further studies are recommended to explore the effect of high serum bilirubin levels on TcB.

Abbreviations

ABE: Acute Bilirubin Encephalopathy; Draeger JM 103: Draeger Jaundice Meter 103; NPV: Negative predictive value; PPV: Positive predictive value; TcB: Transcutaneous bilirubin; TSB: Total serum bilirubin

Acknowledgements

We would like to acknowledge cerebral palsy alliance Australia who through Dr. Greg Powell provided the JM103 TcB device which was used in this study Ms. Kudzi Mateveke who provided initial guide on biostatistical analysis reported in this article and Professor Hilda Mujuru for reviewing the manuscript.

Funding

This research was not funded.

Authors' contributions

GLTC conceived the study, and designed the protocol and coordinated the collection of data and drafted the manuscript. SC participated in coordination of data collection and helped to draft the manuscript. VC performed the biostatistical analysis and generated the figures and legends. All authors read and approved the final manuscript

Competing interests

The authors declare that they have no competing interest.

Author details

[1]Department of Paediatrics and Child Health, University of Zimbabwe-College of Health Sciences, Mazoe Street, Box A178 Avondale, Harare, Zimbabwe. [2]Department of Community Medicine, University of Zimbabwe-College of Health Sciences, Mazoe Street, Box A178 Avondale, Harare, Zimbabwe.

References

1. Greco C, Arnolda G, Boo N-Y, Iskander IF, Okolo AA, Rohsiswatmo R, et al. Neonatal jaundice in low-and middle-income countries: lessons and future directions from the 2015 don ostrow trieste yellow retreat. Neonatology. 2016;110(3):172–80.
2. Knudsen A. The cephalocaudal progression of jaundice in newborns in relation to the transfer of bilirubin from plasma to skin. Early Hum Dev. 1990;22(1):23–8.
3. Keren R, Tremont K, Luan X, Cnaan A. Visual assessment of jaundice in term and late preterm infants. Arch Dis Child-Fetal Neonatal Ed. 2009;94(5):F317–22.
4. Moyer VA, Ahn C, Sneed S. Accuracy of clinical judgment in neonatal jaundice. Arch Pediatr Adolesc Med. 2000;154(4):391–4.
5. Szabo P, Wolf M, Bucher HU, Haensse D, Fauchere JC, Arlettaz R. Assessment of jaundice in preterm neonates: comparison between clinical assessment, two transcutaneous bilirubinometers and serum bilirubin values. Acta Paediatr. 2004;93(11):1491–5.
6. Engle WD, Jackson GL, Sendelbach D, Manning D, Frawley WH. Assessment of a transcutaneous device in the evaluation of neonatal hyperbilirubinemia in a primarily Hispanic population. Pediatrics. 2002;110(1):61–7.
7. Briscoe L, Clark S, Yoxall CW. Can transcutaneous bilirubinometry reduce the need for blood tests in jaundiced full term babies? Arch Dis Child-Fetal Neonatal Ed. 2002;86(3):F190–2.
8. Newman TB, Escobar GJ, Gonzales VM, Armstrong MA, Gardner MN, Folck BF. Frequency of neonatal bilirubin testing and hyperbilirubinemia in a large health maintenance organization. Pediatrics. 1999; 104(Supplement 6):1198–203.
9. Fitzgerald M, Millard C, McIntosh N. Cutaneous hypersensitivity following peripheral tissue damage in newborn infants and its reversal with topical anaesthesia. Pain. 1989;39(1):31–6.
10. Pediatrics AA Of, Obstetricians AC of, gynecologists. Guidelines for perinatal care. Amer academy of Pediatrics; 2002.
11. Yamanouchi I, Yamauchi Y, Igarashi I. Transcutaneous bilirubinometry: preliminary studies of noninvasive transcutaneous bilirubin meter in the Okayama National Hospital. Pediatrics. 1980;65(2):195–202.
12. Yasuda S, Itoh S, Isobe K, Yonetani M, Nakamura H, Nakamura M, et al. New transcutaneous jaundice device with two optical paths. J Perinat Med. 2003;31(1):81–8.
13. Hyperbilirubinemia AA Of PS on, others. Management of hyperbilirubinemia in the newborn infant 35 or more weeks of gestation. Pediatrics. 2004;114(1):297.
14. Raimondi F, Ferrara T, Borrelli AC, Schettino D, Parrella C, Capasso L. Neonatal hyperbilirubinemia: a critical appraisal of current guidelines and evidence. J Pediatr Neonatal Individ Med JPNIM. 2012;1(1):25–32.
15. Bertini G, Pratesi S, Cosenza E, Dani C. Transcutaneous bilirubin measurement: evaluation of Bilitest™. Neonatology. 2008;93(2):101–5.
16. Engle WD, Jackson GL, Stehel EK, Sendelbach DM, Manning MD. Evaluation of a transcutaneous jaundice meter following hospital discharge in term and near-term neonates. J Perinatol. 2005;25(7):486.
17. Kolman KB, Mathieson KM, Frias CA. Comparison of transcutaneous and total serum bilirubin in newborn Hispanic infants at 35 or more weeks of gestation. J Am Board Fam Med. 2007;20(3):266–71.
18. Ho HT, Ng TK, Tsui KC, Lo YC. Evaluation of a new transcutaneous bilirubinometer in Chinese newborns. Arch Dis Child-Fetal Neonatal Ed. 2006;91(6):F434–8.
19. Maisels MJ, Ostrea EM, Touch S, Clune SE, Cepeda E, Kring E, et al. Evaluation of a new transcutaneous bilirubinometer. Pediatrics. 2004;113(6):1628–35.
20. Olusanya BO, Imosemi DO, Emokpae AA. Differences between transcutaneous and serum bilirubin measurements in black African neonates. Pediatrics. 2016:e20160907.
21. Rylance S, Yan J, Molyneux E. Can transcutaneous bilirubinometry safely guide phototherapy treatment of neonatal jaundice in Malawi? Paediatr Int Child Health. 2014;34(2):101–7.
22. Poland RL, Hartenberger C, McHenry H, Hsi A. Comparison of skin sites for estimating serum total bilirubin in in-patients and out-patients: chest is superior to brow. J Perinatol. 2004;24(9):541.
23. Holland L, Blick K. Implementing and validating transcutaneous bilirubinometry for neonates. Am J Clin Pathol. 2009;132(4):555–61.
24. Wainer S, Rabi Y, Parmar SM, Allegro D, Lyon M. Impact of skin tone on the performance of a transcutaneous jaundice meter. Acta Paediatr. 2009;98(12):1909–15.
25. Ebbesen F, Rasmussen LM, Wimberley PDA. New transcutaneous bilirubinometer, BiliCheck, used in the neonatal intensive care unit and the maternity ward. Acta Paediatr. 2002;91(2):203–11.
26. Knudsen A, Ebbesen F. Transcutaneous bilirubinometry in neonatal intensive care units. Arch Dis Child-Fetal Neonatal Ed. 1996;75(1):F53–6.
27. Robertson A, Kazmierczak S, Vos P. Improved transcutaneous bilirubinometry: comparison of SpectR x BiliCheck and Minolta jaundice meter JM-102 for estimating total serum bilirubin in a normal newborn population. J Perinatol. 2002;22(1):12.
28. Samanta S, Tan M, Kissack C, Nayak S, Chittick R, Yoxall CW. The value of Bilicheck as a screening tool for neonatal jaundice in term and near-term babies. Acta Paediatr. 2004;93(11):1486–90.
29. Wong CM, Van Dijk PJE, Laing IA. A comparison of transcutaneous bilirubinometers: SpectRx BiliCheck versus Minolta AirShields. Arch Dis Child-Fetal Neonatal Ed. 2002;87(2):F137–40.
30. Rubaltelli FF, Gourley GR, Loskamp N, Modi N, Roth-Kleiner M, Sender A, et al. Transcutaneous bilirubin measurement: a multicenter evaluation of a new device. Pediatrics. 2001;107(6):1264–71.

20

Incidence and short term outcomes of neonates with hypoxic ischemic encephalopathy in a Peri Urban teaching hospital, Uganda: a prospective cohort study

Hellen Namusoke[1]*, Maria Musoke Nannyonga[2], Robert Ssebunya[2], Victoria Kirabira Nakibuuka[2] and Edison Mworozi[2,3]

Abstract

Background: Hypoxic Ischemic Encephalopathy carries high case fatality rates ranging between 10–60%, with 25% of survivors have an adverse long-term neurodevelopment outcome. Despite the above, there is paucity of data regarding its magnitude and short term outcomes in a low resource setting like Uganda. Therefore we set out to determine the incidence and short term outcomes of Newborns with Hypoxic Ischemic Encephalopathy at St. Francis Hospital, Nsambya.

Methods: This was a Prospective Cohort study conducted between October 2015 and January 2016 at St. Francis Hospital, Nsambya, Kampala- Uganda. Term Newborn babies were enrolled. Umbilical cord arterial blood gas analysis was done for Newborns with low Apgar scores at 5 min. Clinical examination was done on all newborns within 48 h of life, for features of encephalopathy. Neonates with Hypoxic Ischemic Encephalopathy were followed up by a daily clinical examination and a short term outcome was recorded on day seven.

Results: The incidence of Hypoxic Ischemic Encephalopathy was 30.6 cases per 1000 live births. The majority, 10 (43.5%) had mild Hypoxic Ischemic Encephalopathy, followed by 8 (34.8%), 5 (21.7%) that had moderate and severe Hypoxic Ischemic Encephalopathy respectively. A total of (6) 26% died, and (15) 65.2% were discharged within 1 week. Lack of a nutritive suckling reflex (nasogastric feeding), poor Moro reflex, and requirement for respiratory support (oxygen therapy by nasal prongs) were the common complications by day seven.

Conclusions: The burden of Hypoxic Ischemic Encephalopathy is high with a case fatality rate of 26%. There is need to conduct a longitudinal study to determine the long term complications of HIE.

Keywords: Arterial blood gases, Hypoxic ischemic encephalopathy, Intrapartum asphyxia, Newborn, Short term outcomes

* Correspondence: helennankya@yahoo.com
[1]Department of Paediatrics and Child Health, Bethany Women and Family Hospital, P.O box 32022, Clock Tower, Kampala, Uganda
Full list of author information is available at the end of the article

Background

Globally, neonatal mortality accounts for up to 44% of the Under Five Mortality, of which 99% occurs in low and middle income countries [1, 2]. Intrapartum asphyxia and consequential Hypoxic Ischemic Encephalopathy (HIE) is a common cause of potentially avoidable neonatal brain injury and mortality [3]. Birth asphyxia and its complications is the third commonest cause, and contributes to 23% of neonatal mortality in Uganda [4].

Different measures are being taken to reduce neonatal mortality and morbidity. These include preventive measures such as; proper monitoring of labor with a partograph, timely and adequate resuscitation and therapeutic hypothermia of Newborns with HIE to improve outcome [5].

The incidence of HIE is 1.5 per 1000 live births in developed countries and varies between 2.3-26.5 per 1000 live births in developing countries [6, 7]. However, the incidence, and outcomes of HIE is not well documented in most developing countries, including Uganda. Therefore, this study is aimed at determining the incidence, and short term outcomes of HIE among inborn term neonates at a tertiary hospital.

Methods

The study was conducted at St. Francis Hospital, Nsambya, a tertiary hospital providing Neonatal Intensive Care to Kampala and the surrounding districts. The standard of care for HIE at this unit included; Continuous Positive Airway Pressure(CPAP) for moderate and severe HIE to maintain respiratory support, intravenous Phenobarbital and Phenytoin to control seizures as first line and second line therapy respectively. Head cooling, parental nutrition, electroencephalogram (EEG) monitoring and mechanical ventilation were not a standard of care.

This was a prospective cohort study carried out on the labor ward and Neonatal unit of St. Francis Hospital, Nsambya from October 2015 to January 2016.

Inclusion and exclusion criteria

All the following criteria (A + B + C) were required for inclusion in the study:

A. Term newborns delivered at ≥37completed weeks of gestation,
B. Birth weight > 2000 g
C. Delivery at St. Francis Hospital, Nsambya.

Newborns delivered by caesarian section under general anesthesia and those with congenital abnormalities were excluded.

Sample size calculation:

A sample size of 679 participants was calculated for incidence of HIE using a formula for single proportions [8].

This was based on incidence of HIE of 1.8% in Mulago Hospital (similar setting) by Ondoa et al., allowing an error of 1% and confidence interval of 95% [9].

Procedure

At delivery, Apgar score was done at one and 5 min by the attending midwife / research assistant.

A cord arterial blood sample was taken aseptically within 1 hour of delivery for newborns with an Apgar score of less than 7 at 5 min [10]. A heparinized needle was used, and at least 0.2 ml of arterial blood for blood gas analysis was drawn from the umbilical artery. Blood gas analysis was performed using ABL 80 FLEX analyzer within 5 min of sample collection. Clinical examination was done on all newborns within 48 h of life, to assess for features of encephalopathy. These included change in level of consciousness, altered primitive reflexes, tone and autonomic response.

Blood samples for Random Blood Sugar (RBS), C-reactive protein (CRP) were aseptically drawn from the peripheral veins, to rule out hypoglycemia and infection respectively.

All newborns with low APGAR scores (less than 7 at 5 min), intrapartum asphyxia (PH < 7.0, or base deficit ≥12.0 mmol/l) and features of encephalopathy were diagnosed to have HIE. Newborns with HIE were classified into mild, moderate and severe forms using the Modified Sarnat Encephalopathy Grading system (MSEG) as defined by Shalak et al. [11].

Neonates with HIE were managed according to standard operating systems at the unit. These were followed up by a daily clinical examination and short term outcome was recorded on day seven. The short term outcomes of interest included; death, alive without complications or alive with complications (requirement of respiratory support, absence of a nutritive suckling reflex, altered level of consciousness, presence of seizures, altered Moro reflex).

Data management

Coded Data was entered using EPI-DATA version 3.1, and STATA version 11 was used for Statistical analysis. The Chi-square test was used to compare categorical variables and a student t-test for continuous variables with a 95% confidence interval (CI). A P -value of less than 0.05 was significant.

Factors that were statistically significant at bivariate level, and those that are known to be strongly associated with HIE like non-use of partograph to monitor labor, were further analyzed at Multivariate level. This was done using logistic regression fitting models to determine the factors that are statistically and independently associated with HIE. The factors with an adjusted Odds ratio of greater than one and a P-value of < 0.05 were considered statistically significant.

Results

During the study period, 751 newborns were enrolled and 573 newborns excluded (140 were preterm, 32 were still births, 1 had a caesarian delivery under general anesthesia, and 400 did not consent for the study). There were 399 (53%) male and 352 (47%) female participants. The characteristics of the infants and their mothers are shown in Table 1.

Laboratory results for the participants

From this study, 25/751 (3.3%) newborns had low APGAR scores and intrapartum asphyxia as evidenced by either PH < 7.0 or Base deficit of ≥12.0. Two

Table 1 Summary of Maternal and Newborn demographics at St. Francis Hospital that participated in the study

	Frequency (n = 751)	Percentage
Sex of the baby		
Male	399	53
Female	352	47
Baby weight		
< 2.5 kg	14	2
> =2.5 kg	737	98
Age of the mother		
< 20	17	2
20-35	634	84
> =35	100	13
Distance from place of residence to Nsambya Hospital in KM		
< =5	244	32
5-10	237	32
> 10	270	36
Referral case		
Yes	26	4
No	712	96
Fetal heart rate		
< =120	28	4
> 120	723	96
APGAR score at 1 min		
< 7	58	8
> =7	693	92
APGAR score at 5 min		
< 7	25	3
> =7	726	97
Resuscitation done		
Yes	79	11
No	629	89

Newborns with intrapartum asphyxia had hypoglycemia (RBS < 2.5Mmol/l), and infection (CRP > 10 mg/dl).

Incidence of HIE

Of the 751 Newborns enrolled, 58 (8%), and 25 (3%) had low Apgar scores at one and 5 min respectively. All the newborns with low Apgar scores at 5 min had intrapartum asphyxia (as evidenced by low Apgar score, and either PH < 7.0 or Base deficit ≥12.0 mmol/l). A significant proportion of newborns with intrapartum asphyxia [23 of the 25(92%)] got HIE. The proportion of HIE in this study was found to be 3% (24/751); (95% CL: 1.8-4.2). Therefore the incidence of HIE was 30.6 cases per 1000 live births. In this study, 10 (43.5%), 8(34.8%), and 5 (21.7%) had grade I, grade 11 and grade III HIE respectively as shown in Fig. 1.

Factors associated with HIE

The factors that were significantly associated with HIE at Bivariate analysis included: herbal medicine use (COR-3.2, $P = 0.004$), prolonged labour (COR-3.9, P = < 0.001), proloned rupture of membranes (COR-2.6, $P = 0.016$), Referred mothers (COR-3.9, $P = 0.036$), antepartum haemorrhage (COR-4.37, $P = 0.024$) prolonged pregnancy (COR-2.46, $P = 0.025$), Ceasarian delivery (COR-2.3, P = 0.035) and prime parity (COR-2.46, P = 0.025). On the contrary, factors like maternal illness, prolonged pregnancy, and non use of partograph were not significantly associated with HIE in this study as shown in Table 2.

Infants born to mothers with; Antepartum haemorrhage, history of herbal use, refferal and prime parity were significantly associated with HIE at logistic regression as shown in Table 3.

Short term outcome of HIE

Of the 23 participants who got HIE, 6/23 (26%) died. Two thirds (4/6) had grade III HIE, and the rest (2/6) had grade II HIE. The majority, 15/23 (65.2%), were discharged without short term complications, while 2/23 (8.6%) were still admitted with complications by day seven. The complications

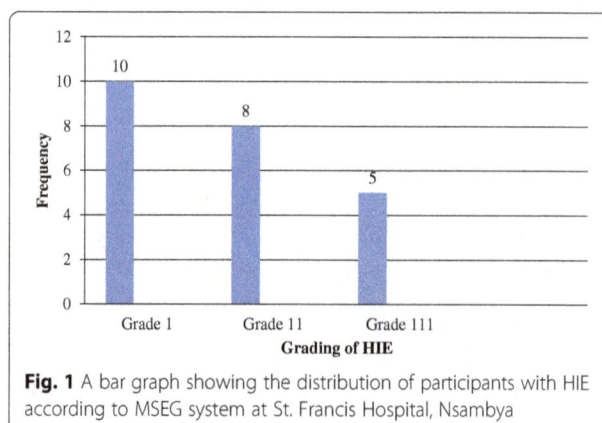

Fig. 1 A bar graph showing the distribution of participants with HIE according to MSEG system at St. Francis Hospital, Nsambya

Table 2 Bivariate table showing factors associated with HIE at St. Francis Hospital, Nsambya

	No HIE n = 728	HIE N = 23	COR(95% C I)	p-value
History of Herbal Use				
No	534(73)	11(48)	1	
Yes	194(27)	12(52)	3.190(1.4-7.2)	0.006
Referral				
No	705(97)	20(87)		
Yes	23(3)	3(13)	3.907(1.1-14.0)	0.036
Antepartum hemorrhage				
No	707(97)	20(87)	1	
Yes	21(3)	3(13)	4.373(1.2-15.7)	0.024
Prime parity				
No	535(74)	13(57)	1	
Yes	188(26)	10(43)	2.461(1.1-5.4)	0.025
Illness during pregnancy				
No	512(70)	20(87)	1	
Yes	216(30)	3(13)	0.301(0.1-1.0)	0.052
Prolonged pregnancy				
No	631(86)	18(78)	1	
Yes	97(14)	5(22)	1.527(0.6-4.1)	0.406
Duration of labor in hours				
< =10	564(77)	9(39)	1	
> 10	164(23)	14(61)	3.991(1.8-8.8)	0.001
Was a partograph used				
No	175(24)	9(39)	1	
Yes	553(76)	14(61)	0.479(0.2-1.1)	0.075
Fetal heart rate				
< =120	24(3)	4(18)	1	
> 120	704(97)	19(82)	0.188(0.1-0.6)	0.004
Prolonged rupture of membranes				
No	450(62)	9(39)	1	
Yes	278(38)	14(61)	2.603(1.2-5.8)	0.02
Mode of delivery				
Normal	508(70)	12(52)	1	
c-section	220(30)	11(48)	2.326(1.1-5.1)	0.035

Table 3 multivariate table showing factors that are independently associated with HIE between at St. Francis Hospital, Nsambya

	COR	P –value	AOR	95% confidence Interval	p-value
Referral case	3.9	0.036	4.058	(1.0-15.7)	0.043
Antepartum hemorrhage	4.373	0.024	5.215	(1.0-26.2)	0.045
Prime parity	2.461	0.025	3.242	(1.3-7.9)	0.01
Illness during pregnancy	0.301	0.052	0.248	(0.1-0.9)	0.031
History of Herbal Use	3.190	0.006	5.291	(2.1-13.4)	0.000
Duration of labor					
> 10 h	3.991	0.001	14.867	(0.8-265.2)	0.066
Use of partograph	0.479	0.075	0.033	(0.0-1.0)	0.048
Caesarian delivery	2.326	0.035	0.091	0.0-161.3	0.529

COR Denotes for Crude Odds Ratio, *AOR* Denotes for Adjusted Odds Ratio

delivered at St. Francis Hospital, Nsambya, Uganda is still high, despite a number of interventions in place. This finding is similar to that reported in developing countries of 2.3-26.5 per 1000 live births by Kurinczuk JJ et al. [6].

This is contraly to the incidence of 39 cases per 1000 live births reported by Chiabi and collegues in Cameroon [12]. There is a high number of refferal cases in Chiabi et al. study of 46.7 and 15.6% from health centres and other hospitals respectively versus 4% found in our study [12]. Therefore there was a high number of complicated deliveries in Cameroon contributing to a high incidence of HIE.

The incidence of HIE in this study was higher than that reported in South Africa (8.5-13.3 per 1000 live births) and India (19.97 cases per 1000 live births) [13, 14]. The lower incidence in South Africa could have been attributed to better monitoring equipment of mothers during labour like cardiotopograph (helps in early

included: poor Moro reflex, lack of a nutritive suckling reflex (nasogastric feeding), and respiratory support (oxygen therapy by nasal prongs). There were 7/23 (30%) with seizures and these were controlled by the fifth day. A surmmary of short term complications of HIE is shown in Fig. 2.

Discussion

Incidence of hypoxic ischemic encephalopathy

The incidence of Hypoxic Ischemic Encephalopathy of 30.6 cases per 1000 live births among Newborn babies

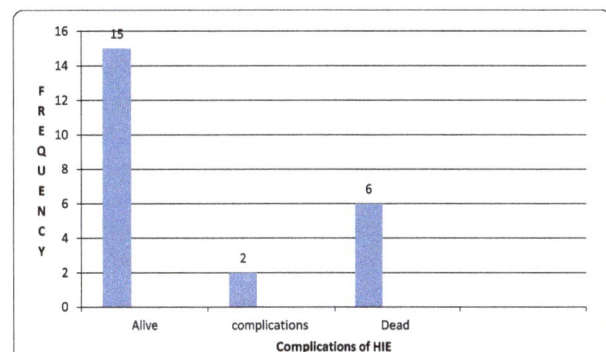

Fig. 2 Bar graph showing summary of short term complications of Hypoxic Ischemic Encephalopathy at St.Francis Hospital, Nsambya

detection of fetal distress for early intervention) which are lacking in the setting.

Factors associated with HIE

Maternal factors such as prime parity, antepartum haemorrhage, referred mother and history of herbal use during labour were significantly associated with HIE.

Prime parity was a significant and common factor associated with HIE in several studies done in Uganda, India, and Saudi Arabia [9, 14, 15]. First time mothers are more predisposed to most antenatal-related-obstetric complications compared to multiparous mothers, and therefore caution should be taken in close monitoring and management of the prime gravidas to prevent complications [16].

On the contrary, factors like prolonged labour, prolonged pregnancy, maternal illness and delayed time between decision making and delivery were significantly associated with HIE in similar studies in Nigeria [17], which was not the case in our study. This could be attributed to the low numbers of mothers noted with the above factors in our study.

Studies by Bikisu et al. in Nigeria and Queresh et al. in Abbottabad [18, 19] showed that abscence of examination and not attending antenatal care were associated with HIE. Similar observations were made in our study where absence of monitoring of labour and being born to a refered mother was associated with HIE.

In addition, use of herbal medicine during pregnancy and labour was significantly associated with HIE (OR-5.2: CL:2.1-13.4, $P = 0.000$). This was however not documented in other studies, probably because it may not be the social practice among mothers in other settings.

Short term outcome of hypoxic ischemic encephalopathy

The study established that 26% of the study participants that got HIE died, of which two thirds was due to grade III HIE. This was similar to a mortality of 26.4% in a prevalence study by Athumani et al. in Muhimbili, Tanzania [20].

These findings slightly differ with a report from a multicenter study by Massaro et al., where 945 Newborns with HIE from different Neonatal Intesive Care Units (NICU) in Washington D.C were followed up for 2 weeks. In this study, 15% of participants died, 85% had complete feeding by discharge, 7.6% required nasogastric feeding, and 6% required supplemental oxygen therapy with < 1% that required tracheostomy [21]. The lower mortality could be explained by the use of therapeutic hypothermia that has been proven to significantly reduce morbidity and mortality from earlier studies [22]. The advanced newborn care in a resourceful setting like the US, was not a practice in this study.

In a South African study, a mortality of 7.8% was reported. This was much lower than that found in our study, though most of the deaths were due to grade three HIE as

was the case in our study [13]. Therapeutic cooling was used as part of the management for those with moderate and severe HIE with better monitoring equipement which was not the case in our study. This may be a contributing factor to the low mortality in this study.

The mortality of 26% noted in this study was higher than that (12.1%) reported in a similar study done in Mulago Hospital in Kampala Uganda [9]. This variation could have been as a result of the lower follow up time of 48 h in a study by Ondoa et al. as compared to the 1 week used for this study.

The level of mortality was slightly lower than that reported in a similar study in India of 31.14% [14]. This may be because the study was carried out during the initiation phase of our neonatal intensive care unit. This has substantially promoted better nursing care.

Strength and limitations

Arterial blood gases were done to confirm evidence of metabolic acidosis in the diagnosis of Hypoxic Ischemic Encephalopathy. However, we are mindful of some limitations like our inability to perform Cranial scans to rule out other possible causes of encephalopathy such as CNS malformations. We were as well unable to do blood cultures to rule out neonatal infections (we used a crp of > 10 mg/dl to diagnose sepsis among participants).This may have contributed to the high incidence of HIE noted. Additionally, there were low numbers of Newborns with HIE which could limit generalisability.

Conclusion

The incidence of Hypoxic Ischemic Encephalopathy at St. Francis Hospital, Nsambya was high at 30.6 cases per 1000 live births. Majority (17/23 (73.9%)) of newborns with Hypoxic Ischemic Encephalopathy were discharged without short term complications by 1 week.

Recommendations

A longitudinal study should be carried out to determine the long term complications of HIE.

Abbreviations

AOR: Adjusted odds ratio; CI: Confidence interval; CNS: Central nervous system; COR: Crude odds ratio; CRP: C- reactive protein; CT: Computerized tomography; EEG: Electroencephalogram; HIE: Hypoxic ischemic encephalopathy; MSEG: Modified Sarnat encephalopathy grading; NICU: Neonatal intensive care unit; RBS: Random blood sugar; WHO: World health organization

Acknowledgements

We send our gratitude to all the research assistants and Nsambya hospital administration for providing the arterial blood gas machine. We acknowledge all the Newborns and their mothers who participated in this study.
A vote of thanks goes to Makerere University School of Public Health: Maternal and Newborn Centre of Excellence and Catholic Scholarship Program -Uganda for funding this study.

We appreciate the efforts of Jjuuko Gerald, Ssebagereka Anthony, Cheptoris Lillian and Pediatricians at Nsambya Hospital towards improving this work.

Funding

This study was funded by Makerere University School of Public Health: Maternal and Newborn Centre of Excellence. The funding body did not have any role in study design, data collection and analysis, interpretation of results and manuscript writing.

Authors' contributions

NH and ME conceived of the study, designed the research protocol, participated in the study, and drafted the manuscript. NVK and NMM supervised and participated in the study. SR participated in writing the manuscript. All authors read and approved the final manuscript.

Authors' information

NH: MBCHB, MMED (PAED), Department of Paediatrics and Child Health, Bethany Women and Family Hospital.
NMM: MBCHB, MMED (Paed), Honorary Lecturer, Department of Paediatrics and Child Health, Mother Kevin Post Graduate Medical School, Uganda Martyrs University- Nkozi.
SR: MBCHB, MMED (Paed), Honorary Lecturer, Department of Paediatrics and Child Health, Mother Kevin Post Graduate Medical School, Uganda Martyrs University- Nkozi.
NVK: MBChB, MMED (Paed) MUK, Cert Neon (SA), Honorary Lecturer, Department of Paediatrics and Child Health, Mother Kevin Post Graduate Medical School, Uganda Martyrs University- Nkozi.
EM: Honorary Lecture Department of Paediatrics and Child Health, Makerere University and Mother Kevin Post Graduate School: Uganda Martyrs University, Nkozi.

Competing interests

The authors declare that they have no competing interests.

Author details

[1]Department of Paediatrics and Child Health, Bethany Women and Family Hospital, P.O box 32022, Clock Tower, Kampala, Uganda. [2]Department of Paediatrics and Child Health, Mother Kevin Post Graduate Medical School, Uganda Martyrs University, Nkozi, Uganda. [3]Department of Paediatrics and Child Health, Makerere University and Mother Kevin Post Graduate School: Uganda Martyrs University, Nkozi, Uganda.

References

1. UNICEF W, World Bank. Levels and trends in child mortality. 2014. Report No.
2. Lawn JE, Cousens S, Zupan J. Lancet neonatal survival steering T. 4 million neonatal deaths: when? Where? Why? Lancet. 2005;365(9462):891–900.
3. Cowan F, Rutherford M, Groenendaal F, Eken P, Mercuri E, Bydder GM, et al. Origin and timing of brain lesions in term infants with neonatal encephalopathy. Lancet. 2003;361(9359):736–42.
4. WHO. Countdown to 2015, stock of Maternal and Newborn survival 2010. World Health Organisation. 2011. Report No.
5. Gunn AJ, Bennet L. Cerebral hypothermia in the Management of Hypoxic-Ischemic Encephalopathy. NeoReviews. 2002;3(6):e116–e22.
6. Kurinczuk JJ, White-Koning M, Badawi N. Epidemiology of neonatal encephalopathy and hypoxic-ischaemic encephalopathy. Early Hum Dev. 2010;86(6):329–38.
7. Lawn JE, Lee AC, Kinney M, Sibley L, Carlo WA, Paul VK, et al. Two million intrapartum-related stillbirths and neonatal deaths: where, why, and what can be done? Int J Gynaecol Obstet. 2009;107(Suppl 1):S5–18. S9
8. Daniel WW. In: BW II, editor. BIOSTATISTICS: a Foundation for Analysis in the health sciences. 7th ed. New York: JOHN WILEY & SONS,INC.; 1999. p. 1999.
9. Ondoa-Onama C, Tumwine JK. Immediate outcome of babies with low Apgar score in Mulago hospital, Uganda. East Afr Med J. 2003;80(1):22–9.
10. American Academy of Pediatrics CoF, Newborn, American College of O, Gynecologists, Committee on Obstetric P. The Apgar score. Pediatrics. 2006; 117(4):1444–7.
11. Shalak LF, Laptook AR, Velaphi SC, Perlman JM. Amplitude-integrated electroencephalography coupled with an early neurologic examination enhances prediction of term infants at risk for persistent encephalopathy. Pediatrics. 2003;111(2):351–7.
12. Chiabi A, Nguefack S, Mah E, Nodem S, Mbuagbaw L, Mbonda E, et al. Risk factors for birth asphyxia in an urban health facility in cameroon. Iran J Child Neurol. 2013;7(3):46–54.
13. Bruckmann EK, Velaphi S. Intrapartum asphyxia and hypoxic ischaemic encephalopathy in a public hospital: incidence and predictors of poor outcome. S Afr Med J. 2015;105(4):298–303.
14. Niladri Sekhar Bhunia NPS. A profile of hypoxic Ischaemic encephalopathy in neonatal intensive care unit. Guwahati. Current Peadiatrics Research: Gauhati Medical College and Hospital; 2015.
15. Itoo BA, Al-Hawsawi ZM, Khan AH. Hypoxic ischemic encephalopathy. Incidence and risk factors in north western Saudi Arabia. Saudi Med J. 2003;24(2):147–53.
16. Robert M, Kliegman REB, Hal B, Jenson, Stanton BF. Kliegman: Nelson textbook of pediatrics. 18th ed. Philadelphia: Saunders, an imprint of Elsevier Inc; 2007.
17. Ugwu GI, Abedi HO, Ugwu EN. Incidence of birth asphyxia as seen in central hospital and GN children's clinic both in Warri Niger Delta of Nigeria: an eight year retrospective review. Global J Health Sci. 2012;4(5):140–6.
18. MSA BGI, Musa A, Adelakun MB, Adeniji AO, Kolawole T. Prevalence and risk factors for Perinatal asphyxia as seen at a specialist Hospital in Gusau, Nigeria. Sub-Saharan Afr J Med. 2015;2(2):64–9.
19. Qureshi AM, ur Rehman A, Siddiqi TS. Hypoxic ischemic encephalopathy in neonates. J Ayub Med Coll Abbottabad. 2010;22(4):190–3.
20. Athumani J. Prevalence and immediate outcome of hypoxic ischemic encephalopathy among infants with birth asphyxia admitted at the neonatal ward of Muhimbili National Rerferal hospital in dares salaam. Official publication of Tanzanian medical students' association. 2007.
21. Massaro AN, Murthy K, Zaniletti I, Cook N, DiGeronimo R, Dizon M, et al. Short-term outcomes after perinatal hypoxic ischemic encephalopathy: a report from the Children's hospitals neonatal consortium HIE focus group. J Perinatol: official journal of the California Perinatal Association. 2015;35(4):290–6.
22. Bona E, Hagberg H, Loberg EM, Bagenholm R, Thoresen M. Protective effects of moderate hypothermia after neonatal hypoxia-ischemia: short- and long-term outcome. Pediatr Res. 1998;43(6):738–45.

21

Infant activity and sleep behaviors in a maternal and infant home visiting project among rural, southern, African American women

Jessica L. Thomson[1]* , Lisa M. Tussing-Humphreys[2], Melissa H. Goodman[1] and Alicia S. Landry[3]

Abstract

Background: Physical inactivity and inadequate amounts of sleep are two potential causes for excessive weight gain in infancy. Thus, parents and caregivers of infants need to be educated about decreasing infant sedentary behavior, increasing infant unrestrained floor time, as well as age specific recommended amounts of sleep for infants. The aims of this study were to determine if maternal knowledge about infant activity and sleep changed over time and to evaluate maternal compliance rates with expert recommendations for infant sleep in a two-arm, randomized, controlled, comparative impact trial.

Methods: Pregnant women at least 18 years of age, less than 19 weeks pregnant, and residing in a lower Mississippi Delta county were recruited between March 2013 and December 2014. Postnatal data was collected from 54 participants between September 2013 and May 2016. McNemar's test of symmetry was used to determine if maternal knowledge changed over time, while generalized linear mixed models and Kaplan-Meier survival curves were used to assess compliance with expert recommendations for infant sleep.

Results: The postnatal retention rate was 85%. Maternal knowledge significantly increased for correct infant sleep position (back) and beginning tummy time by one month of age. Odds of meeting sleep duration recommendations increased by 30% for every one month increase in infant age. Only 20% of the participants were compliant with the back to sleep recommendation for the first 12 months of their infant's life; median time to noncompliance was 7.8 months.

Conclusions: Although baseline knowledge concerning infant activity and sleep was high in this cohort of rural, Southern, African American mothers, compliance with recommendations was not optimal.

Keywords: Infant, Non-confinement time, Sleep duration, African American, Home visiting

Background

The prevalence of excessive body weight in infants and toddlers, defined as weight for recumbent length at or above the 95th percentile on the 2000 Centers for Disease Control and Prevention sex specific growth charts, is approximately 8% in the United States (US) [1]. This is a concern because early excessive weight gain

in infancy leads to increased risks of childhood obesity [2] and adult obesity, notably in African Americans [3]. One potential cause of excessive weight gain in infants is physical inactivity. Methods to increase infant physical activity include limiting the use of devices that restrict movement (e.g., car seats, bouncy seats, and swings) and providing infants with opportunities to move freely. Tummy time, defined as awake and supervised positioning on the stomach, is a form of expert recommended physical activity that allows infants to engage in unrestricted movement necessary to strengthen muscles needed for motor

* Correspondence: jessica.thomson@ars.usda.gov
[1]United States Department of Agriculture, Agricultural Research Service, 141 Experiment Station Road, Stoneville, MS 38776, USA
Full list of author information is available at the end of the article

Infant activity and sleep behaviors in a maternal and infant home visiting project among...

193

development [4]. Thus, it is important for parents and caregivers to recognize the need to decrease sedentary behavior in infants and increase unrestrained floor time, especially in a prone position (e.g., tummy time).

Similar to physical activity, sleep is a basic requirement for healthy development in infants. An inadequate amount of sleep in children has been associated with higher stress and anxiety, difficulty concentrating, and lower academic performance and quality of life/well-being [5]. Further, an inverse association between sleep duration in children and risk of overweight/obesity was found in a meta-analysis of prospective cohort studies [6]. Similarly, evidence from a recent review suggests a link between short sleep duration and insulin resistance in children, potentially leading to type 2 diabetes [7]. Given these adverse associations between short sleep duration and health risks in children, it is essential that parents and caregivers are educated about age specific recommendations for sleep amounts. Educating parents and caregivers about methods for improving sleep quality and increasing sleep duration (e.g., establishing a consistent bedtime routine) [8] also may be necessary to lessen the effects of poor sleep in infancy.

While recent attention has focused on activity and sleep in infants in general, less is known about these behaviors in specific US populations, such as rural, Southern, African Americans. Analysis of secondary and tertiary outcomes in a maternal, infant and early childhood home visiting project afforded such an opportunity. The Delta Healthy Sprouts Project was designed to test the comparative impact of two maternal, infant, and early childhood home visiting curricula on weight status, dietary intake, physical activity, and other health behaviors of women and their infants residing in the rural Lower Mississippi Delta region of the US [9]. Infant activity was a secondary health outcome targeted for improvement. However, preliminary analyses indicated that differences between treatment arms were not significant, likely because the importance of infant activity (e.g., "tummy time" or placing an infant on his or her stomach while awake and supervised) was discussed in both curriculums. Hence, activity and sleep outcomes of the Delta Healthy Sprouts participants' infants, without regard to treatment arm, are described in this paper. Specifically, the objectives were to determine if maternal knowledge and beliefs concerning infant activity and sleep changed over time and to evaluate maternal compliance rates with expert recommendations for infant sleep. The secondary objectives were to explore associations among maternal knowledge and beliefs about infant activity and sleep, and infant activity and sleep behaviors.

Methods

Design

Delta Healthy Sprouts was a randomized two-arm parallel controlled trial. It was designed to evaluate the impact of the Parents as Teachers® (PAT, control) curriculum as compared with a nutrition and physical activity enhanced PAT curriculum (PATE, experimental) on the primary outcomes of maternal gestational weight gain and postpartum weight control and childhood obesity prevention. Participants were randomly assigned to one of the two treatment arms [PAT ($N = 43$) or PATE ($N = 39$)] using a random generator function in SAS® (version 9.4, SAS Institute Inc., Cary, NC) and equal allocation in blocks of 25. Participants were followed for 18 months, starting at approximately 4 months gestation through 12 months postnatal. The Delta State University Institutional Review Board approved the study protocol (number 12–024) and all participants provided written informed consent. The study is registered at clinicaltrials.gov (NCT01746394).

Participants and setting

Recruitment occurred via passive (distribution of flyers and brochures) and active (study staff on site) methods at local health clinics and medical facilities serving pregnant women and at local health fairs. Women also were referred to the study by health clinic/department staff, Special Supplemental Program for Women, Infants, and Children (WIC) nutritionists, social service agencies, and enrolled study participants. Inclusion criteria included: at least 18 years of age; less than 19 weeks pregnant with first, second or third child; singleton pregnancy; and resident of Washington, Bolivar, or Humphreys County in Mississippi. Participant enrollment occurred on a rolling basis; hence baseline data were collected from 82 pregnant women between March 2013 and December 2014.

The target enrollment was 75 women in each of the two arms (control and experimental) of the project. The sample size of 150 women was based on the following assumptions: 20% attrition rate, 15% of infants in the control arm classified as obese in their first year of life, and a 12% difference between treatment arms for percentage of infants classified as obese during their first year of life. Power and sample size calculations for gestational weight gain within the Institute of Medicine recommendations and 12-month postnatal maternal weight loss also were performed [9]. Recruitment was stopped by the study's Principal Investigator prior to reaching these numbers due to unexpected difficulties recruiting pregnant women meeting study criteria. Recruitment was extended as long as possible, but fiscal reasons eventually necessitated the closing of this period. Data collection was completed in May 2016.

Because infant activity and sleep outcomes were the primary focus of this paper, analyses were conducted only for the postnatal cohort (participants who completed the gestational period and had at least one visit in the postnatal period; $n = 54$). Five participants who completed the gestational period but dropped out of the study prior to the postnatal month (PM) 1 visit were excluded from the postnatal cohort. Fig. 1 illustrates the flow of Delta Healthy Sprouts participants through all phases of the study.

Intervention

The PAT control arm of the intervention followed the nationally recognized, evidence-based Parents as Teachers® curriculum which included one-on-one home visits, optional monthly group meetings, developmental screenings, and a resource network for families. The Program seeks to increase parental knowledge of child development, improve parenting practices, provide early detection of developmental delays, prevent child abuse, and increase school readiness [10]. Using the PAT model, Parent Educators provided mothers with evidence-based information and activities during home visits. Materials were

responsive to parental information requests and were tailored to the age of the child (or gestational age of the fetus). Specific to the analyses presented in this paper, Parent Educators discussed putting an infant to sleep on his/her back until 1 year of age, establishing a regular bedtime routine between 2 to 6 months of age, age specific recommended amounts of sleep for infants, and allowing infants to have tummy time and non-confinement time beginning at 1 month of age. Additionally, Safe to Sleep® recommendations [11] were the topic of 3 of the 27 group meetings.

The PATE experimental curriculum of the intervention built upon the PAT curriculum by adding culturally tailored, maternal weight management and early childhood obesity prevention components. The PATE curriculum was guided by the theoretical underpinnings of the social cognitive theory which posits that learning occurs in a social context with a dynamic and reciprocal

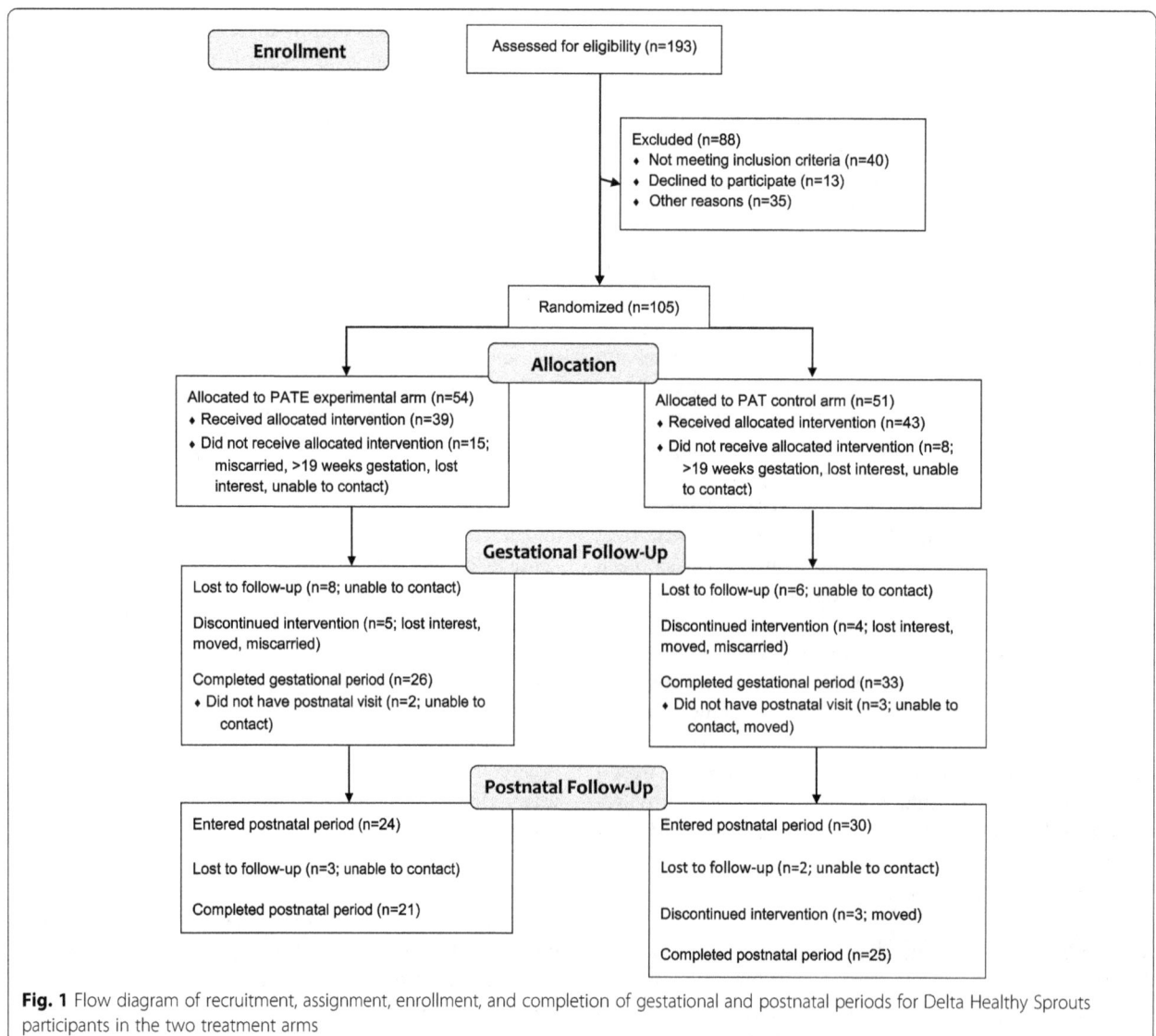

Fig. 1 Flow diagram of recruitment, assignment, enrollment, and completion of gestational and postnatal periods for Delta Healthy Sprouts participants in the two treatment arms

interaction of the person, environment, and behavior [12]. Intervention components aligned with the social cognitive theory included maternal modeling of positive health behavior. The PATE curriculum also was guided by the transtheoretical model of behavior change which integrates key constructs from other theories (i.e., decisional balance, self-efficacy, and process of change) into a comprehensive theory of change that can be applied to a variety of behaviors, populations, and settings [13]. Intervention components aligned with the transtheoretical model of behavior change included provision of information regarding the importance of eating healthfully (for both mother and infant) and being physically active (for both mother and infant) to positively affect attitudes and decisional balance. Additionally, to improve self-efficacy for engaging in these behaviors, discussions about overcoming personal barriers to and encouragement for healthful eating and being physically active were guided by the Parent Educators. Foundational elements from the Diabetes Prevention Program, including a flexible, culturally sensitive, individualized educational curriculum taught on a one-to-one basis, also were incorporated [14]. Further, anticipatory guidance and parenting support principals, elements of the Infant Feeding Activity and Nutrition Trial, were incorporated in the PATE curriculum [15]. Anticipatory guidance involves providing practical, developmentally appropriate, child health information to parents in anticipation of significant physical, emotional, and psychological milestones [16]. Parenting support emphasizes children's psychological and behavioral goals, logical and natural consequences, mutual respect, and encouragement techniques [17].

Intervention components of the PATE arm included appropriate weight gain during pregnancy and weight management after pregnancy, nutrition and physical activity in the gestational (mother) and postnatal (mother and infant) periods, and parental modeling of healthful nutrition and physical activity behaviors. More specific to this paper, lesson topics included tummy and confinement time for infants (PM 1 visit), and family play time and decreased TV time (PM 6 visit). Lessons also included maternal weight gain (gestational) and loss (postnatal) charts for tracking participants' body weight, infant growth charts, hands-on activities, instructional DVDs, and goal setting and barrier reduction for both diet and physical activity. Infants' growth was plotted on World Health Organization (WHO) sex specific reference curves for length-for-age and weight-for-age percentiles.

Both arms of the intervention were delivered in the home to women beginning early in their second trimester of pregnancy by Parent Educators. Parent Educators were African American, college educated women residing in the target communities who had completed the onsite PAT foundational training program that included

methods to build rapport and foster relationships with families and children. Parent Educators also were trained to deliver the nutrition and physical activity lessons and to collect data from participants by PhD level senior staff members. Home visits occurred monthly and were approximately 60–90 min in length for the PAT lessons, and approximately 90–120 min in length for the PATE lessons. The PATE lessons were longer in length due to the additional nutrition and/or physical activity information provided. Approximately 15 to 20 min of these visits were devoted to data collection. Both PAT and PATE participants received the same incentives at every visit. Gift cards were provided at the baseline and first and last postnatal visits. Other incentives included items such as diapers and baby bottles, books, and toys. A comprehensive description of the Delta Healthy Sprouts Project, including additional details regarding study methodology, lesson plan outlines, and Parent Educator training, has been published elsewhere [9].

Measures

Participants' knowledge and beliefs about infant activity and sleep were measured at baseline (gestational month 4 visit) and at study end (PM 12). The child activity knowledge and beliefs scale consisted of four true/false statements that can be found in Table 1. Items on these two scales were based on information provided to the participants during the course of the study. For each item, one point was given if the response was in the desired way (i.e., reflected the current state of knowledge about infant activity and sleep) and 0 points if the response was otherwise. The reliability of this scale was assessed in this study.

Reports of their infants' daily activities were collected from the participants (infants' mothers) at each postnatal visit via electronic surveys. Measures included time spent unconfined and sleeping in a 24-h period, and whether or not the infant was put to sleep on his/her back (back to sleep) and had a regular bedtime. Non-confinement time (e.g., on play mat, in walker, in playpen) was used as a measure of infant physical activity. For this item, the five responses were less than 2 h, at least 2 h but less than 4 h, at least 4 h but less than 6 h, at least 6 h but less than 8 h, and 8 h or more. For infant sleep duration, the six responses were less than 8 h, at least 8 h but less than 10 h, at least 10 h but less than 12 h, at least 12 h but less than 14 h, at least 14 h but less than 16 h, and 16 h or more. For the back to sleep question, the three responses were yes always, yes sometimes, and no. For the regular bedtime question, the three responses were yes, no, and don't know.

Anthropometric measures obtained on the participants at the baseline visit included height which was measured in duplicate using a portable stadiometer (model 217,

Table 1 Delta Healthy Sprouts child activity knowledge and beliefs questionnaire items and responses

Item	Question[c]	Baseline[a]		Study End[b]		Change		
		n	%	n	%	n_1^d	n_2^e	p^f
2a	It is OK to put a baby to sleep on his/her tummy. [F]	58	70.7	44	97.8	29	1	< 0.001
2b	It is OK to keep a baby less than 6 months old in a car seat or bouncy seat for most of the day. [F]	68	82.9	40	88.9	5	5	1.000
2c	Giving a baby tummy time (e.g. time on his/her tummy) should begin by 1 month of age. [T]	38	46.3	43	95.6	22	1	< 0.001
2d	A baby less than 12 months of age needs daily physical activity. [T]	67	81.7	41	91.1	8	2	0.058

[a]Gestational month 4 visit; number and percent of participants who chose correct response, $N = 82$
[b]Postnatal month 12 visit; number and percent of participants who chose correct response, $N = 45$
[c]Letter in brackets indicates correct response to statement; F = false and T = true
[d]Number of participants who chose incorrect response at baseline and correct response at study end (positive change)
[e]Number of participants who chose correct response at baseline and incorrect response at study end (negative change)
[f]P-values for McNemar's test of symmetry for changes from baseline to study end. Bonferroni corrected significance level of $\alpha = 0.013$ used

seca, Birmingham, UK) and weight which was measured using a digital scale (model SR241, SR Instruments, Tonawanda, NY). Both measures were performed without shoes or heavy clothing. Pre-pregnancy body weight was self-reported. Body mass index (BMI) was calculated as weight (kg) divided by height (m) squared where height was averaged if the two measurements differed. Weight also was measured at each of the 17 subsequent (5 gestational and 12 postnatal) visits.

Anthropometric measures obtained on the infants included length and weight which were measured in duplicate if the two measures agreed or in triplicate if the two measures did not agree. For analytic purposes, the measures were averaged. Length was measured using an infantometer (model seca 416, seca, Birmingham, UK). Weight was measured using a digital scale (model SR241, SR Instruments, Tonawanda, NY) with the infant dressed in a diaper only and held in the mother's arms (mother's weight zeroed out). Infant length and weight were measured at each postnatal visit. Weight-for-length percentiles were calculated based on WHO reference growth curves for sex and age [18].

Participants provided self-reported information regarding socio-demographic characteristics (e.g., age relationship status, household size, education, employment, household income, insurance, prenatal care), Supplemental Nutrition Assistance Program (SNAP) and WIC participation, health history, and current health conditions at baseline. At the first postnatal visit, participants provided information regarding birth outcomes (e.g., delivery mode and infant gender, race/ethnicity, birth weight, and birth length). Details regarding other measures and questionnaire data that were collected but are not relevant to the present paper have been published elsewhere [9]. All measures and questionnaires were collected or administered by trained research staff (Parent Educators) using laptop computers loaded with relevant software (Snap Surveys, version 11.20, Snap Surveys Ltd., Portsmouth, NH).

Statistical analysis

Statistical analyses were performed using SAS software. Results were considered significant at $p \leq 0.05$ unless stated otherwise. Descriptive statistics, including means, standard deviations (SD), frequencies, and percentages, were used to summarize participants' socio-demographic and anthropometric characteristics and their infants' birth characteristics. Chi square tests of association or Fisher's exact tests (categorical measures) and two sample t tests or Wilcoxon rank scores with exact p-values (continuous measures) were used to assess differences between postnatal study completers' and non-completers' baseline characteristics. Postnatal completers were defined as participants who had their PM 12 visit. Postnatal non-completers were defined as participants who had at least one visit in the postnatal period but did not complete the PM 12 visit.

To assess the reliability of the child activity knowledge and beliefs scale, the Kuder-Richardson 20 (KR-20) reliability measure was used since the item responses were dichotomous (true/false). KR-20 is analogous to Cronbach's coefficient alpha with dichotomous data. A KR-20 value of 0.7 or above was considered acceptable reliability [19]. To assess changes in the individual items on this scale, McNemar's tests of symmetry (suitable for paired nominal data) were used with Bonferroni correction factors applied ($0.05/4 = 0.013$). Associations between compliance with infant sleep recommendations and participants' knowledge and beliefs about infant sleep were explored with Fisher's exact test.

The National Sleep Foundation's age specific recommendations, which are the result of consensus voting by an expert panel that included members of the American Academy of Pediatrics [20], were used to assess compliance with sleep duration recommendations. These recommendations were 14 to 17 h for newborns (0 to 3 months of age), which corresponded to survey responses 5 and 6 (14 to more than 16 h); 12 to 15 h for infants (4 to 11 months of age), which corresponded to survey response 4 and 5 (12 to less than 16 h); and 11 to 14 h for toddlers (1 to 2 years of age) which corresponded to survey responses 3 through 5 (10 to less than 16 h).

Generalized linear mixed models, using maximum likelihood estimation with the Laplace method, were used to test for significant effects of infant's age (in months) and mothers' knowledge and beliefs about infant activity on infant non-confinement time. These models also were used to test for significant effects of infant's age (in months) and having a regular bedtime on compliance with sleep duration recommendations. Maximum likelihood estimation is an approach for handling missing data with longitudinal (repeated) measures. Infant non-confinement time was modeled using a multinomial distribution (suitable for ordinal measurements) with a cumulative logit function. Compliance with sleep duration recommendations was modeled using a binary distribution with a logit link function. Repeated measurement was modeled as a random effect using an unstructured covariance matrix and random intercepts. Because the item pertaining to keeping a baby in a car/bouncy seat most of the day was the only child activity knowledge and beliefs item that did not change in a positive direction and also because it had the lowest percentage of correct responses at study end, it was included in the infant non-confinement time model. Participants who responded correctly to this item at both baseline and study end were classified as "knowledge correct" and all others were classified as "knowledge incorrect." Education level (less than or a high school education vs. at least some college or technical training) was included in the models as a covariate because it has been associated with infant behaviors [21].

Compliance with putting an infant to sleep on his/her back until 12 months of age and regular bed time were modeled as time-to-event data. The infant's age (in months) at the time the participant first answered "no" or "yes sometimes" to the back to sleep question was used as the time to the event of interest (noncompliance with infant sleep position recommendation). Likewise, the infant's age (in months) at the time the participant first answered "yes" to the regular bedtime question was used as the time to the event of interest. Observations were considered censored if the participant dropped from the study prior to her infant reaching 12 months of age or the infant reached 12 months of age without the respective events occurring.

Kaplan-Meier survival curves using the product-limit method were used to estimate median survival times. Survival analysis represents the most appropriate statistical methods available to handle time-to-event data, especially when censoring is involved [22]. Again maternal education level was included in both models as a covariate. The knowledge item corresponding to correct infant sleeping position (on his/her back) was not included as a covariate in the back to sleep model because of high correct response rates at both baseline and study end. Median survival times and 95% confidence limits were computed using a log-log transformation. Log rank tests were used to test for significant associations of survival time with the covariates.

Results

The postnatal period retention rate was 85% (46/54). The mean number of postnatal visits was 10 (SD 3.2). Presented in Table 2 are maternal baseline socio-demographic and anthropometric characteristics of the postnatal cohort as well as characteristics of infants born to this cohort. The majority of participants were African American (96%), single (89%), receiving WIC (89%), and young (mean age 24 years, SD 4.8). Additionally, mean participant post-pregnancy BMI was in the obese category (31 kg/m^2). The majority of participants' infants were male (57%), fed formula within the first 24 h of birth (89%), and never breastfed (61%). Infant mean gestational age was 39 weeks and infant mean weight-for-height percentile at birth was 52%.

Reliability was insufficient for the child activity knowledge and beliefs scale at baseline (KR-20 = – 0.29). Given the lack of reliability for this scale, questionnaire items were analyzed separately and not summed to create an overall measure of maternal knowledge and beliefs about infant activity and sleep. Summary and change statistics for these individual items are presented in Table 1. At baseline, participants' knowledge and beliefs were generally in agreement with current recommendations with the exception of beginning tummy time at 1 month of age (less than half of the participants responded correctly to this item). Additionally, changes in responses for three of the items were in the direction hypothesized – proportionally more participants who answered the item incorrectly at baseline answered it correctly at study end as compared to participants who answered the item correctly at baseline and incorrectly at study end. Response changes were significant for two of the these three items – putting a baby to sleep on his/her tummy (false response) and tummy time should beginning by 1 month of age (true response). Proportions were approximately equal for the fourth item (keeping a baby in a car/bouncy seat most of the day), suggesting change occurred in both directions (positive and negative).

Median non-confinement time for infants increased steadily from at least 2 h but less than 4 h at PM 1 to 8 or more hours at PM 6. This median level of 8 or more hours of non-confinement time was maintained through PM 12 (data not shown in a table). Results of the

Table 2 Baseline socio-demographic, anthropometric, and birth characteristics of Delta Healthy Sprouts participants and their infants (N = 54)

Characteristic	n	%
Mothers		
Race		
African American	52	96.3
White	2	3.7
Relationship status		
Single[a]	48	88.9
Married	6	11.1
Education level		
≤ High school graduate	24	44.4
≥ Some college/technical	30	55.6
Employment status		
Full time/part-time	21	38.9
Unemployed (looking)	19	35.2
Homemaker/student	14	25.9
Smoker in household	16	29.6
Smoking status		
Current	2	3.7
Stopped before pregnancy	1	1.9
Stopped after became pregnant	1	1.9
Never	50	92.6
Medicaid health insurance	54	100.0
Receiving SNAP	41	75.9
Receiving WIC	48	88.9
Infants		
Male gender	31	57.4
Non-Hispanic ethnicity	53	98.1
Race		
African American	52	96.3
White	2	3.7
Fed formula within 24 h of birth	48	88.9
Ever breastfed	21	38.9
Premature (< 37 weeks gestation)[b]	7	13.0
	Mean	SD
Mothers		
Age (years)	23.6	4.84
Household size	3.9	1.58
Pre-pregnancy BMI[c]	28.9	7.91
Post-pregnancy BMI[d]	30.9	7.70
Infants		
Weeks gestation[b]	38.7	1.69
Birth weight (g)	3132.1	566.37
Birth length (cm)	48.6	2.92

Table 2 Baseline socio-demographic, anthropometric, and birth characteristics of Delta Healthy Sprouts participants and their infants (N = 54) (Continued)

Characteristic	n	%
Birth weight-for-length percentile[e]	51.9	37.45

SNAP Supplemental Nutrition Assistance Program, WIC Special Supplemental Program for Women, Infants and Children
[a]Includes 1 participant who indicated she is divorced
[b]Based on conception date (from online pregnancy calculator and using self-reported due date)
[c]Based on measured height and self-reported weight
[d]Based on weight measured at first postnatal visit
[e]Based on World Health Organization age- and sex-specific growth curves for children

generalized linear mixed models analysis for non-confinement time are presented in Table 3. Both infant age and participant knowledge concerning infant activity were significant explanatory variables in the model. For every one month increase in infant age, the odds of an infant having more non-confinement time increased by 10%. Additionally, infants with "knowledge correct" mothers had 17 times the odds of more non-confinement time as compared to infants with "knowledge incorrect" mothers. Because the confidence limit range for the knowledge variable is wide, this result should be interpreted cautiously.

Percentages of participants infants' who met the National Sleep Foundation age specific sleep duration recommendations ranged from 10% at PM 2 to 87% at PM 12. For 9 out of the 12 study months, the majority (≥ 50%) of infants' sleep duration met the recommended amounts (data not shown in a table). Results of the generalized linear mixed models analysis for meeting sleep duration recommendations also are presented in Table 3. Both infant age and education level were significant explanatory variables in the model. For every one month increase in infant age, the odds of compliance with sleep duration recommendations increased by 30%. Similarly, infants of participants with no more than a high school education had more than twice the odds of compliance with sleep duration recommendations as compared to infants of participants with at some postsecondary education.

Presented in Table 4 are results of the time-to-event analysis for compliance with infant sleep recommendations for the Delta Healthy Sprouts participants' infants. Only 20% of the participants were compliant with the back to sleep recommendation for the first 12 months of their infant's life. Conversely 94% of the participants' infants were put to bed at a regular time at some point in the first 12 months of their life. Median time to non-compliance for the back to sleep recommendation was 7.8 months while median time to compliance for a regular bedtime was 4.2 months. Additionally, participants who did not consistently put their infant to sleep on his/

Table 3 Generalized linear mixed model analysis for activity and sleep outcomes for Delta Healthy Sprouts participants' infants

Outcome	Explanatory variable	OR	95% CL		P
Non-confinement time[a]	Infant age (in months)	1.1	1.06	1.20	< 0.001
	Knowledge correct[b]	17.4	3.31	91.02	0.001
	Knowledge incorrect[b]				
Sleep duration[c]	Infant age (in months)	1.3	1.23	1.40	< 0.001
	≤ High school education	2.2	1.11	4.38	0.024
	> High school education				

OR odds ratio, *CL* confidence limits
[a]Consisted of 5 ordinal responses; education was not a significant covariate
[b]Based on response to keeping an infant in a bouncy/car seat most of the day; item was coded as correct if the response was correct at both baseline and study end and incorrect otherwise
[c]Adherence to National Sleep Foundation age specific recommendations for amount of sleep; regular bedtime was not a significant covariate

her back for the first 12 months of life were as likely to correctly respond to the related child sleep statement (i.e., putting an infant to sleep on his/her tummy; false response) as participants who met the recommendation (97% vs. 100%, Fisher's exact test $p > 0.999$; data not shown in a table).

Discussion

Delta Healthy Sprouts participants' knowledge and beliefs concerning infant activity and sleep behaviors are presented in this paper. Results indicate that participants' knowledge and beliefs about infant activity and sleep at baseline were generally in accordance with expert recommendations with the exception of tummy time. Most participants in this study were aware of expert recommendations concerning putting an infant to sleep on his/her back and providing an infant with daily non-confinement time or physical activity; less than half were aware that tummy time should begin by one month of age. However, at study end, all but one participant responded correctly to the item concerning tummy time. While it is possible that information provided to participants by their infant's pediatrician or other healthcare professional was responsible for the participants' increase in knowledge and beliefs, it is more likely that the increase can be attributed to the PAT Program. In an exploratory study by Koren and colleagues, only 15% and 26%, respectively, of the mothers surveyed immediately and two months postpartum reported receiving information about positioning their infant on his/her abdomen [23]. Further, providers surveyed in this study reported

"random" counseling on tummy time when infants were approximately two to three months of age [23]. Taken together, these results suggest the need for increased awareness among infant caregivers concerning when to begin tummy time.

Similarly, educating parents and caregivers about unrestrained floor time for infants appears needed based on the lack of increased knowledge concerning keeping an infant in a bouncy/car seat most of the day (i.e., confined) in the current study. This is supported by the larger odds of more non-confinement time among infants with "knowledge correct" mothers as compared to infants with "knowledge incorrect" mothers. However, this result should be interpreted cautiously given the small number ($n = 12$) of participants who fell into the "knowledge incorrect" group. Given the success of the Safe to Sleep® public education campaign, a similar nationwide public education campaign to promote recommended awake positioning and adequate unrestrained floor time for infants may be needed to reach all populations within the US, with particular focus on caregivers of infants at highest risk for inactivity and childhood obesity.

Also presented in this paper is Delta Healthy Sprouts participants' compliance with expert recommendations regarding infant sleep. While the majority of infants' sleep duration was compliant with recommended amounts for three-fourths of the study period, the likelihood of compliance increased as the infants became older. Additionally, participants with no more than a high school education were over twice as likely to comply with infant sleep recommendations as compared to

Table 4 Time-to-event analysis for AAP infant sleep recommendations for Delta Healthy Sprouts participants' infants

Recommendation	N	Not Met		Met		Dropped[a]		Survival time			P[b]
		n	%	n	%	n	%	Median	95% CL		
BTS until 12 months	54	38	70.4	11	20.4	5	9.3	7.8	5.6	8.5	0.820
Regular bedtime	54	0	0.0	51	94.4	3	5.6	4.2	3.6	5.1	0.387

AAP American Academy of Pediatrics, *BTS* back to sleep
[a]Participants dropped from the study prior to infant reaching age of recommendation or study end (censored event)
[b]P-value for log rank test for association of survival time with maternal education level

participants with some postsecondary education. This association has not been reported previously in the literature. Contrary to expectations, there was no association between regular bedtime and compliance with sleep duration for the infants in this study, although an association between regular bedtime routine and increased sleep duration had been reported previously [8]. The lack of association in the current study may be due to the majority of infants having a regular bedtime by approximately 4 months of age, compounded with the fact that all infants who remained in the study had a regular bedtime by approximately 12 months of age (i.e., lack of heterogeneity).

At the first postnatal visit, only two infants in this study were not consistently put to sleep on their back. Additionally, approximately half of the infants were consistently put to sleep on their back for the first eight months of their life. All 11 of the participants who put their infant to sleep on his/her back through 12 months of age and all but one of the 34 participants who did not follow this recommendation correctly answered the back to sleep knowledge item. Hence while the mothers in this study were aware of the back to sleep recommendation for their infants, over half of them chose not to follow the recommendation at some point during the first year of their infant's life. Results from previous studies suggest that caregivers may not follow the sleep position recommendation due to reasons involving infant comfort and choking concerns [24]. Additionally, at approximately five to seven months of age, most infants can flip from their back to their stomach. Hence it is probable that mothers in the current study were not as concerned or consistent about proper sleep positioning once their infant was able to flip from back to front. Nonetheless, these results are concerning given racial disparities continue to exist for infant supine sleep (58% and 75% for African American and white populations, respectively) and Sudden Infant Death Syndrome (twice the rate in the African American population as compared to the white population) [24].

The longitudinal design of this study is one of its greatest strengths as is the novel use of time to event analysis for compliance with infant sleep recommendations. Additionally, the population studied is a strength because Southern and African American infants are at increased risk for rapid weight gain and non-supine sleep [3, 24]. Nonetheless data collection was not blinded and therefore a potential source of bias. However, it was not practically, logistically, or financially feasible to have a second set of blinded research staff whose purpose was solely to collect data. The study would have benefited from the use of a measure specific to tummy time and a more refined measure of infant sleep duration (e.g., intervals of one vs. two hours). Finally, arguably the most concerning limitation of this study is its small sample size which may have limited the ability to detect meaningful associations between maternal knowledge and beliefs about infant activity and sleep and infant activity and sleep behaviors.

Conclusions

Baseline knowledge concerning infant activity and sleep recommendations was generally high in this cohort of rural, Southern, African American mothers. However, compliance with recommendations was not optimal suggesting the need for further intervention. Future research designed to improve infant activity and sleep outcomes should consider incorporating methods that not only increase caregivers' knowledge and beliefs, but also positively impact caregivers' actions.

Abbreviations
BMI: Body mass index; KR-20: Kuder-Richardson 20; PAT: Parents as teachers; PATE: Parents as teachers enhanced; PM: Postnatal month; SD: Standard deviation; SNAP: Supplemental nutrition assistance program; US: United States; WHO: World Health Organization; WIC: Special supplemental program for women, infants, and children

Acknowledgements
The authors thank Debra Johnson and Donna Ransome for their research support, including reviewing an earlier version of this paper, and the mothers who participated in this study.

Funding
This work was supported by the United States Department of Agriculture, Agricultural Research Service (Project 6401–53000-003-00D) and in-kind support from the Delta Health Alliance. The views expressed are solely those of the authors and do not reflect the official policy or position of the United States Government.

Authors' contributions
JT had primary responsibility for protocol development, participant screening, enrollment, outcome assessment, data analysis and interpretation, and writing the manuscript. LT-H participated in the development of the protocol, analytical framework for the study, and data interpretation. MG supervised the design and execution of the study, was responsible for enrollment, and contributed to data interpretation. AL was responsible for outcome assessment and contributed to data interpretation. All authors read and approved the final manuscript.

Competing interests
The authors declare that they have no competing interests.

Author details
United States Department of Agriculture, Agricultural Research Service, 141 Experiment Station Road, Stoneville, MS 38776, USA. ²Department of

Medicine and Cancer Center, University of Illinois at Chicago, Chicago, IL, USA. ³Department of Family and Consumer Sciences, University of Central Arkansas, Conway, AR, USA.

References

1. Ogden CL, Carroll MD, Kit BK, Flegal KM. Prevalence of childhood and adult obesity in the United States, 2011-2012. JAMA - Journal of the American Medical Association. 2014;311(8):806–14. https://doi.org/10.1001/jama.2014.732.

2. Taveras EM, Rifas-Shiman SL, Belfort MB, Kleinman KP, Oken E, Gillman MW. Weight status in the first 6 months of life and obesity at 3 years of age. Pediatrics. 2009;123(4):1177–83. https://doi.org/10.1542/peds.2008-1149.

3. Stettler N, Kumanyika SK, Katz SH, Zemel BS, Stallings VA. Rapid weight gain during infancy and obesity in young adulthood in a cohort of African Americans. Am J Clin Nutr. 2003;77(6):1374–8.

4. Institute of Medicine. (2011). Early childhood obesity prevention policies. Goals, Recommendations and Potential Actions. Retrieved from http://www.nationalacademies.org/hmd/reports/2011/early-childhood-obesity-prevention-policies/recommendations.aspx. Accessed 14 Mar 2017.

5. Chaput J, Gray CE, Poitras VJ, Carson V, Gruber R, Olds T, et al. And health indicators in school-aged children and youth 1, *282*(June). 2016; https://doi.org/10.1139/apnm-2015-0627.

6. Ruan H, Xun P, Cai W, He K, Tang Q. Habitual sleep duration and risk of childhood obesity: systematic review and dose-response meta-analysis of prospective cohort studies. Sci Rep. 2015;5(1):16160. https://doi.org/10.1038/srep16160.

7. Dutil C, Chaput J-P. Inadequate sleep as a contributor to type 2 diabetes in children and adolescents. Nutrition & Diabetes. 2017;7(5):e266. https://doi.org/10.1038/nutd.2017.19.

8. Mindell JA, Li AM, Sadeh A, Kwon R, Goh DYT. Bedtime routines for young children: a dose-dependent association with sleep outcomes. Sleep. 2015;38(5):717–22. https://doi.org/10.5665/sleep.4662.

9. Thomson JL, Tussing-Humphreys LM, Goodman MH. Delta healthy sprouts: a randomized comparative effectiveness trial to promote maternal weight control and reduce childhood obesity in the Mississippi Delta. Contemporary Clinical Trials. 2014;38(1) https://doi.org/10.1016/j.cct.2014.03.004.

10. Parents as Teachers National Center Inc. (n.d.). Parents as Teachers. Retrieved April 12, 2017, from http://www.parentsasteachers.org. Accessed 12 Apr 2017.

11. National Institutes Health. (n.d.). " Safe To Sleep ." Retrieved October 30, 2017, from https://www.nichd.nih.gov/sts/Pages/default.aspx. Accessed 30 Oct 2017.

12. Bandura A. Human Agency in Social Cognitive Theory. Annu Rev Psychol. 1989;44(9):1175–84. https://doi.org/10.1146/annurev.psych.52.1.1.

13. Prochaska, J. O., & Velicer, W. F. (1997). The transtheoretical model of health behavior change. American journal of health promotion : AJHP, 12(1), 38–48. Retrieved from http://www.ncbi.nlm.nih.gov/pubmed/10170434.

14. Knowler, W. C., Barrett-Connor, E., Fowler, S. E., Hamman, R. F., Lachin, J. M., Walker, E. A., ... Diabetes Prevention Program Research Group. Reduction in the incidence of type 2 diabetes with lifestyle intervention or metformin. N Engl J Med. 2002;346(6):393–403. https://doi.org/10.1056/NEJMoa012512.

15. Campbell KJ, Lioret S, McNaughton SA, Crawford DA, Salmon J, Ball K, et al. A parent-focused intervention to reduce infant obesity risk behaviors: a randomized trial. Pediatrics. 2013;131(4):652–60. https://doi.org/10.1542/peds.2012-2576.

16. Nowak AJ, Casamassimo PS. Using anticipatory guidance to provide early dental intervention. Journal of the American Dental Association (1939). 1995;126(8):1156–63. https://doi.org/10.14219/jada.archive.1995.0337.

17. Mullis F. Active parenting: an evaluation of two Adlerian parent education programs. J Individ Psychol. 1999;55:359–64.

18. National Center for Health Statistics. (n.d.). WHO Growth Charts. Retrieved May 12, 2017, from https://www.cdc.gov/growthcharts/who_charts.htm. Accessed 12 May 2017.

19. Nunnally JC. Psychometric theory. 2nd ed. New York: McGraw-Hill; 1978.

20. Hirshkowitz M, Whiton K, Albert SM, Alessi C, Bruni O, DonCarlos L, et al. National sleep foundation's sleep time duration recommendations: methodology and results summary. Sleep Health. 2015;1(1):40–3. https://doi.org/10.1016/j.sleh.2014.12.010.

21. Smylie J, Fell DB, Chalmers B, Sauve R, Royle C, Allan B, O'Campo P. Socioeconomic position and factors associated with use of a nonsupine infant sleep position: findings from the Canadian maternity experiences survey. Am J Public Health. 2014;104(3):539–47. https://doi.org/10.2105/AJPH.2012.301061.

22. Hosmer D, Lemehow S. Applied survival analysis: regression modeling of time to event data. New York, NY: John Wiley & Sons; 1999.

23. Koren A, Reece SM, Kahn-D'angelo L, Medeiros D. Parental information and behaviors and provider practices related to tummy time and back to sleep. J Pediatr Health Care. 2010;24(4):222–30. https://doi.org/10.1016/j.pedhc.2009.05.002.

24. Colson ER, Rybin D, Smith LA, Colton T, Lister G, Corwin MJ. Trends and factors associated with infant sleeping position: the national infant sleep position study, 1993-2007. Archives of pediatrics & adolescent medicine. 2009;163(12):1122–8. https://doi.org/10.1001/archpediatrics.2009.234.

22

Immediate postpartum use of long-acting reversible contraceptives in low- and middle-income countries

Margo S. Harrison[1,2*] and Robert L. Goldenberg[1]

Abstract

Globally, data show that many women of reproductive age desire to use modern family planning methods. Many of these women do not have access to modern contraceptives, which is termed their 'unmet need' for contraception. In low- and middle-income countries where total fertility rates can be high and many women have undesired fertility, or wish to increase their inter-pregnancy intervals, access to modern contraceptives is often inadequate.

The puerperium is a unique time for interventions to offer modern contraceptive methods. Having just given birth, women may desire contraceptives to prevent short-interval pregnancy, or further pregnancy, altogether. In high-, middle-, and low-income countries there has been an increased interest in the placement of long-acting reversible contraceptives at or immediately after delivery, regardless of delivery mode. These methods can provide women with highly effective contraception for years, can be manufactured at low cost, are generally well tolerated with a good safety profile, and do not require the user to remember to take them. Oral contraceptives and injectable medications require the patient to present to the clinic during a specific timeframe for follow-up care or a refill, and the clinic may not be proximate, affordable, or have the desired contraceptive in stock.

This document will review the currently published literature on the use of immediate postpartum long-acting reversible contraceptives (placed within two days of delivery) in low- and middle-income countries to report on the prevalence of use and satisfaction rates, and note the lack of data on cost and economic implications. We will also explore data on how future maternal, neonatal, and infant outcomes may be influenced by increased peripartum long-term contraceptive use.

Keywords: Contraception, Long-acting reversible contraception, Immediate postpartum contraception

Background

Long-acting reversible contraception (LARC) includes copper and progesterone-laden intrauterine devices (IUDs) and progesterone-only contraceptive implants, per the World Health Organization (WHO) [1]. LARC is the most effective method of modern contraception and offers the advantages of a rapid return of fertility with removal and are user-independent. Once the devices are placed, the woman does not need to perform any action to support ongoing effective use of the contraceptive [2]. It should be noted that some sources, such as the National Institute for Healthcare Excellence (NICE)

* Correspondence: margo.harrison@gmail.com
[1]Columbia University Medical Center, New York, NY, USA
[2]622 W 168th St, PH 16-29, New York, NY 10032, USA

guidelines from the United Kingdom, include progesterone-only injectable contraceptives in the category of LARC; for the purposes of this review on the use of postpartum LARC in low- and middle-income countries (LMIC), the definition will be restricted to IUDs and implants per the WHO [3].

Intrauterine devices

LARC includes two types of IUDs, the copper and levonorgestrel (LNG) IUDs. The copper IUD is comprised of polyethylene wrapped copper and has been approved by the Food and Drug Administration (FDA) in the United States of America (USA) for use up to ten years. The failure rate over that time period is 1.9 in 100 women [2]. The IUD reduces ovum and sperm transport and viability [2]. The device has minimal side effects, although heavy menstrual bleeding and dysmenorrhea have been cited [2].

The LNG IUD system is approved by the FDA for five years of consecutive use, has a one-year failure rate of 0.2 per 100 women, and prevents pregnancy by altering the function and consistency of cervical mucous, endometrial receptivity, and preventing ovulation in 58–63% of women [2]. The device elutes 20 µg of drug daily and has minimal systemic impact, although headaches, nausea, breast tenderness, depression, and ovarian cyst formation are reported side effects [2]. Additionally, patients have reported discontinuation due to oligo- or amenorrhea, spotting, and irregular bleeding patterns [2].

Contraceptive implant

The contraceptive implant is also a progesterone-only method that elutes etonogestrel over a three-year period and interferes with proper functioning of the hypothalamic-pituitary-ovarian axis while also altering the endometrial lining and cervical mucous [2]. Reported side effects include weight gain, vaginitis, breast pain, acne, headaches, gastrointestinal disturbances, and complications related to implant removal and insertion [2]. Some patients also complain of unpredictable bleeding patterns, which accounts for an 11.3% rate of discontinuation; the typical-use pregnancy rate is reported as 0.05%, which is the effectiveness based on correct and consistent use [2].

Epidemiology

United Nations (UN) data indicate that LARC methods are popular, globally [4]. Sterilization, IUDs, and implants are reported to account for 56% of contraceptive prevalence in 2015, and according to the same UN report, are accounting for a greater share of all contraceptive use with increased prevalence of modern methods around the world [3]. Use of different methods varies by region, however, with the highest use of implants and IUDs in Asia and North America [4].

Postpartum use

Immediate postpartum LARC is defined, per the American College of Obstetrics and Gynecologists (ACOG), as placement of LARC prior to hospital discharge [5]. As ACOG is the professional organization representing obstetrician/gynecologists in the USA, its definition is applicable to a high-income setting where the majority of deliveries occur in facilities. For the purposes of this review, immediate postpartum LARC will be defined as placement of LARC within two days of delivery, regardless of setting or method of delivery, as the IUD can be placed up to 48 h postpartum and the implant can be placed any time if the woman is not breastfeeding;

breastfeeding is not an absolute contraindication as discussed below [6].

Safety

The US Medical Eligibility Criteria for Contraceptive Use, which was developed by the Centers for Disease Control and Prevention (CDC) and the WHO, classifies the safety of contraceptives under various circumstances [7]. Contraceptives are classified as category I through IV. I represents no restrictions to use, II represents a situation in which benefits outweigh risks, III represents a situation in which risks outweigh benefits, and IV represents an unacceptable health risk to the patient of using a given contraceptive in that medical circumstance [7]. Immediate postpartum use (defined by the CDC as placement within ten minutes of placental separation) of the copper IUD is designated as a category I. The LNG IUD is classified as category II because of theoretical concerns regarding the effect of progesterone on breastfeeding, although published data has not supported this concern [2, 7]. IUDs are contraindicated during this time period in women with chorioamnionitis, endomyometritis, or puerperal sepsis [2].

In non-breastfeeding women, the contraceptive implant is category I any time after childbirth, but again, similar to the LNG IUD, is category II for breastfeeding women due to concerns about breastmilk production if placed at less than four weeks postpartum [2]. Again, published data, while not of high quality, does not support this concern in terms of breast milk quality or weight and growth of neonates [2].

LARC does not require antibiotic prophylaxis for placement, can be offered to women with a history of ectopic pregnancy, can be used in an adolescent population, and has very few contraindications. Thus, almost all women are eligible for LARC [2].

Efficacy

According to the CDC, WHO, and ACOG, LARC is safe, but is it also effective? In a high-income population, a large study was performed in almost 7500 women comparing outcomes of participants who were given the contraceptive method of their choice at no cost, including short-acting as well as LARC methods [8]. The unintended pregnancy rate after LARC in the population was 0.27 per 100 participant-years compared to 4.55 in women using pills, patch, or ring. This resulted in a hazard ratio of 21.8 when adjusted for age, education, and history of unintended pregnancy [8]. The authors conclude that LARC is a more effective method of contraception than short-acting methods, including use in adolescent populations [8].

A review of immediate postpartum provision of LARC in high-income settings also found that these methods are safe, effective, and can reduce unmet need for contraception in the postpartum period [9]. The review concludes that IUDs inserted at the time of both vaginal and cesarean deliveries are more likely to be in situ 6–12 months postpartum than those placed at the postpartum visit 4–6 weeks after delivery [9]. They also found longer inter-pregnancy intervals in women using LARC in the immediate postpartum setting, and recommend the use of these methods regardless of impact on breastfeeding [9].

Introduction

The background section of this paper established how LARC is defined, which contraceptives it includes, how it is recommended for use in the immediate postpartum period, and how safe and effective it is when used in real-world settings. Most data on these topics come from high-income countries (HIC). However, the focus of this review is on how LARC is currently being applied in the immediate postpartum setting in LMIC where availability of, access to, and utilization of LARC are less consistent for women in the postpartum setting.

Methods

The objective was to review all literature published from LMIC and summarize the findings. This review, while not a systematic review, did attempt to find all published manuscripts on the use of postpartum IUDs and implants currently in production. The search included the words "postpartum", "IUD", "intrauterine", "implant", and brand names for all devices currently in production. Studies included in the review involved work in sub-Saharan Africa, Southeast Asia, and Latin America. All studies mentioned are included in the references section. Countries are grouped into income categories by the World Bank, which groups WHO member states into income categories based on gross national income per capita. For 2016, LMIC encompasses countries with gross national income per capita between $1006 and $12,235 [10].

Demand and unmet need for modern contraception

Globally, unintended pregnancy contributes significantly to maternal morbidity and mortality, especially in LMIC settings [1]. The WHO estimates that 225 million women around the world desire modern contraception to delay or prevent future childbearing, but do not have access [11]. A review on the determinants of unmet need for family planning in LMIC defines the term as "the proportion of women wishing to limit or postpone childbirth, but not using contraception" [12]. The review found that among 26 quantitative and 8 qualitative studies, the unmet need for family planning in LMIC ranged from 20% to 58% with older age and higher educational

level reducing unmet need, and a higher number of children increasing unmet need [12]. Primary reasons for non-use of modern contraception included an unsupportive partner or health concerns regarding adverse effects of the medications. These findings were not specific to LARC or the postpartum period, but addressed unmet need for modern contraception, generally [12].

Figure 1, reproduced with permission from the United Nations, illustrates the percentage of married or cohabitating women using contraception and with an unmet need for contraception, by region, around the world [4]. Another resource, looking at data from Demographic and Health Surveys (DHS) reported that the average level of unmet need in the 16 countries reviewed was 47% ranging from a high of 82% in Ghana to a low of 23% in Morocco. [13] The WHO identifies sub-groups at highest risk for unmet need for contraception to include adolescents, migrants, urban slum dwellers, refugees, and women in the postpartum period [14].

Of note, delivery in the facility setting appears to be increasing [15]. This finding is inferred from a recent WHO publication reports that between 1990 and 2014 the global average CS rate increased from 12.4% to 18.6% with rates ranging, depending on region, between 6 and 27.2%, and rising at an average rate of 4.4% per year [15]. Interestingly, it is not clear that this increase in facility births has translated to increased placement of postpartum contraception in facility settings, but is a potential point of entry in the healthcare system to target interventions [16].

Reasons for unmet need for contraception in postpartum period in LMIC

The Guttmacher Institute review on unmet need for postpartum contraception in LMIC asserts that the primary reasons given for non-use in this timeframe are the protection afforded to women by lactational amenorrhea and abstinence [13]. Women, for cultural reasons, may not be sexually active in the immediate postpartum period and may experience lactational amenorrhea during breastfeeding [13]. Lactational amenorrhea ranges, on average, from 3 to 4 months to 20 months in sub-Saharan Africa (SSA) [13]. Therefore, the timeframe during which a woman may be considering postpartum contraception varies by population and individual, which can make postpartum family planning programs difficult to design and administer [13].

Another reason unmet need for contraception in the postpartum period is high in LMIC is because postpartum visits are not common, and if women did not deliver in a facility, they will have little interaction with the healthcare system to consider contraception before they become fertile again [17]. Additionally, besides requiring the woman to access the system to obtain LARC, the healthcare system needs to provide the devices. This involves appropriate

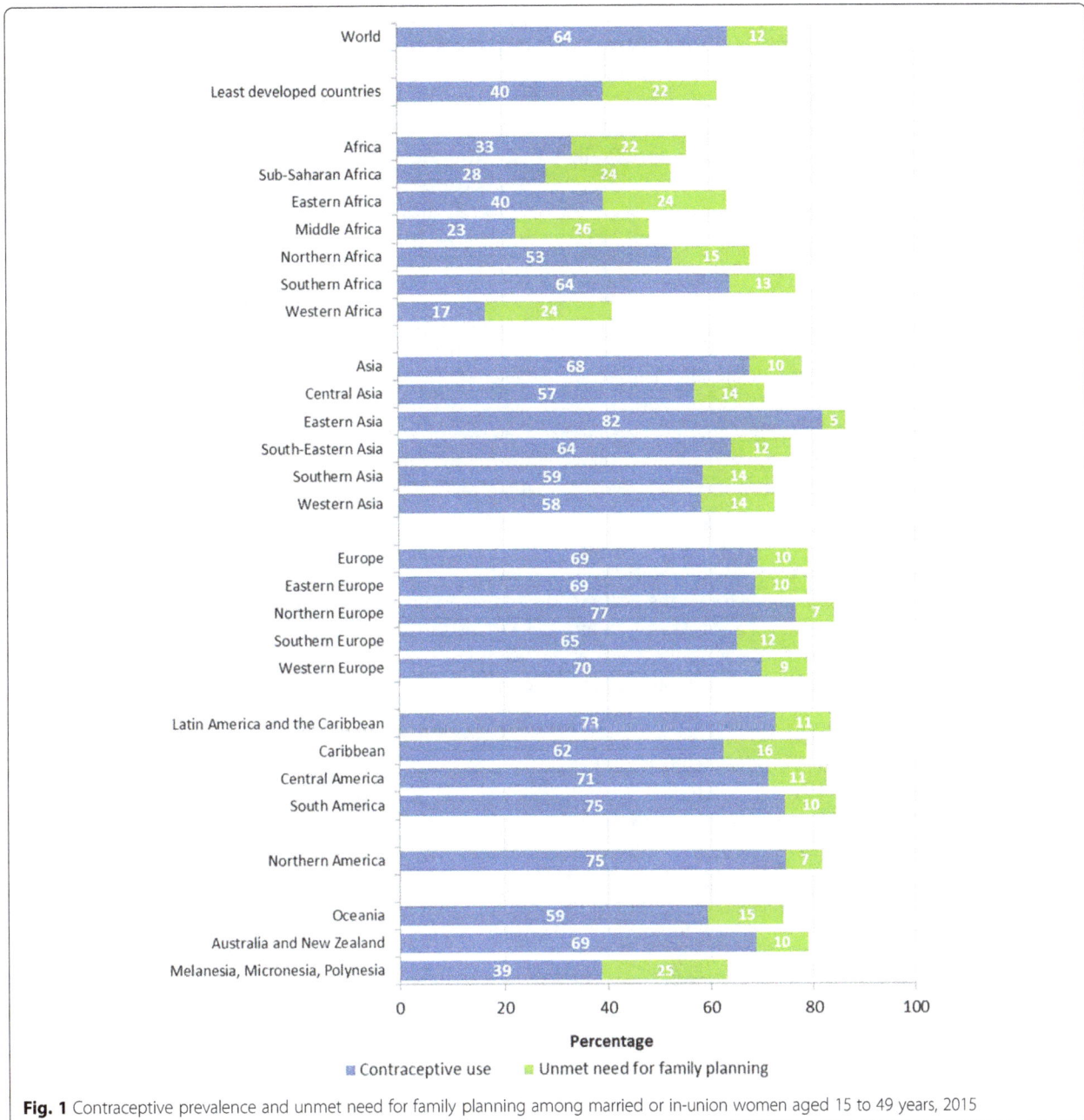

Fig. 1 Contraceptive prevalence and unmet need for family planning among married or in-union women aged 15 to 49 years, 2015

counseling ante- and postnatally, a consistent supply of the devices, and providers that are trained and available to place LARC in the postpartum setting [18]. A recent study from Nigeria found that in the poorest quintile, women had a 35% unmet need for contraception [19]. This finding is largely due to the fact that LARC is not offered in many facilities that poor women frequent and stock-outs are common, which are issues seen in many LMIC [19].

Significance of LARC in LMIC: Implementing strong family planning programs in LMIC is a global health priority. This is reflected in the Millenium Development Goals, goals four and five, which focus on reducing

maternal and child morbidity and mortality, incorporate increasing family planning utilization as an essential method to achieve these aims. [12] Unmet need for contraception results in adolescent, unintended, and short interval pregnancies, as well as unsafe abortion, all of which can result in increased maternal and neonatal mortality [12]. Data has shown that pregnancies conceived less than twenty months following a prior birth are at increased risk of low birth weight, preterm birth, stillbirth, and neonatal and infant mortality [13]. Additionally, a 52-country DHS survey showed that children born less than two years after a sibling have a 60%

increased risk of death at less than one year of age com-pared to those born three to five years after another child [13]. For reasons related to adverse pregnancy and abortion outcomes, as well as the social, educational, and economic impacts of unintended or undesired preg-nancy, contraception in general, and LARC specifically, have an important role to play in LMIC.

Postpartum LARC in LMIC

Utilization

Currently, in LMIC, LARC use is variable. In Nairobi, Kenya's urban slums, a study found that LARC methods were the least adopted methods during the first year postpartum, with only 4% of women opting for implants and even fewer choosing an IUD [20]. However, the study did show that these were the least discontinued methods [20]. Similarly, a study from Ethiopia that inter-viewed almost 900 women in the postpartum setting, found that 1.8% of those currently using contraception had opted for an IUD and 0.2% for an implant [21]. In Malawi, LARC use was higher at 14% with a statistically significant higher continuation rate at 6 months postpar-tum [22]. Studies from Southeast Asia (SEA) show simi-lar utilization rates to SSA. A study from Pakistan looking at use of modern contraceptive methods in post-partum women found that out of the 27% of women who opted for a contraceptive method after delivery, 4.8% chose to use an IUD and 3.1% an implant [23]. A study of 1049 postpartum low-income Indian women found that 162 (15.4%) of them were using contracep-tion; of these, 2.9% had an IUD in situ, and no women were using a contraceptive implant [24]. Overall, from the data reviewed, use of LARC appears to be utilized in less than 15% of postpartum women in LMIC.

Characteristics associated with postpartum LARC utilization

A number of studies have evaluated which characteris-tics make a women more or less likely to utilize postpar-tum contraception, with differing results. A study from Ethiopia found that in 703 participants, characteristics associated with LARC usage were resumption of menses, age < 24 years, interval of 7–9 months post-delivery, and having had antenatal care; about 11% appear to have opted for the implant and about 3% for the IUD [25]. A similar study from Uganda of almost 3300 women found that women who were more likely to utilize postpartum contraception had the following characteristics: higher than a primary level of education, highest wealth status, Protestant, aged 25–29, already had 3–5 children, had been exposed to information about family planning ser-vices via the media, were seen for post-delivery care within 1–2 days of delivery, and had their birth attended by a skilled attendant [26]. This study did not specify the rate of LARC use among the study population. Another

Ugandan study found that the additional characteristics of prior use of contraceptives and partner involvement in the decision-making process were statistically signifi-cant predictors of contraceptive use since delivery, but again did not specify the type of contraceptives utilized [27]. In Pakistan, the characteristics associated with postpartum contraceptive use included women who had delivered in a facility, those who had received informa-tion about birth spacing, those living in a community with high antenatal care utilization rates, and those who lived in less impoverished areas [23]. In India, among 400 participants, characteristics that predicted non-use of postpartum contraceptives were inadequate know-ledge of contraceptive options and fear of side effects [28]. Understanding the specific predictors of use and non-use of postpartum contraceptives, and specifically LARC, in some LMIC settings may help identify targets for interventions to increase uptake in these countries, more generally.

Efficacy

Understanding the safety and efficacy of LARC use in LMIC is essential before programs to increase utilization are implemented. A study from India on postpartum copper IUD placement (after both vaginal and cesarean delivery) found that none of the 434 women who contin-ued to use the IUD were pregnant by 6–18 months post-partum [29]. Continuation rates of the device were 81% by the end of the study [29]. A study from Kenya studied continuation rates of the implant, but did not comment on efficacy in terms of pregnancy rates during the follow-up period; the authors found that of the 97 women who were followed for a year, 79% had continued use of the implant up to that point. [30] A review from the United States Agency for International Development looks at Demographic and Health Surveys and focused on uptake and discontinuation of LARC in LMIC [31]. This document reports that, "On average, within the first year of use, 9 percent of women discontinue using im-plants, 15 percent discontinue IUDs, and 32 percent dis-continue injectables," although this information is not specific to LARC placed in the postpartum period [31].

Side effects

The study previously mentioned from India on postpar-tum copper IUD placement found that in 434 women who received the device, 190 experienced a complication (bleeding 23.5%, expulsion 9%, inability to visualize strings 11.3%) [28]. A recently published study from Uganda where authors conducted focus groups on fac-tors that influenced respondents use of LARC found that women who chose short-acting over long-acting methods cited side effects of LARC as their primary rea-son for doing so, although this was not specific to the postpartum setting [32]. Side effects mentioned were excessive bleeding and lack of periods [32]. In a study of over 1200 Pakistani women who chose LARC methods for contraception, also not specifically in the postpartum setting, found that about 25% of participants complained of side effects related to their device, citing bleeding and pain most commonly [33]. About 30% of patients sought follow-up visits for side effect-related complaints during the twelve-month follow-up period [33]. How side effects from LARC use affect patients in the postpartum setting, specifically, deserves further attention.

Satisfaction

As important to increasing effective family planning programs as are utilization and continuation of postpartum contraceptives, patient satisfaction with the method chosen may be more important. Since many contraceptives have unwanted side effects, finding the right method for a particular women is essential. A study of over 2700 Indian women who opted for a postpartum copper IUD after facility delivery were assessed for their satisfaction immediately status-post placement of the device and six weeks later at their follow-up visit [34]. The mean age of participants was 24 years old, >50% had one living child, and one quarter of the patients had no formal education [34]. 99.6% of the women were satisfied with the IUD at the time of insertion and 92% were satisfied at the six week follow-up visit, at which point the rate of expulsion was 3.6% [34]. A study from Kenya looked specifically at patient's satisfaction with postpartum LARC in the year following device placement, including the implant and both types of IUD [35]. The study was a longitudinal cohort study of 313 women (205 used the subdermal implant, 93 used the LNG IUD, 15 opted for the copper IUD) whose LARC was placed in an interval fashion (6–12 weeks after delivery) and not immediately postpartum within 48 h [35]. The authors declined to publish results for the copper IUD users because they felt the sample size was too small; for the LNG IUD and implant, they found that continuation rates were 89.1% and 91.8%, respectively [35]. 87% of patients reported being 'very satisfied' with the LNG IUD and 75% with the implant at 6 months postpartum; 83.9% and 87.3% were 'very satisfied' after a year, respectively [35]. The authors felt the LNG IUD compared favorably to the implant both in terms of satisfaction and continued use [35]. These results suggest that LARC performs well in LMIC in terms of the patient experience.

Impact on pregnancy outcomes

Studies from HIC have shown that postpartum LARC can positively impact pregnancy outcomes. For example, a prospective observational study of patients in Colorado found that with immediate postpartum implant insertion, there was a 2.6% pregnancy rate one year post-

placement in the intervention group compared to an 18.6% pregnancy rate among the control group [36]. Downstream benefits of using LARC in this population also appeared to include a 2% decrease in preterm birth, which was an unexpected but highly beneficial outcome [36]. This suggests that effective postpartum LARC programs may have an impact on adverse pregnancy outcomes such as preterm birth. While studies from HIC are not the focus of this part of the review, we think it is helpful to summarize the research that has been done in this area to guide future work in LMIC, as studies in this area do not appear to have yet been performed.

Barriers to uptake

We have shown that utilization of postpartum LARC in LMIC overall is poor at rates less than 15%. However, according to the few studies that exist, LARC efficacy is good and satisfaction is high, and there is data from HIC that the impact of the contraceptives on pregnancy outcomes can be beneficial. The next question becomes, what are the barriers to postpartum LARC uptake in LMIC? We have noted that stock-outs, alternative methods of contraception (lactational amenorrhea and abstinence), and poor postpartum healthcare may contribute to poor utilization of postpartum LARC in LMIC. A study from rural Ghana attempted to clarify barriers to IUD uptake. They interviewed pregnant, postpartum, and reproductive-aged women, as well as males and healthcare workers [37]. While not specific to postpartum LARC use, the study found that lack of IUD-specific knowledge, provider discomfort with placement of the device, and poor contraceptive counseling were reasons IUD uptake was poor [37]. The authors recommended that interventions to educate and train providers, increased peer modeling, and improve stocking of IUDs in the community could increase uptake [37]. Incentives to place IUDs, which involve more effort than say an injectable, may also be required.

A study from Rwanda published results of in-depth interviews with women and their partners about barriers to modern contraceptive use postpartum [38]. They concluded that fertility and partner-related factors were associated with non-use of modern contraceptives, especially in the postpartum period because patients had a poor understanding of their fertility during that time [38]. As a result, the authors recommended increasing educational campaigns aimed at couples and increasing information about postpartum contraceptive needs [38]. This is another area that could benefit from more study, especially as it relates specifically to postpartum LARC use in LMIC.

Interventions to increase utilization

This segment of the review focuses on what has been done to improve use of postpartum LARC in LMIC. A number of studies have tried different techniques in both SSA and SEA (Southeast Asia). A review on interventions to improve postpartum family planning use in LMIC found 35 articles focused on interventions to improve postpartum contraception [39]. The authors found eight studies of antenatal interventions and while they felt the data was not of sufficient quality to draw a conclusion, they did suggest "high-intensity" antenatal counseling might affect postpartum contraceptive uptake [39]. All of these studies focused on some type of antenatal counseling program and were conducted in SSA, SEA, and the Middle East.

Eleven studies of postpartum interventions were evaluated, and while again the authors questioned the quality of the evidence, they assert that a single 20-min postnatal counseling session may be able to increase contraceptive uptake [39]. These interventions also focused on postpartum counseling and were conducted all over the world including Latin America, SSA, and Asia.

Combined ante- and postnatal interventions were also reviewed in ten studies. While the authors found that they all showed a substantial impact on contraceptive uptake sometime in the first year postpartum, they questioned whether it was possible to determine which component(s) of the interventions was effective and whether resources were being wasted on combined interventions [39]. These combined interventions were more involved and included not only counseling but home visits, partner counseling, and community mobilization [39]. Studies were included from all major world regions.

The final intervention type they reviewed was the integration of family planning services with other healthcare services, such as childhood immunization programs. [39] They felt that while these interventions had the most potential to be successful, results were not impressive and data were lacking on the effectiveness of these programs. [39] The authors conclude that the "ideal strategy for improving postpartum family planning is to incorporate contraceptive advice and services across the continuum of reproductive healthcare," and that no single intervention or time point was maximally effective at improving postpartum contraceptive uptake [39]. While this review did focus on the postpartum setting, it reviewed all contraceptive methods and was not specific to LARC.

Recently, a review was published on the promotion of intrauterine contraception in LMIC [16]. The authors reviewed and interpreted interventions studied to promote uptake of IUDs in LMIC; based on their narrative review of the literature they concluded that the evidence-base is weak and that no clear strategy exists for increasing utilization in LMIC [16]. They suggest this is due to adverse perceptions of IUDs by providers and patients and that most interventions are not funded by LMIC governments, but rather international organizations [16].

Economic and cost implications for LARC programs in LMIC

The final part of this review is to address the cost and economic implications of scaling up LARC programs in LMIC. Unfortunately, sophisticated cost-effectiveness analyses have not been published from LMIC settings, suggesting this is another area ripe for research. However, NICE has published a clinical practice guideline on the cost-effectiveness of LARC use in the United Kingdom [40]. LARC, in this review, not only included both IUDs and the implant, but the depot medroxyprogesterone acetate injection, as well. The study found that LARC methods were the most effective and least costly, with depot medroxyprogesterone acetate and the LNG IUD being the least cost-effective of the methods studied due to discontinuation, which was a key determinant of their cost-effectiveness [40]. Of note, the incremental cost-effectiveness of the implant, which is considered the most effective LARC method per NICE, as compared to the IUD, which is the cheapest, was £13,206 per unintended pregnancy averted for one year of use [40]. The authors conclude that interventions to improve patient satisfaction and continuation of LARC methods will improve cost-effectiveness even further [40].

Conclusions

The main conclusion of this review is that immediate postpartum LARC has been proven to be a safe and effective means of family planning not only to improve individual health, social, and economic outcomes, but also to achieve global priorities for public health. However, the review does highlight the fact that in each of the different topic areas addressed, there is a lack of high-quality data from LMIC, and that more research needs to be done on making the devices available, promoting programs for large-scale implementation, monitoring and evaluating the impact of LARC on fertility and subsequent pregnancy outcomes, and the cost and cost-effectiveness of such device use in LMIC settings. Additionally, the literature could benefit from more research on the limitations of the use of LARC in LMIC. It may be that these methods are inappropriate for use in such settings given lack of provider availability or training, potential for uterine perforation with placement of IUDs without the opportunity for adequate follow-up, and side effects may be either more pronounced or unacceptable in certain LMIC patient populations. The proof of concept groundwork has been laid that postpartum LARC is acceptable for use in LMIC. Now it is important to invest in the utilization of these products and study if they have the highly beneficial effects on individual and group health, social, and economic outcomes, expected.

Abbreviations

ACOG: American College of Obstetrics and Gynecologists; CDC: Center for Disease Control and Prevention; DHS: Demographic and Health Surveys; FDA: Food and Drug Administration; HIC: High-income countries; IUDs: Intrauterine devices; LARC: Long-acting reversible contraception; LMIC: Low- and middle-income countries; LNG: Levonorgestrel; NICE: National Institute for Healthcare Excellence; SEA: Southeast Asia; SSA: Sub-Saharan Africa; UN: United Nations; USA: United States of America; WHO: World Health Organization

Acknowledgements

With the publication of this document we wish to acknowledge all women in low- and middle-income countries who have an unmet need for postpartum contraception and hope to raise awareness about long-acting reversible contraceptives a method of meeting that need.

Authors' contributions

This manuscript was written and produced by MSH in partnership with RLG. Both authors read and approved the final manuscript.

Funding

This is a non-funded manuscript.

Competing interests

The authors declare that they have no competing interests.

References

1. From evidence to policy: expanding access to family planning – strategies to increase use of long-acting and permanent contraception. WHO Policy Brief, 2012. Access 3.16.17. http://apps.who.int/iris/bitstream/10665/75161/1/WHO_RHR_HRP_12.20_eng.pdf?ua=1
2. Long-acting reversible contraception: implants and interuterine devices. ACOG Practice Bulletin No. 121, 2015.
3. Long acting reversible contraception. Clinical Guideline. NICE 2005. nice.org.uk/guidance/cg30
4. Trends in contraceptive use worldwide, 2015. United Nations Department of economic and social affairs, population division. Access 3.16.17. http://www.un.org/en/development/desa/population/publications/pdf/family/trendsContraceptiveUse2015Report.pdf
5. Immediate postpartum long-acting reversible contraception. ACOG committee opinion, No 671, August 2016.
6. Programming strategies for postpartum family planning. WHO 2013. Accessed 4/3/17. http://apps.who.int/iris/bitstream/10665/93680/1/9789241506496_eng.pdf
7. US Medical Eligibility Criteria for Contraceptive Use. Center for Disease Control and Prevention. MMWR Recomm Rep 2010, 59(RR-4): 1–86.
8. Winner B, Peipert JF, Zhao Q, Buckel C, Madden T, Allsworth JE. At al. Effectiveness of long-acting reversible contraception. N Engl J Med. 2012;366:1998–2007.
9. Goldthwaite LM, Shaw KA. Immediate postpartum provision of long-acting reversible contraception. Curr Opin Obstet Gynecol. 2015;27:460–4.
10. World Bank Country and Lending Groups. Accessed 8/23/17. (https://datahelpdesk.worldbank.org/knowledgebase/articles/906519-world-bank-country-and-lending-groups).
11. Family Planning/Contraception. WHO Fact Sheet. Updated 12/2016. Accessed 3/20/17. http://who.int/mediacentre/factsheets/fs351/en/
12. Wulifan JK, Brenner S, Jahn A, De Allegri MA. Scoping review on determinants of unmet need for family planning among women of reproductive age in low and middle income countries. BMC Womens Health. 2016;16:2.
13. Cleland J, Shah IH, Benova LA. Fresh look at the level of unmet need for family planning in the postpartum period, its causes and program implications. Int Perspect Sex Reprod Health. 2015;41(3):155–62.
14. Unmet Need for Family Planning. WHO Fact Sheet. Accessed 3/23/17. http://www.who.int/reproductivehealth/topics/family_planning/unmet_need_fp/en/
15. Betran AP, Ye J, Moller AB, Zhang J, Gumezoglu AM, Torloni MR. The increasing trend in cesarean section rates: global, regional, and national estimates: 1990 – 2014. PLoS One. 2016;11(2):e148343.
16. Cleland J, Ali M, Benova L, Daniele M. The promotion of intrauterine contraception in low- and middle-income countries: a narrative review. Contraception. 2017;95:519 28.
17. Mbizvo MT, Phillips SJ. Family planning: choices and challenges for developing countries. Best Practice & Research Clinical Obstetrics and Gynaecology. 2014;28:931e943.
18. Canning D, Shah IH, Pearson E, Pradhan E, Karra M, Senderowicz L, et al. Institutionalizing postpartum intrauterine device (IUD) services in Sri Lanka, Tanzania, and Nepal: study protocol for a cluster randomized stepped-wedge trial. BMC Pregnancy and Childbirth. 2016;16:362.
19. Global Health Data Pearls. Excellent family planning progress in Nigeria reported by PMA2020. Global Health Science and Practice. 2017;5(1):28–32.
20. Mumah JN, Machiyama K, Mutua M, Kabiru CW, Cleland J. Contraceptive adoption, discontinuation, and switching among postpartum women in Nairobi's urban slums. Stud Fam Plan. 2015;46(4):369–86.
21. Mengesha ZB, Worku AG, Feleke SA. Contraceptive adoption in the extended postpartum period is low in Northwest Ethiopia. BMC Pregnancy and Childbirth. 2015;15:160.
22. Kopp DM, Rosenberg NE, Stuart GS, Miller WC, Hosseinipour MC, Bonongwe P, et al. Patterns of contraceptive adoption, continuation, and switching after delivery among Malawian women. PLoS One. 2017;12(1):e0170284.
23. Tappis H, Kazi A, Hameed W, Dahar Z, Ali A, Agha S. The role of quality health services and discussion about birth spacing in postpartum contraceptive use in Sindh, Pakistan: a multilevel analysis. PLoS One. 2015;10(10):e0139628.
24. Mody SK, Nair S, Dasgupta A, Raj A, Donta B, Saggurti N, et al. Postpartum contraception utilization among low-income women seeking immunization for infants in Mumbai, India. Contraception. 2014;89(6):516–20.
25. Abera Y, Mengesha ZB, Tessema GA. Postpartum contraceptive use in Gondar town, Northwest Ethiopia: a community-based cross-sectional study. BMC Womens Health. 2015;15:19.
26. Rutaremwa G, Kabagenyi A, Wandera SO, Jhamba T, Akiror E, Nviiri HL. Predictors of modern contraceptive use in the postpartum period among women in Uganda: a population-based cross-sectional study. BMC Public Health. 2015;15:262.
27. Sileo KM, Wanyenze RK, Lule H, Kiene SM. Determinants of family planning service uptake and use of contraceptives among postpartum women in rural Uganda. Int J Public Health. 2015;60(8):987–97.
28. Choudhary D, Pal R, Goel N. Awareness and practice patterns of family planning methods among antenatal women in the Indian community: are we hitting the bull's eye? Biom J. 2015;38:356–8.
29. Mishra S. Evaluation of safety, efficacy, and expulsion of post-placental and intra-cesarean insertion of intrauterine contraceptive devices. J Obstet Gynaecol India. 2014;64(5):337–43.
30. O'Neill E, Tang J, Garrett J, Hubacher D, O'Neill E, Tang J, et al. Characteristics of Kenyan women in a prospective cohort study who continue using subdermal contraceptive implants at 12 months. Contraception. 2014;89(3):204–8.
31. Staveteig S; Mallick L; Winter R. Uptake and discontinuation of long-acting reversible contraceptives (LARCS) in low-income countries. Rockville, Maryland, ICF International, 2015 Sep. 77 p. (DHS analytical studies 54).
32. Tibaijuka L, Odongo R, Welhike E, Mukisa W, Kugonza L, Busingye I, et al. Factors influencing use of long-acting versus short-acting contraceptive methods among reproductive-age women in a resource-limited setting. BMC Womens Health. 2017;17:25. https://doi.org/10.1186/s12905-017-0382-2.
33. Hameed W, Azmat SK, Ali M, Isahaque M, Abbas G, Munroe E et al. Comparing Effectiveness of Active and Passive Client Follow-Up Approaches in Sustaining the Continued Use of Long Acting Reversible Contraceptives (LARC) in Rural Punjab: A Multicentre, Non-Inferiority Trial PLoS ONE 11(9): e0160683. doi:https://doi.org/10.1371/journal. pone.0160683.
34. Kumar S, Sethi R, Balasubramaniam S, Charunat E, Lalchandani K, Semba R, et al. Women's experience with postpartum intrauterine contraceptive device use in India. Reprod Health. 2014;11:32.
35. Hubacher D, Masaba R, Manduku CK, Chen M, Veena V. The levonorgestrel intrauterine system: cohort study to assess satisfaction in a postpartum population in Kenya. Contraception. 2015;91:295–300.
36. Tocce KM, Sheeder JL, Teal SB. Rapid repeat pregnancy in adolescents: do immediate postpartum contraceptive implants make a difference? Am J Obstet Gynecol. 2012;206(481):e1–7.
37. Robinson NA, Moshabela M, Owusu-Ansah L, Kapungu C, Geller S. Barriers to intrauterine device uptake in a rural setting in Ghana. Health Care Women Int. 2016;37(2):197–215.

23

Recent trends, risk factors, and disparities in low birth weight in California, 2005–2014: a retrospective study

Anura W. G. Ratnasiri[1,3*], Steven S. Parry[1], Vivi N. Arief[3], Ian H. DeLacy[3], Laura A. Halliday[2], Ralph J. DiLibero[1] and Kaye E. Basford[3,4]

Abstract

Background: Low birth weight (LBW) is a leading risk factor for infant morbidity and mortality in the United States. There are large disparities in the prevalence of LBW by race and ethnicity, especially between African American and White women. Despite extensive research, the practice of clinical and public health, and policies devoted to reducing the number of LBW infants, the prevalence of LBW has remained unacceptably and consistently high. There have been few detailed studies identifying the factors associated with LBW in California, which is home to a highly diverse population. The aim of this study is to investigate recent trends in the prevalence of LBW infants (measured as a percentage) and to identify risk factors and disparities associated with LBW in California.

Methods: A retrospective cohort study included data on 5,267,519 births recorded in the California Birth Statistical Master Files for the period 2005–2014. These data included maternal characteristics, health behaviors, information on health insurance, prenatal care use, and parity. Logistic regression models identified significant risk factors associated with LBW. Using gestational age based on obstetric estimates (OA), small for gestational age (SGA), appropriate for gestational age (AGA) and large for gestational age (LGA) infants were identified for the periods 2007–2014.

Results: The number of LBW infants declined, from 37,603 in 2005 to 33,447 in 2014. However, the prevalence of LBW did not change significantly (6.9% in 2005 to 6.7% in 2014). The mean maternal age at first delivery increased from 25.7 years in 2005 to 27.2 years in 2014. The adjusted odds ratio showed that women aged 40 to 54 years were twice as likely to have an LBW infant as women in the 20 to 24 age group. African American women had a persistent 2.4-fold greater prevalence of having an LBW infant compared with white women. Maternal age was a significant risk factor for LBW regardless of maternal race and ethnicity or education level. During the period 2017–2014, 5.4% of the singleton births at 23–41 weeks based on OE of gestational age were SGA infants (preterm SGA + term SGA). While all the preterm SGA infants were LBW, both preterm AGA and term SGA infants had a higher prevalence of LBW.

Conclusions: In California, during the 10 years from 2005 to 2014, there was no significant decline in the prevalence of LBW. However, maternal age was a significant risk factor for LBW regardless of maternal race and ethnicity or education level. Therefore, there may be opportunities to reduce the prevalence of LBW by reducing disparities and improving birth outcomes for women of advanced maternal age.

Keywords: Low birth weight, Preterm birth, Prenatal care, Advance maternal age, Maternal health, Health behavior, Small for gestational age

* Correspondence: Anura.Ratnasiri2@dhcs.ca.gov
[1]Department of Health Care Services, Benefits Division, 1501 Capitol Ave, Suite 71.4104, MS 4600, P.O. Box 997417, Sacramento, CA 95899-7417, USA
[3]School of Agriculture and Food Sciences, Faculty of Science, The University of Queensland, Brisbane, Qld 4072, Australia
Full list of author information is available at the end of the article

Background

The terminology currently used to describe infants with a low birth weight (LBW) for a given gestational age varies, including the terms small for gestational age, intrauterine growth restriction, and fetal growth restriction (FGR) [1, 2]. Small for gestational age is defined as a birth weight below the tenth percentile for gestational age [1]. However, some infants with a birth weight below the tenth percentile are normal, and their low weight is due to maternal constitutional factors including weight, height, parity, and ethnicity. These infants do not necessarily have an increased risk for perinatal morbidity and mortality [1, 2]. The term FGR is defined as an antepartum estimated fetal weight less than the tenth percentile for gestational age and its presence may be due to genetic or environmental factors. Most infants with FGR are born small for gestational age. Moderate FGR is defined as a birth weight in the third to tenth percentile, and severe FGR is defined as a birth weight less than the third percentile [1, 2].

The prevalence of LBW is greater in resource-limited countries. While current data show that up to 10% of term infants in developed countries have LBW, that figure is 20% in developing countries [3]. A recent report indicates that 19% of infants in resource-limited areas are born with LBW, and 22% of reported neonatal deaths occur in infants with LBW [3]. In 2012, the Child Health Epidemiology Reference Group evaluated 14 birth cohorts and applied the birth weight standards specified by the International Fetal and Newborn Growth Consortium for the twenty-first Century (INTERGROWTH-21st). Using this definition, LBW was found in 19.3% of live births in low-income and middle-income countries, and 22% of neonatal deaths occurred in infants born small for gestational age [3].

Perinatal mortality increases in infants with LBW, whether they are born at term or preterm [2, 4, 5]. Perinatal mortality increases as birth weight decreases, as shown in a recently published population-based study from Canada, where the highest infant mortality was found in infants with a birth weight less than the fifth percentile, for both term and preterm infants [5]. There are several factors that contribute to increased morbidity and mortality in LBW infants, including congenital malformations, cardiac and respiratory disorders, and perinatal asphyxia [2]. According to the INTERGROWTH-21st standards, infants with LBW are those born weighing less than 2500 g. Intrauterine growth restriction and preterm birth are often associated with LBW. Outcomes associated with LBW include short-term fetal or neonatal morbidity, including respiratory distress syndrome and necrotizing enterocolitis; long-term morbidity, including blindness and cerebral palsy; and early neonatal and infant mortality [6].

In 1995, David Barker first proposed that the fetal environment and early infant health status permanently program the development of the individual into old age, a theory known as the Barker hypothesis, or "fetal origins of adult disease" [7, 8]. Several epidemiological studies have confirmed that LBW is associated not only with developmental issues in surviving infants [9], but with the development of chronic conditions or diseases in adulthood, including coronary artery disease [9–13], stroke, reduced bone mass, dyslipidemia, hypertension, type II diabetes mellitus [14], cancer, osteoporosis, and psychiatric illnesses [8, 15–18]. Despite extensive research devoted to reducing the number of LBW infants, as well as policy statements and clinical and public health practices with the same aim, the prevalence of LBW in the United States has remained unacceptably and consistently high. In addition, racial and ethnic disparities in birth outcomes are well documented in the United States.

Life course health development models may be used to improve public health outcomes, including in the maternal and child health community [19]. As Pies and Kotelchuck (2014) described, there is a need for a framework to address the social determinants and causes of health inequalities and the current facilitators of disparities in maternal and infant health [20, 21].

The aim of this study is to examine the current trends in the prevalence of LBW in California, using the Birth Statistical Master Files (BSMF) compiled by the California Department of Public Health (CDPH), and to identify significant predictors of LBW and racial and ethnic disparities in LBW. By identifying these risk factors and disparities, intervention strategies can be developed to reduce the prevalence of LBW and improve the health of the general population, now and into the future.

Methods

Data sources and study design

We consulted the BSMF, compiled by the CDPH, for the period 2005 through 2014. The study was approved by the California Committee for the Protection of Human Subjects (Protocol ID: 16–10-2759) and the CDPH Vital Statistics Advisory Committee.

In this retrospective cohort study, we collected data on Californian resident births in the years 2005 to 2014. Descriptive statistics were used to characterize all resident births and the prevalence of LBW each year, according to maternal characteristics and perinatal health behavior variables obtained from the BSMF data set.

LBW as a response variable

The response variable in this study was LBW infants. Birth weight was obtained from the birth files and coded as a dichotomous variable to indicate whether the infant was LBW (< 2500 g). Data cleaning was performed before analysis to exclude births with missing information on birth weight and those with any out-of-range values. There were 877 excluded birth records out of 5,267,519 resident births from 2005 to 2014.

Explanatory maternal variables

The explanatory variables considered were maternal socio-demographic status, prenatal health behavior, health insurance status, prenatal care use during the first trimester, and parity [22]. Maternal sociodemographic characteristics included maternal age, education, race and ethnicity, and place of birth and residence. Prenatal health behaviors included smoking during both first and second trimesters and maternal prepregnancy body mass index (BMI). Obesity is commonly classified according to BMI, which is calculated as the individual's weight in kilograms divided by their height in meters squared (kg/m^2). Using the criteria of the World Health Organization, underweight is classified as a BMI < 18.5 kg/m^2, normal weight as 18.5 to 24.9 kg/m^2, overweight as 25.0 to 29.9 kg/m^2; obesity class I as 30.0 to 34.9 kg/m^2, obese obesity class II as 35.0 to 39.9, kg/m^2 and obesity class III as $\geq$ 40 kg/m^2 [23]. The type of health insurance was divided into public (Medi-Cal) and private, considered crude predictors of low and high income, respectively.

Relationship between birth weight and gestational age on fetal growth

Gestational age affects fetal growth and birth weight can be categorized as small for gestational age (SGA) (< 10th percentile), appropriate for gestational age (AGA) (10th to 90th percentile), and large for gestational age (LGA) (> 90th percentile), using new gender specific intra-uterine growth curves based on United States data by Olsen et al. (2010) [24].

We extended these three categories to six categories by characterizing gestational age of 23–41 weeks for singleton births as preterm (< 37 weeks of gestation) and term ($\geq$ 37 weeks of gestation) births: preterm SGA, preterm AGA, preterm LGA, term SGA, term AGA, and term LGA [3]. The preterm AGA and term SGA groups were further extended into with and without LBW (< 2500 g) infants.

Statistical analysis

To identify significant risk factors among the maternal characteristics and perinatal maternal health behaviors associated with LBW, we performed both unadjusted and adjusted logistic regression analysis. The adjusted analysis used multivariable logistic regression, controlling for potential confounding variables in maternal and perinatal health behaviors.

The analysis was extended to study the prevalence of LBW based on all births according to two different interaction scenarios: first, between maternal age and maternal race and ethnicity; and second, between maternal education level and maternal race and ethnicity. Finally, multivariate logistic regression modeling approaches were used to study these two interaction scenarios after controlling for appropriate confounding variables. Multivariate modeling was stratified by maternal age and maternal education level to elaborate disparities in race and ethnicity and to identify the high-risk subgroups. The reference groups for maternal age, race and ethnicity, and education level were the age group 20–24 years, white race, and an education level of a bachelor's degree or higher, respectively. Calculated adjusted odds ratios (AORs) with 95% confidence intervals (95% CI) and p values are presented in the tables.

The logistic regression models were restricted to singleton births. The significance level was set at $p = 0.05$. All analyses were conducted using SAS, version 9.3 (SAS Institute Inc., Cary, NC, USA).

Results

The descriptive statistics for the 5,267,519 resident births that occurred in California during the 10-year period from 2005 to 2014 are listed in Additional file 1: Table S1 in the Supplementary Materials. During this period, the mean maternal age for primiparous women increased by 1. 5 years, from 25.7 years in 2005 to 27.2 years in 2014.

Table 1 shows the prevalence of LBW, according to each variable evaluated. Although the number of LBW infants decreased, from 37,603 in 2005 to 33,447 in 2014, the prevalence of LBW did not change significantly during the study period (6.9% in 2005 to 6.7% in 2014).

Both unadjusted and adjusted logistic regression analyses (Table 2) showed significant differences in the prevalence of LBW within each characteristic studied: maternal age, education level, race and ethnicity, place of birth and residence, demographic region, smoking status, prepregnancy BMI, source of perinatal care payment, first-trimester perinatal care, and parity (all $p < 0.001$).

Maternal age

The prevalence of births in younger women declined over the study period (Additional file 1: Table S1). Births in women younger than 20 years decreased by 41%, from 9.3% in 2005 to 5.4% in 2014. In young adults (age 20–24 years), births decreased by 18%, from 22.9% in 2005 to 18.8% in 2014. In contrast, births in older women increased over the 10-year study period. Births in women aged 40–54 years increased by 20%, from 3.5% in 2005 to 4.3% in 2014; similar trends were observed for women in the age groups 30–34 years and 35–39 years. Table 1 shows the prevalence of LBW according to maternal

Table 1 Total number of low birth weight infants and prevalence according to maternal characteristics and perinatal health behaviors in California for the period 2005–2014

Year	2005	2006	2007	2008	2009	2010	2011	2012	2013	2014
Number of low birth weight infants	37,603	38,460	38,867	37,580	35,774	34,624	33,956	33,657	33,718	33,447
Percentage of low birth weight infants	6.9	6.8	6.9	6.8	6.8	6.8	6.8	6.7	6.8	6.7
Variable										
Maternal age (years)										
< 20	7.7	7.4	7.6	7.5	7.4	7.5	7.3	7.1	7.4	7.2
20–24	6.3	6.2	6.3	6.2	6.1	6.2	6.2	6.2	6.4	6.4
25–29	6.2	6.1	6.1	6.0	6.1	6.0	6.0	6.0	6.1	5.9
30–34	6.6	6.7	6.7	6.6	6.6	6.6	6.5	6.5	6.6	6.4
35–39	7.9	7.9	8.0	8.0	7.8	7.8	7.9	7.7	7.7	7.6
40–54	11.3	11.2	11.0	11.4	11.2	11.1	11.0	10.4	10.9	10.5
Maternal race and ethnicity										
Hispanic	6.2	6.3	6.3	6.1	6.2	6.2	6.2	6.1	6.4	6.3
White	6.5	6.3	6.4	6.4	6.2	6.1	6.1	5.7	6.0	5.7
Asian	7.6	7.7	7.6	7.8	8.1	7.9	7.9	7.9	7.7	7.2
Pacific Islander	7.2	7.5	6.9	6.9	6.3	7.1	7.3	6.5	6.4	6.6
African American	12.8	12.2	12.1	12.4	12.0	12.2	11.8	12.0	11.7	11.8
Multiple race	7.8	7.6	7.8	7.0	7.6	7.7	7.1	7.5	7.3	7.6
American Indian	6.6	6.7	7.5	7.6	6.4	6.8	6.2	6.6	7.0	6.3
Other/unknown	9.1	9.6	10.2	10.0	9.3	10.0	10.1	9.8	10.2	10.0
Maternal education level										
Less than high school diploma	6.6	6.7	6.6	6.5	6.6	6.7	6.6	6.5	6.8	6.9
High school diploma	7.0	6.8	6.7	6.8	6.6	6.6	6.7	6.5	6.7	6.6
Some college or associate degree	6.9	6.9	7.0	6.9	6.7	6.9	6.8	6.7	6.9	6.7
Bachelor's degree or higher	6.8	6.9	7.0	6.9	6.9	6.7	6.6	6.6	6.5	6.2
Unknown	8.2	8.7	8.6	9.0	8.6	8.6	8.9	8.7	9.1	8.8
Maternal nativity										
Foreign-born	6.2	6.3	6.4	6.3	6.4	6.4	6.5	6.5	6.6	6.5
United States-born	7.4	7.3	7.3	7.3	7.1	7.1	7.0	6.8	6.9	6.8
Maternal demographic region										
Central Coast	6.4	6.3	6.1	6.2	6.0	5.8	6.1	5.9	6.2	6.0
Greater Bay Area	6.8	6.9	6.7	6.7	6.8	6.8	6.9	6.9	7.0	6.7
Inland Empire	6.9	6.7	6.9	6.9	6.8	6.8	6.7	6.9	7.1	6.8
Los Angeles County	7.3	7.4	7.4	7.3	7.2	7.3	7.1	6.9	7.0	6.9
Northern and Sierra	6.4	5.9	6.1	6.0	5.4	5.7	6.0	5.8	6.4	6.3
Orange County	6.4	6.4	6.5	6.4	6.6	6.4	6.7	6.3	6.2	6.3
Sacramento area	7.1	7.2	7.1	6.7	6.8	7.2	7.0	6.9	6.8	7.1
San Diego area	6.7	6.5	6.9	6.6	6.6	6.4	6.4	6.3	6.4	6.4
San Joaquin Valley	6.7	6.8	6.8	7.0	6.9	7.0	6.9	6.8	7.1	6.9
Source of prenatal care payment										
Private	6.8	6.8	6.9	6.9	6.8	6.8	6.9	6.7	6.8	6.6
Medi-Cal	6.7	6.7	6.7	6.6	6.6	6.6	6.6	6.6	6.8	6.8
First trimester prenatal care initiation										
Yes	6.7	6.7	6.8	6.8	6.7	6.7	6.7	6.6	6.8	6.6

Table 1 Total number of low birth weight infants and prevalence according to maternal characteristics and perinatal health behaviors in California for the period 2005–2014 *(Continued)*

Year	2005	2006	2007	2008	2009	2010	2011	2012	2013	2014
No	7.6	7.2	6.8	6.6	6.7	6.8	6.8	6.7	6.7	6.8
Parity										
Primiparous	7.2	7.1	7.2	7.1	7.1	7.1	7.1	7.0	7.1	6.9
Multiparous (2–5)	6.5	6.5	6.5	6.5	6.4	6.4	6.4	6.4	6.5	6.4
Multiparous (6–12)	11.1	10.3	10.4	10.4	10.3	10.4	9.9	9.7	10.3	10.5
Plurality										
Singleton births	5.2	5.2	5.3	5.2	5.2	5.3	5.2	5.2	5.3	5.1
Multiple births	56.9	57.1	56.8	56.0	55.4	54.6	54.7	53.8	53.6	52.7
Maternal smoking during both first and second trimesters										
No	N/A	N/A	6.8	6.7	6.7	6.7	6.7	6.6	6.7	6.6
Yes	N/A	N/A	11.3	11.2	11.6	11.4	11.9	12.3	12.5	12.6
Prepregnancy body mass index (kg/m^2)										
Underweight (≤18.5)	N/A	N/A	9.5	9.7	9.7	9.5	9.3	8.8	9.2	9.2
Normal (18.5–24.9)	N/A	N/A	6.7	6.8	6.7	6.7	6.7	6.6	6.8	6.5
Overweight (25.0–29.9)	N/A	N/A	6.3	6.1	6.0	6.2	6.3	6.3	6.3	6.3
Obese I (30.0–34.9)	N/A	N/A	6.6	6.3	6.5	6.7	6.5	6.2	6.5	6.7
Obese II (35.0–39.9)	N/A	N/A	6.8	6.9	7.0	6.6	6.2	6.9	6.8	6.6
Obese III (≥ 40)	N/A	N/A	6.9	7.0	6.5	7.3	6.6	6.9	7.2	6.7

All values are given as percentages, except for the number of low birth weight infants
N/A = Maternal smoking status and the variables needed to compute prepregnancy body mass index were not recorded during 2005 or 2006

characteristics and perinatal health behaviors for each year of the study period.

The unadjusted prevalence and AORs of LBW for singleton births by maternal age is presented in Fig. 1. Women in the oldest age group (40–54 years) were twice as likely to have an LBW infant than women in the 20–24 years reference age group (AOR, 2.01; 95% CI, 1.95–2.06). The 35–39 years age group was 54% more likely to have an LBW infant compared with the reference age group (AOR, 1.54; 95% CI, 1.51–1.56). Women in the 30–34 years age group had a 25% greater chance of having an LBW infant (AOR, 1.25; 95% CI, 1.23–1.27) (Fig. 1 and Table 2). Maternal age was a significant predictor of LBW in California.

Maternal race and ethnicity

Almost 50% of births in California were to women of Hispanic ethnicity, followed by women who were White and Asian. Women of Asian ethnicity accounted for more than 32% of the increase in LBW births, from 11.3% in 2005 to 14.9% in 2014 (Additional file 1: Table S1).

In 2014, the overall prevalence of LBW was 6.7% (Table 1). However, 11.8% of infants born to African American women were LBW compared with 5.7% of those born to White women and 6.3% of those born to Hispanic women (Table 1). In 2014, the prevalence of LBW infants born to African American women was nearly twice that of

White women and 88% greater than in Hispanic women. From 2005 to 2014, the prevalence of LBW births decreased at a slower rate in African American women (7.7%) compared with White women (12.3%).

As shown in Table 2, there were marked disparities in the prevalence of LBW infants born to women of different racial and ethnic groups. African American women had a persistent 2.4-fold prevalence of LBW infants throughout the study period compared with White women (AOR, 2.41; 95% CI, 2.36–2.46).

Compared with White women, Asian women were 80% more likely to give birth to an LBW infant (AOR, 1.80; 95% CI, 1.76–1.83). Pacific Islanders were 50% more likely to give birth to an LBW infant than White women (AOR, 1.50; 95% CI, 1.39–1.62), and Hispanic women were 30% more likely to give birth to an LBW infant than White women (AOR, 1.30; 95% CI, 1.28–1.32) (Table 2).

Interaction between maternal age and maternal race and ethnicity

To identify the association between maternal age and race and ethnicity for LBW, we cross-tabulated the data for LBW according to these two variables. As shown in Fig. 2, the prevalence of LBW was not consistent across maternal age for racial and ethnic groups. African American women had a consistently higher prevalence of LBW compared with other races and ethnicities in

Table 2 Crude and adjusted odds ratio of low birth weight singleton births according to maternal characteristics and perinatal health behaviors in California for the period 2005–2014

Variable	Crude odds ratio		Adjusted odds ratio	
	OR (95% CI)	p value[a]	AOR (95% CL)	p value[a]
Maternal age (years)				
< 20	1.28 (1.26–1.30)	< .001	1.04 (1.01–1.06)	0.001
25–29	0.90 (0.89–0.91)	< .001	1.09 (1.07–1.11)	< .001
30–34	0.92 (0.91–0.94)	< .001	1.25 (1.23–1.27)	< .001
35–39	1.08 (1.06–1.09)	< .001	1.54 (1.51–1.56)	< .001
40–54	1.41 (1.38–1.44)	< .001	2.01 (1.95–2.06)	< .001
20–24 (ref)	Ref		Ref	
Maternal race and ethnicity				
African American	2.57 (2.53–2.62)	< .001	2.41 (2.36–2.46)	< .001
American Indian	1.40 (1.30–1.50)	< .001	1.31 (1.21–1.43)	< .001
Asian	1.53 (1.51–1.55)	< .001	1.80 (1.76–1.83)	< .001
Hispanic	1.27 (1.26–1.29)	< .001	1.30 (1.28–1.32)	< .001
Multiple race	1.45 (1.40–1.49)	< .001	1.41 (1.36–1.45)	< .001
Other/unknown	1.63 (1.58–1.68)	< .001	1.52 (1.45–1.59)	< .001
Pacific Islander	1.40 (1.31–1.50)	< .001	1.50 (1.39–1.62)	< .001
White (ref)	Ref		Ref	
Maternal education level				
Less than high school diploma	1.29 (1.28–1.31)	< .001	1.36 (1.34–1.39)	< .001
High school diploma	1.25 (1.24–1.27)	< .001	1.29 (1.27–1.31)	< .001
Some college or associate degree	1.23 (1.22–1.25)	< .001	1.27 (1.25–1.29)	< .001
Unknown	1.46 (1.43–1.49)	< .001	1.34 (1.29–1.39)	< .001
Bachelor's degree or higher (ref)	Ref		Ref	
Maternal nativity				
United States-born	1.06 (1.05–1.07)	< .001	1.15 (1.13–1.16)	< .001
Foreign-born (ref)	Ref		Ref	
Maternal demographic region				
Central Coast	0.98 (0.95–1.01)	0.246	1.06 (1.03–1.11)	0.001
Greater Bay Area	1.09 (1.06–1.13)	< .001	1.06 (1.02–1.09)	0.001
Inland Empire	1.16 (1.13–1.19)	< .001	1.16 (1.12–1.20)	< .001
Los Angeles County	1.21 (1.17–1.24)	< .001	1.15 (1.11–1.18)	< .001
Orange County	1.02 (0.99–1.05)	0.274	1.06 (1.02–1.10)	0.001
Sacramento area	1.07 (1.03–1.10)	< .001	1.07 (1.03–1.11)	< .001
San Diego area	1.04 (1.01–1.08)	0.006	1.10 (1.06–1.14)	< .001
San Joaquin Valley	1.21 (1.18–1.25)	< .001	1.20 (1.16–1.24)	< .001
Northern and Sierra	Ref		Ref	
Source of prenatal care payment				
Medi-Cal (Public)	1.17 (1.16–1.19)	< .001	1.13 (1.12–1.15)	< .001
Private insurance (ref)	Ref		Ref	
First trimester prenatal care initiation				
No	1.11 (1.10–1.13)	< .001	1.03 (1.02–1.04)	< .001
Yes (ref)	Ref		Ref	

Table 2 Crude and adjusted odds ratio of low birth weight singleton births according to maternal characteristics and perinatal health behaviors in California for the period 2005–2014 *(Continued)*

Variable	Crude odds ratio		Adjusted odds ratio	
	OR (95% CI)	p value[a]	AOR (95% CL)	p value[a]
Parity				
Primiparous	1.40 (1.39–1.42)	< .001	1.57 (1.55–1.58)	< .001
Multiparous (6–12)	1.67 (1.63–1.72)	< .001	1.20 (1.17–1.25)	< .001
Multiparous (2–5) (ref)	Ref		Ref	
Maternal smoking during both first and second trimesters				
Yes	2.11 (2.05–2.16)	< .001	1.98 (1.92–2.04)	< .001
No (ref)	Ref		Ref	
Maternal prepregnancy body mass index (kg/m^2)				
Underweight (< 18.5)	1.58 (1.55–1.61)	< .001	1.49 (1.46–1.52)	< .001
Overweight (25.0–29.9)	0.95 (0.94–0.96)	< .001	0.95 (0.94–0.97)	< .001
Obese I (30.0–34.9)	1.00 (0.99–1.02)	0.919	0.99 (0.97–1.00)	0.118
Obese II (35.0–39.9)	1.04 (1.02–1.06)	< .001	1.01 (0.99–1.04)	0.315
Obese III (≥ 40)	1.08 (1.06–1.11)	< .001	1.02 (0.99–1.05)	0.237
Normal (18.5–24.9) (ref)	Ref		Ref	

AOR adjusted odds ratio, *BMI* body mass index, *CI* confidence interval, *OR* odds ratio

Ref = Reference group

[a] *p* value determined using the χ^2 test

each maternal age group. The wide gap in the prevalence of LBW between African American and White or Hispanic women was consistent for each age group (Fig. 2). Moreover, an almost equivalent higher observed prevalence of LBW was observed for Asian women in the youngest and oldest age groups, resulting in a U-shaped response (Fig. 2). All race and ethnic groups showed rising prevalence of LBW with increasing age, especially from 30 years of age (Fig. 2), but the rate of increase was greatest for American Indian women.

Additional file 1: Table S2 provides the adjusted odds ratios for maternal age for each racial and ethnic group. As indicated in the unadjusted prevalence (Fig. 2), the likelihood of having a LBW infant was greater with increasing

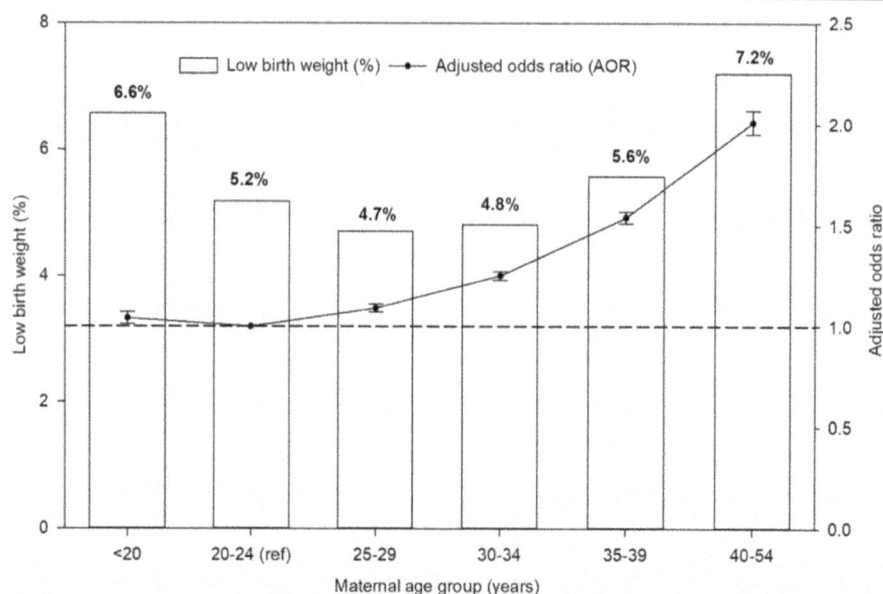

Fig. 1 Unadjusted prevalence and adjusted odds ratios of low birth weight of singleton births by maternal age in California for the period 2005–2014

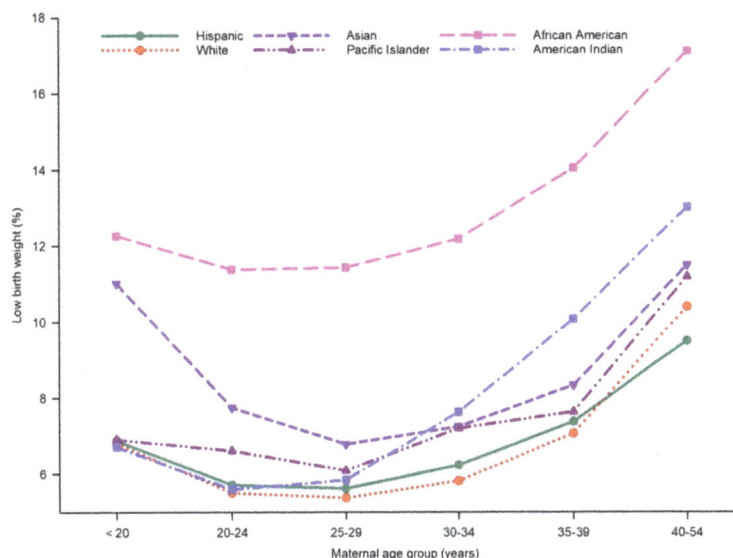

Fig. 2 Unadjusted prevalence of low birth weight by maternal age and maternal race and ethnicity in California for the period 2005–2014

maternal age, mostly from 30 years of age, with the highest prevalence for women in the age group 40–54 years. In contrast to other race and ethnic groups, Asian women were more likely to have LBW infants when they were younger, less than 20 years of age, compared with the reference group - women in the age group 20–24 years. American Indian women with a maternal age of 40–54 years were three times more likely to have LBW infants than the reference age group of 20–24 years (Additional file 1: Table S2).

Maternal education level

In California, births in women with less than a complete high school education decreased by 40%, from 27.3% in 2005 to 16.3% in 2014. During the same period, births in women with a high school diploma as their highest level of education decreased by 12% (Additional file 1: Table S1).

Table 1 shows the prevalence of LBW according to maternal education level. The prevalence of LBW differed in women by education level, although these variations were smaller than those observed for differing age or racial-ethnic group (Table 1). Women with less than a high school diploma had a 36% greater chance (AOR, 1.36; 95% CI, 1.34–1.39) of having an LBW infant than the reference group of women with a bachelor's degree or higher (Table 2).

Interaction between maternal education level and race and ethnicity

To elaborate on the differences in LBW prevalence between maternal educational levels and race and ethnicity, we cross-tabulated the data for LBW accordingly. As shown in Fig. 3, the prevalence of LBW from lower

to higher educational levels differed across racial and ethnic groups (Fig. 2). Unadjusted LBW prevalence was quite similar for women of Hispanic ethnicity, regardless of their educational level, but the magnitude of the disparity varied for other races (Fig. 3). African American women of all education levels had a higher unadjusted prevalence of LBW than women of every other race and education level. The higher prevalence of LBW was most prominent among African American women with a less than high school diploma. However, prevalence of LBW significantly declined with higher educational attainment, with the lowest prevalence among women with a bachelor's degree or higher (Fig. 3).

Additional file 1: Table S3 presents adjusted odds ratios for maternal education level for each racial and ethnic group. Women in most race and ethnic groups with educational level less than a high school diploma were more likely to deliver LBW infants when compared with women having a bachelor's degree or higher, but to a lesser extent for Asian and Pacific Islander women (Additional file 1: Table S3).

Maternal place of birth

From 2005 to 2014, births to foreign-born women decreased by 18%, and births to United States-born women increased by almost 16% (Additional file 1: Table S1). Women born in the United States were 15% more likely (AOR, 1.15; 95% CI, 1.13–1.16) to have an LBW infant than were foreign-born women (Table 2).

Maternal geographic region

Within each year, almost 26% of California births occurred in Los Angeles County, followed by the greater

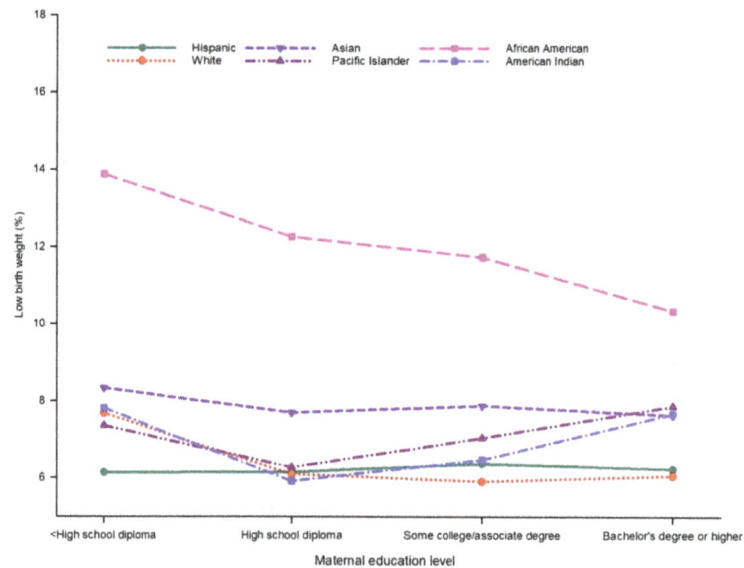

Fig. 3 Unadjusted prevalence of low birth weight by maternal education level and maternal race and ethnicity in California for the period 2005–2014

Bay Area region with slightly more than 17%, and San Joaquin Valley with about 13% of births in the state (Additional file 1: Table S1). Women in the San Joaquin Valley region were 20% more likely (AOR, 1.20; 95% CI, 1.16–1.24) to have an LBW infant compared with those in the Northern and Sierra regions (Table 2).

Perinatal health behaviors

Maternal smoking during both first and second trimesters decreased significantly, by 31%, from 2007 to 2014 (Additional file 1: Table S1). Women who smoked during the first and second trimesters of pregnancy were almost twice as likely (AOR, 1.98; 95% CI, 1.92–2.04) to have an LBW infant than women who did not smoke (Table 2).

The prevalence of LBW births in women who were underweight or of normal weight, based on their prepregnancy BMI, decreased by 9.1 and 6.3%, respectively, from 2007 to 2014. However, the prevalence of LBW births to women who were in the obese I, obese II, and obese III categories increased by 12.0, 21.3, and 26.9%, respectively, from 2007 to 2014 (Table 1). While obesity did not increase the likelihood of LBW, underweight women (prepregnancy BMI < 18.5 kg/m^2) were 49% more likely to have an LBW infant than were women of normal prepregnancy weight (AOR, 1.49; 95% CI, 1.46–1.52) (Table 2).

Insurance type and first-trimester perinatal care

Consistent trends were observed for the percentages of births paid for by Medi-Cal and private insurance. The 2014 figures for California show that 52.7% of births were covered by private insurance and 47.3% were covered by Medi-Cal. Women dependent on Medi-Cal as

their source of perinatal care payment were 13% more likely to have an LBW infant than women with private insurance (AOR, 1.13; 95% CI, 1.12–1.15) (Table 2). Overall, the use of first-trimester perinatal care decreased slightly, from 86.6% in 2005 to 83.2% in 2014.

Birth characteristics

From 2005 to 2014, the prevalence of multiple births was consistent at 3.2% (Additional file 1: Table S1). Parity was consistent over the study period for each of the three groups considered: primiparous, multiparous with 2 to 5 deliveries, and multiparous with 6 to 12 deliveries (Additional file 1: Table S1). Women who were primiparous (AOR, 1.57; 95% CI, 1.55–1.58) or multiparous with 6 to 12 births (AOR, 1.20; 95% CI, 1.17–1.25) were more likely to have an LBW infant than multiparous women with 2 to 5 births (Table 2).

Relationship between birth weight and gestational age on fetal growth

Information on 3,974,973 singleton births in California for the period 2007–2014 was available to elaborate on the relationship between birth weight and gestational age based on OE (Fig. 4). For these births at 23–41 weeks, the 7% of preterm births (< 37 weeks of gestation) comprised of 0.5% preterm SGA, 5.6% preterm AGA, and 1.0% preterm LGA. Among preterm AGA, 49.2% of births were LBW infants while 100% of the preterm SGA births were LBW infants (Fig. 4).

Of the 93% of term births (≥ 37 weeks of gestation), 4.9% were term SGA births, 81.7% term AGA births, and 6.4% term LGA births. Among term SGA births, the

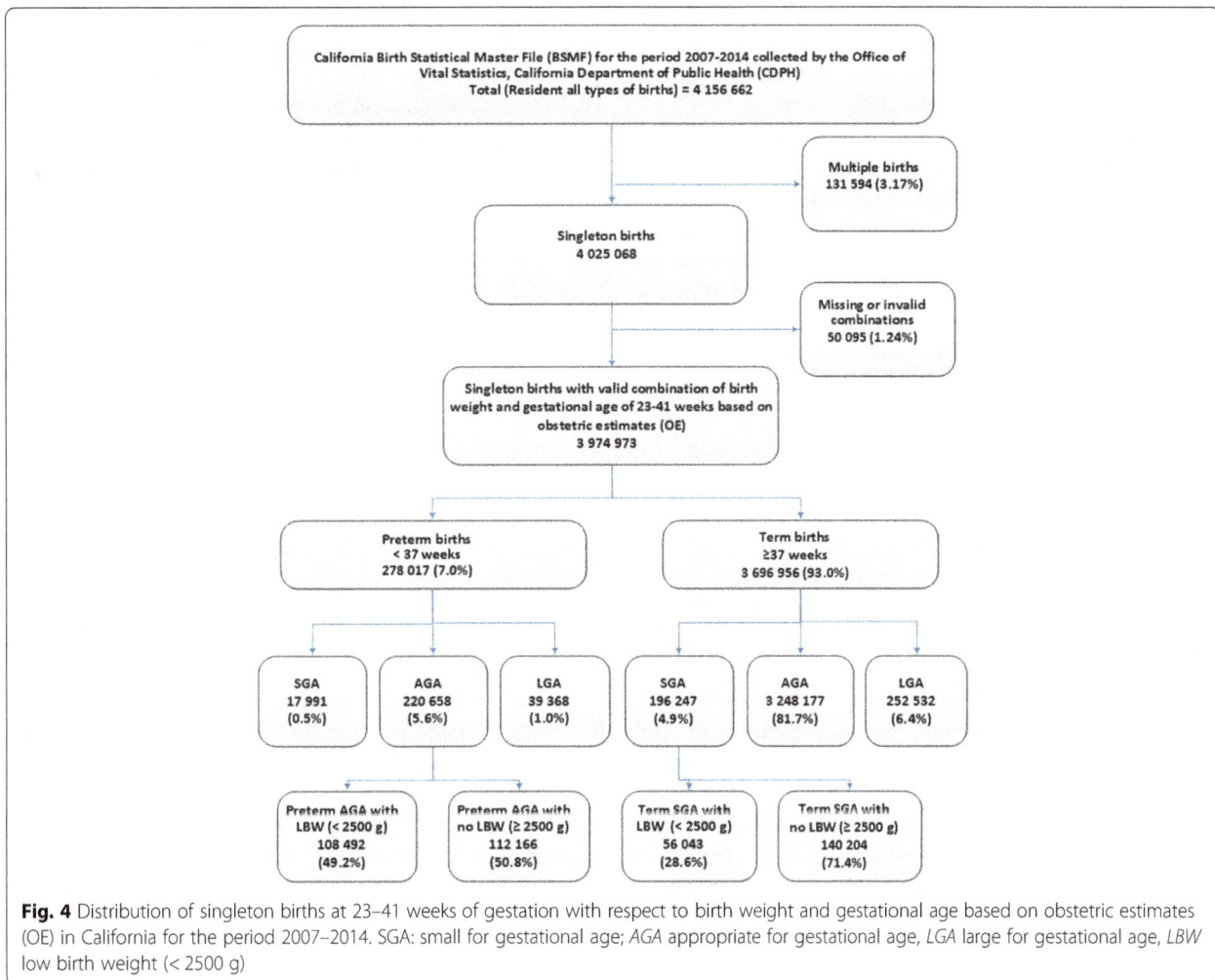

Fig. 4 Distribution of singleton births at 23–41 weeks of gestation with respect to birth weight and gestational age based on obstetric estimates (OE) in California for the period 2007–2014. SGA: small for gestational age; *AGA* appropriate for gestational age, *LGA* large for gestational age, *LBW* low birth weight (< 2500 g)

prevalence of LBW was 28.6% (Fig. 4). Overall, 5.4% of these singleton births at 23 to 41 weeks based on OE of gestational age were SGA infants (preterm SGA + term SGA).

Discussion

This retrospective cohort study, evaluating 5,267,519 resident births that occurred in California from 2005 to 2014, shows that the prevalence of LBW did not change significantly over that 10-year period.

Births to older women, aged from 30 to 54 years, increased over the study period, a trend that is consistent with the steadily increasing national mean maternal age since 2006 [22, 25–28]. The term "advanced maternal age" is used for women who are aged 35 years or greater at the time of delivery; advanced maternal age is considered a major risk factor for poorer pregnancy and perinatal outcomes [29, 30]. Sauer (2015) discussed the underlying reasons for the increased LBW prevalence in women of advanced maternal age [28]. The strong association between maternal age and birth weight reported by other studies was also found in our study [25, 31]. Women 35–39 years

of age were more likely, and women aged 40–54 years were twice as likely, to have an LBW baby compared with women aged 20–24 years. Women aged less than 20 years and aged 40–54 years had a higher prevalence of LBW infants, regardless of their education level. However, Goisis et al. (2017) found that advanced maternal age is not independently associated with the risk of LBW or preterm delivery among women who have had at least 2 previous live births [30].

Disparities in the prevalence of LBW infants between racial and ethnic groups in the United States have been well documented [32, 33]. The persistence of a gap in LBW prevalence between African Americans and Whites is seen throughout the country and continues to be a serious public health problem (Table 1).

The findings of our study are consistent with those of previously published studies that have reported substantial disparities in the prevalence of LBW between women of different racial and ethnic groups. In our study, African American women had a more than 2-fold increase in the prevalence of LBW throughout the study period compared with White women (Table 2). The wide gap in the preva-lence of LBW between African American and White or Hispanic women was consistent for each age group and across the 10-year period of the study.

During 2005, the prevalence of LBW in Hispanic women was 0.3% lower than in White women (6.2% vs. 6.5%). However, the prevalence of LBW was 0.6% greater in Hispanic births compared with births in White women (6.3% vs. 5.7%) in 2014. Therefore, given the increasing number of Hispanic births in California, the findings of this 10-year study provide an alert to the increasing gap in birth weights between Hispanic and White babies.

Overall, the prevalence of LBW when the mother is 40–54 years of age is double that when she is 20–24 years of age. This finding holds true for all groups except for Asian women and those a Multirace origin. Even at the highest education level, African American women had a greater prevalence of LBW compared with other ethnic groups, suggesting persistent disparities based on ethnicity.

The prevalence of United States adults who smoke cig-arettes declined, from 20.9% in 2005 to 16.8% in 2014 [34]. Consistent with national studies, the number of women in our study who smoked tobacco during the first and second trimester decreased between 2007 and 2014 (Table 1). However, pregnant smokers have been reported to be almost twice as likely to have an LBW in-fant than nonsmokers [35]. The latest United States Sur-geon General's Report on Smoking and Health states that tobacco use during pregnancy remains a major pre-ventable cause of disease and death of the mother, fetus, and infant [36]. Women who smoke during pregnancy are more likely to deliver LBW babies, even if the preg-nancy is carried to full term.

Data on maternal smoking and prepregnancy height and weight have been collected in California only since 2007; this study is the first to report trends in prepreg-nancy BMI. The results of our study provide population-based information on BMI for women of childbearing age. The prevalence of births in women who were under-weight or of normal weight, based on prepregnancy BMI, decreased during the study period, but the prevalence of births to women who were in the obese I, obese II, and obese III categories increased significantly (Table 2). Con-sistent with previous studies, ours found that underweight women are more likely to have an LBW infant than women with a normal prepregnancy weight [37, 38]. Our study found no significant association between prepreg-nancy obesity and the risk of having an LBW infant.

The rising prevalence of women in all three obesity classes in California is a public health concern for both women and children. According to a recent Institute of Medicine report, maternal obesity before, during, and after pregnancy poses serious health problems for both mothers and children [39]. Obesity contributes to gestational diabetes

[40–42], preterm delivery [40, 42, 43], fetal injury during de-livery, intrauterine mortality [44], and shorter duration of breastfeeding [45]. The long-term outcomes of maternal obesity include chronic disease such as diabetes, cardio-vascular disease, and premature death. Obesity also carries an increased risk of adverse complications in the subse-quent pregnancy for both mother and baby [40, 44, 46].

This study found significant differences in LBW ac-cording to the maternal place of birth and residence (Table 2). From 2005 to 2014, births in foreign-born women decreased from 46.6 to 38.1%, but they increased for United States-born women, from 53.4 to 61.9%. The former were less likely to deliver an LBW infant, a find-ing that has been reported in previous studies. In a study of mothers in New York City, foreign-born women had lower prevalence of LBW than did United States-born women [32]. Acevedo-Garcia et al. (2005) noted that the effect of being foreign-born on LBW differs according to maternal education and race and ethnicity [47].

We did not encounter any previously published studies that included maternal geographic region as a predictor of having an LBW infant. Our findings show that the preva-lence of LBW differs in different regions of California (Table 2). Infants born in the San Joaquin Valley region are more likely to be of LBW compared with those born in the Northern and Sierra regions. Our study also shows that women who depend on Medi-Cal as their source of perinatal care payment, an indicator of lower socioeco-nomic status, are more likely to have an LBW infant than women who have private health insurance.

Alexander and Korenbrot (1995) reported on the role of perinatal care in preventing LBW. Our results confirm their finding, that attendance at perinatal care during the first trimester is associated with reduced LBW [48].

Maternal parity is a well-recognized predictor of infant birth weight; the lowest birth weights are found in infants born to primiparous women [49]. Our results confirm that parity is a significant predictor of LBW (Table 2). Primiparous and multiparous women with 6 to 12 prior deliveries were more likely to have an LBW infant than were multiparous women with 2 to 5 prior deliveries. This finding is consistent with a study by Hinkle et al. (2014), which found a nonlinear association in which birth weight increased up to parity of 4, then stabilized from parity of 4 to 7 [50].

Both preterm AGA and term SGA births demon-strated a high prevalence of LBW infants. Infants born SGA, whether term or preterm, carry a considerably higher risk of mortality and morbidity in the neonatal period and beyond when compared with AGA infants [3]. The risk is even greater among infants born both preterm and SGA [51].

There are several limitations to this study. Maternal characteristics were restricted to those contained within the BSMF compiled by the CDPH from 2005 to 2014. Maternal age, race and ethnicity, education level, smoking status during pregnancy (usually under-reported), and prepregnancy height and weight were self-reported. Despite these limitations and the inclusion of many possible confounding variables, our study demonstrates significant trends in LBW over a 10-year period in the highly diverse population of California and includes analysis of almost 5 million births.

Conclusions

There was no significant decline in the prevalence of LBW during this 10-year period in California, but maternal age, race and ethnicity, education level, smoking status during pregnancy, and parity are significant risk factors for LBW. Therefore, there may be opportunities to reduce LBW by improving birth outcomes for women giving birth at an advanced maternal age, and by developing public health models to address the identified risk factors and improve the health of the population. The findings of this study illustrate the opportunities to improve fetal, infant, and adult health outcomes, not only in California but throughout the United States. Given the complexity of the etiology of LBW, further research is required on the genetic and epigenetic factors that interact with the social, ethnic, and age-related influences identified in this study.

Abbreviations
95% CI: 95% confidence interval; AGA: Appropriate for gestational age; AOR: Adjusted odds ratio; BSMF: Birth Statistical Master Files; CDPH: California Department of Public Health; FGR: Fetal growth restriction; LBW: Low birth weight; LGA: Large for gestational age; OE: Obstetric estimates; SGA: Small for gestational age

Acknowledgements
The authors thank their friends and colleagues for their critical contributions.

Confirmation
All authors have approved the manuscript for submission.

Authors' contributions
AWGR, KEB, VNA, IHD, and SSP designed the study. Data curation and analysis and review of the literature was performed by AWGR. The study was conducted by AWGR, KEB, VNA, IHD, SSP, LAH, and RJD. Determining and validating the methodology was performed by AWGR, KEB, VNA, and IHD. The first version of the manuscript was written by AWGR, KEB, and SSP. All authors reviewed and approved the final version of the manuscript.

Competing interests
The authors declare that they have no competing interests.

Author details
¹Department of Health Care Services, Benefits Division, 1501 Capitol Ave, Suite 71.4104, MS 4600, P.O. Box 997417, Sacramento, CA 95899-7417, USA. ²Department of Health Care Services, Clinical Assurance and Administrative Support Division, 1501 Capitol Ave, Sacramento, CA 95899-7417, USA. ³School of Agriculture and Food Sciences, Faculty of Science, The University of Queensland, Brisbane, Qld 4072, Australia. ⁴School of Biomedical Sciences, Faculty of Medicine, The University of Queensland, Brisbane, Qld 4072, Australia.

References
1. Battaglia FC, Lubchenco LO. A practical classification of newborn infants by weight and gestational age. J Pediatr. 1967;71:159–63.
2. Malin GL, Morris RK, Riley R, Teune MJ, Khan KS. When is birthweight at term abnormally low? A systematic review and meta-analysis of the association and predictive ability of current birthweight standards for neonatal outcomes. BJOG. 2014;121:515–26.
3. Lee AC, Kozuki N, Cousens S, Stevens GA, Blencowe H, Silveira MF, et al. CHERG small-for-gestational-age preterm birth working group. Estimates of burden and consequences of infants born small for gestational age in low and middle income countries with INTERGROWTH-21st standard: analysis of CHERG datasets. BMJ. 2017;j3677:358.
4. Baer RJ, Rogers EE, Partridge JC, Anderson JG, Morris M, Kuppermann M, et al. Population-based risks of mortality and preterm morbidity by gestational age and birth weight. J Perinatol. 2016;36:1008–13.
5. Ray JG, Park AL, Fell DB. Mortality in infants affected by preterm birth and severe small-for-gestational-age birth weight. Pediatrics. 2017; https://doi.org/10.1542/peds.2017-1881.
6. Goldenberg RL, Culhane JF. Low birth weight in the United States. Am J Clin Nutr. 2007;85:584s–90s.
7. Barker DJ. Fetal origins of coronary heart disease. BMJ. 1995;311:171–4.
8. Calkins K, Devaskar SU. Fetal origins of adult disease. Curr Probl Pediatr Adolesc Health Care. 2011;41:158–76.
9. Barker DJ, Osmond C. Infant mortality, childhood nutrition, and ischaemic heart disease in England and Wales. Lancet. 1986;1:1077–81.
10. Eriksson JG, Forsén T, Tuomilehto J, Osmond C, Barker DJ. Early growth and coronary heart disease in later life: longitudinal study. BMJ. 2001;322:949–53.
11. Leeson CP, Kattenhorn M, Morley R, Lucas A, Deanfield JE. Impact of low birth weight and cardiovascular risk factors on endothelial function in early adult life. Circulation. 2001;103:1264–8.
12. Barker DJ, Osmond C. Low birth weight and hypertension. BMJ. 1988;297:134–5.
13. Barker DJ, Osmond C, Kajantie E, Eriksson JG. Growth and chronic disease: findings in the Helsinki birth cohort. Ann Hum Biol. 2009;36:445–58.
14. Whincup PH, Kaye SJ, Owen CG, Huxley R, Cook DG, Anazawa S, et al. Birth weight and risk of type 2 diabetes: a systematic review. JAMA. 2008;300:2886–97.
15. Boardman JD, Powers DA, Padilla YC, Hummer RA. Low birth weight, social factors, and developmental outcomes among children in the United States. Demography. 2002;39:353–68.
16. Reichman NE. Low birth weight and school readiness. Futur Child. 2005;15:91–116.
17. Barker DJ. The developmental origins of adult disease. J Am Coll Nutr. 2004; 23(Suppl 6):588S–95S.
18. Lahti J, Räikkönen K, Pesonen AK, Heinonen K, Kajantie E, Forsén T, et al. Prenatal growth, postnatal growth and trait anxiety in late adulthood - the Helsinki birth cohort study. Acta Psychiatr Scand. 2010;121:227–35.
19. Halfon N, Larson K, Lu M, Tullis E, Russ S. Lifecourse health development: past, present and future. Matern Child Health J. 2014;18:344–65.
20. Pies C, Kotelchuck M. Bringing the MCH life course perspective to life. Matern Child Health J. 2014;18:335–4.
21. Reichman NE, Hamilton ER, Hummer RA, Padilla YC. Racial and ethnic disparities in low birthweight among urban unmarried mothers. Matern Child Health J. 2008;12:204–15.
22. Montan S. Increased risk in the elderly parturient. Curr Opin Obstet Gynecol. 2007;19(2):110–2.
23. No authors listed. Obesity: preventing and managing the global epidemic. Report of a WHO consultation. World Health Organ Tech Rep Ser. 2000. 894:i–xii.
24. Olsen IE, et al. New intrauterine growth curves based on United States data. Pediatrics. 2010;125(2):e214–24.
25. Hamilton BE, Martin JA, Osterman MJ, Curtin SC, Matthews TJ. Births: Final data for 2014. Natl Vital Stat Rep. 2015;64:1–64.
26. Martin JA, Hamilton BE, Osterman MJ, Curtin SC, Matthews TJ. Births: final data for 2012. Natl Vital Stat Rep. 2013;62:1–68.
27. Kenny LC, Lavender T, McNamee R, O'Neill SM, Mills T, Khashan AS. Advanced maternal age and adverse pregnancy outcome: evidence from a large contemporary cohort. PLoS ONne. 2013;8:e56583. https://doi.org/10.1371/journal.pone.0056583.

28. Sauer MV. Reproduction at an advanced maternal age and maternal health. Fertil Steril. 2015;103:1136–43.

29. Saloojee H, aCoovadia H. Maternal age matters: for a lifetime, or longer. Lancet Glob Health. 2015;3:e342–3. https://doi.org/10.1016/S2214-109X(15)00034-0.

30. Goisis A, Remes H, Barclay K, Martikainen P, Myrskylä M. Advanced maternal age and the risk of low birth weight and preterm delivery: a within-family analysis using Finnish population registers. Am J Epidemiol. 2017;186:1219–26.

31. Manyeh AK, Kukula V, Odonkor G, Ekey RA, Adjei A, Narh-Bana S, et al. Socioeconomic and demographic determinants of birth weight in southern rural Ghana: evidence from Dodowa health and demographic surveillance system. BMC Pregnancy Childbirth. 2016;16:160.

32. Almeida J, Mulready-Ward C, Bettegowda VR, Ahluwalia IB. Racial/ethnic and nativity differences in birth outcomes among mothers in New York City: the role of social ties and social support. Matern Child Health J. 2014;18:90–100.

33. Chang JJ, Tabet M, Elder K, Kiel DW, Flick LH. Racial/ethnic differences in the correlates of mental health services use among pregnant women with depressive symptoms. Matern Child Health J. 2016;20:1911–22.

34. Jamal A, Homa DM, O'Connor E, Babb SD, Caraballo RS, Singh T. Current cigarette smoking among adults - United States, 2005-2014. MMWR Morb Mortal Wkly Rep. 2015;64:1233–40.

35. Inoue S, Naruse H, Yorifuji T, Kato T, Murakoshi T, Doi H. Impact of maternal and paternal smoking on birth outcomes. J Public Health (Oxf). 2017;39:1–10.

36. National Center for Chronic Disease Prevention and Health Promotion (US) Office on Smoking and Health. The health consequences of smoking—50 years of progress: a report of the Surgeon General. https://www.ncbi.nlm. nih.gov/books/NBK179276/ (2014). Accessed 7 Jan 2018.

37. Han Z, Mulla S, Beyene J, Liao G, McDonald SD, Knowledge Synthesis Group. Maternal underweight and the risk of preterm birth and low birth weight: a systematic review and meta-analyses. Int J Epidemiol. 2011;40:65–101.

38. Liu P, Xu L, Wang Y, Zhang Y, Du Y, Sun Y. Association between perinatal outcomes and maternal pre-pregnancy body mass index. Obes Rev. 2016; 17:1091–102.

39. Institute of Medicine (US) and National Research Council (US) Committee to Reexamine IOM Pregnancy Weight Guidelines. In: Rasmussen KM, Yaktine AL, editors. Weight Gain During Pregnancy: Reexamining the Guidelines. The National Academies Collection: Reports funded by National Institutes of Health. Washington (DC): National Academy of Sciences; 2009.

40. Davis EM, Stange KC, Horwitz RI. Childbearing, stress and obesity disparities in women: a public health perspective. Matern Child Health J. 2012;16:109–18.

41. Catalano PM, Kirwan JP, Haugel-de Mouzon S, King J. Gestational diabetes and insulin resistance: role in short- and long-term implications for mother and fetus. J Nutr 2003;133 Suppl 2:1674S–83S.

42. Siega-Riz AM, Viswanathan M, Moos MK, Deierlein A, Mumford S, Knaack J. A systematic review of outcomes of maternal weight gain according to the Institute of Medicine recommendations: birthweight, fetal growth, and postpartum weight retention. Am J Obstet Gynecol. 2009;201:339.e1–14. https://doi.org/10.1016/j.ajog.2009.07.002.

43. Dietz PM, Callaghan WM, Morrow B, Cogswell ME. Population-based assessment of the risk of primary cesarean delivery due to excess prepregnancy weight among nulliparous women delivering term infants. Matern Child Health J. 2005;9:237–44.

44. Viswanathan M, Siega-Riz AM, Moos MK, Deierlein A, Mumford S, Knaack J. Outcomes of maternal weight gain. Evid Rep Technol Assess (Full Rep). 2008;(168):1–223.

45. Hilson JA, Rasmussen KM, Kjolhede CL. Excessive weight gain during pregnancy is associated with earlier termination of breast-feeding among white women. J Nutr. 2006;136:140–6.

46. Gunderson EP, Jacobs DR Jr, Chiang V, Lewis CE, Tsai A, Quesenberry CP Jr, et al. Childbearing is associated with higher incidence of the metabolic syndrome among women of reproductive age controlling for measurements before pregnancy: the CARDIA study. Am J Obstet Gynecol. 2009;201:177.e1–9. https://doi.org/10.1016/j.ajog.2009.03.031.

47. Acevedo-Garcia D, Soobader MJ, Berkman LF. The differential effect of foreign-born status on low birth weight by race/ethnicity and education. Pediatrics 2005;115:e20–e30. doi: 10.1542.peds.2004-1306.

48. Alexander GR, Korenbrot CC. The role of prenatal care in preventing low birth weight. Futur Child. 1995;5:103–20.

49. Shah PS, Knowledge Synthesis Group on Determinants of LBW/PT births. Parity and low birth weight and preterm birth: a systematic review and meta-analyses. Acta Obstet Gynecol Scand. 2010;89:862–75.

50. Hinkle SN, Albert PS, Mendola P, Sjaarda LA, Yeung E, Boghossian NS, et al. The association between parity and birthweight in a longitudinal consecutive pregnancy cohort. Paediatr Perinat Epidemiol. 2014;28:106–15.

51. Katz J, et al. Mortality risk in preterm and small-for-gestational-age infants in low-income and middle-income countries: a pooled country analysis. Lancet. 2013;382:417–25.

24

Simplified antibiotic regimens for treating neonates and young infants with severe infections in the Democratic Republic of Congo: a comparative efficacy trial

Adrien Lokangaka[1*], Melissa Bauserman[2], Yves Coppieters[3], Cyril Engmann[4], Shamim Qazi[5], Antoinette Tshefu[1] and Carl Bose[2]

Abstract

Background: One-quarter of neonatal and infant deaths are due to infection, and the majority of these deaths occur in developing countries. Standard treatment for infection, which includes parenteral treatment only, is often not available in low-resource settings. Infant mortality will not be reduced in developing countries without a reduction in deaths due to infection. We participated in a multi-site trial that demonstrated the effectiveness of three simplified antibiotic regimens compared to standard treatment (The AFRINEST Trial: parent study). For this report, we examined the site-specific data for the Democratic Republic Congo (DRC), the most impoverished of the countries that participated in the study, to determine if outcomes in the DRC were similar to outcomes across all sites.

Methods: The parent study was an individually randomized, open-label, equivalence trial. Infants with clinical signs of severe infection were randomized to receive one of four regimens: 1) injectable penicillin-gentamicin for 7 days (standard therapy; regimen A), 2) injectable gentamicin and oral amoxicillin for 7 days (regimen B), 3) injectable penicillin-gentamicin for 2 days then oral amoxicillin for 5 days (regimen C), or 4) injectable gentamicin for 2 days and oral amoxicillin for 5 days (regimen D). In the DRC, we enrolled 574 infants, of whom 560 met the per-protocol criteria for analysis of treatment effect. The main outcome was treatment failure within the first week of enrollment.

Results: Treatment failure occurred in 52 (9.3%) infants: 17 (11.6%) with the referent treatment regimen, 13 (9.6%) with regimen B (risk difference [RD] -2.0%; CI -9.2% to 5.2%), 13 (9.0%) with regimen C (RD -2.6%; CI -9.6% to 4.4%), and 9 (6.7%) with regimen D (RD -5.0%; CI -11.7% to 1.7%).

Conclusion: As in the parent study, the risk difference between each of the experimental treatments and the reference treatment suggests equivalence. These findings suggest that the conclusion from the parent study, that a simplified antibiotic regimen can be used for the community-based management of possible severe infection in young infants where referral to a hospital for standard care is often not possible, is true in the DRC. We speculate that the widespread use of a simplified, community-based treatment could result in increased coverage with treatment and improved survival in poor areas.

Keywords: Neonatal infection, Simplified antibiotic regimen, Community-based treatment

* Correspondence: adrinloks@gmail.com
[1]Faculté de Médecine, Université de Kinshasa, Kinshasa School of Public Health, PO Box 11850, Kinshasa/Lemba, Democratic Republic of Congo
Full list of author information is available at the end of the article

Background

Reducing child mortality continues to be one of the most vexing challenges in this Sustainable Development Goals era. An estimated 5.6 million children died in 2016; approximately 2.6 million of these deaths occurred in the neonatal period [1]. Of these child deaths, the proportion occurring in neonates and young infants (infants 0–2 months) continues to rise [2]. Evidence-based research, policies, programs and advocacy that target this age group are urgently needed to combat this problem.

Infections are among the leading causes of neonatal and young infant mortality [1]. In 2012, over 0.66 million infants died of serious bacterial infections, such as pneumonia, sepsis, and meningitis [3]. Until 2015, the World Health Organization (WHO) recommended that all neonates and young infants with possible serious bacterial infections (PSBI) be treated in hospitals with injectable antibiotic therapy for 7–10 days [4]. However, this recommendation is difficult to implement in many low-income countries, particularly in rural areas. The Democratic Republic of Congo (DRC), located in central Africa and the fourth most populous African country, is particularly vulnerable to the challenges of implementing these WHO recommendations. In the DRC, nearly all health care in rural areas is provided through health centers that do not typically provide inpatient care. Providers in health centers may refer some patients to their area hospital if inpatient care is advisable and feasible; however, distances from health centers to hospitals vary widely, ranging from less than one mile to 60 miles, the terrain is challenging and obtaining transport poses immense difficulties. For the patient who makes it to a referral hospital, the hospitals are lacking in sufficiently trained health care providers, and equipment and essential medicines are often absent [5]. As a result of these barriers, many infants with PSBI are not taken to hospitals, and if they do get there are either untreated or inadequately treated. These barriers and inadequacies of treatment contribute to the neonatal mortality in these regions.

Because of these barriers to recommended treatment in the DRC and other resource-limited countries, a collaboration of investigators from the WHO and the Universities of Kinshasa and North Carolina participated in a multi-site study (five sites from three countries) that examined the efficacy of four simplified regimens of outpatient antibiotic therapy for the treatment of neonates and young infants with PBSI [6]. The results of the multi-center study (the African Neonatal Sepsis Trial: AFRINEST Trial) were published in the *Lancet* and suggest that these infections could be treated effectively outside of referral hospitals, in health centers or homes [7]. The WHO modified its recommendations for treatment of PSBI based, in part, on the results of this study [8]. However, each of the five sites had unique demography,

geography and healthcare infrastructure that might predict variation in efficacy among sites. The objective of this report is to examine the DRC site-specific data from the multi-site study to determine the comparative efficacy of these treatment regimens in the cohort enrolled in the DRC, the most rural and impoverished of the study sites.

Methods

Study site

Our site was in rural areas of the North and South Ubangi districts in the province of Equateur in northern DRC. The overall population of the study area was roughly 400,000. We included 30 health areas, each served by a health center. Health centers are the primary level facilities staffed by one trained nurse who provides treatment to ill infants.

Study design:

The parent study was a multi-site, individually randomized, open-label, equivalence trial [6].

A. *Eligibility Criteria*

Young infants and neonates (0–59 days old) with signs of PSBI and whose families did not accept or could not access inpatient hospital care for whatever reason were enrolled and randomized. Signs of PSBI included: not feeding well, movement only when stimulated, severe chest indrawing and axillary temperature > 38.0 °C or < 35.5 °C. We excluded infants who had very low weight (< 1500 g) at the time of presentation, had been hospitalized for illness in the previous two weeks or prior to inclusion in the study, any sign of critical illness (unconscious, convulsions, unable to feed at all, apnea, unable to cry, cyanosis, dehydration, bulging fontanel), major congenital malformations inhibiting oral antibiotic intake, active bleeding requiring transfusion, surgical conditions needing hospital referral, and persistent vomiting (vomiting following three attempts to feed the baby within one-half hour).

B. *Surveillance*

We developed an active surveillance system in order to maintain a registry of infants in the study communities. At the beginning of the trial, we used community health workers (CHWs) to conduct a household census in order to identify all births and pregnant women. CHWs repeated the household census every three to four months. We incorporated other methods to discover pregnancies and births: self-reporting of pregnancies to a CHW, identification of pregnant women at antenatal clinics in the community health facilities, and referrals from traditional birth attendants (TBAs) or other key informants.

C. *Enrollment*

CHWs visited the homes of newborns on postnatal days 1, 3, 7, 14, 21, 28, 35, 42, 49 and 60. During these home visits, the CHWs provided standardized advice to the family regarding newborn care, as described in the WHO/UNICEF Joint Statement on home-based care of newborns [6]. At each home visit, CHWs assessed the newborn for signs of illness and counseled the families on recognition of danger signs of infection. Young infants who exhibited danger signs were referred to a health center for evaluation.

All infants who presented with danger signs were evaluated by a study nurse. This assessment was in addition to and independent of an assessment performed by a health center provider, and occurred either in the health center or in the home. If the study nurse confirmed that a danger sign and PSBI was present, the infant was referred to local hospital facility, as recommended in the WHO Integrated Management of Children Illness (IMCI) guidelines [9]. If the family refused to accept hospital referral despite the best efforts of the study nurse, they were considered for enrollment in the study.

D. **Consent**

Consent for study participation was obtained by the study nurse at the health facility or at home in the presence of a witness. Consent included detailed oral communication about the trial and study procedure in the study participant's native language. Illiterate parents were asked to provide a thumbprint on the consent form; literate parents were requested to sign the consent form.

E. *Randomization and Allocation Concealment*

Prior to randomization, infants with PSBI were stratified by age at presentation (< 7 days old and 7 to 59 days old) and assigned to one of four treatment regimens. For allocation concealment, the treatment code for each study infant was sealed in an envelope, one color for each age stratum. Each cluster (a group of health centers) was given envelopes for a set of blocks. When the first infant was enrolled in a cluster in a stratum, the first envelope of the first block for that age stratum was opened, and the infant was treated according to the treatment code inside. When the next infant was enrolled, the next envelope of the block was opened.

F. *Treatment Regimens*

Each patient was randomized to one of four treatment regimens:

- Treatment regimen A (reference treatment): gentamicin (desired range 4–5 mg/kg/day) by intramuscular (IM) injection once daily, and procaine penicillin (desired range 40,000–50,000 units/kg/day) by IM injection once daily for 7 days (14 injections in total)
- Treatment regimen B: gentamicin (desired range 4–5 mg/kg/day) by IM injection once daily and oral amoxicillin (desired range 75–100 mg/kg/day) twice daily for 7 days (7 injections in total)
- Treatment regimen C: gentamicin (desired range 4–5 mg/kg/day) by IM injection once daily and procaine penicillin (desired range 40,000–50,000 units/kg/day by IM injection once daily for 2 days; thereafter oral amoxicillin (desired range 75–100 mg/kg/day) for 5 days (4 injections in total)
- Treatment regimen D: gentamicin (desired range 4–5 mg/kg/day) by IM injection once daily for two days and oral amoxicillin (desired range 75–100 mg/kg/day) twice daily for 7 days; (2 injections in total)

Study outcomes

Treatment failure within day 1–8 following enrollment was the primary outcome and was defined as any one of the following: death, clinical deterioration (hospitalization, emergence of any sign of critical illness, a new sign of severe infection, or re-emergence of a sign of severe infection on day 4 after it had initially disappeared), no improvement in clinical condition by day 4 (if single sign of severe infection was present at enrollment, persistence of the sign, and if multiple signs were present at enrollment, persistence of > 1 sign), no clinical cure by day 8 (persistence of any sign of severe infection on day 8), development of a serious adverse effect to the study antibiotics, or withdrawal of informed consent, any time between days 1–8.

Sample size and analysis plan

The sample size for the parent study was based on an estimated incidence of severe bacterial infection among neonates and young infants of 5%. The analytic plan was to compare failure rates of treatment regimens B, C and D to failure rates following treatment regimen A. Comparisons were made for similarity of effectiveness defined by the upper limit of the 95% confidence interval of the differences in failure rate lying below the similarity margin of + 5%. In the parent study, the required sample for 90% power to demonstrate the similarity of any two treatments assuming that the true failure rates with the reference treatment and the experimental treatment regimens were identical (assumed to be 10%) was estimated to be a total 3040. An additional 560 infants were added to the planned enrollment to allow for failures of adherence to the protocol to allow for both per-protocol and intention-to-treat analyses. Sample size calculations for individual sites were not calculated because there was no a priori intent to perform sit-specific analyses. Therefore, the sample size for the DRC was the number enrolled at this site during the duration of the parent study.

We conducted these single site analyses using STATA version 12.0 (StataCorp, College Station, TX). We analyzed the primary outcome (treatment failure) per-protocol, which is considered a more conservative analysis

than intention to treat (ITT) analysis for equivalence studies. We evaluated the difference in the risk of treatment failure between the reference treatment (regimen A) and all other treatments together with a 95% confidence interval. We report planned investigation of secondary outcomes and comparisons between features of the DRC and the parent study cohort using descriptive statistics only.

Results

From September 17, 2012 to June 28, 2013, we enrolled 574 infants (Fig. 1), 16% of the 3564 infants enrolled in the parent study. Mean maternal age at enrollment was 25 years, and 47% had no formal education. Nearly all (95.3%) attended at least one antenatal clinic visit. Among all infants, 398 (69%) were born in health

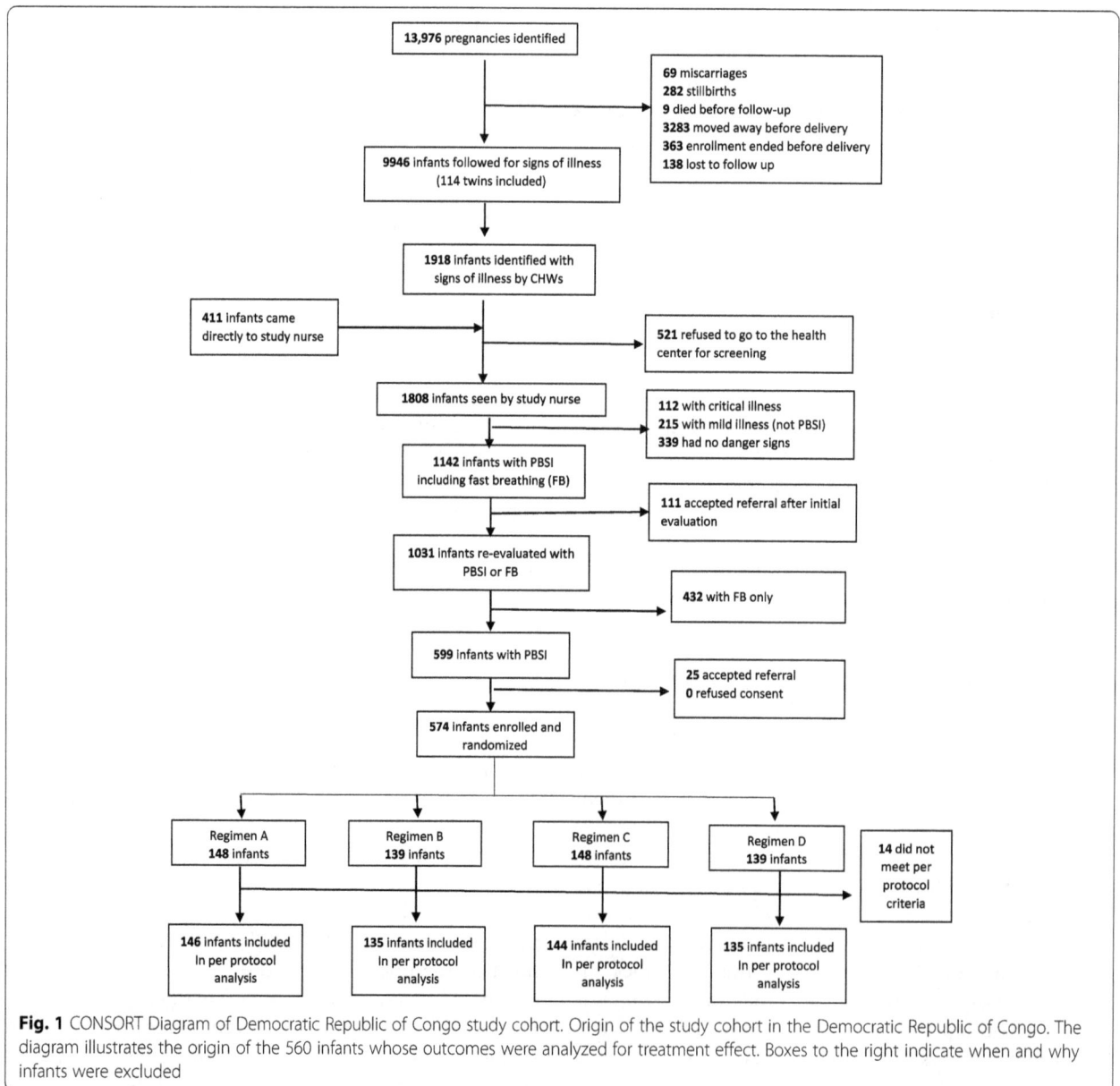

Fig. 1 CONSORT Diagram of Democratic Republic of Congo study cohort. Origin of the study cohort in the Democratic Republic of Congo. The diagram illustrates the origin of the 560 infants whose outcomes were analyzed for treatment effect. Boxes to the right indicate when and why infants were excluded

centers, 66 (12%) in hospitals, and 85 (15%) at home. Compared to all participants in the parent study, participants from the DRC had lower maternal education and more used solid fuel for cooking (Table 1).

In the DRC, the randomization process allocated 148 (25.2%) infants to treatment regimen A, 139 (24.2%) to regimen B, 148 (25.2%) to regimen C, and 139 (24.2%) to regimen D. Enrollment occurred soon after birth for many infants; 198 (34%) were enrolled in their first week of life. Mothers and infants in each group had similar baseline characteristics (Table 2). At enrollment, the most common presenting signs was fever (57.0%). We enrolled 75 infants (13.1%) with two or more signs.

Almost all infants, 98% received all treatment doses as per-protocol analysis, and 97% received all independent outcome assessment visits (Table 3). We excluded 14 infants from our analysis of treatment effect because they did not receive all treatment doses and adequate follow-up as required by the study protocol [6].

Table 1 Demographics for DRC Site compared to AFRINEST study population

	DRC Site	AFRINEST Study Population
	N = 574	n = 3564
Maternal age (years)		
Mean (SD)	25.0 (6.4)	25.9 (5.8)
< 20 years	122 (21%)	440 (12%)
≥ 20 years	385 (67%)	1969 (84%)
Not known	67 (12%)	110 (3%)
Maternal education (years)		
No formal school attendance	271 (47%)	625 (18%)
< 12	292 (51%)	2025 (57%)
≥ 12	11 (2%)	896 (25%)
unknown	0 (0%)	10 (< 1%)
Cooking place and fuel (n)		
Indoor with solid fuel	315 (55%)	1534 (43%)
Outdoor with solid fuel	259 (45%)	771 (22%)
No solid fuel	0	1279 (36%)
Had at least 1 antenatal care visit (n)		
Yes	555 (97%)	3371 (95%)
No	19 (3%)	184 (5%)
Not known	0	9 (< 1%)
Number of previous live births		
1	145 (25%)	847 (24%)
2–3	231 (40%)	1377 (39%)
> 4	198 (35%)	1342 (38%)
Not known	0	8 (< 1%)

Treatment failure occurred in 52 (9.2%) infants (Table 4). When compared to the reference treatment, the risk difference with regimen B was – 2.0% (95% CI: -9.2 to 5.2), with regimen C: – 2.6% (– 9.6 to 4.4), and with regimen D -5.0% (– 11.7 to 1.7) (Table 3). Among treatment failures, 11 infants died; 9 had the appearance of a sign of critical illness; 5 had a new sign of serious infection; and 21 had no improvement in clinical condition by day 4. Treatment failure occurred most commonly on day 4 following enrollment.

Discussion

The AFRINEST Trial, a multi-national study, investigated the safety and effectiveness of simplified regimens for the management of possible serious bacterial infection among infants in resource-poor community settings. This study enrolled 3564 infants in five sites in three countries (Kenya, DRC, and Nigeria) [7]. In the parent study, four week-long treatment regimens were compared. The outcomes of infants treated with three regimens of antibiotics that included combinations of parenteral (intramuscular) and oral antibiotics were compared to outcomes in a reference group treated with daily doses of parenteral antibiotics, the standard care. Treatment failure occurred in 6.8% of infants, but the risk differences between the experimental treatment regimens and the reference treatment were within the pre-specified 5% similarity margin. The conclusion from this study was that treatment with these regimens was equivalent to the standard care.

The purpose of the study reported in this manuscript was to determine whether the results from this multi-national study could be reasonably extrapolated to the DRC. The DRC is a unique environment compared to the other sites for several reasons. First, mothers had less education compared to other sites. Second, the socio-economic status is lower in the DRC. Despite the abundant natural resources of the country, the population of the DRC is among the poorest in the world [10, 11]. According to the 2013 Human Development Report, the DRC ranks last (186th) with a poverty ratio of about 80% [12]. This compares to ranks of 153rd and 145th for Nigeria and Kenya. Third, the DRC has high fertility rates and bigger families. The total fertility rate in the DRC is 6.6, [13] compared to 5.5 in Nigeria [14] and 3.9 in Kenya [15].

As a participant in the multi-national study, we examined the safety and efficacy of simplified antibiotic regimens compared with the reference treatment for the management of neonates and young infants with PSBI among infants enrolled in the study. Our site-specific data demonstrated similarity between each of the experimental treatment regimens and the reference treatment. Treatment failure varied among groups from 11.6% to

Table 2 Baseline characteristics of enrolled infants

Regimen[a]		A	B	C	D
Number of infants enrolled		148	139	148	139
Age at enrollment (days)	Mean (SD)	17 (15)	17 (15)	17 (16)	20 (17)
	< 7 days	54 (36.5%)	46 (33.1%)	55 (37.2%)	43 (30.9%)
	≥ 7 days	94 (63.5%)	93 (66.9%)	93 (62.8%)	96 (69.1%)
Sex	Male	75 (50.7%)	76 (54.7%)	70 (47.3%)	81 (58.3%)
Respiratory rate	Mean (SD)	69 (19)	69 (19)	70 (20)	67 (19)
	< 60	54 (36.5%)	47 (33.8%)	52 (35.1%)	57 (41.0%)
	60–70	27 (18.2%)	21 (15.1%)	26 (17.6%)	16 (11.5%)
	70–79	22 (14.9%)	33 (23.7%)	26 (17.6%)	32 (23.7%)
	80–89	24 (16.2%)	20 (14.4%)	25 (16.9%)	19 (13.7%)
	90–99	8 (5.4%)	9 (6.5%)	9 (6.1%)	8 (5.8%)
	≥ 100	13 (8.8%)	9 (6.5%)	10 (6.8%)	7 (5.0%)
Temperature	< 35.5	6 (4.1%)	8 (5.8%)	12 (8.1%)	12 (8.6%)
	35.5–37.9	39 (26.4%)	47 (33.8%)	44 (29.7%)	33 (23.7%)
	≥38.0–38.9	96 (64.9%)	70 (50.4%)	80 (54.1%)	76 (54.7%)
	≥39.0	7 (4.7%)	14 (10.1%)	12 (8.1%)	18 (12.9%)
Poor feeding		23 (15.5%)	22 (15.8%)	26 (17.6%)	25 (18.0%)
Movement only on stimulation		3 (2.0%)	5 (3.6%)	3 (2.0%)	1 (0.7%)
Severe chest indrawing		33 (22.3%)	40 (28.8%)	32 (21.6%)	31 (22.3%)
Number of signs at enrollment	1	129 (87.2%)	120 (86.3%)	128 (86.5%)	120 (86.3%)
	2	18 (12.2%)	18 (12.9%)	17 (11.5%)	16 (11.5%)
	≥ 3	1 (0.7%)	1 (0.7%)	1 (0.7%)	3 (2.2%)

[a]Regimen A: IM Gentamicin and IM Penicillin × 7 days; Regimen B: IM Gentamicin and oral amoxicillin × 7 days; Regimen C: IM Gentamicin × 7 days and IM Penicillin × 2 days then oral amoxicillin × 5 days; Regimen D: IM Gentamicin × 2 days and oral amoxicillin × 7 days

Table 3 Treatment adherence and follow-up of enrolled infants

Regimen[a]	A	B	C	D
Number of infants enrolled	148	139	148	139
Treatment adherence				
Received all treatment doses as per-protocol	146 (98.6%)	137 (98.6%)	144 (97.3%)	135 (97.1%)
Did not receive all doses, but met per-protocol analysis criteria	2 (1.4%)	1 (0.7%)	4 (2.7%)	4 (2.9%)
Did not meet per-protocol analysis criteria for treatment	0	1[b] (0.7%)	0	0
Follow up by independent outcome assessor				
Received all independent outcome assessment visits	145 (98.0%)	133 (95.7%)	145 (98.0%)	133 (95.7%)
Did not receive all independent outcome assessment visits, but met per-protocol analysis criteria	2 (1.4%)	3 (2.2%)	2 (1.4%)	4 (2.9%)
Did not meet per-protocol analysis criteria for assessment	2 (1.3%)	4 (3.0%)	4 (2.7%)	4 (3.0%)
Included in per-protocol analysis (met both treatment and assessment criteria)	146 (98.6%)	135 (97.1%)	144 (97.3%)	135 (97.1%)

[a]Regimen A: IM Gentamicin and IM Penicillin × 7 days; Regimen B: IM Gentamicin and oral amoxicillin × 7 days; Regimen C: IM Gentamicin × 7 days and IM Penicillin × 2 days then oral amoxicillin × 5 days; Regimen D: IM Gentamicin × 2 days and oral amoxicillin × 7 days
[b]Infant failed to meet both per-protocol treatment adherence and outcome assessment criteria

Table 4 Primary and secondary outcomes in enrolled infants–per-protocol analysis

Regimen[a]	A	B	C	D
Number of infants analyzed	146	135	144	135
Treatment failure n (%)	17 (11.6%)	13 (9.6%)	13 (9.0%)	9 (6.7%)
Risk difference % (95% CI)	referent	-2.0 (− 9.2 to 5.2)	-2.6 (−9.6 to 4.4)	-5.0 (−11.7 to 1.7)
Reason for treatment failure				
Death	1 (0.7%)	2 (1.5%)	6 (4.2%)	2 (1.5%)
Appearance of a sign of critical illness	2 (1.4%)	2 (1.5%)	2 (1.4%)	3 (2.2%)
Appearance of a new sign of serious infection	1 (0.7%)	2 (1.5%)	2 (1.4%)	0
SAE other than death	0	0	0	0
Hospitalization	0	0	0	0
No improvement in clinical condition by day 4	10 (6.8%)	6 (4.4%)	1 (0.7%)	4 (3.0%)
Reappearance of inclusion sign between days 5–8	2 (1.4%)	1 (0.7%)	2 (1.4%)	0
Presence of inclusion sign on day 8	1 (0.7%)	0	0	0

[a]Regimen A: IM Gentamicin and IM Penicillin × 7 days; Regimen B: IM Gentamicin and oral amoxicillin × 7 days; Regimen C: IM Gentamicin × 7 days and IM Penicillin × 2 days then oral amoxicillin × 5 days; Regimen D: IM Gentamicin × 2 days and oral amoxicillin × 7 days

6.7%. Treatment regimen D, which had only two injections of gentamicin, had the smallest proportion of treatment failure. The risk difference in treatment among the three simplified regimens and the reference treatment varied from − 2.0% to − 4.9%. The upper limits of the confidence intervals for all risk differences were less than the pre-specified limit that defined similarity (5%) with the exception of regimen B in which the upper limit of the confidence interval was 5.2%. As expected, the confidence intervals were greater in our smaller tudy population compared to the larger population in the multi-national study. However, it was encouraging to observe that, although the risk of treatment failure for all groups was greater than in the larger study population, all risk differences compared to the referent arm were negative.

Most treatment failures occurred on day 4, and the most common reason for treatment failure was the persistence of the danger signs on day 4. Collectively, these findings are similar to those observed in the multi-national study. In view of these collective similarities with the multi-national, it can reasonably be inferred that treatment regimens for young infants with signs of serious bacterial infection tested in the multi-national study would be equally effective in the DRC.

In response to the publication of the parent study, and a companion study investigating the effectiveness of a simplified antibiotic treatment regimen for fast breathing [16, 17], several respondents expressed concerns about the context, observations and inferences drawn from these studies [18–20]. These concerns included the unexpectedly low mortality rates in all arms of the study, the use of criteria for PSBI that have high sensitivity but low specificity, the inherent over-treatment of infants with viral rather than bacterial infection, and the

potential for emergence of resistance to these antibiotics resulting from the widespread adoption of the simplified regimens. These concerns were addressed in a response by investigators from the parent study [21]. We can only add that the parent study was a pragmatic trial to determine if a simplified alternative to the recommended treatment for PBSI, that is not available to most infants in low resource environments, would be equally effective. Despite the limitations imposed by the study design, the WHO concluded that the evidence was sufficiently compelling to recommend the simplified regimens in low resource settings when the standard treatment is not available [8]. Our site-specific analyses suggest that these recommendations should be adopted in the DRC, and perhaps other similarly impoverished and very low resource environments.

Strengths and limitations

This is the first study in the DRC that compared simplified treatment regimens utilizing oral antibiotic regimens in an outpatient setting for the management of neonatal SBIs. This study was conducted within the context of the existing health structure. However, the protocol was highly supervised; eligibility was confirmed by specially trained study nurses and assessment visits were conducted by the most qualified nurses among them who were not part of the clinical care team. This level of oversight was necessary to ensure the quality of the research but would not typically be available during standard clinical care. Therefore, although the study methodology could be used as a model for capacity-building of the existing health system, scale up might require additional resources. Absent these resources, it is possible that outcomes of simplified treatments might not have compared as favorably to standard treatment. With the support of the WHO, we are currently investigating the feasibility of scale up of simplified regimens in another low-resource area of the DRC. This ongoing study will help address concerns about feasibility. The study was conducted in one of the poorest regions of the country. The confirmation of effectiveness in this area suggests that the effectiveness of these simplified treatments can be generalized to more affluent areas of the country, where scale up might be more feasible.

Although the multi-national study had sufficient statistical power to demonstrate equivalence between treatments, it was not powered for site-specific outcomes. Therefore, our results should be interpreted with some caution. In addition, the relatively low mortality rate among all treatment groups may reflect the intense surveillance of the population. This close surveillance may have resulted in earlier identification of high-risk infants and earlier referral for health care. Later identification might have occurred in the absence of the study resulting in more severe illness at the initiation of antibiotic treatment, and less effectiveness of simplified treatment regimens and higher mortality.

Implications of the results

Community-based treatments are more practical because they do not require inpatient care that is not available to many children in rural areas of the DRC. The most simplified treatment regimen may be particularly useful because it includes primarily on oral treatment. We speculate that the widespread use of this strategy for treating neonates and young infants with PSBI would result in more infants treated more effectively. This, in turn, would reduce mortality among young infants.

Conclusion

Simplified antibiotic regimens for treating infants in rural DRC with PSBI appear to be acceptable, feasible, safe, and effective. Since the most simplified regimen using mainly oral antibiotic and only two injections proved as effective as the WHO-recommended treatment, scaling up this regimen will more likely result in more infants treated effectively and result in reduced mortality in poor areas where hospital care is costly and inaccessible.

Abbreviations

CHW: community health worker; DRC: Democratic Republic of Congo; IMCI: Integrated Management of Child Illness; ITT: Intention to Treat; PSBI: possible serious bacterial infection; TBA: Traditional Birth Attendant; WHO: World Health Organization

Acknowledgements

None

Funding

The study was funded by the Bill and Melinda Gates Foundation through the World Health Organization.

Authors' contributions

AL, SQ, CE, CB, AT conceived of the study. AL, AT performed the data collection. AL, MB, CB analyzed and interpreted the data. AL, MB, CB prepared the manuscript. AL, SQ, CE, CB, AT, YC read and approved the final manuscript.

Competing interests

The authors declare that they have no competing interests.

Author details

[1]Faculté de Médecine, Université de Kinshasa, Kinshasa School of Public Health, PO Box 11850, Kinshasa/Lemba, Democratic Republic of Congo. [2]University of North Carolina at Chapel Hill, Chapel Hill, NC, USA. [3]School of Public Health, Université libre de Belgique (ULB), Brussels, Belgium. [4]University of Washington, Seattle, Washington, USA. [5]World Health Organization, Geneva, Switzerland.

References

1. WHO. Children: reducing mortality. Fact Sheet. http://www.who.int/mediacentre/factsheets/fs178/en/. Accessed 12 Jan 2018.
2. Lawn JE, Cousens S, Zupan J. Lancet Neonatal Survival Steering Team: 4 million neonatal deaths: when? Where? Why? Lancet. 2005;365:891–900.
3. Lawn JE, Blencowe H, Oza S, You D, Lee AC, Waiswa P, Lalli M, Bhutta Z, Barros AJ, Christian P, et al. Every newborn: progress, priorities, and potential beyond survival. Lancet. 2014;384:189–205.
4. World Health Organization. Pocket Book of Hospital Care for Children: Guidelines for the Management of Common Childhood Illnesses, 2nd edition. Geneva: WHO; 2013.
5. Ministere de la Santé et Hygiene Publique. Plan National de Développement Sanitaire 2016–2020. République démocratique du Congo: Ministère de la Santé Publique; 2010.
6. Group AFRINEST. Simplified regimens for management of neonates and young infants with severe infection when hospital admission is not possible: study protocol for a randomized, open-label equivalence trial. Pediatr Infect Dis J. 2013;32(Suppl 1):S26–32.
7. Tshefu, Tshefu A, Lokangaka A, Ngaima S, Engmann C, Esamai F, Gisore P, Ayede AI, Falade AG, Adejuyigbe EA, et al. Simplified antibiotic regimens compared with injectable procaine benzylpenicillin plus gentamicin for treatment of neonates and young infants with clinical signs of possible serious bacterial infection when referral is not possible: a randomised, open-label, equivalence trial. Lancet. 2015;385:1767–76.
8. World Health Organization. Guideline: managing possible serious bacterial infection in young infants when referral is not feasible. Geneva: WHO; 2015.
9. World Health Organization (WHO). Integrated Management of Childhood Illness (IMCI) Chart Booklet. Geneva: WHO; 2008.
10. United Nations Development Programme. Human Development Reports, Congo (Democratic Republic of the). http://hdr.undp.org/en/countries/profiles/COD. Accessed 12 Jan 2018.
11. Sumner A. Global poverty and the new bottom billion: what if three-quarters of the World's poor live in middle-income countries? IDS Work Pap. 2010;2010(349):01–43.
12. UNDP. Human development report 2013: The rise of the South Human Progress in a Diverse World, vol. 125; 2013. p. 1–8.
13. Ministère du Plan et Suivi de la Mise en œuvre de la Révolution de la Modernité (MPSMRM), Ministère de la Santé Publique (MSP) and ICF International. Democratic Republic of Congo demographic and health survey 2013–14: key findings. Rockville, Maryland, USA: MPSMRM, MSP et ICF International; 2014.
14. National Population Commission (NPC) [Nigeria] and ICF International. 2014. Nigeria Demographic and Health Survey. Abuja, Nigeria, and Rockville. Maryland, USA: NPC and ICF International; 2013.
15. Kenya National Bureau of Statistics, Ministry of Health/Kenya, National AIDS Control Council/Kenya, Kenya Medical Research Institute, National Council for Population and Development/Kenya, and ICF International. Kenya demographic and health survey 2014. Rockville, MD, USA: Kenya National Bureau of Statistics, Ministry of Health/Kenya, National AIDS Control Council/Kenya, Kenya Medical Research Institute, National Council for Population and Development/Kenya, and ICF International; 2015.

25

Magnitude and associated factors of postpartum morbidity in public health institutions of Debre Markos town, North West Ethiopia

Asmare Talie[1]*, Abere Yekoye[2], Megbaru Alemu[3], Belsity Temesgen[1] and Yibeltal Aschale[4]

Abstract

Background: Postpartum maternal morbidity is maternal illness that occurs after one hour of expulsion of placenta up to six weeks of childbirth. Though the true burden of this problem is not well known estimates of WHO, UNICEF and UNFPA showed that 1.4 million women experience acute obstetric morbidity annually. Knowledge of magnitude and predicting factors postpartum morbidity is central to understand the extent of the problem and will help as a cornerstone in designing and implementing better preventive strategies.

Objectives: To assess the magnitude and factors associated with postpartum morbidity in public health institutions in Debre Markos town.

Method: Institutional based cross sectional study was conducted in Debre Markos town public health institutions by reviewing delivery charts, delivery records and reporting log books. Total deliveries in each health institution in the previous year were identified and number of records to be included from each institution was determined by probability proportion to size. Systematic sampling technique was employed to select 308 charts for review. Data was collected by trained midwifes using structured checklist; entered by epi info and analyzed using SPSS 20. To present findings descriptive statistics using frequencies, charts and figures were used accordingly. Finally binary and multiple logistic regressions were performed to identify predicting factors.

Results: The magnitude of postpartum morbidity was found to be 101(32.8%). Divorced/widowed women [AOR = 10.920, 95% CI: (2.168, 54.998)], women who didn't have ANC follow up [AOR = 3.710, 95% CI: (1.749, 7.870)], abnormal labour [AOR =3.496, 95% CI: (1.69, 7.22)], women delivered by doctor [AOR =0.111, 95% CI: (0.027, 0.454)] and women who were not attended postpartum visit [AOR =0.088, 95% CI: (0.040, 0.194)] were the factors associated with postpartum maternal morbidity.

Conclusion: Maternal morbidity in Debre Markos health institution was found to be major maternal health issue. Being divorced/widowed, absence of ANC visit, intrapartum abnormalities, delivery attended by skilled professionals and no post-partum visit were important predictors of maternal postpartum morbidity.

Keywords: Postpartum morbidity, Health institution, Magnitude, Debre Markos, Ethiopia

* Correspondence: talieasmare@gmail.com
[1]Department of Midwifery, College of Health Sciences, Debre Markos University, Debre Markos, Ethiopia
Full list of author information is available at the end of the article

Background

Postpartum maternal morbidity is maternal illness that occurs after one hour of expulsion of placenta up to six weeks of childbirth. It is complex, with multiple causes, duration ranging from acute to chronic, severity from transient to permanent with different diagnosis and treatment options [1]. It is major maternal health problem affecting both developed and developing countries on human, social and economic development and associated with poor or nonexistent medical care during labor and after birth [2].

Globally maternal mortality ratio (MMR) declined from 400 maternal deaths per 100,000 live births in 1990 to 210 in 2010, but in Ethiopia MMR increased from673/100,000 live births to 676/100,000 live births [2]. Greater than 60% of maternal deaths worldwide occurred in the postpartum period; of this 45% of postpartum deaths occurred within 1 day of delivery. In developing countries 80% of postpartum deaths caused by obstetric factors which occurred within 1 week of delivery [3].

In developing countries 15-20million women develop disability each year as a result of child birth complications. This is due to lack of skilled birth attendants; most women who experience complications do not receive adequate medical attention to avert serious illness due to failures to recognize the warning signs of complications or fear of poor treatment or high fees at health facilities [4].

Literatures on maternal morbidity showed that severe anemia, delivery at home, low socioeconomic status, and Para three or more are contributing factors for post-partum morbidity in India [5]. In sub-Saharan Africa postpartum morbidity is due to obstructed labour (4%), hypertension disorder (9%), unsafe abortion (4%), infection (10%) and hemorrhage (34%) are causes of postpartum morbidity sub-Saharan Africa [6].

Despite the fact that postpartum morbidity is a serious maternal health problem with lots of contributing factors; very little is known about its magnitude and influencing factors in Ethiopia. Therefore this study aims to close this gap by determining the magnitude and ascertain contributing factors that will help as a foundation in designing preventive strategies.

Methods and materials

Study area and period

The study was conducted in Debre Markos town; a capital city of East Gojam zone located about 300 from Addis Ababa, and 276 km from the Amhara region capital, Bahir Dar. According to the town finance and economic office report, the total population of the town is 101,582 (Male = 49,775, Female 52,806). Regarding public health institution there are 7 health posts, 3 health centers one family guidance association clinic (FGA) and one referral hospital in the town. The gynecology and obstetrics unit of this referral hospital have 20 midwives, two gynecologists and two emergency surgeons with greater than 100 deliveries per month. In the three health centers there are 28 nurses, 11 health officers and 8 midwives with average of 20 deliveries per month in each health center.

Study design

Institution based retrospective cross sectional study was conducted in public health institutions.

Target, source and study population

The target population involves all delivery records in public health institution in Debre Markos town and records of postpartum women who received care in public health institutions of Debre Markos town in the previous year were the source population. The study population contains maternal charts which fulfill inclusion criteria and selected systematically from the source population.

Sample size determination and sampling procedure

Sample size was computed using single population proportion formula by using the following assumption the prevalence (P) of postpartum morbidity as 23.6% [15] with 95% CI and 5% marginal error (d) which gives sample size of 280. By adding 10% contingency for incomplete maternal records the final sample size became 308.Total number of deliveries in each public health institution over the previous one year was identified and population proportion to size was done to determine number of records to be included from each institution. Finally systematic sampling technique using sampling interval of six was used to select records from each institution for review.

Data collection tool and procedure

Eight data collectors who had previous experience in similar assignments participated in data collection by reviewing of mother's charts; delivery records of labour ward and reporting log book. Structured checklist prepared in English was used to collect data after pretested in 5% of maternal cards which were not included in final sample size. The checklist included Socio-demographic factors, maternal health service and obstetric factors of postpartum morbidity. Two data collection supervisors supervised the data collection process regularly.

Variables

Dependent variable

Magnitude of postpartum morbidity.

Independent variable

Socio demographic variables: age, marital status, education, place of residence, ethnicity; Variables related to Maternal Health Service: ANC, place of delivery, birth attendants, number of ANC visit, postpartum care and obstetric factors: obstetric complications, desire for recent pregnancy, maternal HIV status, mode of delivery, Iron supplementation in last pregnancy, duration of labour and parity.

Data entry and analysis

Data was coded and entered to computer using epi info 7 and exported to SPSS version 22 for analysis. Descriptive statistics was used summarize data. All potential variables were entered bivariate logistic regression and those variables with p value < 0.2 were included in multiple logistic regression model to identify predicting factors. Strength of statistical association was measured by AOR with 95% confidence interval and p- value < 0.05 was used to determine statistical significance.

Results

Socio- demographic characteristics

In this study, a total of 308 postpartum women cards were reviewed with 100% response rate. Ninety four (30.5%) were aged between 25 and 29 years. Majority (86.4%) of mothers were married. On the other hand most (95.8%) were Amhara by ethnicity followed by 8 (2.6%) Tigre and 51.6%). (Table 1).

Table 1 Distribution of women by their Socio-demographic characteristics at Debre Markos town public health institutions, North West Ethiopia, April 1, 2015 to March 30, 2016 (n=308)

Variable	Frequency (n)	Percentage (%)
Age of the mother (in years)		
15-19	30	9.8
20-24	86	27.9
25-29	94	30.5
30-34	48	15.6
>=35	50	16.2
Place of residence		
DebreMarkos town	140	45.5
Out of DebreMarkos town	168	54.5
Maternal Education		
No education	141	45.8
Literate	167	54.2
Marital Status		
Unmarried	26	8.4
Married	266	86.4
Divorced/widowed	16	5.2

Obstetric (pregnancy and intrapartum) characteristics

During their most recent pregnancy, 230 (74.7%) of women had ANC follow up of whom only 79 (34.3%) had four ANC visits. Majority of them 210 (68.2%) received iron and folic acid supplementation during pregnancy. Regarding maternal HIV status, 245 (79.5%) were negative followed by 60 (19.5%) and 3 (1%) with unknown and seropositive status respectively. Majority, 193 (62.7%) women were delivered by midwife. The most common complication women encountered during their most recent pregnancy was infection 31 (26.5%) followed bay mal presentation 29 (24.8%) (Table 2).

Postpartum morbidity

The magnitude of postpartum morbidity was found to be 101 (32.8%). Over all morbidities sepsis had the highest prevalence 51 (50.5%) (Fig. 1). The main causes of postpartum sepsis were genitor-urinary tract infection accounted 29(56.9%), wound infections 16 (31.3%) like C/S 6 (37.4%), episiotomy 5 (31.3%), perineal tear 5 (31.3%) and breast complications 6 (11.8%).

Factors associated with postpartum morbidity

Variables considered for multivariate logistic regression analysis were those with a p-value< 0.2 in bivariate analysis and these were place of residence, marital status, ANC service, maternal education, parity, iron supplementation in pregnancy, maternal HIV status, abnormal labour, mode of delivery, birth attendant, past postpartum morbidity and postpartum visit.

After controlling for confounding variables using multiple logistic regression; marital status, ANC service, birth attendant, abnormal labour and postpartum visit showed significant and independent association with postpartum maternal morbidity.

Divorced/widowed women had eleven times higher odds of developing postpartum complications than married women [AOR = 10.920, 95% CI: (2.168, 54.998)]. Women who didn't obtain ANC visit were 3.71 times more likely to develop postpartum morbidity when compared to their counterparts [AOR = 3.710, 95% CI: (1.749, 7.870)]. Women who had labor abnormality in their last delivery were 3.5 times higher odds to develop postpartum morbidity than those who didn't have abnormal labour [AOR =3.496, 95% CI: (1.69, 7.22)].

Women delivered by doctor around 89% less likely develop postpartum complications than women delivered by unskilled birth attendants [AOR =0.111, 95% CI: (0.027, 0.454)]. Similarly, women who delivered by nurse/health officer were 94% less likely developing postpartum morbidity than women delivered by unskilled birth attendants [AOR =0.058, 95% CI: (0.009, 0.361)]. More over; those mothers who hadn't attend postpartum visit were 91.2% less likely to have postpartum morbidity

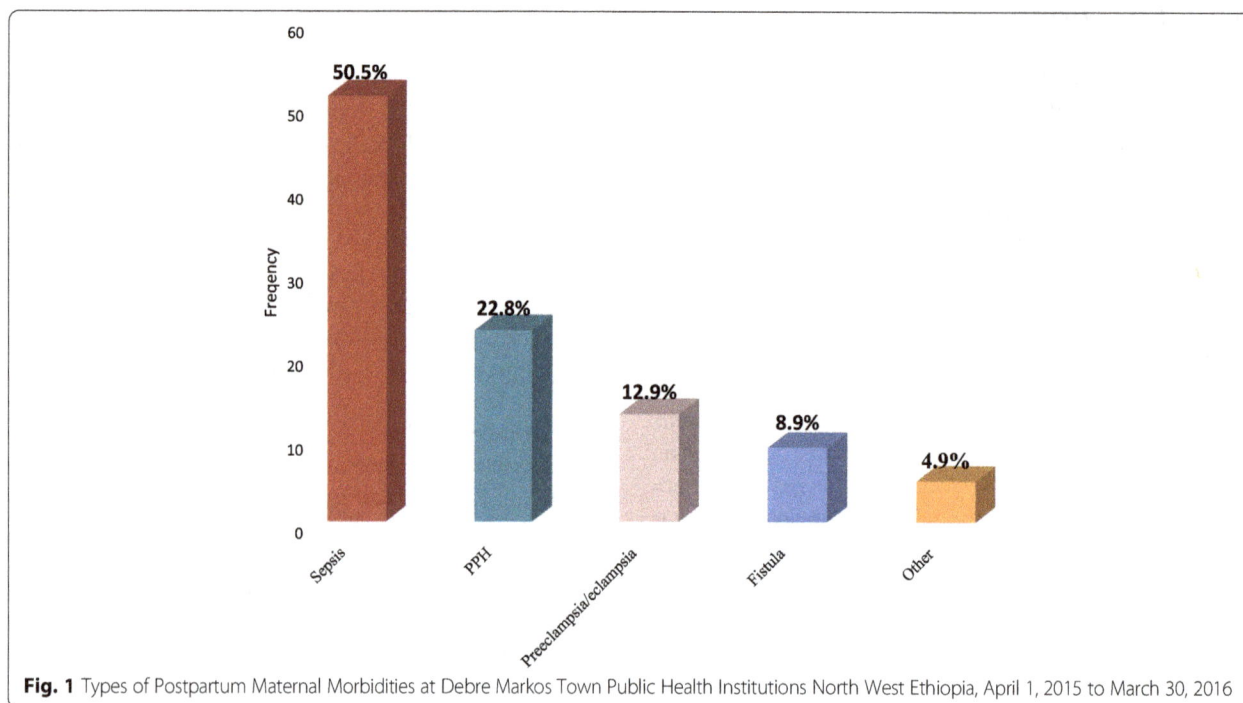

Fig. 1 Types of Postpartum Maternal Morbidities at Debre Markos Town Public Health Institutions North West Ethiopia, April 1, 2015 to March 30, 2016

compared to mothers who had postpartum visit [AOR =0.088, 95% CI: (0.040, 0.194)] (Table 3).

Discussion

This study was carried out to determine magnitude of post-partum morbidity and identify predicting factors in government health institutions in Debre Markos town. Childbirth is a joyful experience for many but unfortunately it can be a difficult period bringing new problems that occurred especially in the first 24 h of child birth and many more may continue to happen lifelong in the days following child birth.

This study showed that magnitude of post-partum morbidity is 32.8%. This finding is consistent with studies done in Pakistan (34.4%), and Bangladesh (30%) [7, 8]. Similar studies in US and India reported higher magnitude of post-partum morbidity; 52 and 52.6% respectively [9, 10]. On the other hand finding of this study is higher when compared to a study done in Gondar (23.6%) [11]. This gap could be because of differences in the study population, study design and study setting. The above studies include only rural residents (study in India), in referral hospital (US) and urban residents and only ANC attendants in (Gondar).Whereas this study was done both rural and urban residents.

Sepsis (50.5%), PPH (22.8%) and hypertension (12.9%) were the three major causes of postpartum morbidity in this study. Many literatures reported conflicting results regarding causes of postpartum

morbidities. Findings of this study were lower when compared to a study conducted in London (PPH 36.4%, HTN 39.4%) and higher than study in Gondar which showed sepsis (6.9%) PPH (14.8%), HTN (9%) [11, 12]. Similar to this finding is an institutional based cross sectional study conducted in India which reported sepsis contribute more than half (51%) of all causes of post-partum morbidity [13].

In this study, marital status showed a significant association with postpartum morbidity. Being divorced/ widowed increase the odds of having postpartum morbidity by a factor 10.92 [AOR = 10.920, 95% CI: (2.168–54.998)]. This result is similar with the study conducted in Nigeria where married women were 72% less likely to have post-partum morbidity [14].

This study confirmed that there is a statistically significant association between ANC service during last pregnancy and occurrence of maternal postpartum morbidity. Mothers who didn't obtain any prenatal care during pregnancy were 3.71 times more likely to develop post-partum morbidity than mothers who had ANC [AOR = 3.710, 95% CI: (1.749, 7.870)].

Consistent to this study is a study done in Pakistan which reported not having prenatal care as risk for postpartum morbidity [7].

The possible explanation might be women who attend antenatal care are screened and get early treatment of pregnancy related complications that predispose to postpartum infections; increase chance of women to deliver in health institutions and also

Table 2 Distribution of women by their obstetric history in DebreMarkos town public health institutions, North West Ethiopia, April 1, 2015 to March 30, 2016 (n=308)

Variable	Frequency (n)	Percentage (%)
Number of ANC visit		
1	64	27.8
2-3	77	33.5
4	79	34.3
>4	10	4.4
Type of complication during this pregnancy		
Anemia	16	13.7
APH	17	14.5
preeclampsia/eclampsia	13	11.1
Infection	31	26.5
Mal-presentation	29	24.8
Other	11	9.4
Place of delivery		
Health center	130	42.2
Hospital	144	46.8
Home	34	11.0
Birth attendant		
Doctor	47	15.3
Midwife	193	62.7
Nurse/health officer	34	11.0
Unskilled	34	11.0
Mode of delivery		
SVD	206	66.9
instrumental delivery	41	13.3
SVD +episiotomy	31	10.1
Cesarean section	30	9.7

more likely to get information from health professionals towards the prevention mechanisms of postpartum morbidity.

Women having intra partum abnormality are susceptible to postpartum infections due to long stay in health institutions, may have frequent vaginal examination; might undergo cesarean section because of (obstructed labour, failed induction/augmentation) and they will have C/S complications. This study showed that, postpartum morbidity was significantly associated & influenced by intra-partum abnormalities. Women who had abnormal labour were more likely to have postpartum morbidity than their counterparts [AOR =3.496, 95% CI: (1.69–7.22)]. Consistent findings were reported from studies done in India, Gondar, Bangladesh and Pakistan [10, 11, 15, 16].

Birth attendant had significant association with postpartum maternal complication. Women delivered by doctor had fewer odds to develop postpartum complications than women delivered by unskilled birth attendants [AOR =0.111, 95% CI: (0.027, 0.454)]. Similarly, women delivered by nurse/health officer less likely to develop postpartum morbidity than women delivered by unskilled birth attendants [AOR =0.058, 95% CI: (0.009, 0.361)]. Consistent results were found from studies done in India, Pakistan, Nigeria and Morocco [5, 7, 14, 17]. This might be related to the fact that skilled birth attendants practice aseptic technique like hand washing and antiseptic materials to provide clean delivery surface, active management of third stage of labour properly applied, utilization of antibiotics during labour and after delivery. In addition to this, mothers delivered by skilled birth attendants are more likely to get information about postpartum danger signs which will increase standard of medical care by preventing postpartum morbidity. Maternal postpartum visit is another predictor of maternal postpartum morbidity. The odds of women who didn't have postpartum visit less likely to have postpartum morbidity when compared to mothers who had postpartum visit [AOR =0.088, 95% CI: (0.040–0.194)]. The possible reason could be majority of women came to those health institutions were when they got postpartum complications.

Strength and limitation
Strength

- Included all governmental health institution in the study area.

Limitation of the study

- Because of lack of standard format about what variables should be documented in every maternal card, some relevant variables were not registered in the clients' document.
- Since the study was an institution based cross sectional study, the results of the study may not show the true picture of the problem in the community.

Conclusion and recommendations
This study confirmed that post-partum morbidity in Debre Markos town public health institutions was high. Divorced/widowed women, women who didn't have ANC service, abnormal labour, delivery attended by Doctor/nurse/health officer and women who didn't have postpartum visit were factors associated with maternal postpartum morbidity. This implies

Table 3 Bivariate and multiple logistic regression analysis of factors associated with postpartum morbidity in DebreMarkos Town Public Health Institutions, April 1, 2015 to March 30, 2016 (n=308)

Variables	Bivariate Analysis			Multivariate Analysis			
	COR	95%CI		P-value	AOR	95%CI	
		Lower	upper			Lower	Upper
Residence							
DebreMarkos	0.304	0.181	0.510	0.131	0.572	0.277	1.181
Out of DebreMarkos	1				1		
Marital Status							
Married	1				1		
unmarried	0.673	0.261	1.738	0.538	0.684	0.204	2.292
Divorced/widowed	9.724*	2.698	35.045	0.004	10.920	2.168	54.998**
Maternal education							
No education	1.897	1.172	3.070	0.867	0.940	0.455	1.943
Literate	1				1		
Parity							
0	0.243	0.076	0.781	0.061	0.157	0.023	1.089
1	0.313	0.154	0.637	0.282	0.552	0.187	1.629
2-4	0.413	0.198	0.860	0.826	1.136	0.362	3.567
>=5	1				1		
ANC follow up							
No	6.268*	3.589	10.945	0.001	3.710	1.749	7.870**
Yes	1				1		
Iron supplementation during pregnancy							
No	4.256	2.547	7.113	0.213	0.443	0.123	1.597
Yes	1				1		
Maternal HIV status							
Negative	1				1		
Positive	1.275	0.114	14.293	0.863	1.349	0.044	41.095
Un known	2.727	1.530	4.859	0.705	1.185	0.493	2.851
Birth Attendant							
Midwife	0.049	0.017	0.146	0.050	0.284	0.081	1.000
Doctor	0.069*	0.021	0.230	0.002	0.111	0.027	0.454**
Nurse/health officer	0.013*	0.003	0.063	0.002	0.058	0.009	0.361**
Unskilled	1				1		
Mode of delivery							
SVD	1				1		
Instrumental delivery	0.442	0.194	1.006	0.042	0.262	0.072	0.952
SVD+ episiotomy	0.437	0.172	1.114	0.173	0.382	0.096	1.523
C/S	1.594	0.737	3.450	0.320	0.355	0.046	2.738
Abnormal Labour							
No	1				1		
Yes	3.524*	2.142	5.796	0.001	3.496	1.692	7.223**
Past postpartum morbidity							
No	1				1		
Yes	5.695	3.167	10.242	0.340	1.582	0.617	4.057
Postpartum visit after this delivery							
No	0.082*	0.042	0.159	0.000	0.088	0.040	0.194**
Yes	1				1		

strategies to reduce maternal mortality and morbidity should give emphasis on access of prenatal care service, early detection and management of intra-partum abnormalities, and educating mothers on benefits of institutional delivery.

Acknowledgements
We would like to express our heartfelt gratitude to our advisor Carmen Robles (PhD, associate prof) who have been a great help to the completion of this research paper.
We would like to extend our heartfelt thanks to each health institutions chart registration room staffs for their support in the data collection process. We would like to thank data collectors for their unreserved and dedicated cooperation.

Funding
This research was funded by Mekelle University College of health Sciences up to data collection and analysis of the result but writing the manuscript was fully covered by the authors themselves.

Authors' contributions
AT designed the study, analysis and drafted the manuscript for publication. AY and MA provided scientific advices on the design of the study, data analysis and throughout the preparation of the manuscript, BT and YA were involved in the design, data collection and preparation of manuscript. All authors read and approved the manuscript.

Competing interests
The author(s) declare that they have no competing interests.

Author details
[1]Department of Midwifery, College of Health Sciences, Debre Markos University, Debre Markos, Ethiopia. [2]Department of Midwifery, College of Health Sciences, MekelleUniversity, Mekelle, Ethiopia. [3]Department of Immunology, Microbiology and Parasitology, College of Health Science, Bahir Dar University, Bahir Dar, Ethiopia. [4]Department of Medical Parasitology, College of Health Sciences, Debre Markos University, Debre Markos, Ethiopia.

References
1. USAID. Maternal Morbidity and Disability: getting the attention it deserves, vol. 2015. London: Parliamentary group on population, development and Reprod Health.
2. World Health Organization. Postpartum care of the Mother& new born practical guide. Geneva: WHO; 2012.
3. United Kingdom. A report on maternal morbidity all party parliamentary group on population, development and Reprod Health. London: Population, Development and Reproductive Health Department; 2009.
4. USAID. Fistula care, Intra Health, Engender Health. Overview of Safe Motherhood and Global Maternal Morbidity and Mortality. Geneva: World Health Organization; 2010.
5. Zanur RZ, Loh KY, Med M. Postpartum morbidity-what we can do. Med J Malaysia. 2006;61(5):651–5.
6. Ferdous J, Ahmed A, Dasjubta SK, et al. Occurrence and determinants of postpartum maternal morbidities and disabilities among women in Matlab. Bangladesh J Health, Population and Nutrit. 2012;30(2):143–58.
7. Federal Democratic Republic of Ethiopia Ministry of Health. Health Sector Development Program IV 2010/11–2014/15. Ethiopia: FMOH, 2010 Oct, 1st.
8. Central Statistical Agency [Ethiopia] and ICF International. Ethiopian Demographic and Health Survey. Addis Ababa, Ethiopia and Calverton. Maryland, USA: Central Statistical Agency and ICF International; 2011.
9. Sebitloane TH. HIV and Post partum mortality /morbidity. Boston: Nelson R Mandela school of Medicine; 2013 Jun.
10. Ashford L. Hidden suffering: Disabilities from Pregnancy and Childbirth in Less Developed Countries. Washington, DC: Population Reference Bureau; 2009.
11. Federal Democratic Republic of Ethiopia Ministry of Health. Basic Emergency obstetric & Newborn Care. 2nd ed. Addis Ababa: FMOH; 2013.
12. Prakash S, Yadav K, Bhardwaj B, Chaudhary S. Incidence of Anemia and its socio-demographic determinants among pregnant women attending for antenatal care: a cross sectional study. Int J Med & Health Res. 2015;1(3):12–7.
13. Lyengar K. Early postpartum maternal morbidity among rural women of Rajasthan, India: A Community-based Study. Int Center for Diarrheal disease research. 2012;30(2):213–25.
14. Department for International Development (DFID). Improving reproductive, maternal and newborn health: Buden, determinants and health systems. 1st ed. UK: Department for International Development; 2010.
15. Tatek A, Bekana K, Amsalu F, Equlenet M, Rogers N. Prospective study on birth outcome and prevalence of postpartum morbidity among pregnant women who attended for antenatal Care in Gondar Town, north West Ethiopia. Andrology-open Access. 2014;3(2):1–125.
16. Ethiopia ministry of finance. Ethiopia MDGs report. 1st ed. Ethiopia: Ministry of finance& economic development; 2012.
17. Callaghan WM, Creanga AA, Kuklina EV. Severe maternal morbidity among delivery and postpartum hospitalizations in the United States. The ACOG. 2012;120(5):29–36.

26

Bacteriological profile and antibiotic susceptibility pattern of common isolates of neonatal sepsis, Ho Municipality, Ghana-2016

Fortress Yayra Aku[1,2], Patricia Akweongo[1], Kofi Nyarko[1], Samuel Sackey[1], Fredrick Wurapa[1], Edwin Andrew Afari[1], Donne Kofi Ameme[1] and Ernest Kenu[1]* ⓘ

Abstract

Background: Globally, 4 million neonates die annually, with one-third of such deaths occurring as a result of infections. In 2011, there were 7.2million deaths in children below 5 years globally, and a proportion of 40% of these deaths occurred in neonates. Sepsis was reported to account for one-third of these deaths. Presently, multidrug antibiotic resistance is rapidly increasing in Neonatal Intensive Care Units (NICUs), particularly in developing countries and poses a threat to public health. The change in these organisms has been reported to vary across regions, between health facilities and even within the same facility. Continuous surveillance is required to inform antibiotic choice for neonatal sepsis management. We identified the common causative organisms of neonatal sepsis and their antibiotic susceptibility pattern in the Ho municipality.

Method: A cross sectional study was conducted in the Ho municipality from January to May, 2016. A semi-structured questionnaire was used to collect socio-demographic data from mothers of neonates with clinically suspected of sepsis. Clinical data of both mothers and neonates were extracted from case notes. A 2 ml volume of blood was also taken from neonates and dispensed into a 20 ml mixture of thioglycollate fluid broth and tryptone soy broth for culture and antibiotic susceptibility pattern determined.

Results: Out of the 150 clinically suspected neonatal sepsis cases, 91 (60.7%) were males. The Median gestational week was 38 (IQR: 36–39) and Median birthweight was 3.0 kg (IQR 2.5–3.4). The prevalence of culture positive sepsis was 17.3% of the 150 suspected cases. A total of 26 different pathogens were isolated, of which gram positive organisms had a preponderance of 18 (69%) over gram negative organisms 8 (31%). *Staphylococcus epidermidis* was the most common 14 (53.8%) isolate identified. There was a single isolate (4%) each of *Proteus mirabilis* and *Escherichia coli* identified. All the isolates identified showed 100% resistance to ampicillin.

Conclusion: The prevalence of culture proven sepsis was 17.3% and *Staphylococcus epidermidis* was the most common isolate identified. Pathogens isolated were resistant to the first line drugs for management of neonatal sepsis. Hence, the need for a review of first line drug for empirical treatment in neonatal sepsis.

Keywords: Neonatal sepsis, Antibiotics, Newborn

* Correspondence: ernest_kenu@yahoo.com
[1]Ghana Field Epidemiology and Laboratory Training Programme and Department of Epidemiology and Disease Control, School of Public Health, University of Ghana, Accra, Ghana
Full list of author information is available at the end of the article

Background

Neonatal sepsis (NS) is a significant contributor of mortality and morbidity in the newborn [1]. It is estimated that globally 4million newborns die yearly with one-third of the deaths caused by infections [2].Various conditions contribute to high neonatal mortality especially in Sub-Saharan Africa of which neonatal sepsis accounts for approximately 26% [3]. In 2008, 22, 672 deaths were estimated to have occurred among neonates in Ghana with neonatal sepsis causing 4923 deaths (21.7%) [4, 5].

Neonatal sepsis refers to a clinical syndrome that is marked by signs and symptoms of infection in the first 28 days of life, with or without isolation of a pathogen [6]. A normal fetus is sterile until shortly before birth since placenta and amniotic sac serve as effective protection against infection. However, at birth, the newborn is exposed to the microbial environment. NS can be categorized as early onset sepsis (EOS) and late onset sepsis (LOS). EOS is defined as onset of signs and symptoms of infection within 72 h of life and may be associated with pathogen isolation or not. In the LOS, signs and symptoms present after 72 h of life [7] and categorization of EOS and LOS is to show the varying causes and pathophysiology of common isolates related to the time of onset of the condition. It is also crucial in prevention and treatment due to aetiological variation.

Some maternal and neonatal factors have been identified to predispose a neonate to sepsis. In a study on neonatal sepsis conducted in 2013 in China, maternal age > 35; mother with affixed occupation; mother of urban residence; caesarean section delivery; and parity were found to influence early onset neonatal sepsis in a univariate analysis [8]. In a similar study conducted at King Edward Memorial Hospital in Western Australia, it was also found that neonates who were born at a lower gestational age (26 weeks ± 1.8) and those who had a lower birth weight (848 g ± 240 g) developed sepsis [9].

Recent reviews of causative agents associated with infants with sepsis in the developing world revealed that in EOS, gram negative organisms predominated in the ratio of 2:1 with *Escherichia coli* being the most commonly isolated pathogen [10]. However, the main causative agent of LOS in neonatal intensive care unit has been reported to be coagulase negative staphylococcus (CoNS). In a study done in the Aga Khan University Hospital NICU Nairobi Kenya, on 152 neonates who presented with sepsis, also found that 58 (38.2%) of them had LOS; and coagulase-negative staphylococcus was the most common isolate both in EOS and LOS [11]. A similar study done in Tanzania, found that *Staphylococcus aureus* was the most common organism isolated from blood culture and pus swab followed by *Klebsiella* species and *Escherichia coli* [12]. A study conducted in Ghana revealed gram positives as the predominant isolate and included coagulase negative staphylococcus (CoNS), followed by *Staphylococcus aureus* and *Streptococcus* species [13].

The main method of diagnosing sepsis is the isolation of causative agents from blood cultures [14]. Since there are no pathognomonic signs and symptoms for sepsis in neonates, it is necessary to carry out investigations in a well set up laboratory that has the capacity to do so [15]. In a study done in Tanzania, clinical signs such as difficulty in feeding, lethargy, convulsion, increase in respiratory rate and cyanosis had a strong association with culture proven early onset sepsis, whiles hypothermia, chest in-drawing, umbilical redness and jaundice were related to late onset form of sepsis (14). In managing sepsis, neonates are given empirical therapy according to the World Health Organization (WHO) Integrated Management of Neonatal and Childhood Illness (IMNCI) algorithm for early detection of severe diseases including severe bacterial infection [15].

Currently at the Volta Regional and Ho Municipal Hospitals' NICUs in the Ho municipality, neonatal sepsis accounts for the highest cause of admission and is managed empirically in line with the WHO recommendation of using ampicillin/cloxacillin and gentamicin as first line antibiotics. There is paucity of published data on neonatal bloodstream infection in Ghana and West Africa [13] and over the period, reports show that neonatal sepsis causative agents differ from region to region and vary from time to time [16]. This change in causative agents coupled with their change in response to commonly used antibiotics and the need for periodic health facility based surveys calls for evidence based data was therefore the basis for our study. This study was done to determine the common isolates of neonatal sepsis and their antibiotic susceptibility pattern to commonly used antibiotics.

Methods

Study design

The study was a hospital based cross-sectional study carried out at two public hospitals in the Ho municipality (Ho Municipal and Volta Regional Hospitals). A 2 ml volume of blood was taken into a universal bottle for culture from neonates clinically suspected of sepsis and admitted at the two NICUs between January and May, 2016 for culture; to determine the common isolates causing sepsis and antibiotic susceptibility pattern of the isolates.

Study population

All neonates and their mothers who delivered by either C-section or spontaneous vaginal delivery and did not receive any antibiotic before the operation were included in the study.

For purposes of this study, neonatal sepsis was defined as neonates presenting with one or more of the following features: presence of fever (≥38 °C) or hypothermia (≤36 °C), convulsions, lethargy, difficulty to feed, difficulty to breathe, hypoglycaemia, vomiting, bulging fontanels, respiratory distress, jaundice and signs of infection on the skin and umbilical pus discharge or hypareamia.

Inclusion and exclusion criteria
All neonates admitted at the NICUs of the two hospitals, who were clinically diagnosed of sepsis by a clinician during the study period, and whose mothers or caretakers consented to be part of the study were included in the study. All neonates admitted at the NICUs of the two hospitals, who were clinically diagnosed of sepsis by a clinician during the study period but died immediately upon arrival before blood culture sample could be obtained, or neonates who were referred to a tertiary facility immediately after assessment were excluded.

Sample size calculation
Using a prevalence of 11%, a total sample size of 150 was calculated using the Cochrane formula [17]. Out of a total of 250 neonates who were in the Neonatal Intensive Care Units (NICU) during the time of the study, 150 who met the inclusion criteria and were randomly recruited.

Data collection
Structured questionnaires were used to collect demographic and clinical details of both neonates and their mothers through interview and review of case notes. Data on the pathogens isolated and their antibiotic susceptibility pattern were also collected after laboratory test was done.

Laboratory investigations
Two millilitres of venous blood was aseptically obtained from the antecubital fossa of each neonate and dispensed into a sterilized universal bottle containing 20 ml of tryptone soy broth to make a 1:10 dilution. In obtaining blood samples, the site was cleaned with isopropyl alcohol concentration of 70% twice before blood was collected. There was strict adherence to microbiological protocol during culture and isolation which included use of sterile loops. In the event of using loops that the authors thought were not sterile enough, isolates were considered as contaminants. Blood culture samples were then transported to the laboratory within 1 h and incubated at 37 °C for 24 h. Each sample was sub-cultured unto commercially prepared blood chocolate agar and MacConkey agar. The sub-cultured agars were incubated at 37 °C and observed for growth. Samples that did not show growth after 24 h were observed for 7 days before

regarded as no growth. Pure colonies of samples that showed growth were taken for gram stain test and biochemical tests using commercially prepared reagents. These tests together with characteristic morphology of pure colonies were used for isolation and identification of pathogens.

Antibiotic susceptibilities of isolated pathogens to the selected antimicrobial agents were determined, using the Kirby Bauer disc diffusion method according to the Clinical and Laboratory Standard Institute [18]. Pure colonies of isolates were emulsified to obtain 0.5 MacFarland standard and inoculated on Muller Hinton agar. Antimicrobial discs were place on the inoculated agar and incubated for 24 h at 37 °C; they were then observed for zones of inhibition, breakpoints identified and determined as susceptible, intermediate or resistant according to the Clinical and Laboratory Standard Institute [18]. All cultures received for neonates after an average of 48 h of onset of sepsis was regarded as delayed.

Data analysis
Case notes were reviewed again and interviews conducted to crosscheck for any anomalies detected. Data collected was checked for completeness and double entry was done. Data was entered into Microsoft Excel and cleaned by crosschecking for missing data, duplicates and outliers. It was then analysed using STATA software version 13.0 (College Station, Texas 77,845 USA). Continuous variables were presented as mean, standard deviation as well as median with inter-quartile range for neonates and their mothers Pathogens isolated from the laboratory investigation and antibiotic susceptibility of the isolates was presented in frequencies and proportions.

Ethical consideration
Approval for this study was obtained from the Ghana Health Service Ethical Review Committee. Permission was also sort from the Municipal Health Directorate and the hospital administration of the respective hospitals. An informed consent was administered to mothers of neonates before participation in the study, and each respondent was given a unique identifier such that data gathered could not be traced back to respondents. Data was kept safe under lock and key and was accessible only to the principal investigator.

Results
Neonatal characteristics
Out of the 150 neonates that were suspected of sepsis and recruited during the study period, 91 (60.7%) were males (Table 1). Majority, 87 (58%) of the mothers of these neonates were delivered by caesarean section. The median gestational week was 38 weeks (IQR: 36–39)

Table 1 Characteristics of neonates with suspected sepsis on admission at NICU, Ho municipality, 2016

Variable	Count (N)	Percent (%)
Sex		
Male	91	60.7
Female	59	39.3
Birth weight		
< 2500 g	35	24.5
≥ 2500 g	108	75.5
Place of birth		
Within study facilities	109	72.7
Outside study facilities	41	27.3
Sepsis category		
Early onset sepsis	81	54
Late onset sepsis	69	46
Gestational age		
≤ 36	41	27.3
37–40	94	62.7
≥ 41	15	10
Length of hospital stay		
≤ 7 days	77	51.3
≥ 8 days	73	48.7
Delivery mode		
SVD	63	42
C/S	87	58
Position of lines		
Central placed	105	70
Peripheral IV catheter	45	30

SVD spontaneous vaginal delivery, *C/S* caesarean section

Table 2 Distribution of maternal socio-demographic characteristics

Variable	Count (N) 150	Percent (%)
Age		
≤ 20	20	13.3
21–30	71	47.3
≥ 31	59	39.3
Marital status		
Married	108	72
Single	41	27.3
Divorced	1	0.7
Residence		
Within Ho Municipality	52	34.7
Outside Ho Municipality	98	65.3
Ethnicity		
Ewes	136	90.7
Akan	9	6
Northern descent	5	3.3
Religion		
Christianity	142	94.7
Islam	6	4
Traditional African Belief	2	1.3
Educational level		
No formal education	12	8
Primary	18	12
JSS	59	39.3
SSS	35	23.3
Tertiary	26	17.3
Employment		
Employed	122	81.3
Unemployed	28	18.7

weeks; and the median birthweight was 3.0 kg (IQR 2.5–3.4) kg. Most of the deliveries, 109 (72.7%) were either at the Volta Regional Hospital or Ho Municipal Hospital; (Table 1). Of the 41 born outside the study facilities, 11 (26.8%) were home deliveries.

Maternal characteristics

The mean age of mothers of the neonates included in the study was (28 ± 6) years with a minimum age of 16 years and maximum 41 years. The number of mothers who resided within the Ho municipality was 52 (34.7%). Most of the mothers were disproportionately Christians, 142 (94.7%) (Table 2).

Common isolates identified

Equal proportions of microorganism were isolated in both early and late onset sepsis. The gram positive isolates identified were *Staphylococcus aureus* and *Staphylococcus epidermidis*. Gram negative organisms include: *Pseudomonas aeruginosa, Escherichia coli, Enterobacter* species

and *Proteus mirabilis* (Table 3). Overall, the commonest microorganism isolated was *Staphylococcus epidermidis* 14 (53.9%), with the greater proportion 9 (69.2%) in early onset sepsis (Table 3). Positive blood cultures were not repeated however, isolates that were considered contaminants by the microbiologist were not included in this study. Lumbar puncture was not done for positive blood cultures in this study.

Antibiotic susceptibility

A total of 44% (66 of 150) of the neonates tested had previously been given antibiotics before their samples were taken.

Based on the antibiotic susceptibility testing of the gram positive organisms isolated from the blood culture, *Staphylococcus epidermidis* showed 100% resistance to ampicillin, and 57% resistance to gentamicin (Table 4).

Table 3 Distribution of isolates of blood culture of neonates with sepsis

Isolate	Early Onset Sepsis		Late Onset Sepsis		
	Count	Percentage (%)	Count	Percentage (%)	Total Count (N)
Gram Positive organism					
Staphylococcus epidermidis	9	69.2	5	38.5	14
Staphylococcus aureus	1	7.7	3	23.1	4
Gram Negative organism					
Escherichia coli	1	7.7	0	0	1
Pseudomonas aeruginosa	2	15.4	2	15.4	4
Enterobacter species	0	0	2	15.4	2
Proteus mirabilis	0	0	1	7.7	1
Total	13		13		26

Of the four *Staphylococcus aureus* organisms isolated, there was a 100% (4/4) resistance to ampicillin, 100% (4/4) resistance to penicillin and 50% (2/4) resistance to gentamicin, (Table 4). However, sensitivity to methicillin was not tested in this study.

A total of eight gram negative organisms were identified in this study, namely *Pseudomonas aeruginosa* (4), *Escherichia coli* (1), *Enterobacter* species (2) and *Proteus mirabilis* (1). *Pseudomonas aeruginosa* showed 75% (3/4) resistance to cefuroxime, 50% (2/4) resistance to cefotaxime, and 25% (1/4) resistance to gentamicin (Table 5).

The percentage resistance of *Escherichia coli* was 100% (1/1) to ampicillin, 100% to cotrimoxazole, 0% to gentamicin, 0% to ceftriaxone and, 0% to cefotaxime (Table 5). *Enterobacter* species showed 100% resistance to ampicillin, 100% resistance to cefotaxime 50% resistance to gentamicin, and 50% resistance to ceftriaxone (Table 5). The resistance of *Proteus mirabilis* was 100% to ampicillin, 100% to cefuroxime, and 0% to cefotaxime (Table 5).

Discussion
Common isolates
Culture results in this study shows that 26 (17.3%) of the suspected neonatal sepsis cases were positive. The results indicate that, gram positive organisms (69%, 18/26) has a preponderance over the gram negative organisms (31%, 8/26). This suggests that majority of the infections were transmitted from handling by health care personnel and family members. Since *Staphylococcus epidermidis*

Table 4 Percentage resistance of gram positive organisms isolated from blood culture

Isolate	Count (N)	AMP	GEN	CRX	COT	PEN	FLU
Staphylococcus epidermidis	14	100	57	64	100	100	100
Staphylococcus Aureus	4	100	50	75	50	100	–

AMP ampicillin, *GEN* gentamicin, *CRX* cefuroxime, *COT* cotrimoxazole, *PEN* penicillin, *FLU* flucloxacillin

and *Staphylococcus aureus* are the major normal flora located on the skin and in the nose respectively, suboptimal hand hygiene by persons who handle neonates, manipulation of peripheral intravenous lines set up on neonates could contribute to the acquisition of these bacteria. Findings from this study, did not correspond to a study done in a Neonatal Intensive Care Unit (NICU) in Bangladesh, where they identified gram negative organisms (78%) to be the most common pathogen of neonatal sepsis [19]. However, in a similar study in Ghana in a tertiary hospital, gram positive organisms had a preponderance over gram negative organisms; similar to findings in this study except that their study had a larger sample size [13].

However, a similar study in a NICU in China, found that gram positive organisms were responsible for a greater proportion of early onset sepsis (83.3%) and late onset sepsis (70%) as compared to gram negative organisms [20], which corroborates the findings of this study. These Findings are also similar to a study in Nigeria which reported a 52.6% proportion of gram positive organisms from blood culture of neonates with sepsis [21].

Staphylococcus epidermidis 9 (64%), was the most common isolate identified of all the bacteria in early onset sepsis (EOS). The same findings were reported in a similar study in Ghana, where *Staphylococcus epidermidis* was the most common isolate in both EOS (59.1%) and LOS (52.8%) in a tertiary hospital [13]. Since reports indicate that, organisms causing EOS are mostly transmitted vertically from the colonized genital tract of mothers, or sometimes through the delivery process, the findings suggest that EOS causing organisms could be transmitted by these means.

In a study in Nepal, results revealed that *Staphylococcus epidermidis* accounted for the greatest proportion (57.3%), followed by (28.1%) of *Escherichia coli*, (11.2%) of *Staphylococcus aureus* and (1.1%) of *Pseudomonas aeruginosa* that were isolated in EOS [22]. This is similar to what was observed in this study. Similar reports were

Table 5 Percentage resistance of gram negative organisms isolated from blood culture

Isolate	Count (N)	AMP	GEN	CRX	COT	CTR	CTX
Pseudomonas aeruginosa	4	100	25	75	75	25	50
Escherichia Coli	1	100	0	0	100	0	0
Enterobacter species	2	100	50	50	50	50	100
Proteus mirabilis	1	100	100	100	100	0	0

I Intermediate susceptibility, *AMP* ampicillin, *GEN* gentamicin, *CRX* cefuroxime, *COT* cotrimoxazole, *CTR* ceftriaxone, *CTX* cefotaxime, *I* intermediate

given in a study done in Tamale Teaching Hospital in Ghana, where 8 (53.3%) of *Staphylococcus* species, 1 (6.7%) *Escherichia coli* [5] and other gram negative organisms of a total of 15 isolates were identified in EOS.

In the late onset sepsis (LOS) cases, majority of the bacteria identified were *Staphylococcus epidermidis* and *Staphylococcus aureus*. Reports in Nepal, indicate that *Enterobacter* species (15%), *Acinetobacter* species *(12%)* and, *Escherichia coli (12%)* were the commonest isolated gram negative organisms in LOS, which contradicts the findings of this study [23]. In addition, a study done in South Africa, identified *Acinetobacter baumannii*, *Klebsiella pneumoniae* and *Escherichia coli* as the predominant gram negative bacteria, together with few *Pseudomonas aeruginosa* and *Enterobacter* species, which is contrary to findings in this study [24]. Considering that, there is a variation of causative organisms of neonatal sepsis, between geographic regions and facilities, the difference in findings in this study could be acceptable. Bacteriological profile of neonatal sepsis causing organisms may vary among countries [25]. Also, composition of these organisms have changed over the last century because of changing trend of antibiotic use and life style [26].

Antibiotic susceptibility

Results of antibiotic susceptibility in the present study indicate that, *Staphylococcus epidermidis*, shows 100% resistance to ampicillin, penicillin, flucloxacillin and cotrimoxazole. This is alarming considering that, either ampicillin or penicillin in combination with gentamicin is recommended as first line drugs for empiric treatment of neonatal sepsis. Though *Staphylococcus epidermidis* shows an approximated average (43%) sensitivity to gentamicin, it indicates that its treatment by first line drugs poses a threat to management of neonates. Neonates may spend longer days on antibiotics and stay longer in hospital as well. This confirms reports in an antibiotic susceptibility test carried out on blood cultures from neonates that, Coagulase Negative *Staphylococcus* including *Staphylococcus epidermidis* showed poor sensitivity (13.5%) to ampicillin [27]. In another study, *Staphylococcus epidermidis* showed 100% resistance to

ampicillin, penicillin and cotrimoxazole [28], which corresponds to the findings of this study. Thus, results in this study could serve as evidence of increasing resistance to commonly used antibiotics.

Staphylococcus aureus, the second gram positive isolate in this study is 100% resistant to ampicillin, and penicillin. The overall high resistance rate exhibited could be attributed to the frequent and unrestricted use of the commonly used antibiotics. Consequently, this could limit future antibiotic choice for treating neonatal infections thereby, affecting survival of septic neonates. In Ghana, resistance rate of 96.4%, and 96.4% to ampicillin, and penicillin respectively was reported [5]; this confirms high resistance rate to these antibiotics identified in this study. Susceptibility to methicillin was not tested in this study, thus sensitivity and resistance to methicillin among neonates was not determined.

We observed a lower resistance (25%) to ceftriaxone and gentamicin. High sensitivity to gentamicin and ceftriaxone by *Pseudomonas aeruginosa* is good for neonatal care. This means that, the use of both drugs in empiric treatment of neonatal sepsis will be effective against *Pseudomonas aeruginosa*. However, the complete resistance to ampicillin, as exhibited by other organisms in this study is devastating. As observed in a study done in India, *Pseudomonas aeruginosa* was 25% resistant to gentamicin, [29] which is comparable to this study.

Enterobacter species showed multidrug resistance (100%) to ampicillin, and cefotaxime. Multidrug resistance in the sick newborn is not a desirable experience for the neonate, family or clinical management staff. The reason is that, it leads to increased cost in terms of money and productive time spent at the hospital by family. Additionally, multidrug resistance of infectious organisms could result in unsuccessful treatment leading to death. Though sensitivity to gentamicin and the third generation cephalosporins (cefuroxime and ceftriaxone) are fairly high, it calls for caution and restriction in its use. As observed in Nepal, *Enterobacter* species had a high multidrug resistance rate (100%) to antibiotics including ampicillin and cefotaxime [23], which is consistent with findings in this study.

The only *Escherichia coli* isolated also exhibits a multidrugresistance to ampicillin, and cotrimoxazole. However, there was no susceptibility to gentamicin and the cephalosporin (cefuroxime, ceftriaxone and cefotaxime). *Escherichia coli* also exhibits multidrug resistance like *Pseudomonas aeruginosa* in this study, which poses a threat to neonatal care in this era of increasing antibiotic resistance. These results are partly consistent, and partly disagrees with a similar study done in Indonesia where *Klebsiella pneumoniae, Escherichia coli, Enterobacter* species and non-fermenting gram negative bacilli were the gram negative organisms isolated; it was reported that, all of them exhibited high resistance to ampicillin, gentamicin and cefotaxime [30].

The single *Proteus mirabilis* organism identified, also exhibits a high level of multidrug resistance but not susceptible to ceftriaxone and cefotaxime. The high level of antibiotic resistance observed is in line with the emerging threat of global antibiotic resistance. One factor accounting for this, could be the indiscriminate use of available antibiotics in the presumptive treatment of neonatal infection. Also, the tendency of clinicians initiating antibiotic therapy before performing blood culture could result in antimicrobial resistance. As observed in this study, blood was obtained from 44% (66 of 150) neonates after the initiation of antibiotic therapy. Thus, it could be a contributing factor to high rates of antibiotic resistance exhibited in this study.

Findings from this study reveal that, all the common isolates of neonatal sepsis show 100% resistance to ampicillin. In addition, all gram positive organisms show 100% resistance to penicillin. However, organisms show appreciable sensitivity to gentamicin, ceftriaxone and cefuroxime. This indicates that "ampicillin/penicillin +gentamicin" combination as the first line of drugs for empiric therapy, needs to be reviewed in terms of ampicillin and penicillin.

Limitations

This study did not determine the selective pressure factors influencing antibiotic susceptibility, but only determined antibiotic susceptibility. Thus factors associated with high antibiotic resistance in this study are not known. The initiation of antibiotic therapy in some neonates prior to obtaining blood culture sample could have reduced culture positivity, hence affecting prevalence of culture proven sepsis in the study. Methicillin was not contained in the multidisc used for the culture, there sensitivity tests for *S. aureus* could not be carried out.

More infants delivered by C-section were included in the study, therefore, the isolated organism isolated are likely to be different. This is because C-section infections maybe hospital acquired and mainly gram negative.

Also, we did not collect data on UTI among mothers. However, only 3 and 12 case notes of mothers contained information on chorioamnionitis and maternal fever. Unavailability of these variables on majority of mothers was a limitation.

Conclusion

The prevalence of culture proven neonatal sepsis in this study is 17.3%. Gram positive organisms were the prevalent neonatal sepsis causing organisms in this study. Of the gram positive organisms, *Staphylococcus epidermidis* was the most common isolate, followed by *Staphylococcus aureus*. *Pseudomonas aeruginosa* was the most common isolate among the gram negative organisms, with single isolates each of *Escherichia coli* and *Proteus mirabilis*. Generally, gram negative bacteria exhibit a better susceptibility rate to gentamicin and ceftriaxone, whiles gram positive organisms are more sensitive to gentamicin. Gentamicin as the first line antibiotic for neonatal sepsis is still quite effective. However, the microorganisms isolated in this study demonstrate an increasing resistance rate. All neonatal sepsis causing organisms were completely resistant to ampicillin and penicillin and hence the need to review the empirical treatment for neonatal sepsis.

Abbreviations
CoNS: Coagulase negative staphylococcus; EOS: Early onset sepsis; LOS: Late onset sepsis; NICU: Neonatal Intensive Care Unit; NS: Neonatal sepsis

Acknowledgements
We would like to appreciate the management of the Volta regional Hospitat and the Ho Municipal Hospital and their neonatal intensive care units for their immense support during data collection, particularly Dr. Lord Mensah, Dr. Amega-Aho, Dr. Larry Kumi, Mrs. Monica Nti and Dr. Agbadi. We are also grateful to the management and staff of the Volta regional hospital laboratory. Gratitude to Ms. Delia Bandoh for her assistance during writing of the manuscript.

Funding
The work was funded by the authors.

Authors' contributions
Conceptualization of idea: FAY, PA. Data collection and analysis: FAY, DA, PA. Drafting of manuscript: FAY, DA, PA, EA, SS, EK. Review and editing: EK, KMN, SS, EA. Finalization manuscript: FAY, DA, EK. All authors read and approved the final manuscript.

Competing interest
The authors declare that they have no competing interests.

Author details
[1]Ghana Field Epidemiology and Laboratory Training Programme and Department of Epidemiology and Disease Control, School of Public Health, University of Ghana, Accra, Ghana. [2]Ghana Health Service, Volta Regional Health Directorate, Ho, Ghana.

References

1. Al-Shamahy HA, Sabrah AA, Al-Robasi AB, Naser SM. Types of bacteria associated with neonatal sepsis in al-Thawra university hospital, Sana'a, Yemen, and their antimicrobial profile. Sultan Qaboos Univ Med J. 2012; 12(1):48–54. Available from: http://www.pubmedcentral.nih.gov/articlerender.fcgi?artid=3286716&tool=pmcentrez&rendertype=abstract

2. Ganatra HA, AKM Z. Neonatal infections in the developing world. Semin Perinatol. 2010;34(6):416–25. Available from: https://doi.org/10.1053/j.semperi.2010.09.004

3. Lawn JE, Cousens S, Zupan J. 4 million neonatal deaths: when? Where? Why? Lancet. 2005;365(9462):891–900. Available from: http://www.sciencedirect.com/science/article/pii/S0140673605710485

4. Black R, Cousens S, Johnson HL, Lawn JE, Rudan I, Bassani DG, et al. Global, regional, and national causes of child mortality in 2008: a systematic analysis. Lancet. 2010;375(9730):1969–87. Available from: https://doi.org/10.1016/S0140-6736(10)60549-1

5. Acquah S, Quaye L, Sagoe K, Ziem J, Bromberger P, Amponsem A. Susceptibility of bacterial etiological agents to commonly-used antimicrobial agents in children with sepsis at the tamale teaching hospital. BMC Infect Dis. 2013;13:89. Available from: http://www.pubmedcentral.nih.gov/articlerender.fcgi?artid=3598494&tool=pmcentrez&rendertype=abstract

6. Verma P, Berwal PK, Nagaraj N, Swami S, Jivaji P, Narayan S. Neonatal sepsis: epidemiology, clinical spectrum, recent antimicrobial agents and their antibiotic susceptibility pattern. International Journal of Contemporary Padiatrics. 2015;2(3):176–80.

7. Shane AL, Stoll BJ. Recent developments and current issues in the epidemiology, diagnosis, and management of bacterial and fungal neonatal sepsis. Am J Perinatol. 2013;30(2):131–41.

8. Jiang Z, Ye G. Factor of early onset neonatal sepsis; 2013. p. 2460–6.

9. Strunk T, Doherty D, Jacques A, Simmer K, Richmond P, Kohan R, et al. Histologic Chorioamnionitis is associated with reduced risk of late-onset sepsis in preterm infants. Pediatrics. 2012;129(1):e134–41.

10. Zaidi AKM, Ganatra HA, Syed S, Cousens S, ACC L, Black R, et al. Effect of case management on neonatal mortality due to sepsis and pneumonia. BMC Public Health. 2011;11(Suppl 3):S13. Available from: http://www.pubmedcentral.nih.gov/articlerender.fcgi?artid=3231886&tool=pmcentrez&rendertype=abstract\nhttp://www.ncbi.nlm.nih.gov/pubmed/21501430\nhttp://www.ncbi.nlm.nih.gov/pmc/articles/PMC3231886/pdf/1471-2458-11-S3-S13.pdf

11. Kohli-Kochhar R, Omuse RG, Revathi G. A ten-year review of neonatal bloodstream infections in a tertiary private hospital in Kenya. J Infect Dev Ctries. 2011;5(11):799–803. Available from: http://www.jidc.org/index.php/journal/article/viewFile/22112734/630\nhttp://ovidsp.ovid.com/ovidweb.cgi?T=JS&PAGE=reference&D=emed10&NEWS=N&AN=2011647840

12. Mhada TV, Fredrick F, Matee MI, Massawe A. Neonatal sepsis at Muhimbili National Hospital, Dar es salaam, Tanzania; aetiology, antimicrobial sensitivity pattern and clinical outcome. BMC Public Health. 2012;12(1):904. Available from: BMC Public Health

13. Labi A, Obeng-nkrumah N, Bjerrum S, Enweronu-laryea C, Newman MJ. Neonatal bloodstream infections in a Ghanaian tertiary hospital: are the current antibiotic recommendations adequate? BMC Infect Dis. 2016;16(1):598. Available from: https://doi.org/10.1186/s12879-016-1913-4

14. Sriram R. Correlation of blood culture results with the sepsis score and the sepsis screen in the diagnosis of neonatal septicemia. Int J Biol Med Res. 2011;2(1):360–8.

15. Kayange N, Kamugisha E, Mwizamholya DL, Jeremiah S, Mshana SE. Predictors of positive blood culture and deaths among neonates with suspected neonatal sepsis in a tertiary hospital, Mwanza-Tanzania. BMC Pediatr. 2010;10:39. Available from: http://www.pubmedcentral.nih.gov/articlerender.fcgi?artid=2889942&tool=pmcentrez&rendertype=abstract

16. WHO. WHO pocket book of Hospital Care for Children. 2005;

17. Charan J, Biswas T. How to calculate sample size for different study designs in medical research. Indian J Psychol Med. 2013;35(2):121–6.

18. CLSI. Performance standards for antimicrobial susceptibility testing; seventeenth informational supplement. 2007.

19. Naher BS, Afroza S, Roy S, Nahar N, Kundu TN. Neonatal Sepsis in A Tertiary Care Hospital: Evaluation of Causative Agents and Antimicrobial Susceptibilities. Bangladesh J. Child Health. 2013;37(1):14–17.

20. Li Z, Xiao Z, Li Z, Zhong Q, Zhang Y, Xu F. 116 cases of neonatal early-onset or late-onset sepsis: a single center retrospective analysis on pathogenic bacteria species distribution and antimicrobial susceptibility. Int J Clin Exp Med. 2013;6(8):693–9. Available from: http://www.ijcem.com/files/ijcem1307017.pdf\nhttp://ovidsp.ovid.com/ovidweb.cgi?T=JS&PAGE=reference&D=emed11&NEWS=N&AN=2013583944

21. Peterside O, Pondei K, Akinbami FO. Bacteriological profile and antibiotic susceptibility pattern of neonatal sepsis at a teaching Hospital in Bayelsa State. Nigeria. 2015;43(3):183–90.

22. Adhikari N, Pk S, Acharya G, Km V. Bacteriological pro fi le and associated risk factors of neonatal sepsis in Paropakar Maternity and Women ' s Hospital Thapathali, Kathmandu Neonatal Sepsis is one of the most common reasons for admission to neonatal units in developing. 2014;16:161–164.

23. Ansari S, Gautam R, Shrestha S, Neopane P, Chapagain ML. Neonatal septicemia in Nepal: early-onset versus late-onset. Int J Pediatr. 2015;2015:379806.

24. Ballot DE, Nana T, Sriruttan C, Cooper PA. Bacterial bloodstream infections in neonates in a developing country. ISRN Pediatr. 2012;2012:1–6.

25. Yunanto A, Margareta Y, Indah D, Pratiwi N. American Journal of Oral Medicine and Radiology Bacteriological Pattern And Antibiotic Susceptibility In Neonatology Ward Ulin General Hospital, Banjarmasin, Indonesia. 2014; 1(1):10–13.

26. Marchant EA, Boyce GK, Sadarangani M, Lavoie PM. Neonatal Sepsis due to Coagulase-Negative Staphylococci. Clin Dev Immunol. 2013;2013.

27. Begum M, Hassan M, Haque ZSM, Jahan N, Chowdhury K, Rob AWS. Study of Bacteriological pathogen causing neonatal sepsis at NICU in Ad-din medical college hospital. Northern International Medical College Journal. 2013;5(1):297–300.

28. Debnath J, Das PK. Bacteriological profile and antibiotic susceptibility pattern of neonatal septicemia in a tertiary care hospital of Tripura. Indian J Microbiol Res. 2015;238–43.

29. Minal T, Vegad MM, Shah PK, Soni S. Study of Gram Negative Organisms in Neonatal Septicaemia and its Antibiotic Susceptibility Pattern. International Journal of Microbiological Research. 2015;6(2):123–29.

30. Viswanathan R, Singh AK, Ghosh C, Dasgupta S, Mukherjee S, Basu S. Profile of neonatal septicaemia at a district-level sick newborn care unit. J Health Popul Nutr. 2012;30(1):41–8. Available from: http://www.pubmedcentral.nih.gov/articlerender.fcgi?artid=3312358&tool=pmcentrez&rendertype=abstract

27

NEC-zero recommendations from scoping review of evidence to prevent and foster timely recognition of necrotizing enterocolitis

Sheila M. Gephart[1*], Corrine Hanson[2], Christine M. Wetzel[3], Michelle Fleiner[4], Erin Umberger[5], Laura Martin[6], Suma Rao[7,8,9], Amit Agrawal[10,11], Terri Marin[12], Khaver Kirmani[4,8], Megan Quinn[1,4], Jenny Quinn[1,13], Katherine M. Dudding[1], Tanya Clay[14], Jason Sauberan[15], Yael Eskenazi[1], Caroline Porter[1], Amy L. Msowoya[16], Christina Wyles[1], Melissa Avenado-Ruiz[17], Shayla Vo[1], Kristina M. Reber[18] and Jennifer Duchon[19]

Abstract

Background: Although decades have focused on unraveling its etiology, necrotizing enterocolitis (NEC) remains a chief threat to the health of premature infants. Both modifiable and non-modifiable risk factors contribute to varying rates of disease across neonatal intensive care units (NICUs).

Purpose: The purpose of this paper is to present a scoping review with two new meta-analyses, clinical recommendations, and implementation strategies to prevent and foster timely recognition of NEC.

Methods: Using the Translating Research into Practice (TRIP) framework, we conducted a stakeholder-engaged scoping review to classify strength of evidence and form implementation recommendations using GRADE criteria across subgroup areas: 1) promoting human milk, 2) feeding protocols and transfusion, 3) timely recognition strategies, and 4) medication stewardship. Sub-groups answered 5 key questions, reviewed 11 position statements and 71 research reports. Meta-analyses with random effects were conducted on effects of standardized feeding protocols and donor human milk derived fortifiers on NEC.

Results: Quality of evidence ranged from very low (timely recognition) to moderate (feeding protocols, prioritize human milk, limiting antibiotics and antacids). Prioritizing human milk, feeding protocols and avoiding antacids were strongly recommended. Weak recommendations (i.e. "probably do it") for limiting antibiotics and use of a standard timely recognition approach are presented. Meta-analysis of data from infants weighing <1250 g fed donor human milk based fortifier had reduced odds of NEC compared to those fed cow's milk based fortifier (OR = 0.36, 95% CI 0.13, 1.00; $p = 0.05$; 4 studies, $N = 1164$). Use of standardized feeding protocols for infants <1500 g reduced odds of NEC by 67% (OR = 0.33, 95% CI 0.17, 0.65, $p = 0.001$; 9 studies; $N = 4755$ infants). Parents recommended that NEC information be shared early in the NICU stay, when feedings were adjusted, or feeding intolerance occurred via print and video materials to supplement verbal instruction.

(Continued on next page)

* Correspondence: gepharts@email.arizona.edu
[1]Robert Wood Johnson Foundation Nurse Faculty Scholar, The University of Arizona College of Nursing, PO Box 210203, Tucson, AZ 85721, USA
Full list of author information is available at the end of the article

(Continued from previous page)

Discussion: Evidence for NEC prevention is of sufficient quality to implement. Implementation that addresses system-level interventions that engage the whole team, including parents, will yield the best impact to prevent NEC and foster its timely recognition.

Keywords: Necrotizing enterocolitis, Very low birth weight, Prevention, Clinical practice guideline, Evidence-based practice, Neonatal intensive care, Infant, Nursing, Parent engagement, Translating Research into Practice Framework, NEC-zero, Practice guidelines, Scoping review,

Neonatal complications increase the cost of prematurity 4–7 fold; [1] but complication rates vary widely among NICUs, especially for those born very low birthweight (VLBW; <1500 g) [2–4]. One of the deadliest complications is necrotizing enterocolitis (NEC), a multi-factorial acquired intestinal disease that is the primary cause of emergency neonatal surgery [5]. NEC involves systemic inflammatory activation and progresses to full intestinal necrosis when severe [6]. NEC survivors can have very long hospital stays [7], require parenteral nutrition long-term, and experience delayed neurodevelopment [8]. Preventing one case of surgical NEC can save up to $250,000 per case, and when not preventable, timely recognition is a priority [9]. Surgery is required in 20–40% of the cases; and up to 50% of those needing surgery will die [4, 6, 10].

Background

As with many neonatal complications, NEC rates vary across NICUs [4, 11–13]. Quality improvement (QI) methods have been shown to reduce rates of NEC [14]. Central to QI is the consistent, measurable implementation of evidence into practice. In 2010, a NEC Clinical Practice Guideline published by the Cincinnati Children's Hospital Guideline Group recommended: 1) preferential feeding of mother's own milk (MOM), 2) providing pasteurized human donor milk (HDM) if MOM is not available, 3) using ibuprofen instead of indomethacin to close a patent ductus arteriosus (a common challenge in prematurity relating to NEC), and 4) administering antenatal steroids to mothers prior to delivery [15]. However, this guideline was not updated because of lack of a team to do so and was retired in 2015 [15]. In response, we sought to fill the gap for a NEC prevention guideline by applying a stakeholder-engaged process to conduct a scoping review and propose implementation recommendations in line with best practices to create trustworthy clinical guidelines [16–19]. To reflect the goal of preventing NEC, ultimately driving its incidence to a goal of zero, the effort was named "NEC-Zero." As parents are the first to notice symptoms and arguably have the most to lose when NEC strikes, they participated as expert stakeholders.

Purpose

The purpose of this paper is to present a scoping review with two new meta-analyses, clinical recommendations, and implementation strategies to prevent and foster timely recognition of NEC. All papers and position statements included in this review defined NEC as Bell's Stage II or greater.

Implementation science framework

To guide efforts, the Translating Research Into Practice (TRIP) implementation science framework was used because of its emphasis on framing evidence-based interventions in intensive care environments in partnership with stakeholders [20–23]. Building on Roger's Diffusion of Innovation theory applied to health [24], the TRIP identifies several factors that impact adoption of evidence-based innovations in practice. Factors include 1) innovation characteristics; 2) communication processes; 3) users; and 4) the social system (see Fig. 1) [20]. The TRIP purports that to be adopted, an evidence-based intervention should be: a) better than usual care; b) compatible with clinicians' values, c) simple, d) trialable in a low risk setting, and e) improve outcomes (process or patient-related). Figure 1 depicts how the TRIP was used to guide this stage of our process.

Methods
Scoping review approach

A stakeholder engaged scoping review was conducted to answer key questions about NEC prevention, timely recognition, implementation strategies and ways to engage parents [25, 26]. Six key steps are typical to scoping reviews: 1) identifying the key questions, 2) finding relevant studies, 3) selecting relevant studies to answer the questions, 4) extracting the data from the studies, 5) summarizing and reporting results, and 6) consulting stakeholders to appraise the literature, propose new resources and provide insights missing from the literature [26–28].

The group of expert stakeholders was selected in four steps. First, a national group of clinical and research experts were invited because they had published significant research and EBP improvement work around NEC. Second, a group of parents who had been impacted by

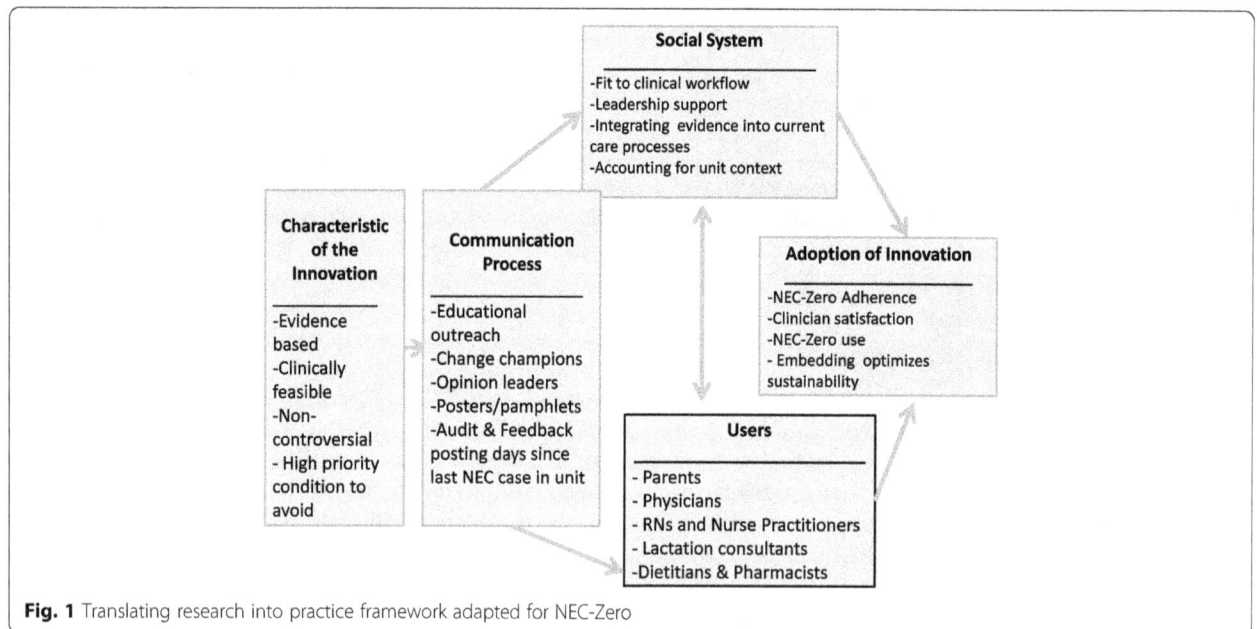

Fig. 1 Translating research into practice framework adapted for NEC-Zero

NEC were recommended by the president of the Preemie Parent Alliance from the NEC Society (E.U.), Graham's Foundation (L.M.), and Hand to Hold (T.C.). Third, a doctorally prepared Clinical Nurse Specialist engaged local stakeholders from the NICUs who intended to implement the recommendations. Finally, at the first meeting all were asked to identify expertise missing from the group, leading to more bedside nurses and a pharmacist joining. Stakeholder characteristics (N = 20) are portrayed in Table 1 and are referred to as "experts" from this point forward.

NEC-zero description

We reviewed evidence for NEC-Zero across four evidence-based facets: 1) preferential human milk feeding; [29–36] 2) adoption of a unit-approved standardized feeding protocol; [37, 38] 3) stewarding medications particularly restricting culture-negative empiric antibiotics to <5 days [39, 40] and avoiding histamine-2 antagonists; [41–43] and 4) adopting a unit-based approach to NEC risk assessment and timely recognition [44, 45]. Withholding feedings during packed red blood cell transfusion was considered [46–48], but evidence was found to be inconclusive. We elected to exclude probiotics from this review due to controversy and lack of standardization in probiotic formulations in the US [49, 50].

Experts participated in six monthly teleconferences. To facilitate communication and ensure all voices were represented, post-meeting surveys were distributed. Meeting minutes were transcribed verbatim and shared with all participants before the next meeting. At the third meeting, subgroups were formed to allow more in-depth appraisal of literature according to each facet of NEC-Zero. Subgroup membership was distributed evenly to ensure equal

representation from nursing, parents, and neonatology. The pharmacist, dietitian, and lactation consultant were specifically asked to be in certain groups (e.g. medication stewardship, feeding protocols, and human milk promotion respectively). When parent voices appeared quiet,

Table 1 Characteristics of NEC Working Group Experts (N = 20)

Characteristic	% (N) or Mean (SD)
Female	80% [16]
Years in Practice (Mean with SD)	18.6 (7.4)
Role	
Registered Nurse (Bedside NICU, Lactation Specialist, Librarian/Nurse, Neonatal Nurse Practitioner or Scientist)	45% [9]
Parent Advocate (Architect, Musician, or Information Specialist)	15% [3]
Pharmacist	5% [1]
Physician (includes Neonatologist, Medical Directors, Scientists)	30% [6]
Registered Dietician	5% [1]
Degree (Highest degree earned)	
Bachelors (B.S., B.S.N.)	20% [4]
Masters (MArch., Med., MLIS, M.S., M.P.H., or M.H.A.)	25% [5]
Doctorate (PharmD, DNP, PhD, or MD)	55% [11]
Geographical Location (United States)**	
Central	15% [3]
Eastern	20% [4]
Mountain	55% [11]
West/Pacific	10% [2]

**Eight states represented over 4 time zones

there was follow-up after the meetings to assure time for them to contribute. Subgroups focused on one of four facets of NEC-Zero and was co-facilitated by a local stakeholder and a national expert. A recommendation template was adapted and served as an outline that assisted with searching, identifying and assessing the state of the current literature. After evaluation, rating and synthesis of the evidence was completed, the four subgroups presented their findings during an all group meeting. The research team actively facilitated the work of the subgroups.

Selection of evidence sources

The literature search was focused to answer key questions [26, 27]. Guidelines, position statements, and studies that focused on the infant born <1500 g and were published in English were included. PubMed, CINAHL, and the Cochrane databases were searched. Targeted internet searches were applied to identify guidelines and position statements from professional organizations (e.g. American Academy of Pediatrics [AAP], American Society for Parenteral and Enteral Nutrition [ASPEN], National Association of Neonatal Nursing [NANN], Society for Breastfeeding Medicine [SBM], and the World Health Organization [WHO]). When the position was very strong, the evidence for the position was described in detail by the organization, and validated with high levels of consensus, an in-depth review of original research was deferred. If no position statement was available, systematic reviews and meta-analyses were evaluated first, followed by individual research studies if no meta-analysis or position statement was available. All participants assisted with critiquing the evidence and coming to consensus on practice recommendations [26, 27].

Experts agreed that clinicians intending to use NEC-Zero practices are likely familiar with GRADE criteria to critique quality of evidence and strength of recommendations [18, 51–53]. Meta-analyses are necessary to consider a body of evidence's quality. In GRADE, observational studies are typically "low" quality but can be upgraded when magnitude of effects are consistent, significantly large (i.e. <0.5 or >2), confounding is accounted for or if there is evidence of a dose response. When a meta-analysis was not available, we combined study results using the Review Manager 5.3 software using random effects modeling. Recommendations are presented as "do it/ don't do it" to reflect a strong recommendation or "probably do it/probably don't do it" to indicate a weak recommendation based on the quality of the evidence and if the quality was upgraded or downgraded (i.e. due to directness, imprecision, consistency of effects or cost balance).

Results

Promoting human milk feeding

The human milk subgroup addressed the evidence for human milk to prevent NEC across four categories: 1)

human milk versus formula feeding; 2) human donor milk (HDM)-derived fortifier compared to cow's milk-derived fortifier; 3) colostrum use for oral care; and 4) implementation strategies to promote human milk in the NICU.

1. Human milk versus formula feeding

Strength of evidence

Position Statements from NANN published in 2015 [54], The AAP in 2012 [55], AWHONN in 2014 [56], and the WHO [57] all promote human milk as the scientifically superior feeding for preterm infants. Specific health benefits for the preterm infant population including lower rates of sepsis, NEC, improved feeding tolerance, improved neurodevelopmental outcomes, lower mortality rates, more responsive immune function, lower rates of Retinopathy of Prematurity and fewer hospitalizations in the first year post-NICU discharge compared to formula feeding. [55] A meta-analysis concluded that if the preterm or low birth weight infant cannot have access to their mother's own milk (MOM), meta-analyses demonstrate that pasteurized HDM demonstrates protection from NEC versus the use of preterm or term formula [58]. Prioritizing the use of MOM over DHM is important because MOM is more bioactive than DHM, contains more immune-supporting human milk oligosaccharides [59] and is more protective against NEC [60].

Recommendations

We agree with the AAP position that all preterm infants should receive human milk and that if MOM is not available, pasteurized DHM is preferred to formula [55]. (High quality, do it).

2. Use of donor human milk (DHM)-based fortifier versus Cow's milk-based fortifier

Strength of evidence

The AAP recommends that human milk be fortified for infants born less than 1500 g [55]. Fortification can be accomplished with adding cow's milk-based fortifier or DHM-based fortifier to human milk. Some refer to a diet that includes MOM, DHM if MOM is unavailable, and DHM-based fortifier as an "exclusive human milk diet." Four studies have evaluated the difference in NEC (defined as Bell's stage II or greater) between the two types of fortified diets [30, 61–63]. When results were pooled from two RCTs [30, 61], lower risks of death, NEC, NEC requiring surgery, and sepsis in infants less than 1250 g was shown with risks rising incrementally as the percentage of cow's milk in an infant's diet increases [64]. Since 2014 when the pooled analysis was published, two more cohort studies have been published [62, 63]. We applied a random effects model to conduct a meta-

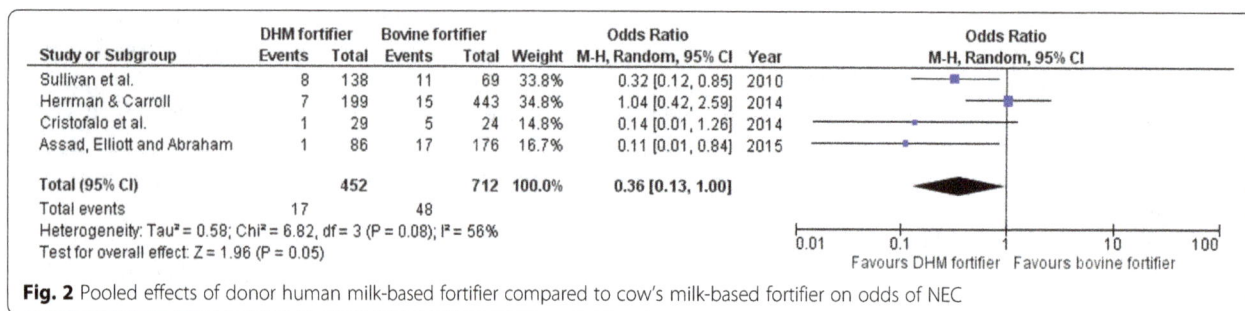

Study or Subgroup	DHM fortifier Events	Total	Bovine fortifier Events	Total	Weight	Odds Ratio M-H, Random, 95% CI	Year	Odds Ratio M-H, Random, 95% CI
Sullivan et al.	8	138	11	69	33.8%	0.32 [0.12, 0.85]	2010	
Herrman & Carroll	7	199	15	443	34.8%	1.04 [0.42, 2.59]	2014	
Cristofalo et al.	1	29	5	24	14.8%	0.14 [0.01, 1.26]	2014	
Assad, Elliott and Abraham	1	86	17	176	16.7%	0.11 [0.01, 0.84]	2015	
Total (95% CI)		452		712	100.0%	0.36 [0.13, 1.00]		
Total events	17		48					

Heterogeneity: Tau² = 0.58; Chi² = 6.82, df = 3 (P = 0.08); I² = 56%
Test for overall effect: Z = 1.96 (P = 0.05)

Favours DHM fortifier   Favours bovine fortifier

Fig. 2 Pooled effects of donor human milk-based fortifier compared to cow's milk-based fortifier on odds of NEC

analysis of the four studies for infants weighing <1250 g at birth (N = 1164) and show that infants fed with DHM-based fortifier had approximately 64% lower odds of NEC compared to those fed with bovine based fortifiers (OR = 0.36, 95% CI 0.13, 1.00, p = 0.05; Fig. 2). Highest protection of DHM-based fortifier was shown in units with high rates of NEC and cost-savings from NEC avoidance may be low if the baseline NEC rate is low. One limitation of the evidence is that it focused on the infant <1250 g and the effect estimate included one. More studies are needed in NICUs with pre-treatment NEC rates that are typical for most NICUs vs. those in the literature in higher rate NEC NICUs. No studies have shown adverse effects of using human milk based fortifiers although adequate growth should be monitored [65].

Recommendations

The subgroup recommends the use of DHM-based fortifier over bovine based fortifier (Moderate quality; probably do it) with prioritized MOM with DHM if MOM is not available. In units with a low baseline incidence of NEC, the cost of DHM-based fortifier may show lower cost-effectiveness compared to those with a high baseline incidence. Greatest effects of DHM-derived fortifier to reduce NEC are shown in units with high baseline NEC incidence.

3. Colostrum as oral immune therapy

Strength of evidence

The use of colostrum for oral care to provide immune therapy in preterm infants was next addressed. Evidence reviewed consisted of 1) a narrative review; [66] 2) three randomized control trials; [33, 67, 68] 3) two cohort studies; [36, 69] 4) a qualitative study; [70] 5) two pilot studies; [32, 35] and 6) a position statement. [54] The studies were typically single site and underpowered to answer questions related to NEC outcomes. However, many of the studies support the safety and feasibility of early colostrum oral care in extremely-low- and very-low-birthweight infants, [32, 33, 35, 36, 68, 69] and specifically in intubated babies [68, 69]. Use of colostrum for oral care impacted other important neonatal outcomes such as reaching full feeding volume earlier [33],

earlier initiation of enteral feedings and better weight gain at 36 weeks corrected gestational age, [36] boosts in immune markers suggesting immune-protection, [68] and a reduction in the length of stay [67]. At least one multi-center RCT is in progress and powered to detect differences in late-onset sepsis, NEC and death outcomes [71]. In one qualitative descriptive study of mothers with infants who had congenital diaphragmatic hernia, strong themes emerged that mothers and family members found meaning in providing colostrum oral care emphasizing that it encouraged them to continue pumping their milk [70]. Although using colostrum for oral care is shown as very low-risk, it is not clear from the studies what the optimal duration or dose is. In the studies reviewed, colostrum oral care was typically started by 48 h of age and continued for 2–5 days. No clinical studies support using DHM for oral care at this time because none are available.

Recommendations

Based upon immune boosting and benefits to promote mother's milk supply, colostrum for oral care is recommended, although its direct effect on NEC has not been shown (Low quality, probably do it).

4. Implementation strategies to promote human milk in the NICU

Strength of evidence

There are a multitude of articles and position statements that unanimously support providing human milk to all infants, but particularly emphasizing the health benefits for infants born early. A recent cost analysis estimated implementation gap burden of failing to provide premature infants with adequate volumes of human milk equates to 1.5 billion dollars annually in the US alone [72]. Implementation guidance is provided by NANN to use a programmatic approach, recommending Spatz's Ten Steps to promote human milk in the NICU [54, 73]. We critiqued the evidence about best implementation strategies to support mothers of premature infants to provide human milk. While the overall effectiveness of human milk promotion programs was shown, few studies were focused on the implementation science behind them. Overall, they showed that to a whole-team approach is needed that systematically and consistently engages mothers with adequate lactation education, pumping support and assessment of adequate milk supply.

Exemplar programs and related resources

Three implementation programs to promote human milk in the NICU were selected as exemplars and reviewed by the subgroup. Each program has videos, education materials, and education content for staff. Measurement of program success have shown by increased breast pumping initiation rates, longer duration of pumping or breastfeeding, higher volumes of milk the infant received, and demonstration that the infant was still receiving human milk at discharge from the NICU [74, 75, 73]. These programs consistently engage parents, moving them from bedside bystanders and validating their essential role on the healthcare team.

Recommendations

The subgroup recommends several steps be adopted to initiate organization-level, provider- level and patient level change to promote human milk and that using a program supports this multi-layered implementation (Table 2) [60, 73, 74]. The strength of these recommendations is based on lower levels of evidence that specifically studied implementation (Low quality, probably do it). More research is needed using high quality designs to assess effective implementation strategies on human milk outcomes.

Engaging parents

Parent subgroup members advised that earlier education about the importance of human milk to help them make an informed decision about providing human milk be given and specific guidance on how to bring in, maintain and monitor milk supply shared. Concerns were raised about delays to initiate pumping, lack of printed education, and materials that did not show women from diverse communities (e.g. African American or Hispanic) breastfeeding. When providing human milk for their vulnerable infant was being presented as a "choice" rather than a necessary medical treatment, they experienced angst at receiving mixed messages from the healthcare team about the importance of human milk. They recommend that lactation education is started before delivery and that they are shown how to set up the breast pump at that time. Fathers were not asked their perspective but mothers were emphatic that supportive partners are critical to the "human milk producing team." In sum, parents recommended 3 key strategies to support them to provide human milk: 1) early and often skin to skin holding, 2) early pumping (i.e. within the first 6 h, preferably within 2 h), and 3) access to lactation support regardless of intention to breastfeed.

Standardized feeding protocols
Strength of Evidence

Standardized feeding protocols (SFPs) address a consistent approach to the: 1) initiation and duration of trophic feeding; [76–79] 2) advancement and fortification of feeding; [77, 80] 3) criteria to stop and specifying how to re-start feedings once held; 4) identification and handling of feeding intolerance; [37, 81, 82] and 5) preferred feeding substance. Patole and deKlerk conducted a meta-analysis in 2005 of 6 observational studies showing reduced risk for NEC of up to 87% for infants <2500 g, when a feeding protocol is in place, even when formula was used within the protocol [38]. Studies were heterogeneous ($p < 0.001$) but when looking at studies similar to each other, pooled risk ratios were more modest (RR 0.71, 95% CI, 0.52 to 0.97) conferring about a 29% reduction in risk for NEC for infants <1500 g. [38] In 2016, our team reviewed papers published since the meta-analysis. When SFPs are used, studies consistently showed lower or unchanged NEC rates [81–86], with some also showing reduced late onset sepsis [83], and fewer days of parenteral nutrition [81, 85]. Weight gain improved after implementing SFPs in some studies [81, 83, 85], and one study showed less occurrence of bronchopulmonary dysplasia [81]. No study showed an increase in NEC rates or any other adverse events. No studies used randomized controlled designs. To pool studies published since 2005 with the Patole and deKlerk meta-analysis, we applied a random effects model combining data from 9 observational studies ($N = 4755$ infants <1500 g) [81, 83–85, 87–91]. Figure 3 shows an overall reduced odds of NEC by 67% (OR = 0.33, 95% CI 0.17, 0.65, $p = 0.001$) with moderate heterogeneity across studies (I [2] = 48%) when SFPs are used. We limited the counts used in this meta-analysis to those infants <1500 g.

Evidence was not conclusive, and more research is needed to identify best strategies for holding feedings when an infant is critically ill (e.g. very hypotensive or receiving prophylaxis for intraventricular hemorrhage with indomethacin), or during packed red blood cell transfusion. Experts did not examine whether continuous or bolus feeding is better. Although further randomized, controlled trials would be useful to increase the quality of evidence supporting SFPs, this type of study will be difficult to justify and conduct in centers that already have SFP in place. Pragmatic multi-site clinical trials that compare effectiveness of one SFP to another using randomized experimental designs could be useful.

Recommendations

We recommend the use of a unit-approved standardized feeding protocol based on the magnitude of their effects to reduce NEC, their low cost, and low risk (Moderate quality, do it). Details of the protocol itself do not appear

Table 2 Recommendations and Implementation strategies for NEC Prevention

Promoting Human Milk

Clinical Recommendations and GRADE	Implementation Strategies
1. Mom's own milk (MOM) is the preferred first line nutrition for preterm infants (except for in cases where it is contraindicated). If no MOM is available, donor human milk (DHM) is preferred over formula. [High quality, do it] 2. DHM-based fortifier is preferred over bovine based fortifier. Benefits of human milk based fortifiers outweigh the risks. Can be cost-effective for the healthcare system, with greater cost savings likely in higher rate NICUs. Impact of human milk-based fortifier on growth is inconsistent across studies and growth should be monitored carefully [Moderate quality, probably do it] 3. There is documented benefit from using colostrum for oral care to boost immune response and to encourage mothers to sustain milk production. (Low quality, probably do it).	Adopt a hospital-based policy to support breastfeeding and providing human milk. Provide education by OBs and Neonatologists when preterm delivery is anticipated about the importance of human milk emphasizing immune as well as nutritional benefit. Reiterate importance of breastmilk for preemies in a parent handbook or pamphlet, translated into commonly spoken languages and written in simple terms. Support initiation of pumping within 6 h after delivery and offer pumping at the bedside when possible. Provide lactation specialist support early (<24 h) and consistently through the stay. Educate staff (e.g. post-partum RNs, NICU RNs, Residents) using diverse training tools. Use huddles to remind staff about human milk education and goals. Provide pumps in the hospital and resources to rent pumps at home. Track initiation of pumping and milk volumes. Use colostrum for oral care. Facilitate regular skin to skin care (aka "kangaroo care"). Offer peer lactation support. Promote non-nutritive breast feeding when the infant is stable. Encourage nutritive breast feeding when appropriate and recommend breast before bottle when possible. Create a breast feeding plan for discharge.

Standardized Feeding Protocols

Clinical Recommendations and GRADE	Implementation Strategies
1. Adopt a unit-approved standardized feeding protocol to reduce inter-provider variation. [Moderate quality, do it]. 2. A multi-disciplinary team should be involved in creating, implementing and monitoring adherence to the protocol.	Consider "Feeding rounds" as a way to audit and feedback on compliance with the feeding protocol. Track initiation of feeds. Track advancement of feeds. Track fortification of feedings. Track growth. Formalize criteria for identifying and managing feeding intolerance. Tie feeding protocol to competencies and ongoing staff education.

Timely Recognition of NEC

Clinical Recommendations and GRADE	Implementation Strategies
1. Early recognition tools can be beneficial in patient safety efforts. Validated tools have been shown to differentiate between infants who get NEC compared to those who do not. [Very low evidence, probably do it]	Consider risk tool to use at the unit level (e.g. GutCheckNEC, NeoNEEDS or eNEC). Use a structured communication script (e.g. Situation-Background-Assessment-Recommendation; SBAR method) to communicate when NEC is suspected and to focus assessment. Educate parents about warning signs of NEC and preventive measures verbally and with printed materials (e.g. pamphlets) written in a way parents can easily understand. Optimal timing for this education is when initiating, advancing, or adding fortification to feeding. Use medically accurate terminology when communicating with parents (e.g. "necrotizing enterocolitis" vs. "tummy problems", etc.) Communicate baby's risk factors to parents and emphasize why human milk is important to help prevent NEC and that they play an important role in NEC prevention. Empower parents and nurses to speak up when concerned.

Medication stewardship

Clinical Recommendations and GRADE	Implementation Strategies
1. Avoid use of H2 blockers within the first 120 days of life (enteral or parenteral) [Moderate quality, don't do it] 2. Restrict empiric antibiotic use to 4 days or less for infants without positive blood cultures or clinical suspicion of infection [Moderate quality, don't do it]	Specify, adopt and automate prescribing guidelines for antibiotics that require a specific number of doses to be ordered. Adopt electronic alerts that warn the clinician that an H2 blocker is ordered and that it increases the risk for NEC. Communicate at handoffs about the date and time antibiotics should be stopped.

Table 2 Recommendations and Implementation strategies for NEC Prevention *(Continued)*

	Collaborate with pharmacists and integrate electronic alerts into electronic health record to remind clinicians to stop unnecessary antibiotics.
	Educate hospital personnel (e.g. neonatology, nursing, physician trainees) on recently published guidelines.
	Participate in antibiotic stewardship and regional collaborative organizations in multidisciplinary teams.
	Evaluate change by measuring the adherence to protocol and the number and % of infants who received prolonged antibiotics or H2 blockers.
	Create and share a report on findings within the local NICU.
	Give feedback to clinicians on their adherence to the medication stewardship guidelines in a way that is timely, individualized, not punitive, and customizable.

as important as reducing inter-provider variation [38, 92]. A SFP should be adopted at the NICU level (i.e. all providers agree to its components) and address: 1) when to initiate and how long to give trophic feeding (typically 10–20 mL/kg/day for 48–72 h); 2) schedules to advance and then fortify feeding (e.g. typically increasing calories by adding fortifier at 22 kcal/oz. after reaching 80–100 mL/kg/day and increasing to 24 kcal/oz. after reaching 120 mL/kg/day); 3) criteria for stopping and restarting feeding (e.g. if a unit decides to hold feeding during blood transfusion, indomethacin, etc.); 4) prioritized fresh human milk (MOM 1st, DHM 2nd, preterm formula 3rd); and 5) criteria to identify, and manage feeding intolerance. Best outcomes across studies appear to be shown when a multi-disciplinary team is involved in creating, implementing and monitoring adherence to the protocol. Guidance on components of effective protocols has been published by ASPEN [77] and the California Perinatal Quality Collaborative [83, 93]. Based on group consensus and recommendations from published papers, [81, 83, 91, 94] several SFP implementation strategies are recommended (see Table 2).

Timely NEC recognition

Beginning signs of NEC occur at approximately 2–4 weeks of age, often when infants have experienced multiple encounters with multiple clinicians [10, 95]. Information relevant to recognizing NEC is contained in many places in the medical record, making it a challenge for clinicians to integrate into their assessments. Nurses and parents often recognize NEC first, but when symptoms are mild or non-specific, treatment delays can occur if communication is unclear or when symptoms are not considered in the context of NEC risk factors [45]. The timely recognition subgroup evaluated biomarkers, bedside monitoring techniques, and information-based tools to assess NEC risk and addressed ways to engage families in the process. Although timely recognition was the goal of the subgroup, based on review of evidence the focus shifted to what was possible to support *timely* recognition because it is not clear from the evidence to what extent early recognition is possible. In other inflammatory disease processes, the longer the time to treatment the more severe the illness becomes and the more difficult it is to treat it.

Strength of evidence

Given the purpose of identifying strategies to adopt in clinical practice, this group evaluated what is currently *most available* and *feasible to implement*. Based on a focused literature search in 2015, several promising noninvasive biomarkers were identified but none appeared widely available for clinical use outside of a research protocol [96, 97]. Bedside monitoring tools to evaluate intestinal perfusion changes did not include guidelines to make them readily implementable [98–100]. Risk scores found in 2015 to promote NEC risk awareness include eNEC™ [45, 101], NeoNEEDS [102], and GutCheck^{NEC} [44, 45]. No tool

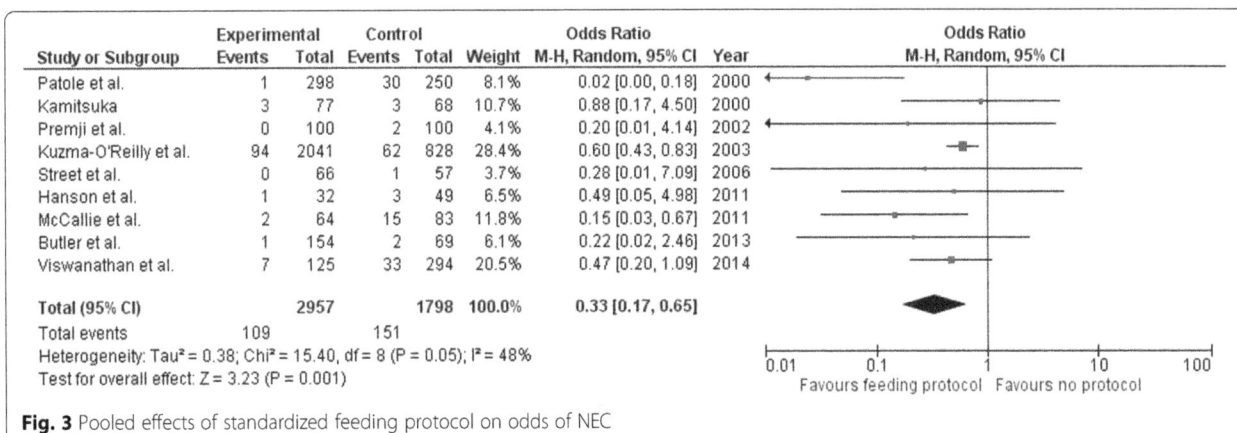

Fig. 3 Pooled effects of standardized feeding protocol on odds of NEC

showed perfect prediction but all showed promise to differentiate between infants who got NEC compared to those who did not. Implementation of NeoNEEDS showed a shift towards fewer severe NEC cases as more "suspected NEC" was identified. eNEC has been clinically tested in a QI project with high inter-rater agreement and positive impact on increasing knowledge of nurses about NEC risk factors [45, 101]. GutCheck^{NEC} was tested with the most infants and showed robust prediction for NEC leading to surgery (AUC = 0.84, 95% CI 0.82–0.84) or death (AUC = 0.83, 95% CI 0.81–0.85) but its ability to discriminate medical NEC was marginal [44, 45].

Much discussion in this group centered on communication strategies and ways to engage parents as timely recognition partners. Review of evidence on communication strategies that support patient safety and rescue protocols showed that structuring communication (e.g. at the change of shift or handoff of care from clinician to clinician or when a nurse calls a physician or NNP) can support clarity and reduce communication failures [103–105]. An international study of families' experiences around NEC communication conducted by the NEC Society identified that information about NEC was most often shared verbally and primarily at the time of diagnosis [106]. Very few parents received anticipatory guidance about warning signs to watch for, preventive strategies they could take, or how different treatments may increase their risk. Parents expressed the great need to be believed when they saw their child "not acting right" and bore the guilt of not advocating for their baby when the outcomes were poor [106]. The subgroup agreed that it would be helpful to have a tool to share with parents but did not want to scare parents or expose them to unnecessary stress and worry. In contrast, parents firmly believed that clinicians should share critical information with parents instead of avoiding doing so for fear of scaring them.

Recommendations

Timely recognition tools can support consistent communication and are shown beneficial in patient safety efforts. Validated tools have been shown to differentiate between infants who get NEC compared to those who do not. Benefits of using them is likely to outweigh risks although more research is needed (Very low evidence, probably do it) [44, 101, 102]. Structuring communication when NEC is suspected in tandem with adopting a risk score was the most implementation-ready strategy to support timely recognition. Such a risk scoring system can also be used to educate staff about NEC risk factors and cue attention to times (e.g. day of life and contexts) when NEC is most prevalent. We recommend that tools like GutCheck^{NEC}, eNEC or NeoNEEDS be coupled with a focused assessment tool that is organized using a Situation-Background-

Assessment-Recommendation (SBAR) format. More research is needed on ways to implement biomarkers and bedside monitoring (e.g. NIRS) into routine practice.

Engaging parents

Parents should be empowered to speak up when they think their baby is not acting right for several reasons including that they know their infant best, they are the most consistent bedside caregiver, and they have the most to lose. Further, parents should be educated on warning signs that signal a change. The group discussed at length the best timing to discuss the symptoms of NEC with parents. The consensus was that discussions could occur when human milk education is given, when feedings are started, advanced, and changed. If signs of feeding intolerance arise, discussions about warning signs of NEC can be addressed. Throughout the discussions, emphasis can be placed on what parents can do to help prevent NEC (e.g. provide human milk) and what the team is doing to watch for it. When parents raise concern that their infant is not acting right, including parent concern as part of a focused assessment tool can support nurse to provider communication. As part of this subgroup's activities, a website was developed to share tools created to engage parents including videos, pamphlets (also in Spanish) and links to diverse family support resources (see http://neczero.nursing.arizona.edu/). A focused assessment tool that combines GutCheck^{NEC} with an SBAR script to support communication when concerns arise is also available at this website.

Medication stewardship

This subgroup worked to address questions related to prolonged antibiotic therapy, barriers to limiting antibiotic therapy, and implementation and monitoring of antibiotic and H2 blocker stewardship to prevent NEC.

Strength of evidence

Three multi-site observational studies in the US (23 NICUs, combined N = 4716 infants) have addressed the role of an extended initial course of antibiotics on risk for NEC [39, 40, 107]. Cotten and colleagues evaluated a prolonged course of antibiotics as a measure of risk associated with each additional antibiotic day with an exclusive focus on infants born weighing <1000 g [39]. The other 2 studies included infants <1500 g with one applying a case-control approach in a single NICU [40], and the second evaluating a cohort of 3 NICUs from a state network over 4 years [107]. Two excluded studies compared those who received no antibiotics compared to those who did for early empiric therapy but did not evaluate the impact of a *prolonged course of* antibiotics [108, 109]. Consistently, all 3 studies showed an increasing odds of NEC or death after 4 days of empiric antibiotics when blood cultures were negative [39, 40, 107]. The decision to restrict antibiotics can address markers of inflammation as well as the presence of a negative blood culture because not all infected babies will have positive blood cultures [110].

Evidence addressed risk of NEC with H2 antagonists came from a systematic review with meta-analysis of 2 cohort studies (N = 11,346, <1500 g) [111]. When pooling the two studies [41, 42], they found significant heterogeneity ($I^{[2]}$ = 73%) but an increased odds of NEC when gastric acid inhibitors (proton pump inhibitors) or H2 receptor blockers (ranitidine, famotidine or cimetidine) were given parenterally or enterally before NEC (OR = 1.78, 95% CI 1.4, 2.27, p < 0.00001). They judged the risk of bias to be low to moderate using the Newcastle-Ottawa scale.

Recommendations

The subgroup recommends judicious antibiotic use to 4 days or less for infants without positive blood cultures or clinical suspicion of infection (Moderate quality, don't exceed 4 days of antibiotics unless highly suspected or proven infection) [39, 40, 107, 112]. When ordering empiric antibiotics, a stop-date or a specific number of doses should be ordered. Use of H2 blockers increases the odds of NEC and sepsis [111] and should be avoided (Moderate quality, don't do it). This group identified ampicillin and gentamicin as the first choice treatment for early onset newborn sepsis [113], restricting higher order cephalosporin use (e.g. cefotaxime and cefepime) to select cases [112]. Preferred duration of therapy was for 48 h to rule out infection based on evidence that showed each additional antibiotic day confers an increased risk of NEC or death [39, 40]. Individual groups may choose to adopt restrictions from longer than 48 h but these should be limited to less than 5 days.

Implementation strategies

The group identified several barriers to implementing a restrictive approach to antibiotics and H2 blockers. These included a concerning clinical presentation, such as respiratory distress, cardiovascular instability, or abnormal lab indices. [114] Using a sepsis calculator may be useful, however current tools are only validated for infants >34 weeks [115, 116]. Clinicians may not be knowledgeable about current recommendations so their practice may not reflect current best evidence. In busy units where attention is focused on cardio-respiratory crises; it is possible that discontinuing antibiotics (a routine task) may be overlooked. If between-shift handoffs are unstandardized, failing to communicate a plan to discontinue antibiotics is more likely. To overcome these barriers, several implementation strategies are described in Table 2.

Discussion

NEC remains a chief threat to the survival and health of premature infants in spite of the evidence available to reduce its incidence. Implementation guidance, toolkits,

and strategies to engage parents are needed to forward improvement efforts. Prioritizing a human milk diet was best supported by evidence, position statements, and stakeholder input. While a specific feeding protocol could not be recommended, the group agreed that using a feeding protocol is evidence-based. Two new meta-analyses conducted as part of this scoping review supported the protective effect of a DHM-based fortifier and feeding protocols to reduce odds of NEC. Avoiding >4 days of antibiotics for the initial empiric course after birth and avoiding any exposure to histamine-2 antagonist medications was recommended.

This scoping review engaged expert stakeholders to review evidence focused on answering key questions and make recommendations to prevent and support timely recognition of necrotizing enterocolitis. Four subgroups reviewed evidence from 11 position statements and 71 research publications. Discussion about the evidence yielded 29 actionable recommendations and guidance on implementation strategies. This approach engaging national experts with local clinicians and parent representatives was consistent with recommendations for designing trustworthy clinical practice guidelines laid out by the National Academy of Medicine and others [16–19]. A geographically diverse expert group yielded a real-world approach to implementation of NEC prevention strategies. Evidence was strongest for promoting a human milk diet, use of a unit-adopted standardized feeding protocol and limiting exposures to unnecessary antibiotics and H2 blockers in early life. Timely recognition continues to be studied as risk tools are refined but the current state of evidence justifies a "probably do it" recommendation because of the potential for benefit, low risk, and support for consistent communication to strengthen patient safety in other areas. In upcoming years, we anticipate more information will be available to support a broad approach to timely recognition. In the meantime, engaging families and structuring assessments and communication when NEC is suspected could strengthen prompt diagnosis and quick action.

Although we reviewed evidence for holding feeding during blood transfusion, the group did not achieve consensus on best approaches because evidence was inconsistent in 2015. Anemia appears to underlie the risk for NEC with transfusion [117, 118]. Transfusion thresholds differ, few have transfusion protocols in place, and addressing confounders that reduce NEC like feeding protocols and human milk exposure is not consistent. Experts recommended that if a neonatal group chose to hold feeding during transfusion, they should agree to *how* they will do so, integrate it into the feeding protocol, and address criteria to restart feeding. The approach taken in the multisite QI project was to hold the feeding only during the transfusion, not advance the feeding volume on the day of the feeding and avoid fortifiers on that day- with significant reduction in the most severe NEC across 8 NICUs [119].

To balance the strengths of this project, we should also address its limitations. Using a scoping review vs. a systematic review approach had the potential to miss important evidence in the literature. We cannot be certain that we included all of the relevant literature. However, we were able to satisfy a diverse group of 20 experts to answer key questions about how to prevent NEC and support its timely recognition using feasible, implementation ready strategies. In an individual NICU's process to adopt evidence-based interventions this work is typically done by <5 busy clinicians who may find our results helpful to their efforts. We did not engage parents specifically whose children did not get NEC as experts, which may have limited the generalizabilty to all parents. However, the processes useful to prevent NEC are also those that support neonatal health broadly (e.g. avoiding excessive antibiotic exposure, promoting a human milk diet and supporting healthy team communication and risk awareness).

Conclusion

Stakeholders maintained engagement when they were organized around the task of answering key questions and agreed to actionable, feasible and evidence-based strategies to foster NEC prevention and timely recognition. Implementation strategies addressed staff education, parent engagement, early discussions, structuring communication, integrating reminders into electronic health record systems, and using audit and feedback mechanisms. Partnering national experts with local experts and ensuring that clinical and parent perspectives were sought yielded balanced, focused, and feasible implementation strategies that any NICU could implement today to drive their incidence of NEC to zero.

Abbreviations

AUC: Area under the curve; CI: Confidence interval; CRP: C-reactive protein; DHM: Donor human milk; FDA: Food and Drug Administration; H2: Histamine-2; HM: Human milk; i-FABP: Intestinal fatty acid-binding protein; NEC: Necrotizing enterocolitis; NICU: Neonatal intensive care unit; NIRS: Near infrared spectroscopy; RCT: Randomized controlled trial; US: United States; VLBW infant: Very low birth weight

Acknowledgements

The authors also wish to acknowledge members of the NEC-Zero working group who are not listed as authors for the time they were able to contribute including Dr. James Moore, Dr. Akhil Maheshwari, Dr. Jordan Leonard, and College of Public Health graduate, Scott Robert Johnson.

Funding

This project was funded by the Robert Wood Johnson Foundation Nurse Faculty Scholars Program (72112) and the Agency for Healthcare Research and Quality (K08HS022908). The content is solely the responsibility of the authors and does not necessarily represent the official views of the Agency for Healthcare Research and Quality or Robert Wood Johnson Foundation.

Authors' contributions

SG conceptualized, led and oversaw all elements of the project, wrote major portions, and meta-analyzed data for feeding protocols and donor human milk derived fortifier. CH co-led the feeding protocol subgroup with KR and EU, drafting the initial feeding protocol section. CW co-led the human milk subgroup with SR and drafted the initial human milk section. MF participated on the human milk subgroup and analyzed the evidence related to oral colostrum care. EU co-led the feeding protocol group and worked with LM and TC to integrate family perspectives. SR co-led the human milk subgroup and drafted the original human milk recommendations. AA co-led the timely recognition group with SG, approving the recommendations proposed. TM participated on the timely recognition group and reviewed the evidence. KK co-led the medication stewardship group with JD. MQ reviewed evidence and participated on the timely recognition group with KD. JS participated on the medication stewardship group and drafted the original summary of evidence on antibiotics and H2 blockers. YE assembled the key questions, recommendations and implementation guidance. CP participated in creating family engagement materials to be included on the website with MA-R, CW, and YE. AM abstracted and analyzed evidence across the studies with SV. KR co-led the feeding protocol workgroup with CH and EU. JD co-led the medication stewardship group with KK, contributing key findings into the manuscript. All authors read and approved the final version of the manuscript.

Competing interests

The authors declare that they have no competing interests.

Author details

[1]Robert Wood Johnson Foundation Nurse Faculty Scholar, The University of Arizona College of Nursing, PO Box 210203, Tucson, AZ 85721, USA. [2]University of Nebraska Medical Center, Omaha, NE, USA. [3]Carle Hospital, Urbana, IL, USA. [4]Banner Health, Cardon Children's Medical Center, Mesa, AZ, USA. [5]NEC Society, Fresno, CA, USA. [6]Graham's Foundation, Canton, GA, USA. [7]Banner Health, Banner University Medical Center-Phoenix, Phoenix, AZ, USA. [8]Phoenix Perinatal Associates, Mesa, AZ, USA. [9]Clinical Assistant Professor and Vice-Chair, Department of Pediatrics, The University of Arizona, Tucson, AZ, USA. [10]Banner Health, Thunderbird Medical Center, Glendale, AZ, USA. [11]Envision Physician Services, Lawrenceville, GA, USA. [12]Augusta University College of Nursing, Athens, GA, USA. [13]NorthBay Medical Center, Fairfield, CA, USA. [14]Hand to Hold, Dallas, TX, USA. [15]Neonatal Research Institute, Sharp Mary Birch Hospital for Women and Newborns, San Diego, CA, USA. [16]Stetson Hills Family Medicine, Glendale, AZ, USA. [17]University of Sonora at Hermisillo, Hermosillo, Mexico. [18]Nationwide Children's Hospital and The Ohio State Wexner Medical Center, Columbus, OH, USA. [19]Columbia University, New York, NY, USA.

References

1. Russell RB, Green NS, Steiner CA, et al. Cost of hospitalization for preterm and low birth weight infants in the United States. Pediatrics. 2007; 120(1):e1–9. doi:10.1542/peds.2006-2386.
2. Schulman J, Stricof RL, Stevens TP, et al. Development of a statewide collaborative to decrease NICU central line-associated bloodstream infections. J Perinatol. 2009;29(9):591–9. doi:10.1038/jp.2009.18.
3. Suresh GK, Edwards WH. Central line-associated bloodstream infections in neonatal intensive care: changing the mental model from inevitability to preventability. Am J Perinatol. 2012;29(1):57–64. doi:10.1055/s-0031-1286182.

4. Yee WH, Soraisham AS, Shah VS, Aziz K, Yoon W, Lee SK. Incidence and Timing of Presentation of Necrotizing Enterocolitis in Preterm Infants. Pediatrics. 2012;129(2):e298–304. doi:10.1542/peds.2011-2022.

5. Fanaroff AA, Stoll BJ, Wright LL, et al. Trends in neonatal morbidity and mortality for very low birthweight infants. Am J Obstet Gynecol. 2007;196(2) doi:10.1016/j.ajog.2006.09.014.

6. Guner YS, Chokshi N, Petrosyan M, Upperman JS, Ford HR, Grikscheit TC. Necrotizing enterocolitis–bench to bedside: novel and emerging strategies. Semin Pediatr Surg. 2008;17(4):255–65. doi:10.1053/j.sempedsurg.2008.07.004.

7. Catlin A. Extremely long hospitalizations of newborns in the United States: data, descriptions, dilemmas. J Perinatol. 2006;26(12):742–8. doi:10.1038/sj.jp.7211617.

8. Rees CM, Eaton S, Pierro A. Trends in infant mortality from necrotising enterocolitis in England and Wales and the USA. Arch Dis Child Fetal Neonatal Ed. 2008;93(5):F395–6. doi:10.1136/adc.2007.136994.

9. Zhang Y, Ortega G, Camp M, Osen H, Chang DC, Abdullah F. Necrotizing enterocolitis requiring surgery: Outcomes by intestinal location of disease in 4371 infants. J Pediatr Surg. 2011;46(8):1575–81. doi:10.1016/j.jpedsurg.2011.03.005.

10. Luig M, Lui K. Epidemiology of necrotizing enterocolitis - Part II: Risks and susceptibility of premature infants during the surfactant era: A regional study. J Paediatr Child Health. 2005;41(4):174–9. doi:10.1111/j.1440-1754.2005.00583.x.

11. Horbar JD, Plsek PE, Leahy K. NIC/Q 2000: establishing habits for improvement in neonatal intensive care units. Pediatrics. 2003;111(4 Pt 2):e397–410.

12. Lake ET, Staiger D, Cheung R, Kenny MJ, Patrick T, Rogowski JA. for Nursing Excellence and Outcomes of Very Low-Birth-Weight Infants. Jama J Am Med Assoc. 2012;307(16):1709–16. doi:10.1001/jama.2012.504.

13. Fitzgibbons SC, Ching Y, Yu D, et al. Mortality of necrotizing enterocolitis expressed by birth weight categories. J Pediatr Surg. 2009;44(6):1072–6. doi:10.1016/j.jpedsurg.2009.02.013.

14. Lee HC, Martin-Anderson S, Lyndon A, Dudley RA. Perspectives on Promoting Breastmilk Feedings for Premature Infants During a Quality Improvement Project. Breastfeed Med. 2013;8(2):176–80. doi:10.1089/bfm.2012.0056.

15. Cincinnati Children's Medical Center. Evidence-Based Care Guideline for Necrotizing Enterocolitis (NEC) among Very Low Birth Weight Infants.; 2010.

16. Graham R, Mancher M, Miller Wolman D, Greenfield S, Steinberg E, editors. Institute of Medicine (US) Committee on Standards for Developing Trustworthy Clinical Practice. In: Clinical Practice Guidelines We Can Trust. Washington (DC); 2011. doi:10.17226/13058.

17. Brouwers MC, Kho ME, Browman GP, et al. AGREE II: advancing guideline development, reporting and evaluation in health care. CMAJ. 2010;182(18):E839–42. doi:10.1503/cmaj.090449.

18. Atkins D, Best D, Briss PA, et al. Grading quality of evidence and strength of recommendations. BMJ. 2004;328(7454):1490. doi:10.1136/bmj.328.7454.1490.

19. Guyatt GH, Oxman AD, Kunz R, et al. Going from evidence to recommendations. BMJ. 2008;336(7652):1049–51. doi:10.1136/bmj.39493.646875.AE.

20. Titler MG, Everett LQ. Translating research into practice. Considerations for critical care investigators. Crit Care Nurs Clin North Am. 2001;13(4):587–604.

21. Moore JE, Titler MG, Kane Low L, Dalton VK, Sampselle CM. Transforming Patient-Centered Care: Development of the Evidence Informed Decision Making through Engagement Model. Womens Health Issues. 2015;25(3):276–82. doi:10.1016/j.whi.2015.02.002.

22. Titler MG. The Evidence for Evidence-Based Practice Implementation. In: Hughes RG, ed. Patient Safety and Quality: An Evidence-Based Handbook for Nurses. Rockville (MD); 2008.

23. Titler MG. Translation science and context. Res Theory Nurs Pract. 2010;24(1):35–55.

24. Valente TW, Rogers EM. The origins and development of the diffusion of innovations paradigm as an example of scientific growth. Sci Commun. 1995;16(3):242–73.

25. Mays N, Roberts E, Popay J. Synthesizing research evidence. In: Fulop N, Allen P, Clarke A, N B, eds. Studying the Organisation and Delivery of Health Services: Research Methods. London: Routledge; 2001:194.

26. Arksey H, O'Malley L. Scoping studies: towards a methodological framework. Int J Soc Res Methodol. 2005;8(1):19–32. doi:10.1080/1364557032000119616.

27. Levac D, Colquhoun H, O'Brien KK. Scoping studies: advancing the methodology. Implement Sci. 2010;5(1):69. doi:10.1186/1748-5908-5-69.

28. Colquhoun HL, Levac D, O'Brien KK, et al. Scoping reviews: Time for clarity in definition, methods, and reporting. J Clin Epidemiol. 2014;67(12):1291–4. doi:10.1016/j.jclinepi.2014.03.013.

29. Lucas A, Cole TJ. Breast milk and neonatal necrotising enterocolitis. Lancet (London, England). 1990;336(8730):1519–1523.

30. Sullivan S, Schanler RJ, Kim JH, et al. An Exclusively Human Milk-Based Diet Is Associated with a Lower Rate of Necrotizing Enterocolitis than a Diet of Human Milk and Bovine Milk-Based Products. J Pediatr. 2010;156(4) doi:10.1016/j.jpeds.2009.10.040.

31. Schanler RJ. Outcomes of human milk-fed premature infants. Semin Perinatol. 2011;35(1):29–33. doi:10.1053/j.semperi.2010.10.005.

32. Rodriguez NA, Meier PP, Groer MW, Zeller JM, Engstrom JL, Fogg L. A Pilot Study to Determine the Safety and Feasibility of Oropharyngeal Administration of Own Mother's Colostrum to Extremely Low-Birth-Weight Infants. Adv Neonatal Care. 2010;10(4):206–12. doi:10.1097/ANC.0b013e3181e94133.

33. Rodriguez NA, Groer MW, Zeller JM, et al. A randomized controlled trial of the oropharyngeal administration of mother's colostrum to extremely low birth weight infants in the first days of life. Neonatal Intensive Care. 2011;24(4):31–5.

34. Lee J, Kim HS, Jung YH, et al. Oropharyngeal colostrum administration in extremely premature infants: An RCT. World Rev Nutr Diet. 2016;114(2):56–7. doi:10.1159/000441922.

35. Montgomery DP, Baer VL, Lambert DK, Christensen RD. Oropharyngeal administration of colostrum to very low birth weight infants: Results of a feasibility trial. Neonatal Intensive Care. 2010;23(1):27–9. www.nicmag.ca

36. Seigel JK, Smith PB, Ashley PL, et al. Early Administration of Oropharyngeal Colostrum to Extremely Low Birth Weight Infants. Breastfeed Med. 2013;8(6):491–5. doi:10.1089/bfm.2013.0025.

37. Gephart SM, Hanson CK. Preventing Necrotizing Enterocolitis With Standardized Feeding Protocols. Adv Neonatal Care. 2013;13(1):48–54. doi:10.1097/ANC.0b013e31827ece0a.

38. Patole SK. Impact of standardised feeding regimens on incidence of neonatal necrotising enterocolitis: a systematic review and meta-analysis of observational studies. Arch Dis Child - Fetal Neonatal Ed. 2005;90(2):F147–51. doi:10.1136/adc.2004.059741.

39. Cotten CM, Taylor S, Stoll B, et al. Prolonged Duration of Initial Empirical Antibiotic Treatment Is Associated With Increased Rates of Necrotizing Enterocolitis and Death for Extremely Low Birth Weight Infants. Pediatrics. 2009;123(1):58–66. doi:10.1542/peds.2007-3423.

40. Alexander VN, Northrup V, Bizzarro MJ. Antibiotic exposure in the newborn intensive care unit and the risk of necrotizing enterocolitis. J Pediatr. 2011;159(3):392–7. doi:10.1016/j.jpeds.2011.02.035.

41. Guillet R, Stoll BJ, Cotten CM, et al. Association of H2-Blocker Therapy and Higher Incidence of Necrotizing Enterocolitis in Very Low Birth Weight Infants. Pediatrics. 2006;117(2):e137–42. doi:10.1542/peds.2005-1543.

42. Terrin G, Passariello A, De Curtis M, et al. Ranitidine is Associated With Infections, Necrotizing Enterocolitis, and Fatal Outcome in Newborns. Pediatrics. 2012;129(1):e40–5. doi:10.1542/peds.2011-0796.

43. Gantz M, Roy J, Guillet R. Analyzing retrospective data with time-varying exposure: A cautionary tale of H2 blockers in ELBW neonates. Am J Perinatol. 2008;25(2):93–100. doi:10.1055/s-2007-1004835.

44. Gephart SM, Spitzer AR, Effken JA, Dodd E, Halpern M, McGrath JM. Discrimination of GutCheckNEC: a clinical risk index for necrotizing enterocolitis. J Perinatol. 2014;34(6):468–75. doi:10.1038/jp.2014.37.

45. Gephart SM, Wetzel C, Krisman B. Prevention and Early Recognition of Necrotizing Enterocolitis. Adv Neonatal Care. 2014;14(3):201–10. doi:10.1097/ANC.0000000000000063.

46. Gephart SM. Transfusion-Associated Necrotizing Enterocolitis. Adv Neonatal Care. 2012;12(4):232–6. doi:10.1097/ANC.0b013e31825e20ee.

47. Christensen RD. Association between red blood cell transfusions and necrotizing enterocolitis. J Pediatr. 2011;158(3):349–50. doi:10.1016/j.jpeds.2010.10.030.

48. Mohamed A, Shah PS. Transfusion Associated Necrotizing Enterocolitis: A Meta-analysis of Observational Data. Pediatrics. 2012;129(3):529–40. doi:10.1542/peds.2011-2872.

49. Alfaleh K, Anabrees J, Bassler D. Probiotics for prevention of necrotizing enterocolitis in preterm infants (Review). Cochrane. 2011;3:1–45.

50. Thakkar HS, Lakhoo K. Necrotizing enterocolitis. Surg. 2016;34(12):617–20. doi:10.1016/j.mpsur.2016.09.004.

51. Guyatt G, Oxman AD, Akl EA, et al. GRADE guidelines: 1. Introduction - GRADE evidence profiles and summary of findings tables. J Clin Epidemiol. 2011;64(4):383–94. doi:10.1016/j.jclinepi.2010.04.026.

52. Owens DK, Lohr KN, Atkins D, et al. AHRQ series paper 5: grading the strength of a body of evidence when comparing medical interventions–agency for healthcare research and quality and the effective health-care program. J Clin Epidemiol. 2010;63(5):513–23. doi:10.1016/j.jclinepi.2009.03.009.

53. Andrews J, Guyatt G, Oxman AD, et al. GRADE guidelines: 14. Going from evidence to recommendations: The significance and presentation of recommendations. J Clin Epidemiol. 2013;66(7):719–25. doi:10.1016/j.jclinepi.2012.03.013.

54. Spatz D, Edwards T. The use of human milk and breastfeeding in the neonatal intensive care unit: NANN position statement #3052. Adv neonatal care. 2015;12(1):56–60. doi:10.1097/ANC.0000000000000313.

55. American Academy of Pediatrics. Breastfeeding and the Use of Human Milk. Pediatrics. 2012;129:e827. doi:10.1542/peds.2011-3552.

56. Association of Women's Health O and NN. AWHONN Position Statement: Breastfeeding. J Obstet Gynecol Neonatal Nurs. 2015;44(1): 145–50. doi:10.1111/1552-6909.12530.

57. WHO/UNICEF. Global Nutrion Target 2025. Breastfeeding policy brief. WHO/ MNH/NHD 14.7. WHO Libr Cat Data. 2014:8. doi:WHO/NMH/NHD/14.7.

58. Q M. Formula versus donor breast milk for feeding preterm or low birth weight infants. Cochrane database Syst Rev. 2014;4(4):CD002971. doi:10.1002/14651858.CD002971.pub3.

59. Marx C, Bridge R, Wolf AK, Rich W, Kim JH, Bode L. Human milk oligosaccharide composition differs between donor milk and mother's own milk in the NICU. J Hum Lact. 2014;30(1):54–61. doi:10.1177/0890334413513923.

60. Meier PP, Johnson TJ, Patel AL, Rossman B. Evidence-Based Methods That Promote Human Milk Feeding of Preterm Infants: An Expert Review. Clin Perinatol. 2017;44(1):1–22. doi:10.1016/j.clp.2016.11.005.

61. Cristofalo EA, Schanler RJ, Blanco CL, et al. Randomized trial of exclusive human milk versus preterm formula diets in extremely premature infants. J Pediatr. 2013;163(6):1592–1595.e1. doi:10.1016/j.jpeds.2013.07.011.

62. Herrmann K, Carroll K. An Exclusively Human Milk Diet Reduces Necrotizing Enterocolitis. Breastfeed Med. 2014;9(4):184–90. doi:10.1089/bfm.2013.0121.

63. Assad M, Elliott MJ, Abraham JH. Decreased cost and improved feeding tolerance in VLBW infants fed an exclusive human milk diet. J Perinatol. 2016;36(3):216–20. doi:10.1038/jp.2015.168.

64. Abrams SA, Schanler RJ, Lee ML, Rechtman DJ. Greater mortality and morbidity in extremely preterm infants fed a diet containing cow milk protein products. Breastfeed Med. 2014;9(6):281–5. doi:10.1089/bfm.2014.0024.

65. Hair AB, Hawthorne KM, Chetta KE, Abrams SA. Human milk feeding supports adequate growth in infants ≤ 1250 grams birth weight. BMC Res Notes. 2013;6:459. doi:10.1186/1756-0500-6-459.

66. Gephart SM, Weller M. Colostrum as Oral Immune Therapy to Promote Neonatal Health. Adv Neonatal Care. 2014;14(1):44–51. doi:10.1097/ANC.0000000000000052.

67. Romano-Keeler J, Azcarate-Peril MA, Weitkamp J-H, et al. Oral colostrum priming shortens hospitalization without changing the immunomicrobial milieu. J Perinatol. 2017;37(1):36–41. doi:10.1038/jp.2016.161.

68. Lee J, Kim H-S, Young HJ, et al. Oropharyngeal Colostrum Administration in Extremely Premature Infants: An RCT. Pediatrics. 2015;135(2):e357–66.

69. Thibeau S, Boudreaux C. Exploring the use of mothers' own milk as oral care for mechanically ventilated very low-birth-weight preterm infants. Adv Neonatal Care. 2013;13(3):190–7. doi:10.1097/ANC.0b013e318285f8e2.

70. Froh EB, Deatrick JA, Curley MAQ, Spatz DL. Making Meaning of Pumping for Mothers of Infants With Congenital Diaphragmatic Hernia. J Obstet Gynecol Neonatal Nurs. 2015;44(3):439–49. doi:10.1111/1552-6909.12564.

71. Rodriguez NA, Vento M, Claud EC, Wang CE, Caplan MS. Oropharyngeal administration of mother's colostrum, health outcomes of premature infants: study protocol for a randomized controlled trial. Trials. 2015;16:453. doi:10.1186/s13063-015-0969-6.

72. Colaizy TT, Bartick MC, Jegier BJ, et al. Impact of Optimized Breastfeeding on the Costs of Necrotizing Enterocolitis in Extremely Low Birthweight Infants. J Pediatr. 2016;175:100–105.e2. doi:10.1016/j.jpeds.2016.03.040.

73. Spatz DL. Ten steps for promoting and protecting breastfeeding for vulnerable infants. J Perinat Neonatal Nurs. 2004;18(4):385–96.

74. Kim JH, Chan CS, Vaucher YE, Stellwagen LM. Challenges in the practice of human milk nutrition in the neonatal intensive care unit. Early Hum Dev. 2013;89(SUPPL2):S35–8. doi:10.1016/j.earlhumdev.2013.08.002.

75. Meier PP, Engstrom JL, Mingolelli SS, Miracle DJ, Kiesling S. The Rush Mothers' Milk Club: breastfeeding interventions for mothers with very-low-birth-weight infants. J Obstet Gynecol neonatal Nurs JOGNN. 2004;33(2):164–74.

76. Bingham EM. Optimizing nutrition in the neonatal intensive care unit: a look at enteral nutrition and the prevention of necrotizing enterocolitis. Top Clin Nutr. 2012;27(3):250–9.

77. Dutta S, Singh B, Chessell L, et al. Guidelines for feeding very low birth weight infants. Nutrients. 2015;7(1):423–42. doi:10.3390/nu7010423.

78. Berseth CL, Bisquera JA, Paje VU. Prolonging small feeding volumes early in life decreases the incidence of necrotizing enterocolitis in very low birth weight infants. Pediatrics. 2003;111(3):529–34.

79. Morgan J, Bombell S, McGuire W. Early trophic feeding versus enteral fasting for very preterm or very low birth weight infants. Cochrane Database Syst Rev. 2013;3:CD000504. doi:10.1002/14651858.CD000504.pub4.

80. Morgan J, Young L, McGuire W. Slow advancement of enteral feed volumes to prevent necrotising enterocolitis in very low birth weight infants. Cochrane Database Syst Rev. 2015;10(12):CD001241. doi:10.1002/14651858.CD001241.pub6.

81. Hanson C, Sundermeier J, Dugick L, Lyden E, Anderson-Berry AL. Implementation, Process, and Outcomes of Nutrition Best Practices for Infants <1500 g. Nutr Clin Pract. 2011;26(5):614–24. doi:10.1177/0884533611418984.

82. Smith JR. Early enteral feeding for the very low birth weight infant: the development and impact of a research-based guideline. Neonatal Netw. 2005;24(4):9–19. doi:10.1891/0730-0832.24.4.9.

83. McCallie KR, Lee HC, Mayer O, Cohen RS, Hintz SR, Rhine WD. Improved outcomes with a standardized feeding protocol for very low birth weight infants. J Perinatol. 2011;31:S61–7. doi:10.1038/jp.2010.185.

84. Viswanathan S, McNelis K, Super D, Einstadter D, Groh-Wargo S, Collin M. Standardized Slow Enteral Feeding Protocol and the Incidence of Necrotizing Enterocolitis in Extremely Low Birth Weight Infants. J Parenter Enter Nutr. 2015;39(6):644–54. doi:10.1177/0148607114552848.

85. Butler TJ, Szekely LJ, Grow JL. A standardized nutrition approach for very low birth weight neonates improves outcomes, reduces cost and is not associated with increased rates of necrotizing enterocolitis, sepsis or mortality. J Perinatol. 2013;33(11):851–7. doi:10.1038/jp.2013.66.

86. Loomis T, Byham-Gray L, Ziegler J, Parrott JS. Impact of Standardized Feeding Guidelines on Enteral Nutrition Administration, Growth Outcomes, Metabolic Bone Disease, and Cholestasis in the NICU. J Pediatr Gastroenterol Nutr. 2014;59(1):93–8. doi:10.1097/MPG.0000000000000314.

87. Street JL, Montgomery D, Alder SC, Lambert DK, Gerstmann DR, Christensen RD. Implementing feeding guidelines for NICU patients < 2000 g results in less variability in nutrition outcomes. J Parenter Enter Nutr. 2006;30(6):515–518. doi:30/6/515.

88. Patole SKK, Kadalraja R, Tuladhar R, Almonte R, Muller R, Whitehall JSS. Benefits of a standardised feeding regimen during a clinical trial in preterm neonates. Int J Clin Pract. 2000;54(7):429–31.

89. Premji SS. A Matched Cohort Study of Feeding Practice Guidelines for Infants Weighing Less Than 1,500 g. Adv Neonatal Care. 2002;2(28):27–36.

90. Kamitsuka MD, Horton MK, Williams MA. The incidence of necrotizing enterocolitis after introducing standardized feeding schedules for infants between 1250 and 2500 grams and less than 35 weeks of gestation. Pediatrics. 2000;105(2):379–84.

91. Kuzma-O'Reilly B, Duenas ML, Greecher C, et al. Evaluation, Development and Implementation of Potentially Better Practices in Neonatal Intensive Care Nutrition. Pediatrics. 2003;111(4):e461. doi:10.1542/peds.111.4.SE1.461.

92. Patole S, McGlone L, Muller R. Virtual elimination of necrotising enterocolitis for 5 years - Reasons? Med Hypotheses. 2003;61(5–6):617–22. doi:10.1016/S0306-9877(03)00251-2.

93. Collaborative CPQ. CPQCC Nutrition Toolkit Appendices.; 2008. https://www.cpqcc.org/qi-tool-kits/nutritional-support-vlbw-infant.

94. Lee Chong H, Kurtin PS, Wight NE, et al. A Quality Improvement Project to Increase Breast Milk Use in Very Low Birth Weight Infants. Pediatrics. 2012;130(6):1679–87. doi:10.1542/peds.2012-0547.

95. Gephart SM, McGrath JM, Effken JA, Halpern MD. Necrotizing Enterocolitis Risk. Adv Neonatal Care. 2012;12(2):77–87. doi:10.1097/ANC.0b013e31824cee94.

96. Gregory KE. Disease Prediction Strategies for Necrotizing Enterocolitis. J Perinat Neonatal Nurs. 2015:5–7. doi:10.1097/JPN.0000000000000088.

97. Nantais-Smith L, Kadrofske M. Noninvasive biomarkers of necrotizing enterocolitis. J Perinat Neonatal Nurs. 2015;29(1):69. doi:10.1097/JPN.0000000000000082.

98. Patel AK, Lazar DA, Burrin DG, et al. Abdominal Near-Infrared Spectroscopy Measurements Are Lower in Preterm Infants at Risk for Necrotizing Enterocolitis. Pediatr Crit Care Med. 2014;15(8):735–41. doi:10.1097/PCC.0000000000000211.

99. Marin T, Moore J, Kosmetatos N, et al. Red blood cell transfusion-related necrotizing enterocolitis in very-low-birthweight infants: A near-infrared spectroscopy investigation. Transfusion. 2013;53(11):2650–8. doi:10.1111/trf.12158.

100. Marin T, Josephson CD, Kosmetatos N, Higgins M, Moore JE. Feeding preterm infants during red blood cell transfusion is associated with a decline in postprandial mesenteric oxygenation. J Pediatr. 2014;165(3):1–9. doi:10.1016/j.jpeds.2014.05.009.

101. Naberhuis J, Wetzel C, Tappenden KA. A Novel Neonatal Feeding Intolerance and Necrotizing Enterocolitis Risk-Scoring Tool Is Easy to Use and Valued by Nursing Staff. Adv Neonatal Care. 2016;16(3):239–44. doi:10.1097/ANC.0000000000000250.

102. Fox JR, Thacker LR, Hendricks-Muñoz KD. Early Detection Tool of Intestinal Dysfunction: Impact on Necrotizing Enterocolitis Severity. Am J Perinatol. 2015;32(10):927–32. doi:10.1055/s-0034-1543984.

103. Gephart SM, Cholette M. PURE Communication: A Strategy to Improve Care Coordination for High-Risk Birth. Newborn Infant Nurs Rev. 2012;12(2):109–14. doi:10.1053/j.nainr.2012.03.007.

104. Gephart SM, McGrath JM, Effken JA. Failure to rescue in neonatal care. J Perinat Neonatal Nurs. 2011;25(3):275–82. doi:10.1097/JPN.0b013e318227cc03.

105. Brady PW, Muething S, Kotagal U, et al. Improving situation awareness to reduce unrecognized clinical deterioration and serious safety events. Pediatrics. 2013;131(1):e298–308. doi:10.1542/peds.2012-1364.

106. Canvasser J, Gadepelli S, Gephart S, Kim J. International Survey of Parental Perspectives of NEC Communication. In: E-PAS. San Diego, CA: Pediatric Academic Societies; 2015:2905.459.

107. Kuppala VS, Meinzen-Derr J, Morrow AL, Schibler KR. Prolonged initial empirical antibiotic treatment is associated with adverse outcomes in premature infants. J Pediatr. 2011;159(5):720–5. doi:10.1016/j.jpeds.2011.05.033.

108. Krediet T, Lelyveld N, Vijlbrief D, et al. Microbiological factors associated with neonatal necrotizing enterocolitis: protective effect of early antibiotic treatment. Acta Paediatr. 2007;92(10):1180–2. doi:10.1111/j.1651-2227.2003.tb02481.x.

109. Tagare A, Kadam S, Vaidya U, Pandit A. Routine antibiotic use in preterm neonates: A randomised controlled trial. J Hosp Infect. 2010;74(4):332–6. doi:10.1016/j.jhin.2009.09.010.

110. Squire E, Favara B, Todd J. Diagnosis of neonatal bacterial infection: Hematologic and pathologic findings in fatal and nonfatal cases. Pediatrics. 1979;64(1):60–5.

111. More K, Athalye-Jape G, Rao S, Patole S. Association of Inhibitors of Gastric Acid Secretion and Higher Incidence of Necrotizing Enterocolitis in Preterm Very Low-Birth-Weight Infants. Am J Perinatol. 2013;30:849–56.

112. Patel SJ, Saiman L, Duchon JM, Evans D, Ferng YH, Larson E. Development of an antimicrobial stewardship intervention using a model of actionable feedback. Interdiscip Perspect Infect Dis. 2012;2012(c) doi:10.1155/2012/150367.

113. Polin RA. Management of Neonates With Suspected or Proven Early-Onset Bacterial Sepsis. Pediatrics. 2012;129(5):1006–15. doi:10.1542/peds.2012-0541.

114. Mukhopadhyay S, Puopolo KM. Clinical and Microbiologic Characteristics of Early-onset Sepsis Among Very Low Birth Weight Infants: Opportunities for Antibiotic Stewardship. Pediatr Infect Dis J. 2017;36(5):477–81. doi:10.1097/INF.0000000000001473.

115. Puopolo KM, Draper D, Wi S, et al. Estimating the probability of neonatal early-onset infection on the basis of maternal risk factors. Pediatrics. 2011;128(5):e1155–63. doi:10.1542/peds.2010-3464.

116. Escobar GJ, Puopolo KM, Wi S, et al. Stratification of Risk of Early-Onset Sepsis in Newborns >=34 Weeks' Gestation. Pediatrics. 2014;133(1):30–6. doi:10.1542/peds.2013-1689.

117. Singh R, Visintainer PF. Association of necrotizing enterocolitis with anemia and packed red blood cell transfusions in preterm infants. J Perinatol. 2011;31(3):176–82. doi:10.1038/jp.2010.145.Association.

118. Patel RM, Knezevic A, Shenvi N, et al. Association of Red Blood Cell Transfusion, Anemia, and Necrotizing Enterocolitis in Very Low-Birth-Weight Infants. JAMA. 2016;315(9):889. doi:10.1001/jama.2016.1204.

119. Talavera MM, Bixler G, Cozzi C, et al. Quality Improvement Initiative to Reduce the Necrotizing Enterocolitis Rate in Premature Infants. Pediatrics. 2016;137(5) doi:10.1542/peds.2015-1119.

28

A retrospective analysis of adverse obstetric and perinatal outcomes in adolescent pregnancy: the case of Luapula Province, Zambia

Albertina Ngomah Moraes[1][*] , Rosemary Ndonyo Likwa[2] and Selestine H. Nzala[2]

Abstract

Background: About three in ten young women aged 15–19 have begun childbearing among the Zambian population, with adolescent pregnancy levels as high as 35% in rural areas. In 2009, Luapula reported 32.1% adolescent pregnancies. The study sought to investigate obstetric and perinatal outcomes among adolescents compared to mothers aged 20-24 years delivering at selected health facilities in Kawambwa and Mansa districts of Luapula.

Methods: A retrospective analysis was carried out of all deliveries to mothers aged between 10 and 24 years for the period January 2012 to January 2013. A total of 2795 antenatal and delivery records were reviewed; 1291 adolescent mothers and 1504 mothers aged 20–24 years. Crude and adjusted odds ratios for the association between maternal age and adverse obstetric and perinatal outcomes were obtained using logistic regression models.

Results: The mean age of the adolescent mothers was 17.5 years. Mothers younger than 20 years faced a higher risk for eclampsia, anaemia, haemorrhage, Cephalopelvic disproportion, prolonged labour and caesarean section. After adjustment for potential confounders, the association between maternal age and adverse obstetric and perinatal outcome diminished. Children born to mothers younger than 20 were at increased risk for low birth weight, pre-term delivery, low Apgar score and neonatal death; the risk for asphyxia, however, tended to increase with age.

Conclusion: The findings demonstrate that adolescent pregnancy increases the risk of adverse obstetric and perinatal outcomes. High rates of adolescent pregnancies in Luapula province are likely as a result of the predominantly rural and poor population. Understanding the factors that contribute to the high levels of adolescent pregnancy in the region will be vital in addressing the situation and subsequently reducing the high obstetric and perinatal morbidity and mortality.

Keywords: Adolescent adverse obstetric perinatal outcome, Luapula, Zambia

Background

Annual global estimates of adolescent pregnancies are placed at around 16 million, about 11% of all births worldwide. An estimated 95% of these pregnancies occur in the developing world with over 50% of women in sub-Saharan Africa giving birth before the age of 20 [1]. Although accounting for only about a tenth of all births in the world, maternal conditions in adolescents produce 23% of the global burden of disability-adjusted life-years (DALYs) and 13% of all deaths from maternal conditions [2].

The majority of adolescent pregnancies are unplanned and unintended. Not only do they impact negatively on the emotional, educational and economic conditions of adolescents, but they are also associated with a high risk pregnancy [3, 4]. Pregnancy often brings a girl's education to an end, sometimes before she finishes primary school. Many adolescents have little power to influence their own futures, let alone those of their children.

* Correspondence: albertina.ngomah@gmail.com
[1]Ministry of Health, Zambia National Public Health Institute, P. O. Box 30205, Lusaka, Zambia
Full list of author information is available at the end of the article

Further, adolescent girls who have sex with older sexually experienced men have a higher risk of contracting HIV [1]. The role of adolescent and youth reproductive health should not be overlooked in our post-2015 bid to *ensure health and well-being for all at all ages, achieve gender equality and empower all women and girls, and ensure inclusive and equitable quality education for all* [5]. Combating problems related to adolescent maternal health will also impact, albeit indirectly, the bid to *end poverty in all its forms* and *end hunger and achieve food security* [6]. By improving the education, skills and prospects of pregnant adolescents, they are enabled to earn income, prevent further unwanted pregnancies and to provide for their families [7].

The framework below (Fig. 1) highlights the socio-economic, demographic and proximate determinants as well as the maternal and perinatal outcomes associated with adolescent pregnancy.

The 2002 United Nations General Assembly Special Session (UNGASS) on Children specified the need to improve care for pregnant adolescents. They declared that women, particularly adolescent expectant mothers, should have ready and affordable access to essential obstetric and perinatal care, well equipped and adequately staffed maternal health care services, skilled attendance at delivery, emergency obstetric care, effective referral and transport to higher levels of care when necessary, postpartum care and family planning in order to promote safe motherhood [8]. Often, adolescents do not receive timely antenatal care (ANC), and they have a higher risk for anaemia, malaria,

HIV and other sexually transmitted infections, obstructed and prolonged labour, fistula, postpartum haemorrhage, mental disorders such as depression as well as pregnancy-related high blood pressure and its complications [9]. Obstructed labour is especially common among young, physically immature women giving birth for the first time. Those who do not die from unrelieved obstructed labour may suffer from fistula, a hole in the birth canal that leaves them incontinent and often social outcasts [10]. Up to 65% of women with obstetric fistula develop this as adolescents [11]. The prevalence of this serious morbidity is particularly high in sub-Saharan Africa. The etiology in almost all cases is neglected obstructed labour [12]. For both physiological and social reasons, mothers aged 15 to 19 are twice as likely to die in childbirth as those in their 20s, and girls under age 15 are five times as likely to die as women in their 20s [13]. Complications of childbirth and unsafe abortions are major factors leading to death in adolescents. Women aged 15–19 account for at least one fourth of the estimated 20 million unsafe abortions and nearly 70,000 abortion-related deaths each year [14].

Babies of adolescent mothers are at higher risk for asphyxia, low birth weight and premature birth thus facing an increased risk of new born health problems [15]. Given that pregnant adolescents are also more likely to smoke and drink alcohol than are older women, this can cause further problems for the child prenatally and after birth [16]. Due to the high rates of HIV/AIDS among adolescent women, children born to young mothers have an increased risk of being born with the virus [17]. Studies

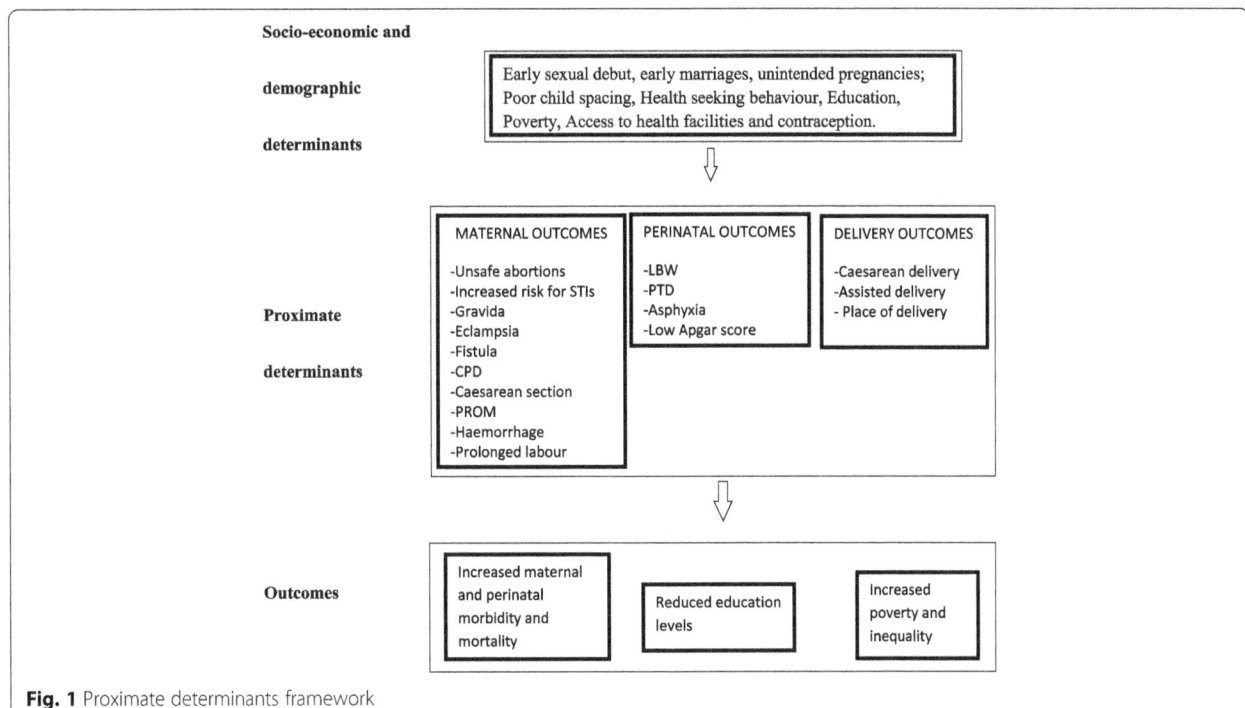

Fig. 1 Proximate determinants framework

have shown rates of new born death to average about 50% higher to adolescent mothers when compared to mothers in their 20s [18]. Furthermore, children whose mothers die are three to 10 times more likely to die. In the first week of life, stillbirths and deaths are 50% higher among babies born to mothers younger than 20 years than among babies born to mothers 20–29 years old [19]. Deaths during the first month of life are 50–100% more frequent if the mother is an adolescent, and the younger the mother, the greater the risk [20].

Among the Zambian population, about three in ten young women aged 15–19 have begun child-bearing. Adolescent pregnancy levels are as high as 35% in rural areas compared with 20% in urban areas; Luapula in particular had 32.1% adolescent pregnancies [21]. Zambia's Adolescent birth rate (ABR) is 141.2 [22], almost three times the global average of 49 per 1000 [23]. According to the 2007 DHS survey [21], at sub-regional level, Luapula province reported the highest rate of first time adolescent pregnancy (8.5%) while Lusaka had the lowest at 3.5% (Fig. 2).

It has been shown that countries with high maternal mortality ratios are generally those countries with high adolescent fertility rates [2]. Zambia's maternal mortality ratio stands at 398 deaths per 100,000 live births [22]. The proportion of adolescent deaths contributing to this figure, however, has not been specifically documented. This is because it is difficult to attain reliable age-specific data in a well-defined population as most data are hospital-based, and the population from which they are derived remains unknown [11]. Unsafe abortions are one of the top five causes of maternal mortality in Zambia. Approximately 30% of maternal deaths are due to unsafe abortions. Induced abortions in girls younger than 18 years account for 25% of maternal deaths [21]. In a 1998 country profile by the Central Statistics Office (CSO), it was shown that around 80% of women admitted to health care facilities with complications from induced abortions were younger than 19. Many abortion-related deaths occur outside of

these health institutions and usually go unreported. Ironically, Zambia has one of the most liberal abortion laws in southern Africa [24]. The infant mortality rate for children born to mothers less than 20 years old is 100 per 1000 live births, compared with 78 per 1000 live births for children whose mothers are 20-29 years old. The perinatal mortality rate for Zambia as a whole is 38 deaths per 1000 pregnancies. Perinatal mortality tends to decrease with increasing length of birth intervals and higher education level of the mother (24 deaths per 1000pregnancies) [21].

The role of maternal age and its effect on adverse obstetric and perinatal outcomes have been the subject of ongoing debate with some studies [25, 26] showing that the associations of adverse perinatal outcomes in adolescents had been confounded mainly by lack of or inadequate ANC and other socio-cultural characteristics. In contrast, other studies did not find statistically significant increase in the risk of adverse outcomes among young adolescents compared with older mothers [27, 28]. Therefore, it is unclear whether adverse obstetric and perinatal outcomes in adolescents are related to maternal age or to other factors such as lack of ANC, education level, poverty, smoking/alcohol use, as well as single parenting.

The aim of this study is to evaluate the obstetric and perinatal outcomes of adolescent pregnancies in Kawambwa and Mansa districts of Luapula Province, Zambia.

Methods

Luapula province is located in the northern part of Zambia. It has 7 districts; the study was restricted to 2 districts- Mansa and Kawambwa. The research was based on data collected from 6 randomly selected health facilities - Mansa General Hospital, Senama Clinic, Buntungwa Clinic, Kawambwa Central Clinic, Mbereshi Mission Hospital and Kawambwa district hospital. These facilities serve as ANC clinics and delivery facilities for the population of Luapula. Data collection was conducted between December 2013 and February 2014.

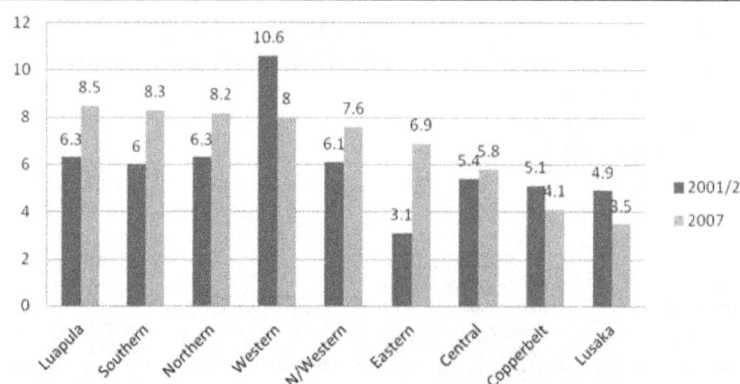

Fig. 2 Adolescent pregnancy by province

The study population was mothers aged between 10 and 24 living in Mansa and Kawambwa districts of Luapula province, Zambia. Inclusion in the study group was restricted to women aged between 10 and 24 years who gave birth between January 2012 and January 2013. Adolescent mothers were categorized into 3 groups: 10-15 years, 16-17 years, and 18-19 years [29].The selection of these three age categories was considered based on the expanded age grouping of adolescence - early adolescence (ages 10–15), middle adolescence (16–17), and late adolescence (18–19) - so as to better capture the age-specific variations in the sexual, marital, and reproductive events among the age groups. Notably, sexuality and sexual activity begin around 10–15 [2] while among the Zambian population, the average age at first sexual intercourse is 17 [22]. A comparison group of 20–24 year old mothers served as the reference group for use in all comparisons in order to assess the association between maternal age and adverse maternal and perinatal outcomes. This age group was considered because it is generally regarded as safe for childbirth and is the peak child bearing age group. Only singleton deliveries were considered in order to eliminate any confounding caused by twin pregnancy.

Of the 3102 records reviewed, 2795 records had information on maternal age and were considered. Data on the number of antennal visits and obstetric and perinatal outcomes was extracted from the ANC and delivery registers at the selected health facilities.

The variables analysed were:

i. Independent variable: maternal age, defined as the age of the mother in completed years at the time of delivery.

ii. Dependent variables: adverse obstetric and perinatal outcomes for both the mother and child. The adverse maternal outcomes evaluated were eclampsia, fistulae, premature rupture of membranes (PROM), cephalopelvic disproportion (CPD), Caesarean section, anaemia, haemorrhage, sepsis, prolonged labour and maternal death. The adverse perinatal outcomes evaluated were LBW (live infant weighing< 2500 g at birth), preterm delivery (live infant delivered at < 37 weeks' gestation), neonatal death (still birth or death occurring during the first 7 days of life), asphyxia and low Apgar scores (< 7) at 5 min.

iii. The potential confounding factors considered in the logistic regression analysis were gravida, marital status, and number of antenatal visits. Gravida was taken to be the number of pregnancies, including current pregnancy, regardless of whether the pregnancies were carried to term. Marital status was dichotomized

between those who had a partner and those who did not have a partner. Antenatal visits were categorised as either poor (no visits), fair (1–2 visits) or good (3–4 visits).

The analysis was carried out using Stata version 11.0. Univariate analysis was performed using the chi-square test. Multiple logistic regression models were constructed in order to control for confounders and assess the independent association between maternal age and adverse obstetric and perinatal outcomes. The rates of adverse obstetric and perinatal outcomes were calculated for each maternal age group. Estimates of the odds ratio (OR) with 95% CI were computed as measures of association between each maternal age group and adverse obstetric and perinatal outcomes under consideration. Logistic regression models were used to control for potential confounding and to derive the adjusted ORs (aORs). Both unadjusted and adjusted odds ratios were reported. Covariates were retained in the final model based on statistical significance.

Results

In total, 2795 delivery records were reviewed, of which 3% ($n = 81$) were 10–15 year olds, 14% ($n = 396$) were 16–17 year olds, 29% ($n = 814$) were 18–19 year olds and 54% ($n = 1504$) were 20–24 year olds (reference group). Mbereshi Mission Hospital had the highest proportion of adolescent pregnancies at 50.7%. The mean age of the adolescent mothers was 17.5 years. Table 1 below shows the distribution of adolescent births by facility.

Maternal characteristics by age group

According to the ANC registers, the ratio of girls with a partner to those without a partner increased with age; 46.9% of those aged 10–15 reported having a partner compared to 71.8% of 15–16 year olds, 84.2% of 18–19 year olds and 94.2% of 20–24 year olds. The majority (97.1%) of adolescents aged 10–15 were gravida 1. Among those aged 16–17 years, 92.2% were gravida 1 with only 0.9% recorded as gravida 3. Similarly, among adolescents aged 18-19 years, the majority (77.8%) were gravida 1 while only 0.2% were gravida 5. Those in the reference group ranged from 32.5% in gravida 1 to 0.1% in gravida 8, with the highest proportion (45.6%) being gravida 2. Most pregnant adolescents attend at least 1 to 2 antenatal visits during their pregnancy. Less than 5% of all age groups, both adolescent and adult, under consideration failed to attend at least 1 antenatal visit. Most adolescent mothers opt to deliver from a health facility- 100% of those aged between 10 and 17, and up to 97.3% of 18–19-year olds. The maternal characteristics by age group are shown in Table 2 below.

A p value < 0.05 was considered statistically significant.

Table 1 Distribution of births to adolescent mothers by facility

	Facility	Total no. Of records reviewed	No. Of births to adolescent mothers	% of adolescent mothers	Mean age of adolescent mothers	SD
1	Buntungwa Clinic	507	234	46.2%	17.6	1.53
2	Kawambwa Central Clinic	429	183	42.7%	17.4	1.02
3	Kawambwa District Hospital	501	247	49.3%	17.3	1.20
4	Mansa General Hospital	744	344	46.2%	17.5	1.08
5	Mbereshi Mission Hospital [a]	142	72	50.7%	17.4	1.30
6	Senama Clinic	472	211	44.7%	17.8	0.91
	TOTAL	2795	1291	46.2%	17.5	1.58

[a]Mbereshi Mission Hospital was under Kawambwa District until 2014 when it was reassigned to Nchelenge District

The association between maternal age and adverse obstetric and perinatal outcomes

Statistical significance in the univariate analysis of the association between maternal age and adverse obstetric and perinatal outcomes was calculated using the chi-square test. Mothers under the age of 16 years were found to have the highest rates of eclampsia, haemorrhage, CPD, prolonged labour and caesarean section compared to their older counterparts. With regards perinatal outcomes, rates of LBW, pre-term delivery and low Apgar score were highest among mothers aged 10–15 years. Significant association was found between maternal age and eclampsia, fistulae, Cephalopelvic disproportion (CPD), Caesarean section, low birth weight (LBW) and perinatal mortality. However, there was no significant association between maternal age and prolonged labour, anaemia, haemorrhage, sepsis, PROM, maternal death, preterm delivery, asphyxia and low Apgar scores. The maternal and perinatal outcomes with corresponding p values are shown in Table 3 below.

Multiple Logistic Regression models of risk factors for adverse obstetric and perinatal outcomes in adolescent mothers

List-wise deletion method was used for missing data in the logistic regression model; only records with available data on each variable were analysed. Compared to mothers aged 20–24, young adolescent mothers were found to face higher odds for eclampsia, anaemia, haemorrhage, sepsis, cephalo-pelvic disproportion, prolonged labour and caesarean section, although not all were statistically significant. The odds of anaemia and sepsis were higher in older adolescents (16–19) but not statistically significant. Young maternal age was associated with higher odds for low birth weight, asphyxia, pre-term delivery, low Apgar score and neonatal death; the odds for asphyxia, however, tended to increase with maternal age.

Logistic regression models were used to control for the selected confounders and to derive the adjusted ORs (aORs), however, this was only possible for certain variables due to the small number of outcomes. These are shown in Tables 4 and 5 below for maternal and perinatal outcomes respectively. When adjusted for confounding, the association between maternal age and adverse obstetric and perinatal outcome diminished. Mothers aged 10–15 still had higher odds of eclampsia, CPD, and prolonged labour Children born to mothers younger than 18 had higher odds of having LBW.

Table 2 Maternal characteristics by age group

	Maternal age group			
	10–15	16–17	18–19	20–24
	N=			
Marital Status	(n = 32)	(n = 176)	(n = 399)	(n = 778)
Partner	15(46.9%)	130(71.8%)	336(84.2%)	733(94.2%)
	17(53.1%)	46(28.2%)	61(15.8%)	45(5.8%)
Gravida	(n = 70)	(n = 348)	(n = 667)	(n = 1255)
1	68(97.1%)	322(92.2%)	519(77.8%)	382(32.5%)
2	2(2.9%)	23(6.9%)	124(18.6%)	536(45.6%)
3	0(0.0%)	3(0.9%)	20(3.0%)	224(14.3%)
4	0(0.0%)	0(0.0%)	3(0.4%)	73(5.1%)
5	0(0.0%)	0(0.0%)	1(0.2%)	24(1.5%)
6	0(0.0%)	0(0.0%)	0(0.0%)	14(0.8%)
7	0(0.0%)	0(0.0%)	0(0.0%)	1(0.1%)
8	0(0.0%)	0(0.0%)	0(0.0%)	1(0.1%)
ANC	(n = 32)	(n = 187)	(n = 408)	(n = 776)
Poor	0(0.0%)	6(3.2%)	10(2.5%)	9(1.2%)
Fair	20(62.5%)	123(65.8%)	262(64.2%)	524(67.5%)
Good	12(37.5%)	58(31.0%)	136(33.3%)	243(31.3%)
Place of Delivery	(n = 22)	(n = 102)	(n = 220)	(n = 400)
	0(0.0%)	0(0.0%)	6(2.7%)	3(0.8%)
Hospital	22(100%)	102(100%)	214(97.3%)	397(99.2%)

Table 3 Rates of adverse obstetric and perinatal outcome by maternal age group

	Maternal age group				
	10–15	16–17	18–19	20–24	p value[a]
Maternal Outcomes					
	n = 42	n = 191	n = 358	n = 654	
Eclampsia (N = 1245)	10(23.8%)	1(0.5%)	4(1.1%)	5(0.8%)	< 0.001
Anaemia (N = 1245)	0(0.0%)	2(1.0%)	3(0.8%)	2(0.3%)	0.513
	n = 50	n = 245	n = 507	n = 915	
Haemorrhage (N = 1717)	3(6.0%)	2(0.8%)	9(1.8%)	16(1.8%)	0.089
	n = 49	n = 209	n = 405	n = 724	
Sepsis (N = 1387)	0(0.0%)	2(1.0%)	4(1.0%)	4(0.6%)	0.751
	n = 22	n = 102	n = 220	n = 400	
Fistulae (N = 744)	0(0.0%)	0(0.0%)	4(1.8%)	19(4.8%)	0.032
PROM[b] (N = 744)	0(0.0%)	1(1.0%)	4(1.8%)	4(1.0%)	0.767
	n = 30	n = 156	n = 369	n = 661	
CPD[c] (N = 1216)	11(36.7%)	29(18.6%)	39(10.6%)	64(9.7%)	< 0.001
	n = 40	n = 217	n = 446	n = 542	
Prolonged labour (N = 1245)	3(7.1%)	8(4.2%)	19(5.3%)	25(3.8%)	0.576
	n = 57	n = 263	n = 554	n = 985	
Caesarean section (N = 1859)	25(43.9%)	70(26.6%)	125(22.6%)	187(19.0%)	< 0.001
	n = 22	n = 102	n = 220	n = 400	
Maternal death (N = 744)	0(0.0%)	2(2.0%)	2(0.9%)	8(2.0%)	0.682
Perinatal outcomes					
	n = 70	n = 332	n = 706	n = 1258	
Low birth weight (N = 2366)	12(17.1%)	52(15.7%)	103(14.6%)	140(11.1%)	0.035
	n = 37	n = 174	n = 416	n = 731	
Pre-term delivery (N = 1358)	2(5.4%)	9(5.2%)	15(3.6%)	18(2.5%)	0.239
	n = 30	n = 156	n = 369	n = 661	
Asphyxia (N = 1216)	0(0.0%)	2(1.3%)	7(1.9%)	4(0.6%)	0.248
	n = 57	n = 263	n = 554	n = 985	
Low Apgar score (N = 1859)	9(15.8%)	38(14.4%)	61(11.0%)	92(9.3%)	0.062
Neonatal death (N = 1859)	4(7.0%)	7(2.7%)	38(6.9%)	39(4.0%)	0.018

[a]chi-square test was used to identify between-group differences. Fischer's exact test was used when the number of outcomes was small
[b]PROM = Premature Rapture of membranes
[c]CPD = Cephalopelvic disproportion

Discussion

The adolescent birth rate was found to be 461.9 per 1000 deliveries to mothers aged between 10 and 19 years, which is three times higher than the national ABR of 141.2 [22]. This is not surprising given that literature has shown that among rural and poor populations the rates of adolescent pregnancy do tend to be higher. The majority (69.2%) of all the adolescent mothers were in their first pregnancy. The youngest mother in the study population was 11 years old at the time of delivery. The findings demonstrate a clear trend of higher risk of adverse outcomes, particularly in mothers below 16 years. Given that adolescent mothers are more likely than older mothers to have sociodemographic characteristics associated with adverse outcomes of pregnancy, the confounding effects of marital status, gravida, adequacy of ANC and place of delivery were accounted for.

The population under consideration for this study allowed for a comparison of adolescent and adult obstetric and perinatal outcomes, something few studies have done. Controlling for confounding factors and the relatively homogeneous population of women studied further strengthen the findings of this study. Unlike most studies on adolescent pregnancy which focus on adolescents aged 15 to 19 years, – with information about pregnancy at younger ages usually only appearing in aggregate statistics

Table 4 Logistic regression models of risk factors for adverse maternal outcomes[a]

Maternal outcomes	Maternal age group	Crude Odds ratio (95% CI)	Adjusted Odds ratio (95% CI)
Eclampsia	10–15	*40.563 (13.094–125.651)*	*30.503 (7.802–119.247)*
(N = 1245)	16–17	0.683 (0.079–5.883)	0.459 (0.049–4.312)
	18–19	1.467 (0.391–5.497)	0.179 (0.019–1.697)
Anaemia	10–15	Non-estimable	Non-estimable
(N = 1245)	16–17	3.450 (0.483–24.652)	7.645(0.439–133.114)
	18–19	2.755 (0.458–16.563)	1.252 (0.093–16.765)
Haemorrhage	10–15	*3.586 (1.010–12.739)*	0.071 (0)
(N = 1717)	16–17	0.463 (0.106–2.025)	Non-estimable
	18–19	1.015 (0.446–2.315)	0.022 (0.001–0.437)
Sepsis (N = 1387)	10–15	Non-estimable	0.466 (0)
	16–17	1.739 (0.316–9.561)	0.475(0)
	18–19	1.796 (0.447–7.218)	0.250(0.013–4.729)
Fistulae (N = 744)	10–15	Non-estimable	Non-estimable
	16–17	Non-estimable	Non-estimable
	18–19	0.371 (0.125–1.106)	Non-estimable
PROM (N = 744)	10–15	Non-estimable	Non-estimable
	16–17	0.980 (0.108–8.865)	1.804 (0.175–18.588)
	18–19	1.833 (0.454–7.404)	0.712 (0.108–4.685)
CPD (N = 1216)	10–15	*5.401 (2.461–11.852)*	1.604 (0.721–3.569)
	16–17	*2.130 (1.320–3.438)*	0.687 (0.416–1.136)
	18–19	1.102 (0.724–1.678)	0.471 (0.301–0.736)
Prolonged labour	10–15	1.488 (0.432–5.126)	2.569 (0.710–9.289)
(N = 1245)	16–17	0.345 (0.119–0.995)	0.397 (0.136–1.155)
	18–19	0.862 (0.479–1.552)	0.928 (0.512–1.682)
Caesarean section	10–15	*3.334 (1.930–5.760)*	0.082 (0.011–0.616)
(N = 1859)	16–17	*1.548 (1.128–2.124)*	0.124 (0.044–0.355)
	18–19	1.243 (0.964–1.605)	0.048 (0.015–0.151)
Maternal death	10–15	Non-estimable	Non-estimable
(N = 744)	16–17	0.980 (0.205–4.687)	1.242 (0.251–6.142)
	18–19	0.449 (0.095–2.136)	0.207 (0.031–1.386)

[a]The covariates included in the logistic regression model were marital status, gravida and ANC

-, this study considered very young maternal age (10-15 years). Data was obtained from the ANC and delivery registers, which consisted of information recorded during ANC visits and immediately following delivery respectively. Some records that did not have available data on each variable were dropped using list-wise deletion (complete case analysis). This meant not all the information collected was used and effectively lowered the sample size and thus the statistical power was reduced and some bias introduced in the estimates. Further bias in the reported estimations was introduced from the use of the maximum likelihood estimation of the logistic model. The study did not take into consideration socio economic indicators such as education and employment status as well as behavioural

risk factors such as maternal smoking and alcohol consumption.

Eclampsia in adolescents is of critical importance considering the untimely access and usage of ANC services which can be used to monitor and manage the condition [11]. If left unchecked, eclampsia poses significant risks to both the mother and baby and can lead to death. According to the findings of this study, adolescent mothers were forty times more likely to develop eclampsia compared to the reference group of mothers aged 20–24 years. This is in line with the findings of other studies [30–32]. It was noteworthy to find that most adolescents do not attend the prescribed 3–4 ANC visits during their pregnancy; at most, they attend an average of 1–2 visits. Given that

Table 5 Logistic regression models of risk factors for perinatal outcomes[a]

Perinatal outcomes	Maternal age group	Crude Odds ratio (95% CI)	Adjusted Odds ratio (95% CI)
Low birth weight (N = 2366)	10–15	1.652 (0.866–3.152)	1.418 (0.417–4.826)
	16–17	*1.483 (1.051–2.092)*	1.455 (0.811–2.611)
	18–19	*1.364 (1.038–1.792)*	0.771 (0.461–1.287)
Pre-term delivery (N = 1358)	10–15	2.263 (0.505–10.142)	0.463 (0.038–5.627)
	16–17	2.161 (0.954–4.895)	0.376 (0.078–1.815)
	18–19	1.482 (0.739–2.972)	0.435 (0.119–1.596)
Asphyxia (N = 1216)	10–15	Non-estimable	Non-estimable
	16–17	2.133 (0.387–11.755)	0.717 (0.051–10.048)
	18–19	3.176 (0.924–10.926)	0.361 (0.028–4.706)
Low Apgar score (N = 1859)	10–15	1.820 (0.865–3.828)	0.034 (0.002–0.401)
	16–17	*1.639 (1.093–2.458)*	0.263 (0.097–0.710)
	18–19	1.201 (0.853–1.690)	0.087 (0.030–0.249)
Neonatal death (N = 1358)	10–15	1.831 (0.631–5.313)	Non-estimable
	16–17	0.663 (0.293–1.500)	Non-estimable
	18–19	*1.786 (1.128–2.828)*	0.025 (0.002–0.265)

OR = 0 no outcome event for the age group
OR = 1 exposure does not affect odds of outcome
OR > 1 exposure associated with higher odds of outcome
OR < 1 exposure associated with lower odds of outcome
[a]The covariates included in the logistic regression model were marital status, gravida, and ANC

adolescent pregnancy has been shown to be high risk, this is far from ideal.

Furthermore, young maternal age was found to be a risk factor for haemorrhage. This may be attributed to an increased risk of placenta abruption in younger mothers [33]. Haemorrhage has been shown to be dangerous, particularly in adolescent mothers presenting with anaemia [34]. This study also found that younger mothers are five times more at risk for CPD than older mothers. In a similar study [35], adolescent mothers had an almost nine times higher risk for CPD than those above 20 years. CPD has been linked to the immaturity of the pelvic bones and birth canal in younger mothers. This immaturity has also been linked to increased risk of prolonged and obstructed labour, episiotomy, and use of forceps [31].

The study also showed an increased risk for prolonged labour and caesarean section before adjustment for confounding. This data is in line with findings of other studies [36, 37]. Caesarean sections today are a timely operative procedure that often save the lives of mothers and babies. Available literature on caesarean sections in adolescents is conflicting with some studies [38, 39] reporting higher rates among adolescents and other reporting lower or similar rates in adolescents compared to older mothers [40, 41] This makes it difficult to draw a clear conclusion, especially given that indications for a caesarean section are quite subjective among obstetricians. Caesarean sections have been linked to intra- and post-operative complications such as placenta previa and placenta accreta, hysterectomy, and bladder and bowel injury [42].

Very little information was available on the levels of fistulae. The complete number of fistulae cases were hard to detect as the only centre in the province where women can access treatment on a regular basis is Mansa General Hospital. Women from all over the province with this condition have to wait for indefinite periods to get access to the service. Some patients are lost to follow up due to being referred from one hospital to another, and in cases where funds are unavailable, this is at their own expense. For the period January 2012 to December 2012, 23 women underwent corrective surgery for Fistulae. Of these, 19 were between 20 and 24, and 4 were aged 18–19 years. The available data, however, does not indicate when the condition developed and is in no way representative of the complete picture.

The maternal mortality rate among adolescent mothers was 3 deaths per 1, 000 live births. In comparison to the findings of a previous study in Mansa [43], this shows a marked decrease in reported mortality, possibly as a result of policies and intervention introduced in the early 2000s to address the high levels of maternal mortality in the country. There was no marked difference in the mortality among adolescent mothers and those aged 20-24 years; both age groups recorded a 2% mortality rate. Literature has shown that the increased risk of maternal death in adolescent mothers has been linked to complications during and following pregnancy and childbirth. These include eclampsia, haemorrhage, sepsis and unsafe abortions. Other complications may exist before pregnancy but are exacerbated during pregnancy [44].

Literature has shown that adolescent mothers continue to grow during pregnancy and are therefore in competition with the developing foetus for nutrients, to the detriment of the foetus [45]. According to the findings of this study, compared with infants born to mothers aged 20 to 24 years, those born to women aged 15 years or younger had about 50% risk of low birth weight. They were also faced with a higher risk of pre-term delivery, low Apgar score and neonatal death. These findings are in line with those of other studies [46–48]. It has been suggested that the higher incidence of low birth weight among adolescent mothers is likely linked to pre-term delivery [49]. Notwithstanding, the risk diminished when it was adjusted for confounders, suggesting that the increased risk of early pre-term delivery, low Apgar score and neonatal death among the youngest adolescents may be explained by the access to ANC, partner status and gravida. Only low birth weight remained a risk factor for young maternal age even with the effect of confounding. This has been shown to be as a result of the competition for nutrients between the growing mother and the foetus and may also be attributed to inadequate weight gain during the pregnancy [50, 51]. However, this was not taken into consideration during this study.

The neonatal mortality rate among adolescents was 38 deaths per 1, 000 live births. Neonatal death was highest among very young mothers (10-15 years old) with 7% mortality recorded, almost double that found among mothers aged 20-24 years. Previous investigations of perinatal mortality in adolescent pregnancy have produced conflicting results. Some studies [31, 36] have found an increased risk of neonatal mortality among adolescent mothers, whereas others found no increase [52, 53].

The high prevalence of adolescent births in the region is likely as a result of the rural setting where high poverty levels and lower educational levels are the order of the day, with 64.91% of the population living in abject poverty, 83.8% literacy rates among 15–24 year olds and a ratio of 0.74 girls to boys in secondary education [54]. The number of adolescents reporting having a partner during ANC was alarming, with as many as 46.9% of 10–15 year olds registered as married in the ANC registers. According to a qualitative study by UNICEF [55], early and forced marriages are rife in Luapula Province, with an estimated incidence of 70% early pregnancy and under-age marriage among adolescents.

The situation is so dire that the Zambian Government has put in place policies that allow adolescents access to a full range of sexual and reproductive health services, including condoms and other means of contraception. The National Population Policy which seeks the reduction of the high levels of fertility, particularly adolescent fertility [56]. Other policies include the National Youth Policy and the National Reproductive Health Policy. However, the concept of adolescent friendly health services (ADFHS) introduced by WHO to define appropriate and convenient health services for adolescents has not been fully implemented in Zambia. Some facilities have youth friendly corners established which serve as entry points of access to care. Although these offer similar services to ADFHS, they target youths as a whole, which comprise different age groups with different health needs and as such adolescents' needs are not specifically targeted [57]. The Saving Mothers Giving Life (SMGL) program, piloted in Zambia in 2012, has intensified efforts to strengthen health services focused on the critical period of labour, delivery and the first 48 h post-partum. Since its launch, the efforts of SMGL have helped improve maternal health outcomes in Zambia. The United Nations Population Fund (UNFPA) launched its manual for healthcare providers from low-and middle-income countries involved in the prevention and management of fistula in August of 2011 and has made great strides, prior to which Zambia did not have a standard training manual. Despite the numerous efforts of government, UNFPA and other stakeholders as well as programs such as SMGL, there is still a clear and pressing need for continued advocacy against teenage marriage as well as at adolescent reproductive health services and school curriculums. One of the major challenges facing the provision of adolescent health services in Zambia is financing. Currently, even though these activities are included in the action plans and budgets, youth friendly services are yet to receive budgetary allocations, and therefore when funds are disbursed, adolescent health activities are not prioritised.

Conclusion

Adolescent pregnancy plays a crucial role in maternal and perinatal health; improvements in reproductive health cannot be complete without improvements in adolescent health. According to current statistics, Zambia's maternal and perinatal mortality rates are amongst the highest in the region. The findings of this study highlight the high levels of adolescent maternal and perinatal mortality and morbidity in Luapula province. This will assist in the promotion of programs and policies advocating for the improvement of adolescent maternal-perinatal health as well as build on the currently available literature.

Adolescent pregnancy, especially in mothers younger than 16 years, increases the risk of adverse obstetric and perinatal outcomes. Efforts to curb the high number of adolescent pregnancies through policy initiatives as well as reproductive health education and better antenatal and obstetric care targeted at adolescents have been shown to play a major role in reducing overall maternal and perinatal morbidity and mortality rates. Despite these efforts and interventions, adolescent pregnancy and its associated adverse outcomes continue to be a problem in the province. Given this trend, it would be imperative to tailor interventions to reduce unintended pregnancies and address adolescent health needs to the specific population. Recognising the existence of avoidable factors that play a key role in the outcomes of adolescent pregnancies, such as access to ANC, must be the first step in designing and implementing intervention programmes. Where possible, evaluations of these interventions that follow the adolescents into adulthood should be performed.

Abbreviations
ADFHS: Adolescent Friendly Health Services; AIDS: Acquired Immuno-Deficiency Syndrome; ANC: Antenatal care; CPD: Cephalopelvic disproportion; CSO: Central Statistics Office; DALY: Disability-Adjusted Life-Years; HIV: Human Immuno-deficiency Virus; LBW: Low birth weight; MDGs: Millennium Development Goals; MMR: Maternal mortality ratio; MoH: Ministry of Health; PROM: Premature rapture of membranes; SMGL: Saving Mothers Giving Life; UNDESA: United Nations Department of Economic and Social Affairs; UNFPA: United Nations Population Fund; UNZABREC: University of Zambia Biomedical Research Ethics Committee; WHO: World Health Organisation; YFC: Youth Friendly Corner; ZDHS: Zambia Demographic Health Survey

Acknowledgements
We wish to thank Prof. Charles Michelo and Dr. Raymond Hamoonga for their editorial input. We also wish to acknowledge the Bloomberg Foundation and the Ministry of Health for their support.

Funding
All costs for data collection and preparation of the manuscript were covered by the corresponding author.

Authors' contributions
ANM conceptualised the study and drafted the manuscript. RNL and SHN contributed substantially to the literature review and manuscript writing. All named authors read and approved the final manuscript.

Competing interests
The authors declare that they have no competing interests.

Author details
[1]Ministry of Health, Zambia National Public Health Institute, P. O. Box 30205, Lusaka, Zambia. [2]Department of Public Health, University of Zambia, P. O. Box 32379, Lusaka, Zambia.

References
1. World Health Organization. Adolescent Pregnancy: Delivering on Global Promises of Hope. Geneva: World Health Organization Press; 2010. p. 3–10.
2. Rosen JE. Position paper on mainstreaming adolescent pregnancy in efforts to make pregnancy safer. Geneva: World Health Organization Press; 2010. p. 16.
3. Moore KA, Myers DE, Morrison DR, Nord CW, Brown B, Edmonston B. Age at first childbirth and later poverty. J Res Adolesc. 1993;3(4):393–422.
4. Geronimus AT, Korenman S. The socioeconomic consequences of teen childbearing reconsidered. Q J Econ. 1992;107(4):1187–214.
5. United Nations General Assembly. Report on the open working group on sustainable development goals. 2015. http://www.asiapacificrcem.org/wp-content/uploads/2015/02/N1450367.pdf. Accessed 2 Oct, 2015.
6. Frost JJ, Forrest JD. Understanding the impact of effective teenage pregnancy prevention programs. Fam Plan Perspect. 1995;1:188–95.
7. Viner RM, Ozer EM, Denny S, Marmot M, Resnick M, Fatusi A, Currie C. Adolescence and the social determinants of health. Lancet. 2012;379(9826):1641–52.
8. United Nations General Assembly Special Session on Children. A world fit for children. 10 May 2002. Plan of Action, B: Goals Strategies and Actions 1. Promoting Healthy Lives, Paragraph 37:1. New York; 2002. Available at https://www.unicef.org/bangladesh/wffc-en_main.pdf. Accessed 16 Aug 2018.
9. UNFPA. State of the World's population. 2004. https://www.unfpa.org/sites/default/files/pub-pdf/swp04_eng.pdf. Accessed 12 Aug 2018.
10. Neelofur-Khan D. Pregnant adolescents - Unmet needs and undone deeds. Geneva: World Health Organization Press; 2007. p. 19–23.
11. Treffers P. Pregnant adolescents-issues in adolescent health and development. Geneva: World Health Organization Press; 2004. p. 33–5.
12. Filippi V, Chou D, Ronsmans C, Graham W, Say L. Levels and causes of maternal mortality and morbidity. 2016. Available at https://www.ncbi.nlm.nih.gov/books/NBK361917/. Accessed 12 Aug 2018.
13. Graczyk K. Adolescent maternal mortality: an overlooked crisis. 2007. http://www.advocatesforyouth.org/storage/advfy/documents/fsmaternal.pdf. Accessed 2 Oct 2011.
14. Grimes DA, Benson J, Singh S, Romero M, Ganatra B, Okonofua FE, Shah IH. Unsafe abortion: the preventable pandemic. Lancet. 2006;368(9550):1908–19.
15. World Health Organisation. Early marriages, adolescent and young pregnancies. 2011. http://apps.who.int/gb/ebwha/pdf_files/EB130/B130_12-en.pdf Accessed 5 January 2018.
16. Scholl TO, Hediger ML, Belsky DH. Prenatal care and maternal health during adolescent pregnancy: a review and meta-analysis. J Adolesc Health. 1994;15(6):444–56.
17. World Health Organisation. Factsheet on Adolescent Health. 2015. Available at http://www.wpro.who.int/mediacentre/factsheets/docs/fs_201202_adolescent_health/en/. Accessed 16 Aug 2018.
18. World Health Organization. World health report 2005: make every mother and child count. 2005. http://www.who.int/whr/2005/whr2005_en.pdf?ua=1. Accessed 5 Oct 2011.
19. Mayor S. Pregnancy and childbirth are leading causes of death in teenage girls in developing countries. BMJ. 2004;328(7449):1152.
20. UNFPA. Adolescent pregnancy - a review of the evidence. 2013. https://www.unfpa.org/sites/default/files/pub-pdf/ADOLESCENT%20PREGNANCY_UNFPA.pdf
21. Central Statistical Office, Ministry of Health, Tropical Diseases Research Centre, University of Zambia, and Macro International Inc. Zambia Demographic and Health Survey 2007. Calverton: CSO and Macro International Inc; 2009.
22. Central Statistical Office (CSO), Ministry of Health (MOH), Tropical Diseases Research Centre, University of Zambia, and Macro International Inc. Zambia Demographic and Health Survey 2013–2014. Rockville: CSO, MOH and Macro International Inc; 2014.
23. United Nations, Department of Economic and Social Affairs, Population Division. Adolescent Fertility since the International Conference on Population and Development (ICPD) in Cairo. 2013. http://www.un.org/en/development/desa/population/publications/pdf/fertility/Report_Adolescent-Fertility-since-ICPD.pdf Accessed 11 Jan 2011.
24. Geloo Z. Diverse factors linked to maternal deaths in Zambia. Washington: Reference Bureau; 2003.
25. Ronsmans C, Khlat M. Adolescence and risk of violent death during pregnancy in Matlab, Bangladesh. Lancet. 1999;354(9188):1448.
26. Tsikouras P, Dafopoulos A, Trypsianis G, Vrachnis N, Bouchlariotou S, Liatsikos SA, Dafopoulos K, Maroulis G, Galazios G, Teichmann AT, Von Tempelhoff GF. Pregnancies and their obstetric outcome in two selected age groups of teenage women in Greece. J Matern Fetal Neonatal Med. 2012;25(9):1606–11.
27. Kwast BE, Liff JM. Factors associated with maternal mortality in Addis Ababa, Ethiopia. Int J Epidemiol. 1988;17(1):115–21.
28. Liran D, Vardi IS, Sergienko R, Sheiner E. Adverse perinatal outcome in teenage pregnancies: Is it all due to lack of prenatal care and ethnicity? J Matern Fetal Neonatal Med. 2013;26(5):469–72.
29. Dixon-Mueller R. How young is "too young"? Comparative perspectives on adolescent sexual, marital, and reproductive transitions. Stud Fam Plan. 2008;39(4):247–62.
30. Kongnyuy EJ, Nana PN, Fomulu N, Wiysonge SC, Kouam L, Doh AS. Adverse perinatal outcomes of adolescent pregnancies in Cameroon. Matern Child Health J. 2008;12(2):149–54.

31. Zabin LS, Kiragu K. The health consequences of adolescent sexual and fertility behaviour in sub-Saharan Africa. Stud Fam Plan. 1998;1:210–32.

32. Arora R, Ganguli RP, Swain S, Oumachigui A, Rajaram P. Determinants of maternal mortality in eclampsia in India. Aust N Z J Obstet Gynaecol. 1994;34(5):537–9.

33. Ananth CV, Wilcox AJ, Savitz DA, Bowes WA, Luther ER. Effect of maternal age and parity on the risk of uteroplacental bleeding disorders in pregnancy. Obstet Gynecol. 1996;88(4):511–6.

34. Ota E, Ganchimeg T, Mori R, Souza JP. Risk factors of pre-eclampsia/eclampsia and its adverse outcomes in low-and middle-income countries: a WHO secondary analysis. PLoS One. 2014;9(3):e91198.

35. Chahande MS, Jadhao AR, Wadhva SK. Study of some epidemiological factors in teenage pregnancy--hospital based case comparison study. Indian J Community Med. 2002;27(3):4.

36. Conde-Agudelo A, Belizán JM, Lammers C. Maternal-perinatal morbidity and mortality associated with adolescent pregnancy in Latin America: cross-sectional study. Am J Obstet Gynecol. 2005;192(2):342–9.

37. Wadhawan S, Narone RK, Narone JN. Obstetric problems in the adolescent Zambian mother studied at the university teaching hospital, Lusaka. Med J Zambia. 1982;16(3):65–8.

38. Bozkaya H, Mocan H, Usluca H, Beşer E, Gümüştekin D. A retrospective analysis of adolescent pregnancies. Gynecol Obstet Investig. 1996;42(3):146–50.

39. Unfer V, Piazze GJ, Di Benedetto MR, Costabile L, Gallo G, Anceschi MM. Pregnancy in adolescents. A case-control study. Clin Exp Obstet Gynecol. 1994;22(2):161–4.

40. Yadav S, Choudhary D, Narayan KC, Mandal RK, Sharma A, Chauhan SS, Agrawal P. Adverse reproductive outcomes associated with teenage pregnancy. McGill J Med. 2008;11(2):141.

41. Hidalgo LA, Chedraui PA, Chávez MJ. Obstetrical and neonatal outcome in young adolescents of low socio-economic status: a case control study. Arch Gynaecol Obstetrics. 2005;271(3):207–11.

42. Clark EA, Silver RM. Long-term maternal morbidity associated with repeat caesarean delivery. Am J Obstetrics Gynaecol. 2011;205(6):S2–10.

43. Nkata M. Maternal deaths in teenage mothers. J Obstet Gynaecol. 1997;17(4):344–5.

44. World Health Organization. Maternal Mortality Factsheet No. 348. 2014. http://www.who.int/mediacentre/factsheets/fs348/en/ Accessed 21 Aug 2014.

45. Scholl TO, Hediger ML, Schall JI, Khoo CS, Fischer RL. Maternal growth during pregnancy and the competition for nutrients. Am J Clin Nutr. 1994;60(2):183–8.

46. Gupta N, Kiran U, Bhal K. Teenage Pregnancies: Obstetric characteristics and outcome. Eur J Obstet Gynecol Reprod Biol. 2008;137(2):165–71.

47. Fraser AM, Brockert JE, Ward RH. Association of young maternal age with adverse reproductive outcomes. N Engl J Med. 1995;332(17):1113–8.

48. Derme M, Leoncini E, Vetrano G, Carlomagno L, Aleandri V. Obstetric and perinatal outcomes of teenage pregnant women: a retrospective study. Epidemiol Biostatistics Public Health. 2013;10(4):e8641-1–e8641-8.

49. Scholl TO, Hediger ML, Salmon RW, Belsky DH, Ances IG. Association between low gynaecological age and preterm birth. Paediatr Perinat Epidemiol. 1989;3(4):357–66.

50. Casanueva E, Roselló-Soberón ME, De-Regil LM, del Carmen AM, Céspedes MI. Adolescents with adequate birth weight newborns diminish energy expenditure and cease growth. J Nutr. 2006;136(10):2498–501.

51. Naeye RL. Teenaged and pre-teenaged pregnancies: consequences of the fetal-maternal competition for nutrients. Pediatrics. 1981;67(1):146–50.

52. Smith GC, Pell JP. Teenage pregnancy and risk of adverse perinatal outcomes associated with first and second births: population based retrospective cohort study. BMJ. 2001;323(7311):476.

53. Satin AJ, Leveno KJ, Sherman ML, Reedy NJ, Lowe TW, DD MI. Maternal youth and pregnancy outcomes: middle school versus high school age groups compared with women beyond the teen years. Am J Obstetrics Gynaecol. 1994;171(1):184–7.

54. United Nations Development Programme. Millennium development goals profile – Luapula province. Lusaka: United Nations Development Programme; 2013.

55. Mann G, Quigley P, Fischer R. A qualitative study of child marriage in six districts of Zambia. Hong Kong: Child Frontiers UNICEF; 2015. Available at https://www.unicef.org/zambia/Qualitative_study_of_child_marriage_in_six_districts_of_Zambia.pdf. Accessed 16 Aug 2018.

56. Ministry of Finance and National Planning. National Population Policy. Lusaka: Ministry of Finance and National Planning; 2007.

57. Ministry of Health. Adolescent health strategic plan 2011–2015. Lusaka: Ministry of Health; 2011.

Permissions

List of Contributors

Zia Ul Haq Gouri
Kothari Hospital and Research Center, Bikaner, Rajasthan, India.

Deepak Sharma
Department of Pediatrics, Pt B.D. Sharma PGIMS, Rohtak, Haryana, India

Pramod Kumar Berwal
Department of Paediatrics, S.P. Medical College, Bikaner, Rajasthan, India

Aakash Pandita
Department of Pediatrics, Government Medical College, Jammu, India

Smita Pawar
Department of Obstetrics and Gynaecology, Fernandez Hospital, Hyderabad, India

Tetsuya Kawakita
Obstetrics and Gynecology, MedStar Washington Hospital Center, 101 Irving Street, 5B45, NW, Washington, DC 20010, USA

Helain J. Landy
Obstetrics and Gynecology, MedStar Georgetown University Hospital, Washington, DC, USA

Paul J. Rozance and William W. Hay Jr.
Perinatal Research Center, Department of Pediatrics, University of Colorado School of Medicine, 13243 E 23rd Ave, MS F441, Aurora, CO 80045, USA

Aparna Sridhar
Department of Obstetrics and Gynecology, David Geffen School of Medicine at University of California Los Angeles, California, USA

Jennifer Salcedo
Department of Obstetrics, Gynecology and Women's Health, University of Hawaii John A. Burns School of Medicine, Hawaii, USA

Jayashree Ramasethu
Division of Neonatal Perinatal Medicine, Department of Pediatrics, MedStar Georgetown University Hospital, Washington DC 20007, USA

Susan Niermeyer
Section of Neonatology, University of Colorado School of Medicine, 13121 E. 17th Avenue, Mail Stop 8402, Aurora, CO 80045, USA

Jane E. Harding
Liggins Institute, University of Auckland, Private Bag 92019, Victoria St West, Auckland 1142, New Zealand

Christopher J. D. McKinlay and Jane M. Alsweiler
Liggins Institute, University of Auckland, Private Bag 92019, Victoria St West, Auckland 1142, New Zealand
Department of Paediatrics: Child and Youth Health, University of Auckland, Auckland, New Zealand

Deborah L. Harris
Liggins Institute, University of Auckland, Private Bag 92019, Victoria St West, Auckland 1142, New Zealand
Neonatal Intensive Care Unit, Waikato District Health Board, Hamilton, New Zealand

J. Geoffrey Chase and Jennifer Dickson
Mechanical Engineering, University of Canterbury, Christchurch, New Zealand

Nguke Mwakatundu Sunday Dominico, Mkambu Kasanga, Fadhili Jamadini, Kelvin Maokola and Donald Mawala
Thamini Uhai Program, Dar es Salaam, Tanzania

Angelo Nyamtema
Thamini Uhai Program, Dar es Salaam, Tanzania
Tanzanian Training Centre for International Health, Ifakara, Tanzania
Saint Francis University College for Health and Allied Sciences, Ifakara, Tanzania

Richard Rumanyika
Thamini Uhai Program, Dar es Salaam, Tanzania
Catholic University of Health and Allied Sciences, Mwanza, Tanzania

Calist Nzabuhakwa
Thamini Uhai Program, Dar es Salaam, Tanzania
Maweni Regional Hospital, Kigoma, Tanzania

Jos van Roosmalen
Thamini Uhai Program, Dar es Salaam, Tanzania
Leiden University Medical Centre, Leiden, The Netherlands
Athena Institute, VU University Amsterdam, Amsterdam, The Netherlands

Zabron Abel
Tanzanian Training Centre for International Health, Ifakara, Tanzania

Deepak Sharma
National Institute of Medical Science, Jaipur, Rajasthan, India

Corinna Binder-Heschl
The Ritchie Centre, Hudson Institute for Medical Research, Melbourne, Australia.

Stuart B. Hooper, Graeme R. Polglase and Euan M. Wallace
The Ritchie Centre, Hudson Institute for Medical Research, Melbourne, Australia.
Department of Obstetrics and Gynaecology, Monash University, Melbourne, Australia.

Douglas Blank
The Ritchie Centre, Hudson Institute for Medical Research, Melbourne, Australia
Neonatal Services, The Royal Women's Hospital, Melbourne, Australia

Andrew W. Gill
Centre for Neonatal Research and Education, The University of Western Australia, Crawley, WA 6008, Australia

Martin Kluckow
Department of Neonatology, Royal North Shore Hospital and University of Sydney, Sydney, NSW 2065, Australia

Arjan B. te Pas
Department of Neonatology, Leiden University Medical Centre, Leiden, The Netherlands

Archana B. Patel
Lata Medical Research Foundation, Nagpur, Maharashtra 440022, India

Sreelatha Meleth, Elizabeth M. McClure and Janet L. Moore
RTI International, Research Triangle Park, North Carolina 27709, USA

Omrana Pasha and Sarah Saleem
Department of Community Health Sciences and Family Medicine, Aga Khan University, Karachi, Pakistan

Shivaprasad S. Goudar
KLE University's JN Medical College, Belgaum, Karnataka, India

Fabian Esamai
Moi University School of Medicine, Eldoret, Kenya

Ana L. Garces
IMSALUD, San Carlos University, Guatemala City, Guatemala

Elwyn Chomba
University Teaching Hospital, Lusaka, Zambia

Linda L. Wright and Marion Koso-Thomas
Center for Research of Mothers and Children, NIH, Rockville, MD 20852, USA

Edward A. Liechty
Department of Pediatrics, Indiana University School of Medicine, Indianapolis, IN 46202, USA

Robert L. Goldenberg
Department of Obstetrics/Gynecology, Columbia University, New York, NY 10032, USA

Richard J. Derman
Department of OB-GYN, Christiana Care, Newark, DE 19718, USA

K. Michael Hambidge
Department of Pediatrics, University of Colorado, Aurora, CO 80045, USA

Waldemar A. Carlo
Department of Pediatrics, University of Alabama at Birmingham, Birmingham, AL 35233, USA

Patricia L. Hibberd
Division of Global Health, Department of Pediatrics, Massachusetts General Hospital, Boston, MA 02114, USA

Lisa M. Tussing-Humphreys
Department of Medicine and Cancer Center, University of Illinois at Chicago, 416 West Side Research Office Building, 1747 West Roosevelt Road, Chicago, IL 60608, USA

Jessica L. Thomson and Melissa H. Goodman
United States Department of Agriculture, Agricultural Research Service, Delta Human Nutrition Research Program, 141 Experiment Station Road, Stoneville, MS 38776, USA

Nefertiti OjiNjideka Hemphill
Department of Kinesiology and Nutrition, 484 West Side Research Office Building, 1747 West Roosevelt Road, Chicago, IL 60608, USA

Alicia S. Landry
Department of Family and Consumer Sciences, University of Central Arkansas, 201 Donaghey Avenue, McAlister 113, Conway, AR 72035, USA

Nega Assefa, Betelhem Belay, Haji Kedir, Desalew Zelalem, Negga Baraki, Melake Damena, Lemessa Oljira and Wondimye Ashenafi
College of Health and Medical Sciences, Haramaya University, Harar, Ethiopia

Melkamu Dedefo
College of Health and Medical Sciences, Haramaya University, Harar, Ethiopia
College of Computing and Informatics, Haramaya University, Harar, Ethiopia

Yihune Lakew
Ethiopian Public Health Association, Addis Ababa, Ethiopia

D. Kumara
Thrive Networks, Oakland, CA, USA

G. Arnolda
Thrive Networks, Oakland, CA, USA
School of Public Health and Community Medicine, Faculty of Medicine, University of New South Wales, Wales, NSW, Australia

L. Moccia
Thrive Networks, Oakland, CA, USA
Amici della Neonatologia Trentina, Trento, Italy

H. M. Nwe
Department of Paediatrics, University of Medicine (1), Yangon, Myanmar

D. Trevisanuto
Amici della Neonatologia Trentina, Trento, Italy
Children and Women's Health Department, Medical School University of Padua, Padua, Italy

A. A. Thin
Mandalay Children's Hospital (300), Mandalay, Myanmar

A. A. Thein
Department of Neonatology, University of Medicine (1), Yangon, Myanmar

T. Defechereux
Department of Surgery, Liege University Hospital, Liege, Belgium

Spencer McClelland, Maria Teresa Benedetto-Anzai, Teresa Cheon and Yuzuru Anzai
NYU Langone Medical Center, Department of Obstetrics and Gynecology, 800 2nd Avenue, Suite 815, New York, NY 10017, USA

Naomi Gorfinkle
Johns Hopkins University School of Medicine, 4 South Broadway, Baltimore, MD 21231, USA.

Alan A. Arslan
NYU Langone Medical Center, Division of Epidemiology, Departments of Obstetrics and Gynecology, Environmental Medicine, and Population Health, 650 First Ave, Rm. 532, New York, NY 10016, USA

Alice Gong, Judith Livingston and Kathleen Matula
Department of Pediatrics, The University of Texas Health Science Center at San Antonio, 7703 Floyd Curl Dr. San Antonio, Texas 78229, USA

Yvette R. Johnson
Cook Children's Hospital, 1500 Cooper St., Dodson Specialty Building, 2nd Floor, Fort Worth, TX 76104, USA

Andrea F. Duncan
The University of Texas Health Science Center-Houston, 6431 Fannin St., Houston, Texas 77030, USA

Thomas P. Sartwelle
Deans and Lyons, LLP, Houston, TX, USA

James C. Johnston
1150 N Loop 1604 W, Ste 108-625, San Antonio, TX 98110, USA
Global Neurology Consultants, Auckland, New Zealand

Berna Arda
Department of Medical Ethics, University of Ankara, Ankara, Turkey.

Caroline J. Chantry and Daniel Tancredi
Department of Pediatrics, University of California Davis Medical Center, 2516 Stockton Blvd, Sacramento, CA 95817, USA

Aubrey Blanton, Véronique Taché and Laurel Finta
Obstetrics and Gynecology, University of California Davis Medical Center, Sacramento, CA, USA.

Gwendoline Lilly Tanyaradzwa Chimhini and Simbarashe Chimhuya
Department of Paediatrics and Child Health, University of Zimbabwe-College of Health Sciences, Mazoe Street, Harare, Zimbabwe.

Vasco Chikwasha
Department of Community Medicine, University of Zimbabwe-College of Health Sciences, Mazoe Street, Harare, Zimbabwe

Hellen Namusoke
Department of Paediatrics and Child Health, Bethany Women and Family Hospital, Clock Tower, Kampala, Uganda

Maria Musoke Nannyonga, Robert Ssebunya and Victoria Kirabira Nakibuuka
Department of Paediatrics and Child Health, Mother Kevin Post Graduate Medical School, Uganda Martyrs University, Nkozi, Uganda

Edison Mworozi
Department of Paediatrics and Child Health, Mother Kevin Post Graduate Medical School, Uganda Martyrs University, Nkozi, Uganda
Department of Paediatrics and Child Health, Makerere University and Mother Kevin Post Graduate School: Uganda Martyrs University, Nkozi, Uganda

Jessica L. Thomson and Melissa H. Goodman
United States Department of Agriculture, Agricultural Research Service, 141 Experiment Station Road, Stoneville, MS 38776, USA

Lisa M. Tussing-Humphreys
Department of Medicine and Cancer Center, University of Illinois at Chicago, Chicago, IL, USA

Alicia S. Landry
Department of Family and Consumer Sciences, University of Central Arkansas, Conway, AR, USA

Robert L. Goldenberg
Columbia University Medical Center, New York, NY, USA

Margo S. Harrison
Columbia University Medical Center, New York, NY, USA
622 W 168th St, PH 16-29, New York, NY 10032, USA

Steven S. Parry and Ralph J. DiLibero
Department of Health Care Services, Benefits Division, 1501 Capitol Ave, Suite 71.4104, MS 4600, Sacramento, CA 95899-7417, USA

Anura W. G. Ratnasiri
Department of Health Care Services, Benefits Division, 1501 Capitol Ave, Suite 71.4104, MS 4600, Sacramento, CA 95899-7417, USA
School of Agriculture and Food Sciences, Faculty of Science, The University of Queensland, Brisbane, Qld 4072, Australia

Laura A. Halliday
Department of Health Care Services, Clinical Assurance and Administrative Support Division, 1501 Capitol Ave, Sacramento, CA 95899-7417, USA

Vivi N. Arief and Ian H. DeLacy
School of Agriculture and Food Sciences, Faculty of Science, The University of Queensland, Brisbane, Qld 4072, Australia

Kaye E. Basford
School of Agriculture and Food Sciences, Faculty of Science, The University of Queensland, Brisbane, Qld 4072, Australia
School of Biomedical Sciences, Faculty of Medicine, The University of Queensland, Brisbane, Qld 4072, Australia

Adrien Lokangaka and Antoinette Tshefu
Faculté de Médecine, Université de Kinshasa, Kinshasa
School of Public Health, Kinshasa/Lemba, Democratic Republic of Congo

Melissa Bauserman and Carl Bose
University of North Carolina at Chapel Hill, Chapel Hill, NC, USA

Yves Coppieters
School of Public Health, Université libre de Belgique (ULB), Brussels, Belgium

Cyril Engmann
University of Washington, Seattle, Washington, USA

Shamim Qazi
World Health Organization, Geneva, Switzerland.

Asmare Talie and Belsity Temesgen
Department of Midwifery, College of Health Sciences, Debre Markos University, Debre Markos, Ethiopia

Abere Yekoye
Department of Midwifery, College of Health Sciences, MekelleUniversity, Mekelle, Ethiopia

Megbaru Alemu
Department of Immunology, Microbiology and Parasitology, College of Health Science, Bahir Dar University, Bahir Dar, Ethiopia

Yibeltal Aschale
Department of Medical Parasitology, College of Health Sciences, Debre Markos University, Debre Markos, Ethiopia

Albertina Ngomah Moraes, Rosemary Ndonyo Likwa and Selestine H. Nzala
Ministry of Health, Zambia National Public Health Institute Lusaka, Zambia

Index

www.ingramcontent.com/pod-product-compliance
Lightning Source LLC
Chambersburg PA
CBHW080454200326
41458CB00012B/3971